CERVICAL CANCER AND HUMAN PAPILLOMAVIRUS

HEARING

BEFORE THE

SUBCOMMITTEE ON CRIMINAL JUSTICE, DRUG POLICY AND HUMAN RESOURCES

OF THE

COMMITTEE ON GOVERNMENT REFORM

HOUSE OF REPRESENTATIVES

ONE HUNDRED EIGHTH CONGRESS

SECOND SESSION

MARCH 11, 2004

Serial No. 108–206

Printed for the use of the Committee on Government Reform

Available via the World Wide Web: http://www.gpo.gov/congress/house
http://www.house.gov/reform

U.S. GOVERNMENT PRINTING OFFICE

96–225 PDF WASHINGTON : 2004

For sale by the Superintendent of Documents, U.S. Government Printing Office
Internet: bookstore.gpo.gov Phone: toll free (866) 512–1800; DC area (202) 512–1800
Fax: (202) 512–2250 Mail: Stop SSOP, Washington, DC 20402–0001

COMMITTEE ON GOVERNMENT REFORM

TOM DAVIS, Virginia, *Chairman*

DAN BURTON, Indiana
CHRISTOPHER SHAYS, Connecticut
ILEANA ROS-LEHTINEN, Florida
JOHN M. MCHUGH, New York
JOHN L. MICA, Florida
MARK E. SOUDER, Indiana
STEVEN C. LATOURETTE, Ohio
DOUG OSE, California
RON LEWIS, Kentucky
JO ANN DAVIS, Virginia
TODD RUSSELL PLATTS, Pennsylvania
CHRIS CANNON, Utah
ADAM H. PUTNAM, Florida
EDWARD L. SCHROCK, Virginia
JOHN J. DUNCAN, JR., Tennessee
NATHAN DEAL, Georgia
CANDICE S. MILLER, Michigan
TIM MURPHY, Pennsylvania
MICHAEL R. TURNER, Ohio
JOHN R. CARTER, Texas
MARSHA BLACKBURN, Tennessee
PATRICK J. TIBERI, Ohio
KATHERINE HARRIS, Florida

HENRY A. WAXMAN, California
TOM LANTOS, California
MAJOR R. OWENS, New York
EDOLPHUS TOWNS, New York
PAUL E. KANJORSKI, Pennsylvania
CAROLYN B. MALONEY, New York
ELIJAH E. CUMMINGS, Maryland
DENNIS J. KUCINICH, Ohio
DANNY K. DAVIS, Illinois
JOHN F. TIERNEY, Massachusetts
WM. LACY CLAY, Missouri
DIANE E. WATSON, California
STEPHEN F. LYNCH, Massachusetts
CHRIS VAN HOLLEN, Maryland
LINDA T. SANCHEZ, California
C.A. "DUTCH" RUPPERSBERGER, Maryland
ELEANOR HOLMES NORTON, District of Columbia
JIM COOPER, Tennessee

——— ———

———

BERNARD SANDERS, Vermont (Independent)

MELISSA WOJCIAK, *Staff Director*
DAVID MARIN, *Deputy Staff Director/Communications Director*
ROB BORDEN, *Parliamentarian*
TERESA AUSTIN, *Chief Clerk*
PHIL BARNETT, *Minority Chief of Staff/Chief Counsel*

SUBCOMMITTEE ON CRIMINAL JUSTICE, DRUG POLICY AND HUMAN RESOURCES

MARK E. SOUDER, Indiana, *Chairman*

NATHAN DEAL, Georgia
JOHN M. MCHUGH, New York
JOHN L. MICA, Florida
DOUG OSE, California
JO ANN DAVIS, Virginia
EDWARD L. SCHROCK, Virginia
JOHN R. CARTER, Texas
MARSHA BLACKBURN, Tennessee

ELIJAH E. CUMMINGS, Maryland
DANNY K. DAVIS, Illinois
WM. LACY CLAY, Missouri
LINDA T. SANCHEZ, California
C.A. "DUTCH" RUPPERSBERGER, Maryland
ELEANOR HOLMES NORTON, District of Columbia

——— ———

EX OFFICIO

TOM DAVIS, Virginia

HENRY A. WAXMAN, California

J. MARC WHEAT, *Staff Director*
ROLAND FOSTER, *Professional Staff Member*
NICOLE GARRETT, *Clerk*
SARAH DESPRES, *Minority Counsel*

CONTENTS

	Page
Hearing held on March 11, 2004	1
Statement of:	
Coburn, Tom A., M.D., Muskogee, OK; Freda Bush, M.D., FACOG, Jackson, MS; John Thomas Cox, M.D., Santa Clara, CA; Margaret Meeker, M.D., Traverse City, MI; and Jonathan M. Zenilman, M.D., Baltimore, MD	92
Thompson, Ed, M.D., Deputy Director for Public Health Services, Centers for Disease Control and Prevention; Edward L. Trimble, M.D., Gynecologic Oncologist, National Cancer Institute National Institutes of Health; and Daniel G. Schultz, M.D., Director, Office of Device Evaluation, Center for Devices and Radiologic Health, Food and Drug Administration	38
Weldon, Hon. Dave, a Representative in Congress from the State of Florida	25
Letters, statements, etc., submitted for the record by:	
Coburn, Tom A., M.D., Muskogee, OK, prepared statement of	95
Cox, John Thomas, M.D., Santa Clara, CA, prepared statement of	107
Cummings, Hon. Elijah E., a Representative in Congress from the State of Maryland, prepared statement of	12
Meeker, Margaret, M.D., Traverse City, MI, prepared statement of	119
Schultz, Daniel G., M.D., Director, Office of Device Evaluation, Center for Devices and Radiologic Health, Food and Drug Administration, prepared statement of	74
Souder, Hon. Mark E., a Representative in Congress from the State of Indiana, prepared statement of	4
Thompson, Ed, M.D., Deputy Director for Public Health Services, Centers for Disease Control and Prevention, prepared statement of	41
Trimble, Edward L., M.D., Gynecologic Oncologist, National Cancer Institute National Institutes of Health, prepared statement of	61
Waxman, Hon. Henry A., a Representative in Congress from the State of California, prepared statement of	18
Weldon, Hon. Dave, a Representative in Congress from the State of Florida, prepared statement of	27
Zenilman, Jonathan M., M.D., Baltimore, MD, prepared statement of	123

CERVICAL CANCER AND HUMAN PAPILLOMAVIRUS

THURSDAY, MARCH 11, 2004

HOUSE OF REPRESENTATIVES,
SUBCOMMITTEE ON CRIMINAL JUSTICE, DRUG POLICY AND
HUMAN RESOURCES,
COMMITTEE ON GOVERNMENT REFORM,
Washington, DC.

The subcommittee met, pursuant to notice, at 11:05 a.m., in room 2247, Rayburn House Office Building, Hon. Mark E. Souder (chairman of the subcommittee) presiding.

Present: Representatives Souder, Cummings, Waxman, Davis, Norton, Sanchez, and Ruppersberger.

Staff present: J. Marc Wheat, staff director and chief counsel; Roland Foster, professional staff member; Nicole Garrett, clerk; Phil Barnett, minority staff director; Sarah Despres and Tony Haywood, minority counsels; Jean Gosa, minority assistant clerk; and Naomi Seiler, minority staff assistant.

Mr. SOUDER. Good morning. Thank you for being here.

Today's hearing will examine the latest medical science regarding cervical cancer and ongoing Federal efforts to treat the disease and prevent infection from the virus that causes it.

Each year in the United States, over 12,000 women develop cervical cancer and more than 4,000 women die of the disease. By way of comparison, about the same number of women die from HIV/AIDS ever year.

In 2001, cervical cancer was estimated to be the 12th most commonly new diagnosed cancer among women in the United States. According to the American Cancer Society, non-invasive cervical cancer may be four times as widespread as the invasive type.

Experts agree that the infection by certain strains of human papillomavirus [HPV], is the primary cause of nearly all cervical cancers. HPV infection is also associated with other cancers and more than 1 million pre-cancerous lesions.

About 20 million Americans are currently infected with HPV. An estimated 5.5 million Americans become infected with HPV every year, and 4.6 million of these are acquired by young Americans between the ages of 15 and 24.

In 1988, Dr. Stephen Curry from the New England Medical Center said HPV "is rampant. If it weren't for AIDS, stories about it would be on the front page of every newspaper."

Fifteen years later, most Americans still have never heard of HPV, and most are unaware of the dangers the virus can pose or how to protect themselves against infection, and it is still rampant.

On Monday of this week, researchers reported that an alarming one-third of women in a recent study were found to be infected with a strain of HPV linked to cervical cancer.

In January of this year, the Centers for Disease Control and Prevention issued its first-ever comprehensive HPV prevention report. The CDC report states: "Because genital HPV infection is most common in men and women who have had multiple sex partners, abstaining from sexual activity (i.e., refraining from any genital contact with another individual) is the surest way to prevent."

It continued: "For those who choose to be sexually active, a monogamous relationship with an uninfected partner is the strategy most likely to prevent future genital HPV infections. For those who choose to be sexually active but who are not in a monogamous relationship, reducing the number of sexual partners and choosing a partner less likely to be infected may reduce the risk of genital HPV infection."

The CDC reports that "The available scientific evidence is not sufficient to recommend condoms as a primary prevention strategy for the prevention of genital HPV infection."

The CDC's findings echo a 2001 report entitled "Scientific Evidence on Condom Effectiveness for Sexually Transmitted Disease (STD) Prevention" prepared by the National Institute of Allergy and Infectious Diseases in consultation with the Food and Drug Administration, the U.S. Agency for International Development, and CDC, which evaluated all published data on latex condoms and STD prevention and concluded that "there was no evidence that condom use reduced the risk of HPV infection."

These scientific findings are important because Public Law 106–554, signed by President Clinton on December 21, 2000, requires the CDC to educate the public and health care professionals about HPV prevention and directs the FDA to "reexamine existing condom labels . . . to determine whether the labels are medically accurate regarding the overall effectiveness or lack of effectiveness of condoms in preventing sexually transmitted diseases, including HPV."

Because of the lack of awareness of HPV, there has been much confusion about the virus. I would like to emphasize two important points.

First, not everyone infected with HPV will develop cancer, but those with persistent, high risk strains of HPV are at increased risk. And second, while treatment can prevent the progression of cervical cancer, treatment should not be confused with HPV prevention. Treatment is often invasive, unpleasant, and costly, and does not include the necessity for additional treatments or adverse side effects.

Today I look forward to learning what efforts Federal agencies are taking to protect the public against HPV and cervical cancer, and, in particular, what actions the CDC is undertaking to promote the agency's HPV recommendations.

I also look forward to an update on the status of Federal programs to diagnose and treat cervical cancer and to develop an effective HPV vaccine. Congress has passed a number of laws over the past decade to increase access to testing and treatment. Because deaths from cervical cancer are largely preventable, it is vitally important that women have access to and are routinely screened for HPV and cervical cancer, and, if necessary, treated.

Finally, I look forward to hearing from the experts on our second panel, who are on the front lines every day treating patients with HPV and learning what advice they may have for Federal policymakers for improving efforts to educate, prevent, and treat HPV and cervical cancer.

Thank you all for being here today, and we look forward to your testimony and insights on this very important issue.

[The prepared statement of Hon. Mark E. Souder follows:]

Subcommittee on Criminal Justice,
Drug Policy and Human Resources

Opening Statement of Chairman Mark Souder

"Cervical Cancer and HPV"

March 11, 2004

Good morning and thank you all for being here.

Today's hearing will examine the latest medical science regarding cervical cancer and ongoing federal efforts to treat the disease and prevent infection from the virus that causes it.

Each year in the United States, over 12,000 women develop cervical cancer and more than 4,000 women die of the disease. By way of comparison, about the same number of women die from HIV/AIDS every year.

In 2001, cervical cancer was estimated to be the 12th most commonly new diagnosed cancer among women in the U.S. According to the American Cancer Society, non-invasive cervical cancer may be 4 times as widespread as the invasive type.

Experts agree that infection by certain strains of human papillomavirus (HPV) is the primary cause of nearly all cervical cancers. HPV infection is also associated with other cancers and more than one million pre-cancerous lesions.

About 20 million Americans are currently infected with HPV. An estimated 5.5 million Americans become infected with HPV every year and 4.6 million of these are acquired by young Americans between the ages of 15 and 24.

In 1988, Dr. Stephen Curry from the New England Medical Center in Boston said HPV "is rampant. If it weren't for AIDS, stories about it would be on the front page of every newspaper."

Fifteen years later most Americans still have never heard of HPV and most are unaware of the dangers the virus can pose or how to protect themselves against infection and it is still rampant.

On Monday of this week, researchers reported that an alarming one-third of women in a recent study were found to be infected with a strain of HPV linked to cervical cancer.

In January of this year, the Centers for Disease Control and Prevention issued its first-ever comprehensive HPV prevention report. The CDC report states:

"Because genital HPV infection is most common in men and women who have had multiple sex partners, abstaining from sexual activity (i.e. refraining from any genital contact with another individual) is the surest way to prevent infection.

"For those who choose to be sexually active, a monogamous relationship with an uninfected partner is the strategy most likely to prevent future genital HPV infections. For those who choose to be sexually active but who are not in a monogamous relationship, reducing the number of sexual partners and choosing a partner less likely to be infected may reduce the risk of genital HPV infection."

The CDC report notes that "The available scientific evidence is not sufficient to recommend condoms as a primary prevention strategy for the prevention of genital HPV infection."

The CDC's findings echo a 2001 report entitled "Scientific Evidence on Condom Effectiveness for Sexually Transmitted Disease (STD) Prevention" prepared by the National Institute of Allergy and Infectious Diseases of the National Institutes of Health in consultation with the Food and Drug Administration, the U.S. Agency for International Development and CDC, which evaluated all published data on latex condoms and STD prevention and concluded that "there was no evidence that condom use reduced the risk of HPV infection."

These scientific findings are important because Public Law 106-554, signed by President Clinton on December 21, 2000, requires the CDC to educate the public and health care professionals about HPV prevention and directs the FDA to "reexamine existing condom labels ... to determine whether the labels are medically accurate regarding the overall effectiveness or lack of effectiveness of condoms in preventing sexually transmitted diseases, including HPV."

Because of the lack of awareness about HPV, there has been much confusion about the virus. I would like to emphasize two important points.

First, not everyone infected with HPV will develop cancer, but those with persistent, high risk strains of HPV are at increased risk.

And second, while treatment can prevent the progression of cervical cancer, treatment should not be confused with HPV prevention. Treatment is often invasive, unpleasant, and costly and does not preclude the necessity for additional treatments or adverse side effects.

Today, I look forward to learning what efforts federal agencies are taking to protect the public against HPV and cervical cancer, and in particular, what actions the CDC is undertaking to promote the agency's HPV prevention recommendations.

I also look forward to an update on the status of federal programs to diagnose and treat cervical cancer and to develop an effective HPV vaccine. Congress has passed a number of laws over the past decade to increase access to testing and treatment. Because deaths from cervical cancer are largely preventable, it is vitally important that women have access to and are routinely screened for HPV and cervical cancer, and, if necessary, treated.

Finally, I look forward to hearing from the experts on our second panel who are on the frontlines every day treating patients with HPV and learning what advice they may have for federal policy makers for improving efforts to educate, prevent and treat HPV and cervical cancer.

Thank you all for being here today. We look forward to your testimony and insights on this very important issue.

Mr. SOUDER. I would now like to yield to our distinguished ranking member, Mr. Cummings.

Mr. CUMMINGS. I want to thank you, Mr. Chairman, for holding this hearing today on this women's health issue, cervical cancer.

Fifty years ago, cervical cancer was a leading cause of cancer death among women in the United States and around the world. Thanks to advances in cancer screening and treatment, the threat of mortality from cervical cancer has been dramatically reduced in the United States. Still, thousands of women are newly diagnosed each year and the American Cancer Society estimates that nearly 4,000 women will die from it in 2004.

The risk of illness and death from cervical cancer is spread unevenly among women in the United States. Despite improved screening rates enabled by congressionally authorized CDC screening programs, unequal access to screening remains a problem that contributes to significant disparities in cervical cancer rates along the lines of race, educational level, income, and age.

Women who belong to racial and ethnic minority groups are disproportionately represented among the new cases of cervical cancers. Asian, African-American, and Hispanic women have significantly higher mortality rates from cervical cancer than White women; women with less than a high school education are less likely to have testing than more highly educated women; and despite the peak in incidence of cervical cancer among women 40 to 55 years old, women in this age group are less likely to have been screened than a younger woman.

As chairman of the Congressional Black Caucus, I am particularly disturbed that African-American women are 60 percent more likely to have cervical cancer and 33 percent more likely to die from it as compared to White women.

The great tragedy in the American Cancer Society's estimates of thousands of lives that will be lost is that these deaths are indeed avoidable. The Department of Health and Human Services notes in its Healthy People 2010 initiative that the likelihood of cervical cancer survival is nearly 100 percent if early detection is followed by appropriate treatment and followup. But cost remains a barrier to access to Pap tests and DNA tests for HPV that, when used together, can accurately determine whether a woman is or is not at risk for cervical cancer or precursor conditions.

Any discussion of cervical cancer must involve HPV because genital HPV infection is a necessary precursor for cervical cancer. But, too often, discussions about HPV devolve into discussions of the merits of abstinence-only education. Some of my colleagues believe abstinence-only education is the answer to transmission of HPV and STDs in general, despite the lack of evidence that such programs are effective and the accumulating body of evidence to the contrary.

I expect that we will hear a lot of discussion today about condoms and the CDC's recent report finding that condom use is not supportable as a primary prevention strategy for genital HPV transmission. Far more relevant to the lives of women at risk of cervical cancer is CDC's finding in the same report that condom use is effective in reducing the risk of cervical cancer. This finding speaks to the bottom line question, which is: How do we effectively preserve and protect the lives of women?

HPV, when it doesn't lead to cervical cancer, is not life-threatening. An estimated 75 to 80 percent of Americans will have an HPV infection at some time during their lifetime. In the vast majority of cases the infection will resolve spontaneously. A tiny percentage will be at risk of developing cervical cancer or pre-cancerous conditions, however. Identifying these women and, where necessary, providing treatment is critical.

The most important message that can come out of today's hearing is that cervical cancer can be prevented, detected, treated, and cured, and that health screening and condom use are essential components of a sound, realistic public healths strategy for combating cervical cancer and the spread of sexually transmitted disease. Until we have done all we can to expand access to screening and treatment, and until there is evidence that abstinence-only education programs are effective, conversations about condom efficacy for HPV will continue to be an unconstructive sidebar to the important matter of erasing the threat of cervical cancer.

Indeed, it is worth keeping in mind that we made enormous strides in reducing cervical cancer deaths even as the so-called sexual revolution was occurring. Ensuring that cervical cancer death rates continue to go down for women in all parts of American society is what matters most. The only certain way to do that is by devoting more resources to what we know works: providing screening and treatment for women at risk. This should remain the foundation of a public health strategy for cervical cancer that puts health and wellness before religious and social ideology, and science before politics.

Thank you again, Mr. Chairman, for holding a very important hearing. I sincerely hope that we will have an opportunity to listen to our witnesses very carefully and make progress with regard to this illness that affects so many women in our country.

I yield back.

[The prepared statement of Hon. Elijah E. Cummings follows:]

Opening Statement of

Representative Elijah E. Cummings, D-Maryland-7
Ranking Minority Member

Subcommittee on Criminal Justice, Drug Policy and Human Resources
Committee on Government Reform
U.S. House of Representatives
108th Congress

Hearing on "Cervical Cancer and Human Papillomavirus (HPV)"

2247 Rayburn House Office Building

March 11, 2004

Mr. Chairman,

Thank you for holding this hearing on a very important women's health issue: cervical cancer.

Fifty years ago, cervical cancer was the leading cause of cancer death among women in the United States and around the world. Thanks to advances in cancer screening and treatment, the threat of mortality from cervical cancer has been dramatically reduced in the United States. Still, thousands of women are newly diagnosed each year and the American Cancer Society estimates that nearly 4,000 women will die from it in 2004.

The risk of illness and death from cervical cancer is spread unevenly among women in the United States. Despite improved screening rates enabled by congressionally authorized CDC screening programs, unequal access to screening remains a problem that contributes to significant disparities in cervical cancer death rates along the lines of race, educational level, income, and age.

Women who belong to racial and ethnic minority groups are disproportionately represented among new cases of cervical cancer; Asian, African American, and Hispanic women have significantly higher mortality rates from cervical cancer than white women; women with less than a high school education are less likely to have testing than more highly-educated women; and, despite the peak incidence of cervical cancer among women 40-55 years-old, women in this age group are less likely to have been screened than younger women.

As Chairman of the Congressional Black Caucus, I'm particularly disturbed that African American women are 60% more likely to have cervical cancer and 33% more likely to die from it, as compared to white women.

The great tragedy in the American Cancer Society's estimates of thousands of lives that will be lost is that these deaths are avoidable. The Department of Health and Human Services notes in its Healthy People 2010 initiative that the likelihood of cervical cancer survival is nearly 100% if early detection is followed by appropriate treatment and follow-up. But cost remains a barrier to access to Pap tests and DNA tests for HPV that, when used together, can accurately determine whether a woman is or is not at risk for cervical cancer or precursor conditions.

Any discussion of cervical cancer must involve HPV because genital HPV infection is a necessary precursor for cervical cancer. But, too often, discussions about HPV devolve into discussions of the merits of abstinence-only education. Some of my colleagues believe abstinence-only education is the answer to transmission of HPV and STDs in general, despite the lack of evidence that such programs are effective and the accumulating body of evidence to the contrary.

I expect that we will hear a lot of discussion today about condoms and the CDC's recent report finding that condom-use is not supportable as a primary prevention strategy for genital HPV transmission. Far more relevant to the lives of women at risk of cervical cancer is CDC's finding in the same report that condom-use *is* effective in reducing the risk of cervical cancer. This finding speaks to the bottom line question, which is, how do we effectively preserve and protect the lives of women?

HPV when it doesn't lead to cervical cancer is not life-threatening. An estimated 75 to 80 percent of Americans will have an HPV infection at some time during their lifetime. In the vast majority of cases, the infection will resolve spontaneously. A tiny percentage will be at risk of developing cervical cancer or pre-cancerous conditions, however. Identifying these women and, where necessary, providing treatment is critical.

The most important message that can come out of today's hearing is that cervical cancer can be prevented, detected, treated, and cured, and that health screening and condom-use are essential components of a sound, realistic public health strategy for combating cervical cancer and the spread of sexually transmitted diseases.

Until we have done all we can to expand access to screening and treatment, and until there is evidence that abstinence-only education programs are effective, conversations about condom efficacy for HPV will continue to be an unconstructive sidebar to the important matter of erasing the threat of cervical cancer.

Indeed, it is worth keeping in mind that we made enormous strides in reducing cervical cancer deaths even as the so-called sexual revolution was occurring. Ensuring that cervical cancer death rates continue to go down for women in all parts of American society is what matters most. The only certain way to do that is by devoting more resources to what we know works: providing screening and treatment to women at risk. This should remain the foundation of a public health strategy for cervical cancer that puts health and wellness before religious and social ideology, and science before politics.

Thank you, again, Mr. Chairman, for holding a very important hearing. I sincerely hope that it will lead to further advances toward eliminating cervical cancer as a cause of illness and death for women in the United States.

Mr. SOUDER. Thank you.

I would now like to recognize Mr. Waxman. I was going to recognize you next, because you are the senior ranking member on the full committee. Then I would go over to this side.

Mr. WAXMAN. Well, you are all very kind to let me proceed with my opening statement.

I am pleased to be here with the members of this subcommittee.

When it comes to human papillomavirus [HPV], public health policy must start with a single question: How can we reduce the rate of cervical cancer in the United States?

And this is a critical question because HPV causes cervical cancer and cervical cancer kills nearly 4,000 women in this country every year.

So I think to address this question we have to look at what works.

First, evidence demonstrates that the Pap test works. It is a simple test that can find precancerous lesions, pointing the way for treatment that can prevent invasive cervical cancer from ever developing.

It is a tragedy that about half the women with newly diagnosed cervical cancers have never had a Pap test. Expanding access to this service is an important public health priority.

Second, evidence demonstrates that condoms work to prevent cervical cancer. The CDC has found that condom use is associated with lower rates of cervical cancer. It is critically important that the public be aware of this potentially life-saving information.

Third, evidence demonstrates that comprehensive education can reduce sexual risk-taking that may lead to sexually transmitted diseases like HPV. These education programs typically stress the importance of abstinence, but also provide information on other options as well.

It is important to look at the question of how we can reduce the rate of cervical cancer in this country. I am concerned, however, that today's hearing will not focus, as it should, on this question. Instead, I am concerned that this hearing will, instead pursue a different question entirely: how the science of HPV can be used to advance the ideological agenda of abstinence only education.

This is neither a useful question, nor a new one. For years, those who have argued that teenagers should not be taught about the full range of options available to prevent unwanted pregnancy and sexually transmitted diseases, including abstinence and the proper use of condoms, have used the example of HPV to try to undermine public confidence in any other approach other than abstinence.

The main argument is to point out again and again and again that condoms are not proven to reduce the number of HPV infections. Therefore, the argument goes, condoms should carry warning labels and, ideally, should not be used at all.

Well, it is true that condoms have not been proven to reduce the risk of HPV infection. However, what is more significant is that condoms are associated with less cervical cancer, which is, after all, the key reason we care about HPV infection.

Moreover, and this is very important, condoms, when used consistently and correctly, are very effective in preventing HIV infection, and can also reduce the risk of transmission of other sexually transmitted diseases, such as gonorrhea and chlamydia, as well as prevent unwanted pregnancies. Anything that undermines the effectiveness of condoms for these uses will have serious public health consequences. Are condoms perfect? Of course not. But reality requires us not to measure public health strategies against perfection, but rather to ask a key question: compared to what?

There are those on this committee and in this Congress who insist that abstinence-only education is the solution to teen pregnancy and sexually transmitted diseases because "abstinence works each time."

Well, the evidence, however, indicates that abstinence-only education works rarely, if at all. Independent reviews have failed to find any significant impact of abstinence-only education on real outcomes. And recently, for example, an independent study commissioned by the Minnesota Health Department found that sexual activity doubled among junior high school students who participated in an abstinence-only program. And earlier this week, a study of 12,000 teens presented to the National STD Prevention Conference found that those who pledge to remain virgins until marriage have the same rate of sexually transmitted diseases as those who do not take this pledge.

These studies are inconvenient for those who want to argue exclusively for abstinence-only approaches to public health problems, and I am concerned that we will not hear much about them at the hearing today.

So I urge my colleagues on this committee and in this Congress not to let wishful thinking take the place of facts. We must listen to experts, not try to pressure them to saying what we expect to hear. We must hear the evidence, not be bound by preconceived agendas.

And to do all this well, we must start with the right question: How can we reduce the rate of cervical cancer in the United States?

I thank you, Mr. Chairman, for this hearing, and I thank the witnesses particularly for coming and participating, and I look forward to their testimony.

[The prepared statement of Hon. Henry A. Waxman follows:]

Statement of Rep. Henry A. Waxman, Ranking Minority Member
Committee on Government Reform
Hearing on "Cervical Cancer and Human Papillomavirus (HPV)"

March 11, 2004

When it comes to Human Papillomavirus, known as HPV, public health policy must start with a single question: How can we reduce the rate of cervical cancer in the United States?

This is the critical question for HPV because HPV causes cervical cancer. And cervical cancer still kills nearly 4,000 women in this country every year.

To address cervical cancer, we must be guided by evidence of what works.

First, evidence demonstrates that the Pap test works. This simple test detects precancerous lesions, pointing the way for treatment that prevents invasive cervical cancer from ever developing. As the CDC recommended in its report to Congress: " Regular cervical cancer screening for all sexually active women and treatment of precancerous lesions remains the key strategy to prevent cervical cancer."

It is a tragedy that about half of the women with newly diagnosed cervical cancer have never had a Pap test. Expanding access to this service is a public health priority.

Second, evidence demonstrates that condoms work to prevent cervical cancer. The CDC has found that condom use is associated with lower rates of cervical cancer. It is critically important that the public be aware of this potentially life-saving information.

Third, evidence demonstrates that comprehensive education can reduce sexual risk-taking that may lead to sexually transmitted diseases like HPV. These education programs typically stress the importance of abstinence but also provide information on other options as well. The CDC, Substance Abuse and Mental Health Services Agency and the National Campaign to Prevent Teen Pregnancy have reviewed many of these programs and found them to be effective.

It *is* important to look at the question of how we can reduce the rate of cervical cancer in the United States. I am concerned, however, that today's hearing will not focus, as it should, on this question. Instead, I am concerned that this hearing will instead pursue a different question entirely -- how the science of HPV can be used to advance the ideological agenda of abstinence-only education.

This is neither a useful question, nor a new one. For years, those who have argued that teenagers should not be taught about the full range of options available to prevent unwanted pregnancy and sexually transmitted diseases, including abstinence and the proper use of condoms, have used the example of HPV to try to undermine public confidence in any other approach besides abstinence.

The main argument is to point out, again and again, that condoms are not proven to reduce the number of HPV infections. Therefore, the argument goes, condoms should carry warning labels, and ideally, should not be used at all.

It is true that condoms have not been proven to reduce the risk of HPV infection. However, what is more significant is that condoms are associated with less cervical cancer – which is, after all, the key reason we care about HPV infection.

Moreover, and this is very important, condoms, when used consistently and correctly, are very effective in preventing HIV infection, and can also reduce the risk of transmission of other sexually transmitted diseases such as gonorrhea and chlamydia as well as prevent unwanted pregnancies. Anything that undermines the effectiveness of condoms for these uses will have serious public health consequences

Are condoms perfect? Of course not. But reality requires us not to measure public health strategies against perfection, but rather to ask a key question: compared to what?

There are those on this Committee and in this Congress who insist that abstinence-only education is the solution to teen pregnancy and sexually transmitted disease, because "abstinence works each time."

The evidence, however, indicates that abstinence-only education works rarely, if at all. Independent reviews have failed to find any significant impact of abstinence-only education on real outcomes. Recently, for example, an independent study commissioned by the Minnesota Health Department found that sexual activity doubled among junior high school students who participated in an abstinence-only program. And earlier this week, a study of 12,000 teens presented to the National STD Prevention Conference found that those who pledge to remain virgins until marriage have the same rates of sexually transmitted disease as those who do not take this pledge.

These studies are inconvenient for those who want to argue exclusively for abstinence-only approaches to public health problems. I am concerned that we will not hear much about them at the hearing today.

But I urge my colleagues on this Committee and in this Congress not to let wishful thinking take the place of facts. We must listen to experts, not try to pressure them into saying what we expect to hear. We must hear the evidence, not be bound by preconceived agendas.

To do all this well, we must start with the right question: How can we reduce the rate of cervical cancer in the United States?

I thank the witnesses for coming, and I look forward to their testimony.

Mr. SOUDER. Thank you.

Ms. Davis, do you have an opening statement?

Ms. DAVIS. Yes, Mr. Chairman. Thank you so much for holding this hearing on what I think is a very important issue. And you have already stated, as others have, the statistics of the number of new cervical cancer cases, and how many women in America die from cervical cancer. And I will just tell you that the percentage of women dying in Africa with HPV is even higher than the percentage here in the United States, where we sent condoms over to protect them from AIDS, but don't bother to tell them they could die from HPV; and I am really concerned about this alarming news.

And my colleagues have said that CDC has not proven that condoms prevent HPV, but they have proven that they might help. Well, this is not about a social ideology or a religious ideology, it is about informing women, letting them know. And to let our young girls and the women think that they are protected from these diseases by saying condoms are fine, go ahead, use them, when truly the only way they can be protected is abstinence, and that is not an ideology, it is a fact. And to hear the argument that if we let the American public know that condoms don't protect you from HPV, then people will stop using condoms, to me that explanation is totally unacceptable. We are still putting women at risk because we are not letting them know that HPV is a factor, it is a problem.

And I am looking forward to hearing the testimony of the witnesses and trying to get some of the facts, and I really, truly appreciate your having this hearing. Thank you, Mr. Chairman.

Mr. SOUDER. Thank you.

Ms. Norton, thank you for being here. Would you like to make an opening statement?

Ms. NORTON. Thank you, Mr. Chairman, for shedding light on an important precursor to cervical cancer. I do want to say to my good chairman of the Civil Service Subcommittee, I don't think anybody here was making or would make the argument that women should not be informed of their risks that HPV bring, as well as other risks. My goodness, HPV is very, very common. Eighty percent of sexually active people show HPV. Obviously, not all HPV leads to cancer, or we would really have a cancer epidemic on our hands, but the fact that it is a precursor or means that you could get cancer is very important information.

The CDC report that has been referred to here seems to me has made clear that condoms should not be the major strategy for preventing HPV infection. That is important information to shout from the hilltops. But the CDC report was also clear that condoms reduce cervical cancer. So what we have here is what we have often in medical science, we have a preventative that doesn't prevent everything, and we better tell people about it.

Let me go on record right now as being for a better condom. Perhaps the first thing we ought to be doing is encouraging research so you get a condom that people will use and that, in fact, prevents HPV. And I say so because we all know that condoms are here to stay; they are one of the oldest, one of the cheapest, and one of the most effective methods of birth control and of disease prevention. That is a fact. They ought to be improved, because something so cheap and something so generally effective is not going to be wiped out even by telling people about the risk of HPV, and certainly not by a very important hearing.

I was impressed with the study that Mr. Waxman referred to and my staff had brought to my attention, that the teens who pledged to be abstinent showed the same rate of sexually transmitted diseases as those who did not. These are teens, in good faith, trying to do what is right. Interestingly, one of the problems, according to the study, was the so-called virginity pledgers were less likely to use condoms. Here we come back to abstinence only and to the failure to understand what we must do to in fact be where we want to be. All children, all children should abstain from sex. And disease is only one of a dozen reasons why no child should be engaged in sex. This society has failed utterly to make that point, and I don't think that anyone believes we will ever be truly successful there.

The other point, of course, is that adults should be monogamous. I regret to say we have failed to make that point as well.

With these two giant failures on our hands, we need to talk about abstinence, and we need to talk about it clearly so that children understand why. That, yes, it is for religious and moral reasons; yes, it is for preserving yourself for a mate; and, yes, it is for preventing disease, which may have a greater effect than some other reasons. But all together the information needs to be transmitted.

But if we are going to have a hearing today on cervical cancer, we certainly must say that whether you abstain or not, every woman should have a Pap smear. If you want to look at why we have reduced the incidents of cervical cancer over the last several years, you will turn to the Pap smear. So we have to have a range of interests if we are truly interested in cervical cancer.

And I thank you, Mr. Chairman.

Mr. SOUDER. Thank you.

I would now like to ask unanimous consent that all Members have 5 legislative days to submit written statements and questions for the hearing record, and that any answers to written questions provided by the witnesses also be included in the witness. Without objection, it is so ordered.

I also ask unanimous consent that all exhibits, documents, and other materials referred to by Members and the witnesses may be included in the hearing record, and that all Members be permitted to revise and extend their remarks. Without objection, it is so ordered.

Our first panel is composed of our colleague, Dr. Dave Weldon, a representative from Florida. Welcome home, former member of this subcommittee.

It is the tradition of this committee to administer an oath, but we do not do that for Members of Congress, because we already took the oath.

So you will now be recognized for 5 minutes. Thank you for taking the time to join us today.

STATEMENT OF HON. DAVE WELDON, A REPRESENTATIVE IN CONGRESS FROM THE STATE OF FLORIDA

Mr. WELDON. Thank you very much, Mr. Chairman. It is certainly a pleasure to be in what was previously, I believe, my hearing room when I was on the committee. And thank you very much for calling this hearing; it is a very, very important subject. And I certainly want to thank the ranking member as well, Mr. Cummings.

Sexually transmitted diseases are one of the most important health issues facing our Nation today. According to the CDC, 3 million new cases of chlamydia, 1 million new cases of herpes, 5 million cases of trichomoniasis, and 5.5 million new cases of HPV occur every year. Unfortunately, women and adolescents seem to bear disproportionately the burden in this epidemic.

Just recently, the Alan Guttmacher Institute's perspective on sexual and reproductive health published data demonstrating that almost half of all STD infections were among 15 to 24-year-olds; and HPV, trichomoniasis, and chlamydia accounted for 88 percent of all these new cases.

What is worse is that our agencies entrusted to protect public health have been slow to act effectively to prevent further spread of these costly and harmful infections. After over a decade of increases in HPV incidence, the Centers for Disease Control and Prevention only just recently determined an effective prevention policy for HPV.

The CDC's recent report states "Because genital HPV infection is most common in men and women who have had multiple sexual partners, abstaining from sexual activity (i.e., refraining from any genital contact with another individual) is the surest way to prevent infection." While the CDC is to be commended for promoting abstinence as a sure means to avoid HPV infection, it has taken a long time for this common sense and science-based conclusion to be reached.

Other agencies have been quick to spend some $6 billion on research to advance methods of identifying and treating cervical cancer, but little on true primary prevention and risk avoidance. I believe this inattention to abstinence as a positive public health approach is only a symptom of a larger, more troubling phenomenon, a phenomenon that places science behind politics and social agendas. That phenomenon I am describing promotes the notion that technology can effectively mitigate our problems and that individual behavior is fixed-particularly with respect to sexual activity.

Doctors like myself are great friends of technology because it allows us to help millions who are sick and in need of treatment. Technology is good medicine because it aids in diagnosis and treatment, and can help reduce risks and costs. Nonetheless, technology is still no match to that simple ounce of prevention. Eating properly can stave off obesity and all its consequences like diabetes and heart disease; not smoking can prevent emphysema and lung cancer; and avoiding excessive alcohol can prevent liver disease. An equally important message today is avoiding sexual promiscuity can prevent not only unplanned pregnancies, but a host of incurable diseases, some of which lead to cancer and death.

We have known for years that STDs, including HIV/AIDS and HPV, are closely associated with promiscuous sexual behavior, but most of our public health approaches have sought to employ intervention modalities that reduce the rate of infection instead of true preventive strategies. Instead of seeing reductions in HIV and AIDS, chlamydia and HPV, we have seen significant increases year after year. In fact, after hundreds of millions of dollars to eliminate syphilis, an easily preventable and treatable infection, we are now seeing syphilis incidences on the rise, particularly in many communities where specific prevention efforts were implemented. This is because we have not been engaging in true prevention; we have, in reality, been engaging in risk reduction programs. Unfortunately for millions of young people, this has resulted in neither prevention nor risk reduction, as the rate of these STDs has continued to increase.

Certainly, as a physician who has practiced full-time for 15 years before coming to Congress, and who still sees patients, I have seen on a personal level the consequences of what we are talking about today. The heartache of infertility caused by chlamydia scarring of the fallopian tubes, chronic recurring cycles of pain from herpes, and even disability and death from HIV and from metastatic cervical cancer due to HPV.

As a policymaker and as a physician, my objective is to see fewer STD infections. Currently, the predominant method to achieve that objective is clinical. The clinical approach seeks to screen and counsel as many people as possible, and to provide them with a condom in the hopes of reducing STD infections. Certainly, many of these pursuits are worth continuing and expanding aggressively.

However, as a physician, I can only see one patient at a time. A much better public health approach, particularly for behavioral risks, is to reduce the need for patients to enter my office in the first place. That is why education is so important.

My former colleague, Tom Coburn, introduced legislation that became law mandating that the CDC and the FDA educate the public about the risk of contracting chlamydia and other STDs through sexual contact. I have seen little evidence to indicate the CDC and the FDA are in compliance with this important law. Even in the area of public education, Federal programs are, for the most part, doing very little to prevent people from coming into my office.

Mr. Chairman, I believe that we need to continue to aggressively promote accurate information to all young people and adults on the true efficacy of the condom in preventing the transmission of sexually transmitted diseases and, as well, the best methods for preventing these diseases in the first place.

I thank you. I will submit my entire written statement for the record, and I would be very happy to field any questions.

[The prepared statement of Hon. Dave Weldon follows:]

Testimony of Congressman Dave Weldon
before the Subcommittee on Criminal Justice, Drug Policy and Human Resources
Hearing on Cervical Cancer and Human Papillomavirus (HPV)
March 11, 2004

Thank you Chairman Souder and Ranking Member Cummings for addressing this important public health issue.

Sexually Transmitted Diseases are one of the most important health issues facing our nation because our nation is facing an epidemic of STDs. According to the CDC, 3 million new cases of Chlamydia, 1 million new cases of herpes, 5 million cases of trichomoniasis, and 5.5 million new cases of HPV occur each year.

Unfortunately, women and adolescents seem to bear a disproportionate share of the STD epidemic. Just recently, the Alan Guttmacher Institute's *Perspectives on Sexual and Reproductive Health* published data demonstrating that almost half of all STD infections were among 15-24 year olds and HPV, trichomoniasis and Chlamydia accounted for 88% of all new cases.

What is worse is that our agencies entrusted to protect public health have been slow to act effectively to prevent further spread of these costly and harmful infections. After over a decade of increases in HPV incidence, the Centers for Disease Control and Prevention only just recently determined an effective prevention policy for HPV.

The CDC's recent report states: "Because genital HPV infection is most common in men and women who have had multiple sex partners, abstaining from sexual activity (i.e. refraining from any genital contact with another individual) is the surest way to prevent infection."

While the CDC is to be commended for promoting abstinence as a sure means to avoid HPV infection, it has taken a long time for this common sense and science based conclusion to be reached. Other agencies have been quick to spend some $6 billion on research to advance methods of identifying and treating cervical cancer but little on true primary prevention and risk avoidance.

I believe that this inattention to abstinence as a positive public health approach is only a symptom of a larger, more troubling phenomenon. A phenomenon that places science behind politics and social agendas.

That phenomenon I am describing promotes the notion that technology can effectively mitigate our problems and that individual behavior is fixed – particularly with respect to sexual activity.

Doctors are great friends of technology because it allows us to help millions who are sick and need treatment. Technology is good medicine because it aids in diagnosis and treatment and it can help reduce risks and costs.

None the less technology is still no match for that simple ounce of prevention.

Eating properly can stave off obesity and all its consequences like diabetes and heart disease. Not smoking can prevent emphysema and lung cancer, and avoiding excessive alcohol can prevent liver disease. An equally important message today is avoiding premarital sex can prevent not only unplanned pregnancies but a host of incurable diseases some of which can lead to cancer and death.

We have known for years that STDs, including HIV/AIDS and HPV, are closely associated with promiscuous sexual behavior. But most of our public health approaches have sought to employ intervention modalities to reduce the rate of infection instead of true prevention strategies. Instead of seeing reductions in HIV/AIDS, Chlamydia, and HPV, we have seen significant increases year after year.

In fact, after hundreds of millions of dollars to eliminate syphilis, an easily preventable and treatable infection, we are now seeing syphilis incidents on the rise, particularly in many of the communities where specific "prevention" efforts were implemented. This is because these have not been true prevention; they have in reality been "risk reduction" programs. Unfortunately, for millions of young people they have resulted in neither prevention nor risk reduction as the STD rates of those who followed these recommendations have sky-rocketed.

Certainly as a physician who practiced full time for 15 years before coming to congress and who still sees patients, I have seen on a personal level the consequences of what we are talking about today. The heart ache of infertility caused by Chlamydia scaring of the fallopian tubes, chronic recurring cycles of pain from herpes, and even disability and death from things like metastatic cervical cancer due to HPV and as well HIV and AIDS.

Yes, the sexual revolution of the 60's and the 70's and the continuing efforts by some to normalize teen sex is hurting our young people, permanently scarring them, and yes, even killing some of them..

As a policy maker and a physician, my objective is to see fewer STD infections. Currently, the predominant method to achieve this objective is clinical. The clinical approach seeks to screen and counsel as many people as possible and provide them with a condom in the hopes of reducing STD infections.

As a physician I can only see one patient at a time. A much better public health approach – particularly for behavioral risks - is to reduce the need for patients enter my office in the first place.

That is why education is so important. My former colleague Tom Coburn introduced legislation that became law mandating that CDC and FDA educate the public about the risk of contracting Chlamydia (or HPV?) through sexual contact.

I have seen little evidence to indicate the CDC and FDA are in compliance with this important law.

Even in the area of public education, federal programs are for the most part doing little to prevent people coming into my office.

That is because many groups are relying on the condom, and the data on condom efficacy is quite clear. In the age group of primary concern (the xx to 24 year olds) the condom has limited efficacy, and for some of these diseases, the effectiveness of the condom in preventing disease transmission has never been established. Indeed the pathophysiology of some of these STDs indicates that a condom is not likely to be effective in preventing transmission.

They have preemptively given up by assuming that there is no way to change sexual behavior, particularly among young people. Instead, the objective of many NGOs that partner with the CDC is to reduce not eliminate incidents of unintended pregnancy, HIV/AIDS, and STDs.

I remain astounded by the notion within the public health community and employed by NGOs, like Advocates for Youth and the American College of Obstetrics and Gynecology, that the normalization of adolescent sexual activity is a positive public health objective.

The evidence is clear that teenage sexual behavior is inherently harmful these children. If our goal is to prevent adolescents from contracting STDs, then we should work to educate them fully about the risks associated with sexual activity and seek to eliminate adolescent sexual behavior. This is the only way to achieve the public health objectives we are seeking.

The conflict over risk elimination versus risk reduction has come to a head with the epidemic of Human Papillomavirus and its significant contribution to the increase of cervical cancer.

The scientific evidence is clear that condoms provide little protection from infection by HPV. Yet agencies and organizations are fighting to keep that fact from the public, particularly the young people who are most at risk. This is in the face of nearly 5,000 women who die from cervical cancer each year.

Education is vital to preserve the health of women and adolescents. And I believe federal prevention and education programs should start emphasizing risk avoidance, not simply risk reduction.

It will be hard because of the political and social agendas that have invested so much in risk reduction. But as we look at the entirety of sexual behavior and the impact on the health of adolescent and women, it seems clear that the policies of the past have failed to achieve fewer infections despite years of effort and billions of federal dollars in support of the risk reduction approach.

Mr. Chairman, my hope is that this hearing and the diligent oversight of the subcommittee will continue to fight for the health of women and adolescents. Lives are at stake.

Thank you very much and I would be glad to answer any questions you might have.

Mr. SOUDER. Thank you. I appreciate your comments very much. I think it is very important that we aren't defeatists. The primary role of this subcommittee is really to work with narcotics issues, and clearly in narcotics we work at prevention in the schools, we work at interdiction, we work at eradication. We have all sorts of things, in addition to treatment questions. And if we just said, oh, well, we can't stop drug abuse, we better just treat the victims, we would have a tremendous problem. And we are seeing the same challenge here with HPV.

We have heard twice referred to in opening statements this study that recently came out. Yesterday the New York Times reported that most teenagers who pledge to remain abstinent until marriage did not keep this pledge. When compared to those teens who chose condoms, the teens who took the pledge were more likely to delay the age of sexual debut; they were more likely to be married at a younger age; they were more likely to be virgins when they married. They were also less likely to be infected with three STDs that the researchers used as markers. I would note that the researchers did not screen the study subjects for HPV. Despite the lower STD rates of those who took the virginity pledges, as compared to those who chose safe sex, opponents of abstinence education claim this study proves that abstinence education is a failure.

Could you comment on these findings and this conclusion that we have already heard here this morning?

Mr. WELDON. Well, let me start out by saying I have not seen the study in question. From what I gather, it appears to be a followup from an earlier study published by the same author, which was looking at 12,000 teenagers and showed a significant delay on the onset of sexual activity of 18 months. As I understand it, though, based on the numbers he did report, there was a reduction in the incidence of sexually transmitted diseases in the group that took the pledge. In Whites it was 2.8 percent versus 3.5 percent; Hispanics, 6.7 percent versus 8.6 percent; and in the Black community it was 18.1 percent versus 20.3 percent.

Clearly, the trend is a lower incidence, and what I think we need here is more research on this subject. But the fact that sexual activity was delayed significantly I think should not be discounted. Many of the people who are criticizing abstinence, I don't think they would recommend that I, as a physician, stop telling my patients to stop smoking because it is bad for you simply because the majority of them continue to smoke. As a matter of fact, in clinical practice it was determined that when doctors do that, a certain percentage do actually quit; and though it is very small and many doctors get discouraged, so they stop telling their patients to stop smoking, when you multiply that over hundreds of thousands of dollars over the millions of people in this country, the end result, and this is what the public health officials concluded, you can prevent hundreds of thousands of people from going on to develop lung cancer or emphysema, even though the response rate was fairly low.

Now, what I think this study is actually telling us is that you need more followup with these young people. But certainly to give up on the notion that abstinence works in preventing the onset of teen sexual activity, abstinence education, flies contrary to what the science is actually telling us. Certainly there is some very excellent data on this issue out of Africa in Uganda, that you can significantly delay the onset of sexual activity through abstinence education programs.

Mr. SOUDER. So in effect, if I understand what you are saying, if this would be like a high school class took a no smoking pledge without background or other types of things, no followup with it, you would have some who might actually follow through, which is a gain.

Mr. WELDON. Right.

Mr. SOUDER. But you would have some who wouldn't, some who might do it less frequently, some who might not change their behavior at all. But you certainly gained in two different groups from the pledge. What you are saying is the study didn't prove any failure of abstinence education, or even of the pledge. In fact, the pledge, from their own data, did work, but that it didn't work 100 percent. And what that should suggest is that a broader abstinence education program might even get more results than just a pledge.

Mr. WELDON. I am not sure I would go as far as what you just said. I think the way I would interpret this agrees initially with what you said, that some kids will delay the onset of sexual activity. The way I interpret this is that more research is needed, and if you are going to have an effective intervention, you may need to have some kind of significant followup from the original pledge.

Mr. SOUDER. We certainly find that true in alcohol, tobacco, and in other narcotics, that you have to have more than just an initial pledge. That would be no surprise.

Mr. WELDON. Absolutely. Absolutely.

Mr. SOUDER. Mr. Cummings.

Mr. CUMMINGS. Just to piggy-back on what was just said, when you say followup, what do you mean?

Mr. WELDON. Well, I am not intimately expert on the True Love Waits, the pledge program, but the researcher that has been tracking these kids, he was originally at Columbia and I think he is now at Yale, Dr. Berman. He originally published some data 3 years ago that showed this was working very, very effectively in getting kids to delay the onset of sexual activity. And what he did was a very nice followup study which showed, yes, they did delay, but if you actually do a surveillance study, at least in the three markers that he used, you see only a very small reduction in the incidence of these diseases in the pledge takers.

And so my question is does that mean we throw the whole concept out the window? And I say no. We need to go back and look at is there a way to make the program better, is there a way to make the program work better?

But the other point I was trying to make is if you see a 1 percent reduction in the incidence of these diseases, if you translate that over the entire population of the United States, from this study, then you may be getting into hundreds of thousands of kids that are avoiding these diseases. So does that mean we abandon it? And I would say no. I would say more research is badly needed in this, but I think it is certainly an accurate statement to be telling these kids that the best way to prevent these diseases is through abstaining from sexual activity and, in particular, abstaining from having multiple sexual partners. The data is actually the more partners you have, the more likely you are to acquire these diseases. And when you look at the fact that some of the diseases they can contract can be fatal, I think it is a message that is definitely worth giving our young people, because we are telling them the truth.

Mr. CUMMINGS. Well, I want to go back to something Ms. Norton said, because I don't want us to be confused here. I don't see that there is anything wrong with saying you should abstain. I think the question becomes for that person who does not decide to abstain. I have gone into high schools, and I remember one time I went to a middle school, and I thought I was pretty hip.

Mr. WELDON. I thought you were too.

Mr. CUMMINGS. And I was telling these young people that it is very difficult to progress when you have a baby on your back. And after the thing was over, and this was in middle school, some kids came to me and said, Mr. Cummings, we like you and everything, but you don't know, but a lot of these folks are already involved in sexual activity, and you really didn't sound too hip up there. And I continue to say those things, but while we may want a certain thing, I think we also have to deal with a dose of reality, too, in some other instances. And I think that is one of the points Ms. Norton was making. And I use the analogy that when my 21-year-old daughter was 3 years old, she used to like to play hide and go seek. And she would come up to me and she would put her hand up to her face, and she would say, daddy, you cannot find me; and she was right in front of me. And I think we have to deal with the reality that as much as we might like to see our young people abstaining, that simply is not always the case, and so then I think you then have to say, OK, if they are not abstaining, then what advice do you give.

Mr. WELDON. Well, that is a great question. I think, as a policymaker, that should be the purview of local school districts, parents, teachers, churches to get engaged on that issue. The primary concern that I have had for years is an over-aggressive emphasis on a condom as a solution to the problem ignores the scientific fact that compliance with condom use amongst 15 to 24-year-olds is extremely poor. You can't take the condom data based on HIV discordant couples in their 30's and 40's, where you are talking about one spouse has it, one doesn't, where you get compliance rate with condom use at 99 percent, you cannot take that data and extrapolate it to these kids, the ones we are really talking about now, because that is when they contact HPV, it smolders for years, and then it becomes cervical cancer later in life.

And so I think you need to give the kids the full message, and the full message is that the condom, No. 1, is not a sure way to prevent some of these diseases; and the best way to prevent all these diseases is through abstinence, understanding that a significant number of them will not be able to comply. At least we should give them the message.

Mr. CUMMINGS. Thank you.

Mr. SOUDER. Mrs. Davis.

Mrs. DAVIS. I think Dr. Weldon just said what I would say. It is very disturbing to me that you have 4.6 million of the 9 million new STD cases were 15 to 24. And, to me, when we send the money down to the local schools, or what have you, to make the condoms available to these kids, and that is what they are, kids, and, yes, reality is they are sexually active, but I think we need to, to quote Ms. Norton, we need to yell it from the top of the rooftops that these condoms we are sending down to you don't protect you. And I don't think we are doing that. I think what we are doing is saying, well, you should abstain, but just in case you can't, here is the condom. And we don't tell them what the possible effects will be using the condom, so they have a false sense of security. So I think we are sending the wrong message when we use taxpayer dollars to give condoms out to these kids and we don't tell them, by the way, you are probably going to be dead maybe at age 24 by cervical cancer, but we are giving you the condoms, so go do your thing. To me, abstinence is the only way.

Mr. WELDON. If I could just add one more thing. You know, this is a social problem that goes beyond sex education. There are some dynamics here that we have little or no control over, specifically, some of the messages that come through our culture, particularly on the television, in the movies, out of Hollywood, and the truth is the sexual revolution is a bit of a lie in that totally unfettered sexual liberty indeed can lead to significant disability and death and poverty, as Mr. Cummings was alluding to with the burden of trying to raise a child as a single mother. However, we have first amendment issues there that run contrary to us trying to constrain those kinds of bad messages getting out in our culture.

Mr. SOUDER. Would the gentlelady yield to me for a second?

I wanted to followup with your smoking example. I have certainly been to schools where the majority of the kids were smoking, and increasing numbers in some schools, particularly younger ages and young girls. And I certainly favor more treatment for the results of that smoking, but I don't back off my message because it is going younger and increasing. I don't understand the philosophy that says we should not deliver the primary message.

Mr. WELDON. Well, you are absolutely right. And I haven't looked at the more recent data, but as I understand it, smoking rates are going down.

Mr. SOUDER. Overall.

Mr. WELDON. Overall. And the incidents of smoking-related diseases in some categories, I believe, appears to be trending downward. And when you think about it, this is a phenomenon that we are finally starting to see based on 30 or 40 years of effort in the public health arena, which began with the little labels on the cigarette boxes and now employs some very, very sophisticated Madison Avenue-type messaging going out to young people, a lot of the money for that coming through this tobacco settlement.

I believe if we earnestly apply ourselves, we can turn this problem around. Certainly, to turn our back on it and ignore it would be a tragedy. And to continue to do what we have been doing in the past is equally a tragedy, because the rates are going up. And so we need to step back and say what we are doing is not working; we need to try something new. And I think the abstinence messaging, and if you look at the experience in Uganda, where I think you had a very nice national program to get out a message of abstinence and you did see a significant reduction in at least HIV that was tracked, I think there is plenty of reason to continue to pursue this agenda.

And if you read the news reports on that study that has been quoted by some of the people on the minority side, published in the New York Times, if you read deep into the study, people acknowledge that we need more research on this issue, and I think we certainly do. And the people who are giving an abstinence message need to really look at this research very, very closely and see how they can modify their message, expand their message in a way so that it can be more effective.

Mr. SOUDER. Any further questions?

Ms. Norton.

Ms. NORTON. You know, there is a developing consensus here, I think, that the more people, including young people, know, the better off they are. I happen to be really for telling them about disease because I think you might frighten them away from sex, and particularly since I believe that young people should not have sex. Of course, when we are talking about abstinence, we better be careful here that we are talking about young people, yes, but we are also talking about adults here. And, of course, the message of abstain doesn't make a lot of sense in today's adult world.

So if you are telling them that condoms don't work, for example, should you also tell them that abstinence doesn't also work? Also sometimes doesn't work?

Mr. WELDON. Well, abstinence is 100 percent effective when it is practiced 100 percent of the time.

Ms. NORTON. Yes, the day it is practiced. How about the next day when it is not?

Mr. WELDON. That is a scientific fact. Ms. Norton, I did physical exams on elderly women going into nursing homes, and maybe this is a different era, who confessed to me that they had never had sex in their entire life. People can abstain. It is something that actually goes on. It may be totally disbelieved by Hollywood.

Ms. NORTON. Well, you are not advocating abstinence for adults, are you?

Mr. WELDON. Well, here is what I really wanted to say. If you look at the success in the condom in preventing the transmission of diseases like gonorrhea, syphilis, and they haven't studied HPV, but the data on gonorrhea and syphilis is pretty clear in this age group that we are talking about.

Ms. NORTON. What age group are you talking about, sir?

Mr. WELDON. Fifteen to 24-year-olds. The efficacy on the condom in preventing the transmission of gonorrhea from the man to the woman is, I think, about 40 percent or 50 percent; and from the woman to the man it is slightly better, 60 percent, in that range. And I think the syphilis data is somewhat similar. And I don't want to get into the excruciating details of the path of physiology of the transmission of these diseases, but I think we owe it to young people to tell them those facts, that the data on the efficacy of the condom is not 100 percent.

Now, part of the problem, and this is something else that we need to explain to young people, with this issue of how well these things work is that it is very hard to get into 100 percent compliance mode. They will use the condom some of the time.

Ms. NORTON. And they will use abstinence some of the time.

Mr. WELDON. Well, basically, anybody who is engaging in being sexually promiscuous is just not being abstinent.

Ms. NORTON. How about having sex once and getting HPV? I mean, the notion of calling everybody who falls off the wagon for abstinence promiscuous is, I think, an insult to human nature. Sometimes people fail. We all fail sometimes.

Mr. WELDON. I am not doing that. What I am talking about is if you look at who gets these diseases, the correlation is the increased number of sexual partners you have. OK? As you have more sexual partners, you are much more likely to contact HPV, HIV, and a whole host of other diseases. And if you are doing it without, obviously, the use of any type of contraceptive or a condom, the incidence rates go much, much higher.

Ms. NORTON. The notion of letting the information flow is something that, particularly on this part of the isle, we have been for sometimes meeting, if I may say so, concerns on the other side of the isle when business comes and says they don't want certain kinds of things on labels. So, indeed, I would like to ask you do you think it would be a good thing to put on the labels of condoms that it does not prevent HPV?

Mr. WELDON. Yes, I do. And I think it would also be appropriate to put the label that it is not 100 percent effective in preventing the transmission of gonorrhea and syphilis. That would be another reasonable thing to put on there.

Ms. NORTON. You know, I knew that if we kept this up, Mr. Weldon, you and I could find our points of agreement. We just found it. Thank you very much.

Mr. SOUDER. Thank you.

We have been joined by Congresswoman Sanchez from California, and I will yield to her for any statement and questions.

Ms. SANCHEZ. Thank you very much. I just want to have a brief sort of comment, and then I will get ahead to my question.

I think sort of the analogies that are being drawn here, between smoking and sex and abstinence, I don't think the messages need to be mutually exclusive, either or. I think when you arm young people, and there are responsible young people, and educate them about abstinence, and if abstinence is practiced 100 percent, it is 100 percent effective. However, for those who don't practice abstinence, to suggest condom use may reduce significantly their chances of contracting a sexually transmitted disease, I think that is also valid. It is like saying, OK, look, I don't want to buy my kid a motorcycle and say go ride the motorcycle, but if my kid is 18, has saved up the money and bought the motorcycle, I don't want to just say wear a helmet and you will be safer. While that is true, I would want my kid, if he or she bought a motorcycle, I would want to say, OK, you need a helmet you need to take training classes, you need to understand all of the risks involved. And I think with condom use, yes, it probably is sporadic among kids that are 15 to 24 years old, because they are not given all of the information about the proper way to use it and the small risks associated with the fact that they can contract sexually transmitted diseases through improper use or for whatever failures.

But from everything that I understand, the most important risk factor for cervical cancer is not the presence of HPV infection, but it is really a failure to receive timely Pap screening and followup care. So I am interested in knowing what your thoughts are on this, because we seem to have sort of focused in on HPV and condom use, but from everything that I have read and everything that I have heard, HPV is not the biggest determinant of who will ultimately fall victim to cervical cancer.

Mr. WELDON. Well, I am not a gynecologist, I am a general internist, and so I only did probably three or four Pap smears a day in my clinical practice, where gynecologists, and I think you are going to hear from Tom Coburn, did maybe 40 or so a day in their clinical practice. And I promoted it in all of my patients in the age group at risk, to have it done every year.

The new findings have been that HPV is the cause of cervical cancer, and this has precipitated a tremendous amount of discussion within the public health community and at CDC, and as well, obviously, in the halls of Congress about primary prevention. Because when you are doing Pap smears, you are doing surveillance; you are saying we know there are millions of women out there who now have this virus, so we are going to do surveillance and we are going to catch it early using the Pap smear technology, and respond in a way that prevents them from developing metastatic cervical cancer and dying early. And we need to continue to do that, and we need to continue to do that aggressively.

Mr. Cummings' comments about access to timely health care are extremely important. We need to do more in that arena as well. But I think it is very, very interesting, can we do more in the arena of primary prevention? And what has emerged is data that suggests that you do not prevent the transmission of this disease by wearing a condom. And when I say disease, I am talking about HPV. The condom does appear to lower the incidence of cervical cancer in the group of women who are affected with HPV.

So I think what Ms. Norton was referring to, full disclosure to young people is the way we really should be going, that is the path we should be going down, and telling these kids all the facts and not just assuming a posture of, well, we can't change behavior, and give them condoms and, therefore, we will lower the incidence of these conditions. I think we need to go several steps beyond that.

The message that I have always liked has been the Ugandan message, which is try to abstain from sex and be faithful in marriage. If you cannot do those things, then, minimally, you should wear a condom, even knowing that the condom is not 100 percent effective for preventing many of these diseases.

Ms. SANCHEZ. Might I suggest a radical notion? That perhaps those two messages, in addition to you might want to get regular Pap smears and screening, could be a three-pronged attack toward trying to reduce the overall incidences of cervical cancer for many women in this country.

Mr. SOUDER. Mr. Ruppersberger.

Mr. RUPPERSBERGER. Excuse me for not being here. A lot of committee hearings today, and after my questions I have to go to another committee hearing. I know you understand that.

Mr. SOUDER. Right.

Mr. RUPPERSBERGER. We are on the same side of the isle sometimes.

Mr. SOUDER. Mr. Ruppersberger, Congressman Weldon has a similar problem, so if you could just ask short questions.

Mr. RUPPERSBERGER. I will be very quick.

First, and I am not sure whether you can answer this question, is the rate of sexual activity or STDs among teenagers who have received abstinence-only education lower than among teenagers who have received comprehensive sex education? Would you be able to answer that question?

Mr. WELDON. The one thing I can tell you is that the teens that received abstinence education appear to delay the onset of sexual activity. And so the way you asked me that question, you get into the science of how you want to measure what you are talking about, and one of the measures that were used in one of the studies we were talking about previously, looking years later at the prevalence of certain sexually transmitted diseases, the difference between the abstinence group and those who didn't receive abstinence did not appear to be significant.

So I am not sure I can answer your question exactly, but it is a very well established fact that children who receive an abstinence-based education message will delay the onset of sexual activity as much as 18 to 24 months, which I think is a worthwhile accomplishment.

Mr. RUPPERSBERGER. Well, it is my understanding the median age of marriage for women is 25 years of age, and for men I believe is 26, and that 90 percent of Americans are sexually active before age 25. Now, with that in mind, is it safe to base public health policy on strategies that require behavior that is so far outside today's normal cultural norms? And I think that is an important question, because we need to cut through all our ideological issues, wherever we are, and get to the bottom line on how we deal with the issue.

Mr. WELDON. Yes, I think there is a good rationale for providing teenagers an abstinence message, and one of the reasons is the female genital tract in teenagers is anatomically slightly different than in adults. Teenagers are much more prone to complications of sexually transmitted diseases, and so to abandon a message for teenagers simply because we don't expect adults to fully comply I think is misguided.

Mr. RUPPERSBERGER. Well, I agree with you. I don't debate that with you, I agree with you on that.

Mr. SOUDER. Thank you very much.

Thank you for staying and taking the questions this morning.

Mr. WELDON. Pleasure.

Mr. SOUDER. If the second panel could come forth. Dr. Ed Thompson, Deputy Director for Public Health Services, Center for Disease Control and Prevention; Dr. Edward Trimble, Gynecologic Oncologist, National Cancer Institute, National Institutes of Health. And if you could remain standing as you come forward, because we will also do the oath in a minute. Dr. Daniel Schultz, Director of the Office of Device Evaluation, Center for Devices and Radiologic Health, Food and Drug Administration.

If you would each raise your right hand.

[Witnesses sworn.]

Mr. SOUDER. Let the record show that each of the witnesses responded in the affirmative.

Well, thank you all for coming to this wonderfully non-controversial subject.

Dr. Thompson, we appreciate it, and we will have you give your testimony first.

STATEMENTS OF ED THOMPSON, M.D., DEPUTY DIRECTOR FOR PUBLIC HEALTH SERVICES, CENTERS FOR DISEASE CONTROL AND PREVENTION; EDWARD L. TRIMBLE, M.D., GYNECOLOGIC ONCOLOGIST, NATIONAL CANCER INSTITUTE NATIONAL INSTITUTES OF HEALTH; AND DANIEL G. SCHULTZ, M.D., DIRECTOR, OFFICE OF DEVICE EVALUATION, CENTER FOR DEVICES AND RADIOLOGIC HEALTH, FOOD AND DRUG ADMINISTRATION

Dr. THOMPSON. Thank you, Mr. Chairman. I am Dr. Ed Thompson, Deputy Director for Public Health Services.

Mr. SOUDER. I think you are going to have to, just like we are struggling with the mics, get as close as you can.

Dr. THOMPSON. I will try to swallow it. Here, how about that?

I am the Deputy Director for Public Health Services of the Centers for Disease Control in Atlanta. It my privilege to represent the CDC here today. I have two goals. One is to provide you with information, and the second is as I always do at hearings of this sort, I intend to convince you that southerners do not speak slowly.

Members of the committee and Mr. Chairman, we appreciate your holding this hearing, and we appreciate the depth of your understanding that has been reflected in the comments that you have already made about this complex issue. We have little additional knowledge to bring to you on this subject, and we acknowledge that. All of us are troubled by the number of sexually transmitted diseases and infections occurring in this country, and this problem is most disturbing when it occurs, as it too often does, among America's youth. We are absolutely convinced, and it is clear to us, that the first line of defense against STDs for this particular population is abstaining from sexual activity. We appreciate the committee's interest in the health of America's youth, and women in particular, and we welcome this opportunity to discuss CDC's activities with regard to prevention of cervical cancer and human papillomavirus infection.

As has been clearly noted, although HPV infection is known to be associated with a number of diseases, the one of, by far, the greatest public health importance is cancer of the uterine cervix, for which HPV has a causal relationship. Cervical cancer, as has been noted, and as my colleagues from the National Cancer Institute can elaborate on, can be prevented largely through screening and early detection and treatment of precancerous lesions. And when it does occur, with screening and early treatment, the success rate of treatment for cervical cancer is in excess of 90 percent.

If you will take note of the chart to my left, this shows, in the large bar, which, if it were not cut in half to fit the screen, would go above the ceiling of this room. We see the number of human papillomavirus infections occurring in American women annually in excess of 2 million. And then we see a bar representing the number of cervical cancer diagnoses occurring each year in this country, and a bar representing, for the year for which this chart was prepared, the number of cervical cancer deaths. As noted, that number of cervical cancer cases is in excess of 10,000, and the number of deaths is approximately 4,000.

Now, the important thing that this chart shows, however, is that in spite of the preventability and the treatability of cervical cancer, we still have over 10,000 occurrences and approximately 4,000 deaths. Even more important, of these women, approximately one half have never been screened, and an additional 10 percent have not been screened within the last 5 years.

If you will look at the next chart that we are putting up over here, this shows you information from CDC's behavioral risk factor surveillance system, and it indicates clearly that as we continue to find that millions of American women still are not receiving adequate screening for cervical cancer and its precursors, this is the number of women or the percentage of American women who have been screened for cervical cancer in the last 3 years, and it has not only not reached 100 percent by a long shot, it has continued relatively the same over the last decade.

HPV infection is, as has been noted, the most common sexually transmitted infection in the United States, and, as noted, approximately 20 million Americans are infected at any given point in time, and about 5.5 million new infections do occur each year.

As illustrated on the next chart, a recent estimate suggests that as many as 80 percent of sexually active American women will have developed HPV infection at least at some point by the time they reach age 50. And you see that graphically depicted here.

A genital HPV infection is transmitted primarily through sexual intercourse, and since it is almost always asymptomatic, the usual source of transmission is someone who has no idea he or she is infected. The most important risk factor for HPV infection is clearly the number of sexual partners. For both men and women, the risk of acquiring a genital HPV infection generally increases with increasing numbers of lifetime male sex partners.

CDC has been involved in a variety of clinical laboratory and epidemiological studies of genital HPV infection for over 20 years. Public Law 106–554 included new provisions for CDC with regard to HPV, and since the enactment of that law we have undertaken additional activities. These have included sentinel surveillance to determine the prevalence in various age groups and populations of specific types of HPV; the collection of additional national prevalence and surveillance information using CDC's National Health and Nutrition Examination Survey [NHANES]; the initiation of several formative research activities to assess knowledge and attitudes of the public and of HPV-infected individuals about HPV; and the completion of formative research to develop a survey to assess knowledge, attitudes, and practices of health care providers regarding HPV diagnosis and treatment.

The status of these activities and timeline for this completion were outlined in August 2003 in a report to Congress titled "Human Papillomavirus: Surveillance and Prevention Research." A copy of that report was sent to the committee, along with the written testimony we provided to you early this week.

Now, the photograph that you see here shows one of many CDC laboratory activities conducted on HPV. CDC has conducted laboratory research on clinical outcomes of HPV disease, prevalence and risk factors for HPV, biological markers of cervical cancer and HPV, and development of sensitive HPV diagnostic tools.

CDC's National Breast and Cervical Cancer Early Detection Program provides cancer screening for under-served and uninsured women. Approximately one-half of the women receiving services through this program are from racial and ethnic minority populations. Since its inception, this program has identified over 55,000 women with cervical cancer precursors, and approximately 1,000 with cervical cancer.

In January of this year, CDC submitted a report to Congress titled "Prevention of Genital HPV Infect," summarizing available science and making recommendations about strategies to prevent HPV infection and cervical cancer. A copy of that report was provided to the committee as well, along with the testimony that you have received.

I can summarize the recommendation from that report if it is the committee's pleasure. If not, I would like to thank the committee again for this opportunity to describe CDC's activities with regard to HPV and cervical cancer, and I am prepared to answer any questions the members may have at the appropriate time.

[The prepared statement of Dr. Thompson follows:]

Testimony
Before the Subcommittee on Criminal Justice, Drug Policy, and Human Resources
Committee on Government Reform
United States House of Representatives

CDC's Human Papillomavirus (HPV) and Cervical Cancer Prevention Activities

Statement of

Ed Thompson, M.D.
Deputy Director for Public Health Services
Centers for Disease Control and Prevention,
U.S. Department of Health and Human Services

SAFER • HEALTHIER • PEOPLE

For Release on Delivery
Expected at 11:00 AM
on Thursday, March 11, 2004

Good Morning. I am Dr. Ed Thompson, the Deputy Director for Public Health Services of the Centers for Disease Control and Prevention (CDC) at the Department of Health and Human Services' (HHS). Thank you Mr. Chairman and members of both sides for holding this hearing, for your abiding interest in this subject, and for providing a forum for us to discuss these complex and challenging issues. All of us are troubled by the number of sexually transmitted diseases (STD) cases and infections in America. This problem is most disturbing when it occurs –as it too often does - among our nation's youth. It is absolutely clear, for this population in particular, that abstaining from sexual activity is the first line of defense against STD. We appreciate the commitment that members of this Committee have to protecting the health of the nation's youth and women in particular and welcome this opportunity to present our considerations on the prevention of one specific sexually transmitted infection, genital human papillomavirus (HPV) and its most dramatic complication, cervical cancer.

I. Cervical Cancer Overview

Although HPV infection has been found to be associated with a number of diseases, the one that is by far the greatest public health importance is cancer of the uterine cervix. A large body of scientific research over the past 20 years has shown that HPV is one of the causes of developing cervical cancer. Cervical cancer can be largely prevented through screening and early detection and treatment of precancerous abnormalities of the cervix. Decades ago, cervical cancer was one of the most common and deadly cancers in women in the United States. In the past 40 years, widespread cervical cancer screening using the Papanicolaou (Pap) test, and treatment of precancerous cervical abnormalities have resulted in a dramatic decrease in the occurrence of cervical cancer and associated mortality. The purpose of screening with the Pap test is to detect cervical abnormalities that can be treated, thereby preventing progression to invasive cervical cancer, and also to detect invasive cervical cancer at a very early stage. Progression from cervical cancer precursor lesions to invasive cancer is usually a slow process, estimated to take 10 to 15 years. If detected early and managed promptly, survival rates for cervical cancer are over 90%.

In 2004, the American Cancer Society estimates that 10,520 women will be diagnosed with cervical cancer and 3,900 women will die from it. Approximately half of these women will have never been screened, and an additional 10% of these women will not have been screened within the past five years. CDC's Behavioral Risk Factor Surveillance System continues to find that millions of American women still do not receive adequate screening for cervical cancer and its precursors. The most important factors associated with inadequate cervical cancer screening include absence of a usual source of health care, lack of health insurance, and immigration to the United States in the last 10 years. Other factors include older age, low income, low level of education, presence of chronic disabilities, and Asian and American Indian/Alaska Native race/ethnicity. Death rates from cervical cancer in the United States are higher among foreign-born women than women born in the United States. Therefore, the largest gain in reducing the occurrence of cervical cancer and deaths could be achieved by increasing screening rates among women who have never or rarely been screened.

Each year, cervical cancer treatment costs the United States about $2 billion. However, one of the best prevention methods for cervical cancer, the pap test, is an extremely cost effective measure at $4,535 per year of life saved.

II. Clinical Outcomes of Genital HPV Infection

Human papillomavirus is a family of more than 100 types of virus that infects skin cells and mucous membranes. The types are selective in what kind of cells they infect. Approximately 70% of HPV types infect the skin in various parts of the body, where the most common problem they cause is warts. The other 30% primarily target genital areas. Genital HPV infection can cause genital warts and cervical cell abnormalities that produce abnormal Pap tests, and is also associated with various types of anogenital cancers, the most important of which is cancer of the cervix. Most genital HPV infections do not cause disease, but instead remain asymptomatic and clear up on their own without treatment, usually within one year. Genital HPV types are designated as high- or low- risk, depending on the health effects that may result from infection. Low- risk types can cause genital warts or benign low-grade abnormalities in cervical cells, but are not associated with cervical cancer. In addition to problems in the genital area, low-risk genital types can sometimes occur in other parts of the body. For example, recurrent respiratory papillomatosis, a very rare disease of the respiratory system, can be caused by transmission of low-risk HPV during birth. High-risk types, primarily types 16, 18, 31, and 45, can cause low-grade cervical cell abnormalities, high-grade cervical cell abnormalities that are precursors to cancer, and invasive cervical cancer itself. HPV infection has also been associated with cancers of the anus, vulva, vagina, and penis, although each of these is much less common than cervical cancer, with the exception of anal cancer in homosexual men. The association of high risk genital type HPV with nongenital cancers has also been studied and current evidence indicates a possible role in a subset of head and neck and esophageal cancers. In addition, while a few studies suggest a possible association of HPV with cancer of the prostate, the findings are not consistent and the most recent studies do not indicate that HPV is associated with these cancers. To reiterate, the vast majority of both high-risk and low-risk types of genital HPV infections usually clear up without treatment and cause no long-term medical consequences, probably as a result of the body's immune response.

III. Prevalence of and Risk Factors for HPV

Genital HPV infection is the most common sexually transmitted infection for both men and women in the United States. About 20 million Americans at any given point in time are currently infected, and about 5.5 million people become newly infected each year. A recent Duke University estimate suggests that about 80% of sexually active men and women will have acquired genital HPV by age 50. Genital HPV infection is primarily transmitted through sexual intercourse. Most infections are asymptomatic, so the usual source of transmission is an individual who has no idea he or she is infected. The most important predictor of infection for women is young age, followed by number of sex partners. For men, the leading risk factor is number of partners. For both women and men, the risk of acquiring a genital HPV infection generally increases with increasing numbers of lifetime male sex partners. In addition, another factor that increases a woman's risk of HPV infection is the sexual activity of her partner. Several studies have indicated that for a woman, the greater the number of partners that her partner has had, the greater her risk for acquiring HPV--even if she only has sex with that one individual.

IV. CDC Activities to Address Genital HPV Infection, HPV Disease, and Cervical Cancer

a) CDC HPV Clinical, Epidemiologic, and Prevention Activities

CDC has been involved in the study of genital HPV infections for more than 20 years. Activities have included a variety of clinical and epidemiological studies of genital HPV infection. These efforts were refocused in 1999 with a report of an External Consultants' Meeting on *Prevention of Genital HPV Infection and Sequelae,* which detailed an extensive list of recommendations for public health prevention activities and research evaluation priorities (Attachment A). The following year, Congress passed Public Law 106-554, which included new provisions for CDC concerning HPV. Since the law's enactment, CDC has implemented the following activities:

- Initiated sentinel surveillance activities in collaboration with six health departments throughout the country to determine the prevalence in various age groups and populations of specific types of HPV infection in the United States.

- Initiated collection of additional HPV prevalence and surveillance information in nationally representative population samples, using CDC's National Health and Nutrition Examination Survey, that will provide specific information on HPV 16, one of the most common high-risk types of HPV associated with cervical cancer.

- Initiated several formative research activities to assess knowledge and attitudes of the public and HPV-infected individuals about HPV healthcare-seeking and sexual behaviors and HPV information needs.

- Completed formative research to develop a provider survey that will assess knowledge, attitudes and practices regarding HPV diagnoses and treatment. The provider survey will assess perceptions, practice barriers, and facilitators regarding HPV risk assessment, testing, treatment, counseling, and partner services.

In August 2003, the status of these activities and a timeline of their completion were outlined in a Report to Congress, Human Papillomavirus: Surveillance and Prevention Research (Attachment B).

b) HPV Laboratory Studies

CDC has conducted laboratory research on clinical outcomes of HPV disease, prevalence and risk factors for HPV, biological markers of cervical cancer and HPV, and development of sensitive HPV diagnostic tools. Examples of this research include development of:

- A national registry to describe the course of recurring respiratory papillomatosis (an infection involving the vocal cords of children and adults);
- Novel methods of HPV detection and evaluation by analysis of HPV 16 genetic changes, gene expression, and host/immune response;
- Novel biomarkers to improve early detection of cervical neoplasia with funding from the National Cancer Institute (CDC will also be initiating a study of cervical cancer in Appalachian women in Southern Ohio that will examine HPV factors in the context of socio-biologic background.); and
- Standardized methods for HPV detection, typing and serology to facilitate vaccine development, use, and evaluation, and novel noninvasive methods to monitor HPV immunity by testing saliva.

c) CDC Activities to Prevent Cervical Cancer

The Breast and Cervical Cancer Prevention Mortality Act of 1990 authorized CDC to establish the first national program to increase access to and use of breast and cervical cancer screening services. Now in its 13th year, CDC's National Breast and Cervical

Cancer Early Detection Program provides cancer screening for uninsured and underserved women, particularly low-income women, older women, and women of racial/ethnic minorities. Specifically, the program provides pelvic examinations and Pap tests, along with clinical breast examinations and mammograms. It also funds post-screening diagnostic services such as surgical consultation and biopsy and colposcopy. Through this program, CDC currently funds all 50 U.S. states, the District of Columbia, four U.S. territories, and 13 American Indian/Alaska Native organizations to support activities at the state, tribal, territorial and national levels in the following areas: screening; tracking, follow-up and case management; quality assurance; public and professional education; evaluation and surveillance; and partnership development.

The program provides health care services to women who are at or below 250% of the federal poverty level, uninsured or underinsured, and ages 18 to 64 for Pap testing and 40 to 64 for mammograms. To date, almost 1.75 million women have been screened. The program has provided women with more than four million screening examinations, through which approximately 14,446 women with breast cancers, 55,210 women with precancerous cervical lesions, and 1,020 women with cervical cancers have been diagnosed. Fifty percent of the women screened are from racial/ethnic minority populations.

CDC also collects data through the Behavioral Risk Factor Surveillance System (BRFSS) to monitor the frequency of Pap tests. BRFSS is a telephone survey conducted by all state health departments, the District of Columbia, Puerto Rico, the Virgin Islands, and Guam with assistance from CDC. The primary focus of these surveys has been on behaviors linked with chronic diseases that are the leading causes of death. This information is essential for planning and conducting public health programs at national, state, and local levels and evaluating these programs to ensure they are effective.

Finally, in 2002, NCI and CDC collaborated on the publication of the *U.S. Cancer Statistics 2000 Incidence* report for the first time in history. Produced in cooperation with the North American Association of Central Cancer Registries, this report provides state-specific data and regional level data for cancer cases diagnosed in 1999 including cervical cancer. The same report was produced in 2003 highlighting cancer cases diagnosed in 2000. In 2004, for the first time, this report will include mortality data as well as incidence (occurrence of new cancer cases) data. With availability of broad-based cancer incidence data, we can better identify, understand and address variations in the occurrence of new cancer cases and work to reduce health disparities among different population groups.

V. Prevention Strategies for HPV & HPV disease:

a) Prevention Strategies for Genital HPV Infection

Prevention of genital HPV infection is important for reducing the prevalence of genital warts and abnormal Pap tests as well as cervical cancer. The traditional public health strategy for preventing STD in a community has four components: shorten the duration of infectiousness of those who are infected, reduce the efficiency or likelihood of transmission of infection, limit the number of persons who are exposed to the person while they are infected, and locate and intervene with exposed persons before they become infectious. This is essentially the same approach used in limiting the spread of other infectious diseases (such as TB) unless there is a vaccine or other measure to reduce overall susceptibility in the population. The following is a discussion of how these strategies can be applied to genital HPV infection.

Reducing Duration of Infectiousness - The most common approach to reducing the infectiousness of many STD is treatment with an antibiotic that cures the infection. In contrast to many STD, there is no effective cure for genital HPV. Treatment for HPV is limited because it is not directed to the HPV itself. Instead, treatment includes removing lesions (genital warts or abnormal cells) through cryotherapy, electrocautery, laser therapy, surgical excision, or topical pharmacologic agents. The limited data that are available indicate that such therapies can reduce but probably do not eliminate infectiousness.

Reducing the Likelihood of Transmission – The second approach to halt spread of disease is to reduce the ability of the infection to be transmitted from an infected person to another person who is not yet infected. For STD, the most common approach to reduce transmission likelihood has been physical barriers such as condoms. Many studies have evaluated the effectiveness of condoms in preventing genital HPV infection; however, all have significant methodologic limitations which make their interpretation difficult. Presently, the effect of condoms in prevention of HPV infection is unknown. While some published studies of HPV infection have found evidence of reduced risk associated with condom use, most published studies on genital HPV infection and condom use have not shown a protective effect of condoms. However, available studies suggest that condoms reduce the risk of the clinically important outcomes of genital warts and cervical cancer (see January 2004 CDC HPV Report to Congress). One possible explanation for the protective effect of condoms against warts and cancer is that condom use could reduce the quantity of HPV transmitted or decrease the likelihood of re-exposure, thereby decreasing the chance of developing clinical disease. An alternative explanation is that condom use may reduce exposure to a co-factor for cervical cancer, such as chlamydia or genital herpes, thereby reducing the chance of developing cervical cancer. The available scientific evidence is not sufficient to recommend condoms as a primary prevention strategy for the prevention of genital HPV infection. There is evidence that indicates that the use of condoms may reduce the risk of cervical cancer.

Reduction of Sexual Behavior Risk – The third approach to preventing transmission of infectious disease is to limit the number of persons exposed to an individual while they are infected. Because genital HPV infection is most common in men and women who have had multiple sex partners, abstaining from sexual activity (i.e., refraining from any genital contact with another individual) is the surest way to prevent infection. For those who choose to be sexually active, a monogamous relationship with an uninfected partner is the strategy most likely to prevent future genital HPV infections. For those who choose to be sexually active but who are not in a monogamous relationship, reducing the number of sexual partners and choosing a partner less likely to be infected may reduce the risk of genital HPV infection.

Intervene with Exposed Persons Before They Become Infectious - "Contact tracing," or partner notification is an important element in controlling some other STD such as syphilis and HIV. However, genital HPV infection is so prevalent that most partners of persons found to have HPV infection are infected already, so notification will not necessarily identify uninfected exposed persons in whom infection can be prevented. In addition, as mentioned previously, no curative therapy is available for HPV infection. Finally, in the vast majority of people, genital HPV infection is cleared by the body's immune system. For all these reasons, partner notification is not thought to be a useful strategy for preventing transmission of genital HPV infection.

Vaccines - In contrast to other prevention approaches, vaccines are effective in preventing the spread of an infectious disease by reducing overall susceptibility in uninfected partners. A variety of HPV vaccines may provide immunity to a combination of high-risk and low-risk HPV types are under investigation. The goal of a HPV vaccine is to prevent genital warts, cell abnormalities and cervical cancer. So far, results from studies are encouraging. In one trial, an HPV-16 vaccine given to adolescent girls who were negative for HPV-16 DNA at the beginning of the study demonstrated 91% efficacy in preventing HPV-16 infection and essentially complete protection (100% efficacy) in preventing persistent HPV-16 infection and cervical cancer precursors. Trials of other HPV-16 vaccines and vaccines with multiple HPV types are underway and are likely to provide an important new approach for prevention of genital HPV infection within the next several years. Other types of research are also important for laying the groundwork for vaccine programs. Evaluations of economic feasibility, patient acceptability, and predictions about the number of cervical cancer deaths that could be averted have been promising. CDC is working with partners such as the Advisory Committee on Immunization Practices to identify information needed for public health recommendations concerning vaccinations, and with the World Health Organization to identify markers for HPV DNA to monitor population immunity. CDC and its partners are also evaluating non-invasive methods of detecting HPV infection such as in saliva. Clearly, the combination of an effective vaccine with currently used or recommended methods of prevention would provide optimal protection against HPV infection and consequences.

CDC has prepared a Report to Congress on Prevention of Genital HPV Infection. (Attachment C). This report summarizes available science and makes a series of recommendations about the strategies most likely to be effective in preventing future infections of genital HPV infection and cervical cancer. I would like to summarize the recommendations from that report. First addressing strategies for individuals and secondly addressing strategies for public health agencies.

Individual Strategies

1) The surest way to eliminate the risk for future genital HPV infections is to refrain from any genital contact with another individual.

2) For those who choose to be sexually active, a long-term, mutually monogamous relationship with an uninfected partner is the strategy most likely to prevent future genital HPV infections. However, it is difficult to determine whether a partner who has been sexually active in the past is currently infected. Partners less likely to be infected include those who have had no or few prior sex partners.

3) For those choosing to be sexually active and who are not in long-term mutually monogamous relationships, reducing the number of sexual partners and choosing a partner less likely to be infected may reduce the risk of genital HPV infection. Partners less likely to be infected include those who have had no or few prior sex partners.

4) While available scientific evidence suggests that the effect of condoms in preventing HPV infection is unknown, condom use has been associated with

lower rates of the HPV-associated diseases of genital warts and cervical cancer. The available scientific evidence is not sufficient to recommend condoms as a primary prevention strategy for the prevention of genital HPV infection. There is evidence that indicates the use of condoms may reduce the risk of cervical cancer.

5) Regular cervical cancer screening for all sexually active women and treatment of precancerous lesions remains the key strategy to prevent cervical cancer.

6) In the future, receiving a safe and effective HPV vaccine to help prevent genital HPV infection as well as the HPV-associated diseases of genital warts and cervical cancer would be an important prevention measure. However, an effective HPV vaccine would not replace other prevention strategies.

Public Health Strategies

1) Promote increased cervical cancer screening among never and rarely-screened women and appropriate follow-up of those with abnormal Pap tests.

2) Work with public and private partners to increase awareness about prevention of genital HPV infection and cervical cancer among health care providers and in the general public.

3) Collaborate with private industry to promote and accelerate the development of a safe and effective HPV vaccine;

4) Continue epidemiologic, laboratory, and behavioral research on genital HPV infection including studies of the prevalence of HPV in the United States, research on the attitudes and concerns of women diagnosed with HPV infection (e.g., concerns about cancer or about transmission), and surveys of provider knowledge and practices regarding HPV.

b) CDC Strategies to Address Cervical Cancer

CDC's strategies to address the cervical cancer burden include providing services to underserved women, providing outreach to women who have not been screened with the last three years, and developing educational materials to assist states with their public awareness/education and outreach efforts. Public education and outreach involve the design and delivery of clear and consistent messages about cervical cancer and the benefits of early detection using a variety of methods and strategies to reach priority populations. States receive funds to create and disseminate educational resources to women, especially those who are rarely or never screened.

CDC recently developed a cervical cancer fact sheet entitled *Basic Facts on Screening and the Pap Test*. This fact sheet is written at the sixth grade reading level and addresses the basics of cervical cancer and testing. The purpose of the fact sheet is to encourage women to be screened, as early detection is the key to reducing morbidity and mortality related to cervical cancer. It is available in print and on the Internet at http://www.cdc.gov/cancer/nbcccepd/bccpdfs/cc_basic.pdf.

Lastly, while CDC does not provide funding for treatment services, Congress passed the Breast and Cervical Cancer Prevention and Treatment Act of 2000 to address this issue. The Act provides Medicaid services for women screened through the National Breast and Cervical Cancer Early Detection Program if they are U.S. citizens or qualified aliens in States that elect to participate. According to the Centers for Medicare and Medicaid Services, 49 states and the District of Columbia have received approved Medicaid amendments to participate in this program.

VI. Conclusion

In closing, I would like to thank the Subcommittee again for this opportunity to describe CDC's critical activities and its strategies to prevent future genital HPV infection and cervical cancer.

I am prepared to answer any questions that members may have.

Mr. SOUDER. Thank you very much. You did prove southerners can talk really rapidly, but not like we Yankees.

Dr. Trimble.

Dr. TRIMBLE. Chairman Souder, on behalf of Dr. Andrew von Eschenbach and the National Cancer Institute, we would like to thank you for this opportunity to testify on HPV and cervical cancer. I am Edward Trimble, an obstetrician-gynecologist and gynecologic oncologist working at the National Cancer Institute.

A hundred years ago, cervical cancer was the leading cause of cancer deaths among women in the United States. Since the identification and adoption of effective screening for cervical cancer with the Pap smear, based on our understanding of the natural history of precancerous changes in the cervix, we have been able to reduce both incident and death rates from cervical cancer dramatically in the United States and elsewhere in the developed world.

Over the past century, we have learned much about the natural history of cervical neoplasia or abnormal cell growth. We have learned that cervical cancer is preceded by precancerous changes in the cervix. We have learned that treatment of these precancerous changes can prevent the development of cancer. We have learned that a Pap smear taken from the cervix can identify these precancerous changes. More recently, we have identified the human papillomaviruses as the major cause of cervical cancer. Studies also suggest that HPVs may play a role in cancers of the anus, vulva, vagina, and penis, and some cancers of the throat. There are more than 100 types of HPVs, of which only 30 can be transmitted by sexual contact. HPV is one of the most common sexually transmitted viruses. Only rarely does an infection with high-risk HPV develop into pre-cancer or cancer. The majority of HPV infections go away on their own and do not cause any abnormal cell growth.

The NCI has made a strong commitment to understanding the causes of cervical cancer and the relationship of HPV viruses to the development of cervical cancer. In fiscal year 2003, we spent $79 million for research on cervical cancer. We have funded extensive research to understand why most adults exposed to the HPV virus do not develop cancer or any other health problems resulting from that infection. NCI scientists have developed a new vaccine approach to prevent infection with HPV and are also working to develop a therapeutic vaccine to protect women already infected with the virus from developing cancer. In addition, NCI has worked extensively to improve the reliability of Pap tests, to evaluate new methods of screening for cervical cancer, and to combine testing for HPV with Pap tests. NCI is also committed to working to improve treatment for women diagnosed with cervical cancer. In 1999, we issued a clinical announcement to alert women and their doctors of a major treatment advance, combining chemotherapy and radiation in cervical cancer. NCI investigators are also working to preserve fertility in women with early cervical cancer, as well as to reserve bladder, bowel, and sexual function after treatment for cervical cancer. Finally, we have increased our support for research to address the gaps in the delivery of treatment research advances to all populations. We are building long-term relationships between research institutions and community-based programs to learn more about the causes of cancer disparities across the United States and develop ways to eliminate these disparities. In the future, as part of NCI's challenged goal to eliminate the suffering and death due to cancer by 2015, we plan to continue our close collaboration with our sister agencies, to make available effective vaccines for HPV, to reduce the emotional and economic costs of screening for cervical cancer, to improve the accuracy of screening, and to find more effective treatment for cervical cancer.

My written testimony contains additional details on our research program. I would be happy to answer any questions you might have.

[The prepared statement of Dr. Trimble follows:]

Testimony
Before the Subcommittee on Criminal Justice, Drug Policy, and Human Resources
Committee on Government Reform
United States House of Representatives

NIH Research on Human Papillomavirus and Cervical Cancer

Statement of

Edward L. Trimble, M.D., M.P.H.

Gynecologic Oncologist,
National Cancer Institute,
National Institutes of Health,
U.S. Department of Health and Human Services

For Release on Delivery
Expected at 11:00 AM
on Thursday, March 11, 2004

Chairman Souder and members of the House Subcommittee on Criminal Justice, Drug Policy and Human Resources, on behalf of Dr. Andrew von Eschenbach and the National Cancer Institute, would like to thank you for this opportunity to testify on HPV and cervical cancer. I am Dr. Edward Trimble, a gynecologist oncologist working in the Cancer Therapy Evaluation Program of the National Cancer Institute.

One hundred years ago, cervical cancer was the leading cause of cancer deaths among women in the United States. Since the identification and adoption of effective screening for cervical cancer with the Pap smear and based on our understanding of the natural history of precancerous changes in the cervix, we have been able to reduce both incidence and death rates from cervical cancer dramatically in the United States.

Over the past century, we have learned much about the natural history of cervical neoplasia or abnormal cell growth. We have learned that cervical cancer is preceded by precancerous changes in the cervix. We have learned that treatment of these precancerous changes can prevent the development of cancer. We have learned that a Pap test taken from the cervix can identify precancerous changes. More recently, we have identified human papillomaviruses (HPVs) as the major cause of cervical cancer. Studies also suggest that HPVs may play a role in cancers of the anus, vulva, vagina, and penis, and some cancers of the oropharynx (middle part of the throat including the soft palate), the base of the tongue, and the tonsils. There are more than 100 types of HPVs, of which only 30 types can be transmitted by sexual contact. HPV is one of the most common of the sexually transmitted viruses. Rarely can an infection with high risk

HPV develop into precancer or cancer. The majority of HPV infections go away on their own and do not cause any abnormal cell growths.

The NCI has made a strong commitment to understanding the causes of cervical cancer and the relationship of HPV viruses to the development of cervical cancer. In fiscal year 2003, NCI spent $79 million for research on cervical cancer. NCI has funded extensive research to understand why most adults exposed to the HPV virus do not develop cancer or any other health problems resulting from that infection. NCI scientists have developed a new vaccine approach to prevent infection with HPV and are also working to develop a therapeutic vaccine to protect women already infected with the virus from developing cancer. In addition, NCI has continuously worked to improve the reliability of Pap tests, to evaluate new methods of screening for cervical cancer, and to combine testing for HPV with Pap tests. NCI is also committed to working to improve treatment for women diagnosed with cervical cancer. In 1999, the NCI issued a clinical announcement to alert women and their doctors of a major treatment advance, combining chemotherapy and radiation therapy in cervical cancer. NCI investigators are also working to preserve fertility in women with early cervical cancer, as well as to preserve bladder, bowel, and sexual function after treatment for cervical cancer. Finally, NCI has increased its support for research to address the gaps in the delivery of research advances to all populations. NCI is building long-term relationships between research institutions and community-based programs to learn more about the causes of cancer disparities in minority communities and to develop ways to eliminate these causes.

As part of the National Cancer Institute's Challenge Goal *to eliminate the suffering and death due to cancer by 2015,* we are working to discover, develop, and deliver the interventions that will prevent many cancers, detect and eliminate many others, and modulate the behavior of the remainder so that, ultimately, no one has to suffer and die as a result of this disease. To this end, NCI is supporting research studies on HPV and cervical cancer as they align with Discovery, Development and Delivery.

DISCOVERY

The Guanacaste Study of HPV Natural History is being conducted in the Guanacaste Province, an area in Costa Rica with a very high incidence rate of cervical cancer. Cervical cancer is the leading cause of cancer death in regions without effective cytology programs and screening. This study involves women who live in a region where there is a lack of effective cervical cytology programs and screening. This prospective study of HPV infection and cervical neoplasia is based on the recruitment and 7-year follow-up of a random sample of approximately 10,000 women 18+ years of age, residing in Guanacaste. The study has permitted several studies of HPV infection, cytology, cervicography, and the whole spectrum of cervical neoplasia. The epidemiologic risk factors for each stage of neoplasia have been identified, controlling for the central role of type-specific HPV infection. Follow-up of the cohort at six month to yearly intervals depending on disease status is complete and data analysis will examine the origins of precancer and cancer.

The **Genetic Supplementation Study** is nested within the Guanacaste Study (see above) in Costa Rica. It is a case control study intended to systematically evaluate the role of both viral variants and host immune response genes in cervical carcinogenesis. Biological specimens are being collected from women enrolled in the Guanacaste Study and detailed genotyping of the viral genome as well as genotyping of genetic polymorphisms in the genome of those women will be performed. A major focus will be the study of immune genes, particularly those known to interact with HPV and an assessment of genes potentially modifying other HPV cofactors.

The **Study to understand Cervical Cancer Early Endpoints and Determinants (SUCCEED)** is a study to comprehensively assess biomarkers of risk for each progressive stage of cervical neoplasia (normal, HPV-infected, precancer, cancer) and to discover a new set of biomarkers that can distinguish those at highest risk of cervical cancer from those with benign HPV infection. Over 1000 women will be recruited into the study and a subsequent 2-year prospective component will be conducted to validate the most promising candidate biomarkers and their key outcomes for HPV clearance, persistence, and progression to precancer.

The **Alternatives in Women's Health Care Immunology Study (nested within ALTS, described under Delivery)**, has enrolled approximately 900 women in a prospective study to identify biomarkers associated with permissive versus protective immune response to low-grade cervical lesions. Women with low-grade cervical disease are being followed at six month intervals for two years. Cellular and immunological parameters at entry will be correlated with progression, persistence or regression of low-grade lesions during follow-up.

A longitudinal study of **HPV Infection and Cervical Neoplasia in Sao Paulo, Brazil** was conducted on 2404 women, in which cervical specimens from Pap smears were tested for cytology and HPV genotyping every 4-6 months over a period of 8 years. Actuarial and non-actuarial analyses were used to measure time and rates of lesion progression and regression according to status and type of HPV infection. The study found that precursor lesions of the cervix persist longer and progress more quickly in women with oncogenic HPV infections than in women with non-oncogenic infections or without HPV. The study concluded that testing cervical lesions for oncogenic HPVs may help identify those lesions that are likely to progress rapidly. Results of this study are published in: *N.F. Schlecht, R.W. Platt, E. Duarte-Franco, M.C. Costa, J.P. Sobrinho, J.C.M. Prado, A. Ferenczy, T.E. Rohan, L.L. Villa, E.L. Franco 2003 Human Papillomavirus Infection and Time to Progression and Regression of Cervical Intraepithelial Neoplasia JNCI 95: 1336-43.*

DEVELOPMENT

A high priority of the NCI is to prevent cervical cancer by developing a vaccine that prevents and treats HPV infection and premalignant disease. There is growing evidence that a VLP-based (virus-like particle) HPV vaccine will be effective in preventing genital HPV infection. A large randomized **Vaccine Trial** is planned in Costa Rica to evaluate the efficacy of two virus-like particle (VLP)-based prophylactic human papillomavirus (HPV) vaccines developed at NCI. Volunteers in the trial will be screened for cervical disease at entry and will receive three VLP or three placebo vaccinations over the course of six months. Participants will be followed for four years and information collected on side effects of the vaccine (safety), immune reduction by the vaccine, and the occurrence of cervical disease.

Another high priority area is the development of affordable, second-generation DNA-based tests for the diagnosis of HPV infection. A partnership with the Gates Foundation and the Program for Appropriate Technology in Health (PATH) is an initiative, still in the planning stages, to create a low-cost test in two to three years for field testing.

Optical Technologies for Cervical Neoplasia is a Program Project Grant, sponsored by the **Cancer Imaging Program/National Cancer Imaging Program (CIP/NCI)** that uses a method of technology assessment that will guide the development of new and existing optical technologies to detect and diagnosis early cervical cancer. Evaluation of these optical technologies will provide improved screening and detection methods for cervical intra-epithelial neoplasia that are both sensitive and cost-effective in both developing and developed countries. The relationship between optical signatures and the underlying cancer biology is not well understood. Preliminary studies demonstrate that this imaging approach accurately detects the intracellular changes that occur as cells become abnormal and can be applied to developing mathematical models for distinguishing normal and neoplastic tissue. Recent clinical trials have shown that the imaging technique is feasible for use in large populations and can be adapted for simple, inexpensive imaging systems for use in screening trials worldwide. NCI investigators will continue to develop this promising new technology in a large randomized trial comparing fluorescence and reflectance screening with standard cervical cancer screening techniques.

Rapid Access to Preventive Intervention Development (RAPID) provides funding and resources to develop agents that prevent, reverse, or delay cancer development. RAPID is designed to quickly move novel preventive molecules, such as HPV vaccines for cervical cancer, from the laboratory into clinical studies.

The **Gynecologic Cancer Intergroup (GCIG)** is an organization of international cooperative groups for clinical trials in gynecologic cancers that is identifying active treatments for cervical cancer.

DELIVERY

The **ASCUS/LSIL Triage /Study for Cervical Cancer (ALTS)** is a clinical trial to find the best way to help women and their doctors decide what to do about abnormal Pap test results that are diagnosed in about three million women in the United States each year. ASCUS stands for atypical squamous cells (abnormal cells lining the cervix) of undetermined significance and LSIL for low-grade squamous intraepithelial lesions. Most of these abnormalities are mild and will go away without treatment, but some may signal a precancerous condition or, rarely, cancer.

The motivation for this trial was to use the information about the role of HPV to design better treatment and prevention strategies to reduce the burden of cervical cancer and its precursors. The study consisted of three management strategies: (1) immediate colposcopy of all women; (2) repeat cytology with colposcopy only if the results show a high grade lesion; and (3) HPV testing and repeat cytology in combination, with referral to colposcopy if either the HPV test is positive or the cytology shows a high grade lesion. Four Clinical Centers - University of Alabama, Birmingham AL; Magee-Womens Hospital, Pittsburgh PA; University of Oklahoma, Oklahoma City OK; and University of Washington, Seattle WA - enrolled approximately 5,000 women with a recent diagnosis of ASCUS or LSIL. Participants were followed at six month intervals for a total of 2 years and the efficacy and cost-effectiveness of the different strategies in the early detection of high-grade lesions were compared.The findings were as follows:

- HPV testing is sensitive in detecting underlying precancerous lesions among women with a Pap test diagnosis of ASCUS

- Neither cytology nor HPV testing is useful for triaging women with a Pap test diagnosis of LSIL

- A single colposcopic-directed biopsy procedure is not completely sensitive in detecting precancers

The **Bethesda System for Cervical Cytology** was developed under the auspices of the NCI to provide a coherent framework for reporting Pap test results. Currently over 90% of cytology laboratories in the U.S. and many countries internationally use this system. The standardized terminology has facilitated correlation among different research studies and has become the basis for professional societies to develop patient management guidelines.

The **Portland Kaiser Cohort Study** has enrolled almost 24,000 women obtaining a routine Pap smear screening at any of the seven Portland Kaiser-Permanente clinics for the purpose of conducting a prospective study of HPV infection and cervical neoplasia. This is a companion study for the Guanacaste Study (described above under Discovery). The enrollment phase has yielded a prevalent case-control comparison which has demonstrated that HPV is the primary risk factor for cervical intraepithelial neoplasia. The study also has shown that HPV testing can be used to clarify borderline Pap smears. The full cohort based on up to 10-years of follow-up showed the usefulness of combined Pap tests to improve the detection of cervical cancer. The use of HPV DNA testing as an adjunct to Pap tests was approved in 2003 by the Food and Drug Administration, and several groups have modified screening recommendations accordingly.

The **Cancer Research Network** is a consortium of researchers affilitated with eleven major not-for-profit HMOs that is providing the mechanism for NCI to quickly obtain better data on patterns of cancer care from multiple perspectives. One of their recent findings indicates that the majority of breast and cervical cancer cases appear to be associated with an absence of screening and failures in detection.

For the purpose of **broadening our understanding of the causes of cancer disparities,** the NCI has implemented a partnership demonstration project in eight states to increase screening for breast and cervical cancer among women who have never or rarely been screened (in collaboration with CDC, USDA and ACS). Despite a three-fold reduction in cervical cancer mortality nationwide, many counties from Maine through Appalachia, many of the southeastern states, the Texas/Mexico border, and in the Central Valley of California have experienced higher cervical cancer mortality rates. To address these high rates, the partnership will use NCI analyses of county mortality rates to identify high-rate counties and will work to train staff of CDC's Breast and Cervical Cancer Early Detection Program; USDA's Cooperative State Research, Education, and Extension Service; ACS's regional cancer control programs; and NCI's Cancer Information Service to increase screening among high-risk women.

In the future, NCI plans to continue its close collaboration with its sister agencies in DHHS to make available effective vaccines for HPV to reduce the emotional and economic cost of screening for cervical cancer, to improve the accuracy of screening, and to find more effective treatment for cervical cancer.

Mr. SOUDER. Thank you very much.

Dr. Schultz.

Dr. SCHULTZ. Good morning, Mr. Chairman and members of the subcommittee. I am Dr. Dan Schultz, Director of the Office of Device Evaluation in the Center for Devices and Radiological Health at the FDA. I am pleased to speak today about FDA's implementation of Public Law 106–554 with respect to the labeling of condoms.

FDA has conducted an extensive literature and labeling review. Based on these reviews, we are developing a draft guidance document on condom labeling and proposed rule which would make the guidance a special control for condoms.

FDA regulates all medical devices in the United States, including condoms. Since 1987, FDA has issued a series of guidance documents that addresses specific elements of condom labeling related to protection against sexually transmitted diseases. The typical condom package contains a front panel on the external box that is referred to as the principal display panel. Current FDA guidance recommends that the display panel of the package for condoms include a statement regarding contraception and a statement on STD risk reduction, and that labeling emphasize the need for proper use.

Public Law 106–554, enacted in December 2000, directs the Secretary of HHS to determine whether the labels are medically accurate regarding the overall effectiveness or lack of effectiveness of condoms in preventing sexually transmitted diseases, including HPV. Although the interest of this hearing targets HPV, we complied with the law by exploring the labeling regarding other STDs as well.

To fully accomplish this task, we conducted a comprehensive systematic review of the published literature and other relevant information, and are now looking at how the results from this review might impact condom labeling. Our basic conclusions are as follows.

One, the protection a condom may provide against different STDs will vary depending on the transmission vectors of a particular STD, the specific infectivity of the virus or bacteria, and the biological mechanisms of progression from infection to disease. The law asks particularly about HPV infection, which can manifest as lesions, symptomatic or asymptomatic, on a man's penis, scrotum, a woman's vulva, cervix, or either's peri-anal areas. Because condoms do not cover all these areas, they may not provide the same protection as they do against STDs transmitted through bodily fluids like HIV or gonorrhea.

Two, condoms are highly effective against HIV and other STDs that are transmitted by genital secretions.

Three, studies on STDs characterized by genital ulcers, such as genital herpes and syphilis, are inconclusive as to whether condoms lower the risk of these diseases. We believe that the condom will provide some measure of protection when it covers the lesion or ulcer.

Four, clinical studies evaluating the relationship between condoms and HPV-related disease have not been consistent. However, even though the biologic mechanism has not been conclusively demonstrated, women whose partners use condoms seem to be at reduced risk for genital warts and cervical cancer compared to women whose partners do not use condoms. Therefore, there does appear to be a benefit from condom use for prevention of HPV-related disease.

As a result of these findings, CDRH has developed a regulatory plan to provide condom users with a consistent labeling message about STDs and the protection they should expect from condom use. FDA is preparing new guidance on condom labeling to address these issues. FDA anticipates proposing to amend the classification regulations for condoms to make such labeling guidance a special control.

FDA is also committed to helping bring safe and effective technologies to the market, including new tests for the detection of HPV and improved methods of evaluating Pap tests. FDA is reviewing a number of investigational new drug applications for vaccines for the prevention of HPV infections, several of which are in advanced clinical development. In addition to efforts directed at HPV infection, treatment of cervical cancer is a very active field for clinical research, and several novel technologies are currently being evaluated for the treatment of this disease.

In conclusion, FDA is working to present a balanced view of condom performance, being careful neither to overstate effectiveness, nor to discourage use where it is appropriate.

Mr. Chairman, I want to reiterate that FDA is committed to monitoring closely the body of scientific evidence related to the degree in which male condoms offer any protection from HPV, HPV-related disease, and other STDs. We will continue to exercise our regulatory responsibilities to ensure accurate, clear, and understandable labeling in accordance with the best available science. I am happy to answer any questions that you may have.

[The prepared statement of Dr. Schultz follows:]

Testimony
Before the Subcommittee on Criminal Justice, Drug Policy, and Human Resources
Committee on Government Reform
United States House of Representatives

FDA's Implementation of Public Law 106-554

Statement of

Daniel G. Schultz, M.D.
Director,
Office of Device Evaluation
Center for Devices and Radiologic Health,
Food and Drug Administration,
U.S. Department of Health and Human Services

For Release on Delivery
Expected at 11:00 AM
on Thursday, March 11, 2004

INTRODUCTION

Good morning, Mr. Chairman and Members of the Subcommittee. I am Dr. Daniel Schultz, Director of the Office of Device Evaluation in the Center for Devices and Radiological Health (CDRH) at the Food and Drug Administration (FDA or the Agency). I am pleased to speak today about FDA's implementation of Public Law (P.L.) 106-554 with respect to the labeling of condoms. Specifically, FDA has complied with P.L.106-554, by reexamining existing condom labeling to determine whether the labels are medically accurate, regarding the overall effectiveness or lack of effectiveness of condoms in preventing sexually transmitted diseases (STDs), including human papilloma virus (HPV). FDA has conducted an extensive literature and labeling review. Based on these reviews, we are developing a draft guidance document on condom labeling and correlating proposed rule, which would make the guidance a special control for condoms.

REGULATORY BACKGROUND

FDA is responsible for protecting the public health by assuring the safety, efficacy, and security of drugs, biological products, food, cosmetics, medical devices, and products that emit radiation. We do this by keeping abreast of public health issues, writing regulations that further protect the American people, and enforcing those regulations and the statutes that govern us. This hearing specifically touches on our medical device regulatory authorities. As defined by Federal law, the term "device" covers several thousand health products, ranging from simple articles such as tongue depressors and heating pads, to cutting-edge and complex devices such as pacemakers, lasers, and imaging technologies. The Medical Device Amendments of 1976 to the Federal Food, Drug, and Cosmetic Act gave FDA specific authority to regulate the safety and effectiveness of medical devices.

Using a risk-based classification framework, FDA places every medical device into one of three "classes" depending on the degree of regulatory control needed to provide reasonable assurance of safety and effectiveness. Devices posing the lowest risk, such as elastic bandages, are placed in Class I (General Controls). These general controls include the classification process itself, establishment registration and premarket notification, Quality System Requirements for manufacturing, provisions regarding adulteration and misbranding, recordkeeping, and reporting of adverse events. If general controls alone do not reasonably ensure the safety and effectiveness of a device, but FDA can identify an additional measure or measures that would provide that assurance -- "special controls" – FDA places that type of device into Class II (Special Controls), e.g., laparoscopes. Such Class II devices generally pose higher risks than Class I devices. They are then subject to the general controls that also apply to Class I devices, plus one or more of a wide range of special controls that the Agency may designate. These special controls may include performance standards, postmarket surveillance, patient registries, guidance documents, labeling, and/or clinical studies which, taken together with the general controls, are sufficient to provide a reasonable assurance of safety and effectiveness of the device. When FDA cannot be assured that the combination of general controls and special controls is sufficient to reasonably ensure safety and effectiveness of a medical device – generally higher risk devices – such devices are placed into Class III (Premarket Approval), e.g., the newer generation of global endometrial ablation systems. Premarket Approval (PMA) requires manufacturers to submit an application to FDA, which is then subject to careful scientific review to provide reasonable assurance of the safety and effectiveness of the device. FDA approval of a PMA application is necessary before a Class III device may be marketed. Once approved for marketing, Class III devices also remain subject to the general controls already described.

REGULATION OF CONDOMS

Condoms are Class II medical devices.[1] Presently, FDA addresses condom labeling with general device labeling regulations (21 CFR part 801), as well as two specific labeling regulations, one on condom expiration dating (21 CFR 801.435) and another on user warnings about allergic reactions to natural rubber latex (21 CFR 801.437). In

[1] FDA has not to date specified any measures as special controls for condoms. Condoms were devices marketed before the passage of the Medical Device Amendments of 1976, and as such, were classified into Class II as part of the initial classification of all existing devices. At that time, the statute anticipated that mandatory performance standards would be established to govern each Class II device type. This proved to be an overwhelming task for FDA, and in 1990, as part of the Safe Medical Devices Act of 1990 (P.L. 101-629), Congress changed the definition for Class II devices to make them subject to special controls—a wider range of measures than mandatory performance standards. FDA is working to specifically identify special controls for devices that were classified into Class II prior to the 1990 statutory change. While not presently designated as special controls, however, there are several existing requirements and recommendations for condom labeling that address specific safety and effectiveness issues that condoms pose.

addition, dating back to 1987, FDA has issued a series of guidance documents that address specific elements of condom labeling related to protection against STDs.

It is important to recognize that latex condoms for men are a well-made medical device that laboratory studies have shown to provide an essentially impermeable barrier to particles the size of STD pathogens. FDA has oversight responsibility to ensure that condoms are manufactured properly, and manufacturers - in turn - follow quality system regulations, including design controls, to ensure that their products do what they are intended to do: protect against pregnancy and sexually transmitted diseases. Condoms manufactured today meet performance standards for strength and freedom from holes (leakage). These standards ensure a minimum level of performance with respect to condom strength and barrier properties, characteristics that we believe are tied to what a condom is intended to do. To encourage conformance with these standards, FDA has officially recognized these standards and integrated them into both its premarket and postmarket device programs.

The typical condom package contains a front panel on the external box that is referred to as the "principal display panel." The "principal intended action" of any device must be stated on this display panel. In addition, every condom box includes more detailed information: directions for use and other important information on an insert or printed on the inside of the box.

Current FDA guidance recommends that the principal display panel of the primary retail package for condoms include a "principal intended action" statement regarding contraception and a second statement on STD risk reduction such as the one below:

Protection against sexually transmitted diseases (STDs):
If used properly, latex condoms will help to reduce the risk of transmission of HIV infection (AIDS) and many other sexually transmitted diseases.

In addition, our current guidance recommends that the package insert for condoms contain the following expanded statement:

If used properly, latex condoms will help to reduce the risk of transmission of HIV infection (AIDS) and many other sexually transmitted diseases, including chlamydia infections, genital herpes, genital warts, gonorrhea, hepatitis B, and syphilis.

AGENCY ACTIVITIES RELATED TO CONDOM LABELING

In 2001, FDA began a systematic and comprehensive review of the medical literature and key studies underlying the 2001 workshop[2] summary report and related

---

[2] The June 2000 workshop was led by the National Institute of Allergy and Infectious Disease, in partnership with the National Cancer Institute, National Institute of Child Health and Human Development, the Centers for Disease Control and Prevention, the U. S. Agency for International Development, FDA, and other

conclusions, as well as many other clinical studies on the subject that have been published since the workshop. In short, our analysis of available studies and related reports on this topic have led us to a number of findings, which are consistent with both the 2001 workshop summary and the recent Centers for Disease Control and Prevention (CDC) Report to Congress on Genital HPV Infection. Our basic conclusions are as follows:.

- Depending on the transmission vector(s) of a particular STD, the specific infectivity of the virus or bacteria, and the biological mechanisms of progression from infection to disease, the protection a condom may provide against different STDs will vary. P.L. 106-554 asks particularly about HPV infection, which can manifest as lesions – symptomatic or asymptomatic - on a man's penis or scrotum, a woman's vulva or cervix, or either's perianal areas. Because condoms do not cover all of these areas, they may not provide the same protection as they do against STDs transmitted though bodily fluids, like HIV or Gonorrhea. These same factors noted above, namely transmission vectors, infectivity, and biological mechanisms, also limit the ability to properly conduct well-controlled clinical studies that are necessary to more clearly determine condom effectiveness.

Federal agencies.

- Correct and consistent use of condoms can reduce the risk of sexual transmission of HIV (the virus that causes AIDS). We also believe that condoms, when used consistently and correctly, can reduce the risk of other STDs that are transmitted by genital secretions (such as semen or vaginal fluids), and these include gonorrhea, chlamydia, and trichomoniasis.]

- Scientific studies on STDs characterized by genital ulcers, e.g., genital herpes and syphilis, are inconclusive as to whether the risk of these diseases is lowered for condom users. However, based on what we do know about the transmission vector for these diseases, we believe that the condom will provide some measure of protection when it covers the ulcer.

- Clinical studies evaluating the relationship between condoms and HPV-related disease have not been consistent. However, even though the biological mechanism has not been conclusively demonstrated, women whose partners use condoms seem to be at reduced risk for genital warts, as well as at reduced risk for cervical cancer - compared to women whose partners do not use condoms. Therefore, there does appear to be a benefit from condom use for prevention of HPV-related disease.

AGENCY ACTIVITIES RELATED TO IMPLEMENTATION OF P.L. 106-554

P.L.106-554, enacted in December 2000, directs the Secretary of Health and Human Services to do the following review:

> *The Secretary of Health and Human Services, shall reexamine existing condom labels that are authorized pursuant to the Federal Food, Drug, and Cosmetic Act to determine whether the labels are medically accurate regarding the overall effectiveness or lack of effectiveness of condoms in preventing sexually transmitted diseases, including HPV.*

FDA has carefully reexamined existing condom labeling to determine whether the labels are medically accurate regarding the overall effectiveness of condoms in preventing STDs, including HPV. Although the interest of this hearing targets HPV, we complied with the law by exploring the labeling regarding other STDs as well. To fully accomplish this task, Agency staff have conducted a comprehensive systematic review of the published medical literature on condoms and STDs. Given the enormous scope of this effort, we have just completed this literature review and are now looking at how the results from this review might impact condom labeling.

Based on the review of the current condom literature, CDRH has developed a regulatory plan to provide condom users with a consistent labeling message about STDs and the protection they should expect from condom use. FDA is preparing new guidance on condom labeling to address these issues, with the target of publishing that guidance as a draft for public comment later this year. FDA also anticipates proposing to amend the classification regulations for condoms, to make such labeling guidance a special control for condoms.

NEW TECHNOLOGIES TO HELP DETECT AND PREVENT HPV INFECTION

In 2004, the American Cancer Society estimates that 10,520 women will be diagnosed with cervical cancer and 3,900 women will die from it. However, with proper screening, cervical cancer is avoidable and, if caught early, curable. Regular cervical cancer screening for all sexually active women and treatment of precancerous lesions remains the key strategy to prevent cervical cancer.[3]

FDA is committed to help bring safe and effective technologies to the market quickly. As noted in the testimony of CDC and NIH, there are many strains of HPV. In 1995, FDA approved the first DNA test for detection of HPV. In 1999, we approved an improved version of the test, the HC2 High-Risk HPV DNA Test, which can identify 13 of the most frequently occurring high-risk types of HPV associated with the development of cervical cancer. On March 31, 2003, the Agency approved expanded use of this test, so it now can now be used, in conjunction with a Pap test, for screening women over the age of 30. In addition, since the mid-1990s, FDA has reviewed and approved several automated and computerized systems to allow for better slide

[3] January 2004 "Report to Congress: Prevention of Genital Human Papillomavirus Infection," prepared by the Centers for Disease Control and Prevention.

preparation and more rapid screening of Pap tests. These devices are now widely used in clinical laboratories to aid in Pap test screening.

In addition, FDA's Center for Biologics Evaluation and Research (CBER) is currently working with manufacturers to bring preventive HPV vaccines to market. CBER convened an FDA Vaccines and Related Biological Products Advisory Committee meeting, in November 2001, to address endpoints for HPV vaccine efficacy trials. CBER staff have also presented at WHO meetings on HPV vaccine development, where the focus was also cervical cancer-related indications. Currently, CBER has a number of investigational new drug applications (INDs) for vaccines for the prevention of HPV infection, several of which are in advanced clinical development.

In addition to efforts directed at HPV infection, treatment of cervical cancer is a very active field for clinical research and several novel technologies are currently being applied for the treatment of this disease. CBER has more than a dozen INDs under review, for treatment of cervical cancer.

CONCLUSION

P.L. 106-554 directs FDA to look at condom labeling, not only with respect to their "overall effectiveness" in preventing STDs, but also with respect to their "lack of effectiveness." Since we have completed our literature review, we are exploring new opportunities to best inform condom users about important limitations of the device.

FDA is working to present a balanced view of the risks and benefits in condom labeling, being careful to neither encourage device use in circumstances where it may not be medically appropriate, nor to discourage device use in circumstances where it is.

Mr. Chairman, I want to reiterate that FDA is committed to monitoring closely the body of scientific evidence relating to the degree to which male condoms provide protection from HPV, HPV-related disease, and other STDs. We will continue to exercise our regulatory responsibilities appropriately in accordance with the best available science. I am happy to answer any questions you might have.

Mr. SOUDER. Thank you.

I wanted to start with Dr. Thompson at CDC. Could you put the first chart back up again?

What do you estimate would be the number of women with abnormal Pap smears who require invasive treatment? Do you have any idea? You have high risk, general infections, the diagnosis, but do you have any idea of the number of women with abnormal Pap smears who require invasive treatment?

Dr. THOMPSON. Certainly. Virtually any woman with an abnormal Pap smear certainly requires medical attention. How many of those will require invasive treatment versus observational treatment and other types of treatment I would not be able to speculate on, although there might be some knowledge of that with my colleagues from the National Cancer Institute.

Mr. SOUDER. Do you have any idea of that?

Dr. TRIMBLE. Our surveillance methods do not capture pre-invasive disease very well, so our best sources cannot give you information.

Mr. SOUDER. Obviously, a cancer diagnosis is very severe. Part of the question is in how much we stress things related to HPV. In the category that I just was referring to, as far as invasive treatment, can that be painful, when somebody is doing that? In other words, is that something you would rather not have, presumably? In other words, we definitely don't want to get death, but what I am trying to say here, because this is a sexually transmitted disease that many people don't talk about or aren't familiar with, and we are looking at cervical cancer and you say, well, that is very extreme. But how hard we hit prevention is like are there a larger group of people even more than 12,000, and 4,000 who are exposed to invasive procedures that could in fact be painful, and we don't even know the number of them. So we don't even know the scope of the problem of what we have to prevent. Because we are not trying to just prevent cancer if in fact there are other painful things that could be avoided.

Dr. THOMPSON. I would not disagree with that at all. The important message that the chart is intended to convey is that two of those bars should not appear at all. We can prevent virtually all cervical cancer, and almost any cervical cancer death represents a failure of the system.

Mr. SOUDER. But the sole goal isn't to prevent cancer, because, while we want to prevent cancer, and obviously saving life is a primary, that would be, like I mentioned earlier, when we deal with a narcotics issue, is saying our sole goal is to prevent overdose deaths of heroin, as opposed to merely somebody who beats his wife, has other kinds of problems related to heroin. The problem with HPV is beyond just cervical cancer, it is a huge problem that we need to address, but it has somewhat of a difference here, how we focus on prevention as opposed to just treatment. Are those numbers just available or you just don't know them?

Dr. TRIMBLE. We have no national surveillance system for capturing the number of Pap smears done each year in the United States. The data that Dr. Thompson cited is based on a telephone survey, so it was restricted, obviously, to women with telephones.

So we don't know for sure the number of Pap smears done each year in the United States.

Mr. SOUDER. So you don't know how many abnormal either?

Dr. TRIMBLE. We can estimate it based on some large samples. We know that, obviously for women who undergo a Pap smear, it is an uncomfortable procedure, as I think any woman in this room would be able to tell you. Women who are found to have an abnormal Pap smear then will undergo a repeat gynecological examination and colposcopy, which is uncomfortable, and can be painful if biopsies are taken. But I can't tell you the number of, let us say, colposcopies done each year in the United States; there is no data source for that.

Mr. SOUDER. Obviously, I have had a number of friends who would have preferred not to have gone through that procedure; not necessarily related to HPV, but there are other things here other than just the final stages that we prefer to avoid if we can.

And given that premise, I also wanted to ask Dr. Thompson, how do you see the CDC, then, proceeding with HPV prevention, both to avoid the ones you have on the chart and also this probably much larger interim group that has precancerous lesions and other things that need to be treated?

Dr. THOMPSON. Well, we have a number of activities, some of which are already underway, and others will be guided now by some of the findings that we have made from this new report. I think as the report reflects, there is a need to educate providers more about some of the things that we have learned in this report. There is a need to educate the public to a greater degree about human papillomavirus, its relationship to cervical cancer, and the fact that it does require a variety of followup measures such as Pap smear screening; but, in addition, it can be prevented by certain behavioral decisions if the person chooses to make those decisions. And we are in the process of, in some cases, already reflecting in our documents for the public this new information. The other cases we are in the process now of gathering information about people's current knowledge so we can tailor messages to that current knowledge and so we can deliver it in ways that people will understand it and take it to heart.

Mr. SOUDER. Several members here referred, in a kind of a side comment way, to this, and so I wanted to clarify this question in a number of ways. The CDC HPV prevention report claimed that "The use of condoms may reduce the risk of cervical cancer." The first part of this question is how many of the studies on HPV showed that there was a possible reduction in cervical cancer?

Dr. THOMPSON. There were three studies that were identified, among the published studies, that addressed this particular issue, and of those, if my recollection is correct, five identified a reduction in the risk of cervical cancer that was associated with consistent condom use, or at least with condom use as best it was measured by the survey. Of those five, two were statistically significant. So you have some statistically significant findings and a definite trend in all of the studies.

Mr. SOUDER. I missed what you said. There were five?

Dr. THOMPSON. I have been corrected, there were nine. And of those, seven showed positive results, but only two of those were statistically significant.

Mr. SOUDER. And when you say statistically significant, at what range, minimal significance or very statistically significant?

Dr. THOMPSON. The typical study value that we use, and I can't speak to these in particular, is at the 95 percent confidence level.

Mr. SOUDER. Ninety-five percent confidence level, which would be 5 percent deviation. And then how significant was that 95 percent? In other words, you are confident that there was a statistical differential. Was it like a 1 percent difference or two? We heard earlier, when we were talking about the abstinence education, that it was statistically significant, and it was also a 30 percent differential between those who signed the pledge and not. So there are two parts. The statistical question is statistically significant; and then now that we have granted a statistically significant, was it a major, minor?

Dr. THOMPSON. How large was the difference itself?

Mr. SOUDER. Yes.

Dr. THOMPSON. In some cases the difference was small; in other cases the difference was relatively large and it showed a pretty substantial preventive impact.

Mr. SOUDER. OK, if you can give us maybe some followup data.

Dr. THOMPSON. If you would like the exact numbers, we can provide you those in followup.

Mr. SOUDER. I just need it for the record.

Of those who were found, what proportion of the women and girls are likely to require treatment for precancerous? You don't necessarily have that in those studies or do you have that?

Dr. THOMPSON. If you would clarify just a little bit what you are asking. Of the women in the studies how many required additional followup and treatment?

Mr. SOUDER. Yes.

Dr. THOMPSON. We don't have that information.

Mr. SOUDER. You don't have that. That is what we were talking about earlier. Is there any evidence that the women who use condoms do not develop cervical cancer?

Dr. THOMPSON. Yes. In the studies I just referred to, that was the end point that was being evaluated, cervical cancer.

Mr. SOUDER. And we have already addressed are there other threats to that.

I heard the discussion both in the written testimony and your verbal that you are working toward things, but I wanted to make sure that it is in the record. I ask it to Dr. Schultz. Is there currently an effective vaccine to prevent HPV infection or cervical cancer?

Dr. SCHULTZ. Not to the best of my knowledge. But there may be other people who are more able to answer that question.

Mr. SOUDER. Dr. Trimble.

Dr. TRIMBLE. The Merck Corp. has presented the results of a phase 3 randomized trial demonstrating that they were able to prevent infection with HPV–16. So that was a prophylactic trial targeted at one of the subtypes, the subtype which is the most common cause of cervical cancer.

Mr. SOUDER. So it is being developed, but it is not on the market.

Dr. TRIMBLE. Right. The study has been published. They are currently studying a multivalent vaccine targeting additional three subtypes to HPV–16, but my understanding is nowhere in the world is there an HPV vaccine that is licensed and on the market.

Mr. SOUDER. How many subtypes are there?

Dr. TRIMBLE. There are more than 100 subtypes of HPV.

Mr. SOUDER. So if this vaccine were effective, it would address, potentially, three of them.

Dr. TRIMBLE. Four, actually. It is HPV–16 and 18, which are the most common cancer-causing viruses, as well as 6 and 11, which are most commonly associated with genital warts but not cancer.

Mr. SOUDER. Is there currently a microbicide that is available that would prevent transmission of HPV?

Dr. TRIMBLE. Not to my knowledge.

Dr. THOMPSON. There is not one currently licensed for use.

Mr. SOUDER. Dr. Schultz, you agree with that?

Dr. SCHULTZ. I would agree that there is nothing currently indicated for the prevention of that disease.

Mr. SOUDER. Do you believe condoms provide complete protection?

Dr. SCHULTZ. No, I don't think they provide complete protection. I think a lot of people have addressed that question, and we would agree that they provide some protection, but not complete protection.

Mr. SOUDER. Do you agree with that, Dr. Trimble?

Dr. TRIMBLE. Yes, we concur with the CDC's review of the issue.

Mr. SOUDER. I was a little confused, and I want to make sure because, Dr. Schultz, in your testimony you used "appear" and other things that were less decisive, and my understanding from your testimony, our current guidance recommends that the package insert for condoms contain the following statement: "If used properly, latex condoms will help reduce the risk of transmission of HIV infection and many other sexually transmitted diseases, including" and then you list about seven. Does that FDA guidance for condom labeling contradict the FDA scientific studies for this reason: that earlier you also said that some of the studies on STDs, I think it was the statement before that, were inconclusive? So if the studies are inconclusive, why would you list some of them as far as that it will help?

Dr. SCHULTZ. I think the answer is that when those statements were formulated, we had a certain body of data to look at. I think what we have tried to do, again, over the last 3 years, along with our colleagues in the other agencies, is to examine that data more closely, which is why we are currently engaged in the effort that we are, to see about ways to improve that labeling. So I am not sure I can answer your question any better than that, but I think that we believe that the statements do have some value. We think that there are better ways and more informative ways to provide that information.

Mr. SOUDER. Because, at a minimum, anything beyond "may" seems a pretty big stretch at this point. Would you agree?

Dr. SCHULTZ. I think that there are some areas where the word "may" is a stronger may, and then there are some areas where the word "may" is probably a weaker may. And, again, I think that is our goal, is to try to see if we can do a better job differentiating between those and providing, again, more informative information to the user.

Mr. SOUDER. I wanted to clarify for myself; I think Mr. Cummings isn't here right now. Did I understand you to say, Dr. Thompson, that over 50 percent of the cervical cancer cases were minority?

Dr. THOMPSON. No. No, what I said, that in CDC's Breast and Cervical Cancer Screening Program, which is aimed primarily at under-insured and uninsured women, where you will find a lot of minorities, that approximately half the women served by that program are racial and ethnic minorities. We do not have figures, at least at hand, and I am not sure we have them at all, as to what percentage of the women found to have cervical cancer or cervical cancer precursors in that program are minorities and which are not. We can get those figures for you, but I would caution that since this is a safety net program, meant only to serve those women who have no other source of cervical cancer screening, that it is not going to reflect the larger U.S. population.

Mr. SOUDER. What would be interesting is if a percentage is 40 percent African-American is the rate of cervical cancer higher than 40 percent. In other words, do they have a rate proportionate to the number of people being served that are disproportionately hitting certain communities, because that would suggest where we have to do outreach targeting. Not that there wouldn't be a higher incidence in the population as a whole, but what is the incidence relation to their proportion of the people being screened?

Dr. THOMPSON. These figures do exist, and, if you would like, we will provide you with those.

Mr. SOUDER. I think that would be helpful for the committee.

Dr. Schultz, in the labeling, which is one of the reasons, if not the primary reason, we are having this hearing, because some of us have been concerned, why has it taken so long? It has been nearly 4 years since we first passed legislation in Congress; there have been lots of studies coming that we do all kinds of labeling things that we put on, and then if additional information comes, you might have to adjust it. But there seems to be a certain body of information that has been here and it has been 4 years since we passed the act. Why has this taken so long?

Dr. SCHULTZ. I think that is a fair question, and I think that the best answer that I can give you, Mr. Chairman, is that we felt that this was a very important request and something that we needed to pay careful attention to. I think what we have heard today, and as is included in all of our testimony, there have been a number of studies, a number of meetings, a number of interactions that have occurred in those 3 years. We are certainly committed to looking at this and making the requisite changes, but we felt that our first responsibility was to attempt to gather the information and do it in a systemic and comprehensive way. So I would agree with your statement. I think that we have done that now, and our plans are to move ahead.

Mr. SOUDER. Well, I don't pretend to be as informed on these subjects as Dr. Coburn and Dr. Weldon, who were very active in this original piece of legislation, though I supported their efforts. One does 200 and one may do 4 Pap smears. I do zero. So I don't intend to be somebody who is expert on it, but I find it frustrating when people are dying and many others are going through painful treatments, and others are getting diseases they are going to have the rest of their life, it takes 4 years to respond, when we have many other labeling type requests that also are very complicated, that required lots of research, that are very delicate, that are politically controversial, but seem to move faster than 4 years.

And one thing I would like for our record, you said there were meetings, there were different processes. We would like that for the record. We are an oversight committee. Part of our job is very specific. This committee is supposed to see that the laws of Congress are enforced by the executive branch. There was a time period that allowed the development of the studies, but that, to be generous, would be probably 2 years, not 4 years. And we want to see this move forward, but we would also like to see the evidence, as we have asked of the last administration, when we had lots of conflicts as a Republican. But also as a Republican administration, we want to see the evidence that the meetings took place, what they were, when they were, and why this process is taking so long.

Would any of you like to hear anything here? Because I am going to go vote and then we will be back, and I know Mr. Cummings is planning to be back too. Anything you would like to add?

With that, I am going to assume that we are done with this panel, and we will move to the panel. If Mr. Cummings, when he comes back, has any questions, if you could remain.

Just a second, let me find out how many votes there are before I ask you to do that.

I think, since he is not here, we are going to go ahead and dismiss, because we have three votes, so it will be quite a while. Thank you very much for coming. He will submit any written questions, Mr. Waxman and any of the other Members who do. Thank you for your time.

[Recess.]

Mr. SOUDER. The subcommittee now stands reconvened.

And if the third panel will come forth, Dr. Tom Coburn, a former Member of Congress, from Muskogee, OK; Dr. Freda Bush from Jackson, MS; Dr. John Cox from Santa Barbara, CA; Dr. Barbara Meeker from Traverse City, MI; Dr. Jonathan Zenilman from Baltimore, MD.

I am going to briefly recess the subcommittee again.

[Recess.]

Mr. SOUDER. The subcommittee is reconvened.

If you could each stand and raise your right hand.

[Witnesses sworn.]

Mr. SOUDER. Let the record show that each of the witnesses responded in the affirmative.

I thank you each for coming, and if I can again say for the record, in addition to Dr. Coburn from Muskogee, OK; Dr. Bush from Jackson, MS; Dr. Cox from Santa Barbara, CA; Dr. Meeker from Traverse City, MI; and Dr. Zenilman from Baltimore, MD. We thank each of you for coming and participating in our discussion today, and we will start with Dr. Coburn.

STATEMENTS OF TOM A. COBURN, M.D., MUSKOGEE, OK; FREDA BUSH, M.D., FACOG, JACKSON, MS; JOHN THOMAS COX, M.D., SANTA CLARA, CA; MARGARET MEEKER, M.D., TRAVERSE CITY, MI; AND JONATHAN M. ZENILMAN, M.D., BALTIMORE, MD

Dr. COBURN. Mr. Chairman, thank you. I need to make some corrections. I am not a member of the American Academy of Otorhinolaryngology, but the American Academy of Otorhinolaryngolic Allergy. And I need to make that correction.

I am happy to be here. I am going to summarize my testimony and ask that my written testimony be made part of the record.

This is a disease that is very dear to my heart. I have delivered in excess of 3,500 babies, close to 4,000. I have handled every complication of sexually transmitted disease there can be, and there is no question that we have an uncontrolled epidemic in this country, worse now than when this bill was offered, and it is not being dealt with appropriately by the Government and the agencies in regard to that.

And I want to just describe an 18-year-old girl this last month who came in for treatment from me who has had one sexual partner. It hasn't been 10 or 15 years since she was exposed to this virus, she became sexually active at the age of 16. And through her testing and Pap smear, she ended up losing a good portion of her cervix to prevent her from having invasive cancer. That is not the end of the story, because what in fact it will do is decrease her likelihood of ever achieving a pregnancy, and, if she does achieve a pregnancy, increase the likelihood of pre-term delivery, which the average pre-term delivery in this country now costs us as a Nation about $200,000. So this disease is not without consequences.

I think it is also very important that we not just limit it to the sexually transmitted disease aspect of it, because there is a new study out just this year. Twenty to 25 percent of all head and neck cancers now are associated with this virus, can be directly associated with exposure of this virus. Rectal carcinoma, especially in the gay population, is 100 percent attributable to this virus. So there is tremendous costs associated with this virus that we need to look at and ask why the Government hasn't responded in the way it should in terms of prevention.

And I also interestingly note, and I think this is part of the culture that needs to be looked at, when we hear the CDC mentioned, we don't ever hear the complete name of the CDC mentioned anymore; it is the Center for Disease Control. We heard Dr. Thompson, who I have a great deal of respect for, but the fact is the Center for Disease Control is not their name. It is the Center for Disease Control and Prevention. And although they dropped the name of Prevention, in this case they dropped that aspect of the responsibility, because they failed miserably in terms of the prevention of this disease.

I also would make a couple comments outside of my written testimony. We heard several times today about statistically significant reduction in cancer of the cervix associated with condoms. There are 20 studies in that. Two may show, and the word is "may"; it is not does, it is not "is," it is not "will", it is may show a reduction. There are 15 that statistically say there is no reduction in cervical cancer. So it is important to have a balanced look. There are two that may show a reduction.

The other thing that I would say is what Congresswoman Norton had to say is right on. We need access for the women in this country to make sure they are screened. There is no question about that. And there is no question that the minority population has the greatest risk for not being screened. Of the two cancers of the cervix in my practice in the last 2 years who have gone on to die were both minority women who presented late with an advanced stage of the disease.

Finally, I would make a point that the CDC did not address. There is over 1.350 million procedures done every year in this country for cervical dysplasia, and that ranges all the way from just doing a simple microscopic exam with biopsies of the uterine cervix, to cryotherapy, to laser surgery, to what we call leap electrical excision, to hysterectomy. And those aren't even counted in the numbers that the CDC are looking at. So the minimum we are spending, the minimum we are spending in this country on this disease on a gynecological aspect is $3 billion. That doesn't have anything to do with all the late stage carcinoma of the vulva, which is out there that CDC isn't following. Nobody is looking at a young lady who gets treated by HPV and then 35 years later ends up with a carcinoma of the vulva, of the reproductive system; and nobody has gone back and nobody has looked forward to see what that cost is. So if you look at the overall cost of what we are paying in terms of health care dollars for the lack of prevention for HPV, what we see is a cost greater than what HIV is costing this Nation; and we ought to talk about it frankly.

And then the final point that I would make, as my time is just about out, is our young people aren't stupid. They may make immature decisions, they may make wrong decisions, but to say we should not give them every bit of information about this disease, and to say that a condom shouldn't be labeled appropriately to warn them that this will not protect them, and the fact that a condom, in the best hands of an adolescent, fails about 13 to 20 percent of the time for pregnancy, so it is not a cure-all that we hear so blatantly stated; and in terms of sexually transmitted disease it is even less than that, of many of the other diseases.

So I would like to see the committee look at the total aspect of this disease, also to follow the public law that I authored before I left Congress, and to hold accountable the CDC and the FDA. To think that the FDA may not, and I thought it was very peculiar. I thought may meant may, I didn't know may meant strong or soft or weak. I thought may meant may. And the fact is condoms do not offer significant protection against this virus, and the packaging ought to label it, because our children have a right to know. If they want to make a bad decision, they will. And I routinely advise patients in my practice that if they are going to be sexually active, and if they are going to be outside of monogamous relationships, they ought to always use a condom. I am not anti-condom, but I am pro-truth and pro-science. And this isn't a bias, this is interrupting a health pattern that costs us dearly, impacts lives tremendously, and the social and emotional costs of this disease cannot be measured.

And with that I thank you.

[The prepared statement of Dr. Coburn follows:]

Prepared Testimony of the Honorable Tom A. Coburn, M.D. Before the Subcommittee on Criminal Justice, Drug Policy and Human Resources

"Cervical Cancer and Human Papillomavirus"

March 11, 2004

Chairman Souder, Ranking Member Cummings, distinguished members of the Subcommittee, I am grateful for the opportunity to address the Subcommittee regarding cervical cancer and human papillomavirus (HPV). I commend the Subcommittee for its continued efforts to promote awareness about HPV and cervical cancer.

Observations from My Medical Practice

I am a practicing physician and a member of the American Academy of Family Physicians and the American Academy of Otorhinolaryngology. I have been practicing medicine for 18 years. My patients represent a broad segments of the population, including those covered under Medicaid and Medicare.

During my nearly two decades treating patients I have seen an every growing number affected by sexually transmitted diseases. In particular, I have been performing an increasing number of procedures to treat HPV infection.

I want to relate to you the story of one recent patient of mine. She is an 18-year-old girl who has had only one sexual partner. She is now infected with HPV. To prevent the onset of invasive cervical cancer, a large portion of this young girl's cervix had to be removed. As a result she is less likely to be able to become pregnant in the future and more likely to have a premature infant if she does become pregnant. And despite already undergoing invasive treatment, she remains at risk for future complications and additional surgeries.

This girl and the others that I am caring for every day in my medical practice are the real faces of those affected by HPV. What we are confronting is not an isolated epidemic.

The National HPV Epidemic

HPV is the most common sexually transmitted disease in the United States. About 24 million Americans are currently infected with HPV according to the National

Cancer Institute and an estimated 5.5 million Americans become infected with HPV every year. With 4.6 million of these HPV infections acquired by those aged 15 to 24, HPV accounts for over half of all new sexually transmitted diseases among young Americans. On March 8, 2004, researchers from the Colorado Health Sciences Center reported that more than 30 percent of women in a recent study were found to be infected with a strain of HPV linked to cervical and anal cancer. In comparison, 18.7 percent of men carried HPV-16, one of 10 high-risk strains of the virus.

Over 1,350,000 women will have invasive procedures each year just to assess the status of their abnormal pap smears secondary to HPV. According to the American Cancer Society, every year over 12,000 new cases of invasive cervical cancer are diagnosed and more than 4,000 women die of the disease. And non-invasive cervical cancer is estimated to be four times as widespread as the invasive type.

HPV is also associated with oral cancer, cancers of the vagina, penis, anus, head and neck, more than one million pre-cancerous lesions, and genital warts. In addition, HPV has been detected in some prostate tumors. An infected mother may transmit HPV to her newborn with affected children facing prolonged, difficult treatment for respiratory papillomatosis.

Federal Health Agencies Ignore Scientific Data

During my tenure in Congress (1995- 2001), I heard from other practicing physicians all across the nation confronting the same epidemic of HPV and other STDs that I was seeing in my own medical practice. Few of my patients with HPV, or the patients of my colleagues, had ever heard of the virus and were unaware of its health risks.

A growing library of scientific data demonstrated that HPV was linked to a number of serious health conditions, with over 99 percent of all cervical cancers associated with HPV infection.

Likewise, scientific data concluded that condoms provided no protection against HPV infection. "Behaviors such as beginning sexual intercourse at an early age-- especially age 16 or younger-- and having many sexual partners increase the chance that a woman will develop an HPV infection in the cervix," according to the National Cancer Institute. Those with multiple sexual partners or who had partners with multiple sexual partners enhance their risk for pervasive HPV infection by increasing the likelihood of exposure to HPV, as well as repeated exposure and re-infection, regardless of condom use.

Therefore, those who chose to have multiple sexual partners believing they were being protected by following the advice of the Centers for Disease Control and Prevention (CDC) to use condoms, were actually placing themselves and their partners at increased risk for HPV infection.

Studies had indicated for years that promiscuity was associated with cervical cancer and that contrary to CDC dogma, condoms did not protect against the cervical cancer virus. Then an April 1- 3, 1996 National Institutes of Health Consensus Development Conference Statement on Cervical Cancer stated "Primary prevention of HPV infection will require (1) directing education efforts toward adolescents and health care providers regarding the strong causal link between acquisition of HPV as a sexually transmitted disease and development of cervical cancer and its precursors, (2) encouraging delayed onset of sexual intercourse, (3) developing an effective prophylactic vaccine, and (4) developing effective vaginal microbicides. The data on the use of barrier methods of contraception to prevent the spread of HPV is controversial but does not support this as an effective method of prevention."

Regardless of these scientific findings and recommendations, the CDC ignored the NIH consensus statement and continued to focus almost exclusively on promoting condom use and regular PAP tests.

As a family physician/obstetrician, I cannot understate the importance of regular PAP test for women and I support federal efforts that encourage and provide access to such tests.

As an HPV prevention message, however, this approach was designed to fail, as it has. Promoting condom use did nothing to control the rampant spread of HPV since condoms cannot prevent HPV infection. PAP tests and treatment certainly are responsible for the dramatic decline in cervical cancer deaths, but likewise do not and cannot prevent HPV infection. CDC has confused disease management with disease prevention.

Treatment is often invasive, unpleasant, and costly and does not preclude the necessity for additional treatments or adverse side effects.

Cervical cancer is treated using surgery, radiation and chemotherapy; sometimes two or more methods are used. The most common types of surgery include cryosurgery, laser surgery, cone biopsy, simple hysterectomy, radical hysterectomy and pelvis lymph node dissection, and pelvic exenteration. Radiation therapy may involve external radiation or internal radiation (radioactive materials implanted in the tumor).

Treatment for cervical dysplasia—a premalignant or precancerous change in the cells of the cervix that may progress to cancer—include surgery, cone biopsy, cryosurgery, laser surgery, and electrosurgery.

The direct medical cost of treating a patient with cervical cancer is $9,200 to $13,360, while surgery to remove a precancerous lesion is $1,100 to $4,360. The financial burden of HPV in the U.S. has been estimated to range from $1.6 billion to $6 billion annually, making HPV one of the most costly sexually transmitted diseases after HIV/AIDS.

It is a cruel distortion of the word "prevention" to tell women and young girls that the tremendous physical, emotional and financial costs of treatment for HPV infection are a cost worth bearing as a consequence of federal health agencies intentional distortion and cover-up of scientific data related to HPV.

Armed with personal stories of women suffering the physical and emotional consequences of HPV infection from my own medical practice and supported by the best available scientific data, I repeatedly asked the CDC and the Food and Drug Administration (FDA) to take action to educate the public about HPV. Yet both CDC and FDA continued to maintain that condoms do prevent HPV or that perhaps more research was necessary to determine what level of protection condoms do provide.

In a February 19, 1999 letter to the House Commerce Committee on which I served, Dr. Richard D. Klausner, then-Director of the National Cancer Institute (NCI), stated, "condoms are ineffective against HPV." The science in this regard is so clear that Dr. Klausner concluded "additional research efforts by NCI on the effectiveness of condoms in preventing HPV transmission are not warranted."

On March 16, 1999, the House Commerce Committee's Subcommittee on Health and the Environment held a hearing a hearing entitled "Women's Health: Raising Awareness of Cervical Cancer." At this hearing, CDC continued to argue that condom use does protect against HPV. When asked in a follow up letter to NCI to "explain the difference in conclusions made by CDC and NCI," Dr. Douglas Lowy, Deputy Director of NCI's Division of Basic Sciences, explained that "the NCI conclusion that condoms are ineffective against HPV infection is based on the results of several long term studies that have failed to show that barrier contraceptives prevent cervical HPV infection, dysplasia, or cancer." NCI provided a number of published studies to support this lack of protection but was unable to explain CDC's claims, suggesting that perhaps CDC had confused HPV with HIV.

When the expert testimony of the Nation's premier health agency and published scientific data still failed to convince CDC and FDA that condoms do not protect against HPV, I asked Dr. Klausner to convene a panel of experts to review the available data and issue a consensus statement. On June 12-13, 2000, in Herndon, Virginia, representatives from the National Institute of Allergy and Infectious Diseases, FDA, CDC and the U.S. Agency for International Development gathered to evaluate the published data on latex condoms and STD prevention.

The panel's report entitled "Scientific Evidence on Condom Effectiveness for Sexually Transmitted Disease (STD) Prevention" issued in April 2001 "concluded that there was no evidence that condom use reduced the risk of HPV infection." The panel, furthermore, found that based on a meta-analysis of published studies, condoms could reduce the risk of HIV infection for men and women and the risk of gonorrhea for men only. In regards to the remaining STDs, the panel concluded "there was insufficient evidence from the epidemiological studies on these diseases to draw definite conclusions about the effectiveness of the latex male condom in reducing the transmission of these diseases."

Yet a month after the release of the panel's report, the CDC website posted a fact sheet entitled "Condoms and Their Use in Preventing HIV and Other STDs" that read "The correct and consistent use of latex condoms during sexual intercourse- vaginal, anal, or oral- can greatly reduce a person's risk of acquiring or transmitting most STDs, including HIV infection, gonorrhea, chlamydia, trichomonas, human papilloma virus infection (HPV), and hepatitis B."

The Passage of a Federal HPV Law

With my pleas ignored, I authored legislation directing the CDC and FDA to take actions to educate the public with "medically accurate information" about HPV. I was disappointed when groups that claimed to advocate for women's health, such as the American College of Obstetricians and Gynecologists (ACOG), opposed my proposal and fought to keep the public misinformed about HPV.

The HPV law was approved by Congress as a component of the Consolidated Appropriations Act of 2001 and became Public Law 106-554 with the signature of President Bill Clinton on December 21, 2000. In a Statement of Administration policy, President Clinton stated, "The Administration supports the goal of better informing the public about HPV and the fact that the use of condoms may not fully prevent HPV transmission."

The law directed CDC to develop a report outlining the "best strategies to prevent future infections, based on the available science." CDC was also directed to conduct a number of studies to determine the prevalence of specific types of HPV infection in various regions of the U.S., the impact of HPV diagnosis on patients, the level of HPV knowledge of physicians and the public. Upon the completion of these studies, CDC is to "develop and disseminate educational materials for the public and health care providers regarding HPV and its impact and prevention."

The law directs the FDA to "reexamine existing condom labels ... to determine whether the labels are medically accurate regarding the overall effectiveness or lack of effectiveness of condoms in preventing sexually transmitted diseases, including HPV."

Finally, the law requires that all educational and prevention material printed by the Department of Health and Human Services (HHS), CDC, FDA, and other HHS agencies, contractors, grantees and subgrantees "that are specifically designed to address STDs including HPV shall contain medically accurate information regarding the effectiveness or lack of effectiveness of condoms in preventing the STD the materials are designed to address."

Enactment of the Law

I quickly learned that it would require more than passing a law to convince CDC and FDA to take action to educate the public about HPV.

The law is clear that the CDC and other government agencies and partners must provide "medically accurate information regarding the effectiveness or lack of effectiveness of condoms" in preventing HPV and other sexually transmitted diseases. Yet in a July 2001 "Dear Colleague" letter to its partners, the CDC issued inaccurate information regarding the effectiveness of condoms. The CDC stated "epidemiological studies have generally not demonstrated an association between condom use and the risk of HPV infection, but these studies are inconclusive because of limitations in how they were designed. Again, these limitations would generally lead to an underestimation of the protective effect." The inaccurate claim that studies are "inconclusive" is repeated several times in the CDC letter. The CDC letter also provides what is labeled "Theoretical Basis for Protection" that claims "consistent and correct use of latex condoms would be expected to protect against transmission of genital ulcer diseases and HPV in some, but not all, instances." This is medically inaccurate and does not reflect the available clinical science.

A progress report was required to be made to Congress within a year of enactment of this law, which would have been December 21, 2001. The report, dated "August 2003," was delivered to Congress on September 12, 2003, nearly two years overdue.

The CDC was required by law to "develop a final report not later than three years after such effective date [before December 21, 2003], including a detailed summary of the significant findings and problems and best strategies to prevent future infections, based on the available science." CDC released a timetable in September 2003 projecting that this report would not be released in compliance with the legally sanctioned date, but rather in 2007, four years after the due date set by law.

Congress approved the HPV law precisely because federal health agencies had failed to educate the American public about the health risks of HPV and how it can be prevented and now these same agencies were continuing their cover-up of the HPV epidemic, now in violation of federal law.

Because of this continued resistance, I requested the Inspector General of the Department of Health and Human Services "conduct a thorough investigation to determine why Public Law 106-554 has been both misinterpreted and largely ignored by CDC and the FDA and to make recommendations to ensure that these agencies immediately comply with the directives and intent of this law" and to "determine if federal agencies and organizations receiving federal funds are providing medically accurate information about HPV."

But only after pressure was applied to CDC by this Subcommittee and other Congressional offices, did the agency finally issue the HPV prevention report on January 30, 2004, a month past the deadline set by law.

The CDC report, entitled "Report to Congress: Prevention of Human Papillomavirus Infection" finally acknowledges that the CDC's long held positions on HPV and condoms were incorrect. Specifically, the CDC report states:

> "Because genital HPV infection is most common in men and women who have had multiple sex partners, abstaining from sexual activity (i.e. refraining from any genital contact with another individual) is the surest way to prevent infection. For those who choose to be sexually active, a monogamous relationship with an uninfected partner is the strategy most likely to prevent future genital HPV infections. For those who choose to be sexually active but who are not in a monogamous relationship, reducing the number of sexual partners and choosing a partner less likely to be infected may reduce the risk of genital HPV infection. ...
>
> "The available scientific evidence is not sufficient to recommend condoms as a primary prevention strategy for the prevention of genital HPV infection. ...
>
> "Regarding other possible prevention approaches, no data indicate that treatment of clinical lesions or use of microbicides will prevent transmission of infection."

The FDA has yet to act to ensure that condom labeling is medically accurate to reflect the lack of effectiveness of condoms in preventing HPV infection as required by the law. The FDA's failure to inform consumers about the lack of effectiveness of condoms in preventing HPV undermines that agency's mission of ensuring that products are safe and effective.

Recommendations

Continued oversight by this Subcommittee is essential to ensure that CDC and FDA fully comply with the federal HPV prevention and education law and to ensure that the public is given medically accurate information about HPV.

With 4.6 million young people under the age of 25 expected to contact this disease, more than 4,000 women projected to die as a result of cervical cancer and up to $6 billion to be spent on HPV care all within a single year, turning back the HPV epidemic should be among the highest of CDC's priorities. CDC must take immediate action to aggressively promote the findings and prevention recommendations contained within its January 2004 HPV prevention report. This includes promoting the value of delaying sexual debut and avoiding promiscuity. Recent studies have found that young Americans are ready to hear this message and are already choosing abstinence. *The New York Times* reported on March 7, that "More than half of all male high school students reported in 2001 that they were virgins, up from 39 percent in 1990." The trends are similar for female students, who are even more likely than boys to report that they are virgins, according to the data reported in the *New York Times*.

In addition to efforts to support healthy behaviors, Congress and the National Institutes for Health should continue to support the research and development of an effective HPV vaccine.

Finally as a physician I believe that the history of stonewalling, cover-up and erroneous statements regarding HPV put forth by CDC and FDA over the past decade have compromised these agencies' credibility and endangered the public's health. This is unfortunate since so many look to these agencies for sound scientific advice and guidance.

I thank this Subcommittee for its continued leadership in protecting the public's health by ensuring that science is not manipulated, suppressed or distorted to advance a political rather than public health agenda.

###

Mr. SOUDER. Thank you very much.

Dr. Bush.

Dr. BUSH. Thank you, Mr. Chairman, for the opportunity to speak here today to this very important issue. I am Dr. Freda McKissick Bush from Jackson, MS. I have been practicing obstetrics and gynecology for the last 21 years, and I have been in women's health for about 35 years helping women to have positive childbirth experiences, because I think it is great to be a woman, but also helping them make good choices for their gynecologic health.

Through the years, the hidden epidemic of human papillomavirus [HPV], has been a challenge to them achieving that ideal. HPV is the most prevalent of all viral sexually transmitted infections, as we have heard this morning, and it is estimated that 5.5 million women are infected by HPV every year in the United States, 3.5 million have abnormal Pap smears; 13,400 are diagnosed with cervical cancer, and 4,100 die.

Of the more than 100 HPV strains identified, around 35 can infect the human genital tract. Infection with benign strains that do not cause cancer may lead to genital warts, which may be associated with itching, burning, or pain. In contrast, most infections with cancer-causing strains may have no symptoms at all. Unlike non-sexually transmitted viral infections such as the common cold, influenza, or measles, that only last a week or two, HPV infections can last for months, and occasionally for years.

Recent estimates indicate that 50 to 75 percent of sexually active adults are HPV-positive. In general, that puts sexually active people at risk for HPV. This includes age at onset of sexual activity, at least age, less than 16 years; multiple sexual partners; sex with partners who engage in high-risk sexual behavior; adolescent and young adult females are biologically more susceptible to HPV disease because their cervix has not yet matured. So you have younger people getting infected and suffering greater consequences because of the immaturity of their bodies.

The incubation period between HPV infection and the development of genital warts ranges from 30 days to 9 months. These changes resulting from cancer-causing strains are usually not visible to the naked eye. Once a person is infected, the virus persists for an average of 8 months. Approximately 10 to 12 percent of women will have persistent infections. The persistence of infection has been identified as a significant risk factor for the development of cervical dysplasia and cancer.

With current Pap smear screening technology, it is possible to sort abnormal specimens into low-and high-risk categories. Patients with high-risk types require microscopic evaluation of the cervix to identify the abnormal areas so that cervical biopsies can be obtained for pathologic evaluation.

In the United States, more than 50 million Pap smears are evaluated annually. The question was asked earlier what does this translate into as far as pre-cancerous lesions. According to the American Cancer Society, 1.2 million Pap smears have low-grade squamous interepithelial lesions; 300,000 have high-grade lesions. Sadly, 13,400 cases of cancer are diagnosed.

Approximately two-thirds of males whose female sexual partners are diagnosed with cervical dysplasia have microscopic HPV lesions of the penis. Infection of the penis or anus with high-risk HPV types predisposes these men to cancer of those organs.

Because HPV is a viral infection, no curative treatment is available. In 2000, a national panel was convened by NIH to investigate condom effectiveness. This panel found that condoms do not provide any protection for HPV infection in females, although it may reduce the risk for HPV-associated diseases. Because genital warts and asymptomatic HPV infection may be outside the area covered by a condom, consistent and correct condom use leaves a significant chance for transmitting these and other sexual diseases.

Obviously, the best way to prevent transmission of any sexually transmitted infection is to abstain from sexual intercourse outside a long-term mutually monogamous relationship such as marriage. Ad Health, the nationwide adolescent health study, found that the best deterrent to sexual activity among adolescents involved parental influence, moral and religious training, community influences, and appropriate peer influences.

In conclusion, HPV is a preventable disease. You must initiate methods to track the incidence and prevalence of disease. We must take steps to stop the alarming increase in this disease among teens and young adults. We must stop promoting methods that are known to have high failure rates in preventing HPV transmission, notably the condom, and be honest in informing young people about this fact. We must continue to emphasize highly effective methods of prevention, namely abstinence, whenever possible.

Thank you, again, for the opportunity to continue to promote health.

Mr. SOUDER. Thank you. And we will make sure that NIH, FDA, and CDC get your number, since they didn't appear to have those numbers at a congressional hearing meant to discuss that subject, which was a tad frustrating.

Dr. BUSH. Yes, sir.

Mr. SOUDER. Dr. Cox.

Dr. COX. My name is Tom Cox. I would like to thank you for having me here today. I have been a gynecologist for 30 years. I am the director of the Women's Clinic at the University of California-Santa Barbara. For the last 16 years my primary interest has been in studies on the natural history of HPV and cervical cancer, and on the best options of prevention of cervical cancer, including writing national guidelines for both primary screen and management.

I had the privilege of testifying before the House Subcommittee on Health and the Environment on HPV in 1999, and at that time I mentioned the tremendous progress this country has made in reducing cervical cancer rates as a result of Pap screening. In 1949, the year that the Pap screening was introduced to this country, the 2004 equivalent of 50,000 cases of cervical cancer occurred. This rate is 12,200 this last year and is solely, but steadily, declining.

Since 1999, there has been a real "sea change" in cervical cancer screening recommendations and in management of women with abnormal Pap tests. New recommendations have been issued that focus on detection of the cause of cervical cancer, and we all know that to be HPV, and not solely on the often subjective cervical cellular changes in cytology. Improved screening and improved management of abnormal Pap tests, and the promise of an effective vaccine against the most important of the oncogenic HPV types are moving us toward the eventual elimination of cervical cancer. In the near term, better targeting of high-risk populations could translate into further progress in reducing cervical cancer.

By high-risk populations, I am referring particularly to the majority of women who get cervical cancer who have either never had a Pap test or have had one or more Paps, but have not had them at recommended intervals. A substantial commitment to understanding the reasons for failure to attend screening and facilitation of access to health services is necessary in order to overcome these barriers. As far as I am concerned, this is where our focus today should be, because this is something we can truly do something about.

Cervical cancer not infrequently strikes women of late childbearing age, disrupting families and society much more than many other cancers that occur with highest frequency in the elderly. The fact that cervical cancer can be prevented in most circumstances makes these deaths especially tragic. Wise investment by Government in a program of cervical cancer prevention is, therefore, both morally right and economically sound.

As we have heard repeatedly today, infection with HPV does not mean a woman will eventually get cancer. The reality is that the vast majority of sexually active Americans will be infected with HPV at some point in their lives, but only a small proportion of women infected with HPV will see it progress to cervical cancer. Most commonly, the immune system suppresses or eliminates HPV, usually within 6 to 24 months, and although HPV must be present for cervical cancer to develop, the converse is not true. The good news is that cervical cancer is nearly entirely preventable because the progression from pre-cancer to cancer typically takes years or even decades, during which time persistent infections leading to pre-cancer can be detected by Pap screening or HPV testing, and subsequently treated.

So given the complexities of the HPV-cervical cancer link, what are the appropriate public health messages? I would argue that policymakers and public health practitioners have an obligation to be both realistic and pragmatic. The median age for marriage in the United States continues to rise for both men and women. By 2000, the median age for first marriage was 25 years for women and 27 years for men. The median age of puberty is 13. Throughout history, virginity, at least for women, until marriage has been secured primarily by either very early marriage of women, soon after puberty, or by sequestering women in strictly controlled separation of sexes until marriage. Neither option would be acceptable in this country; hence, 90 percent of Americans engage in sex prior to marriage. So although abstinence messages for young people make good sense, abstinence until marriage as the sole message is irresponsible.

I would urge those individuals influential in making public policy to avoid fear-based messages that overstate the risk of HPV and understate the protection provided by condoms, particularly for other STDs, particularly for HIV. Disparaging condoms threatens to undermine the tremendous progress that we have made in lowering teen pregnancy rates and in reducing the risk of transmission of far deadlier STDs such as HIV. Instead, the most helpful public health message for the prevention of cervical cancer is to encourage women to get appropriate screening and recommended followup care.

Again, thank you for the opportunity to address these issues. I firmly believe that the war against HPV and cervical cancer can and will be won in my lifetime, but it will not be won by hyperbole, but rather by providing the best protective cervical screening available for all women and by providing HPV vaccines to all children once these vaccines become available.

My written testimony contains additional details. I would be pleased to answer any questions that you may have.

[The prepared statement of Dr. Cox follows:]

Statement of J. Thomas Cox, MD
Regarding
Hearing on Human Papillomavirus and Cervical Cancer

Chairman Souder, members of the House Subcommittee on Criminal Justice, Drug Policy and Human Resources, my name is John Thomas Cox, MD. I am Director of the Women's Clinic at the University of California in Santa Barbara, Past-Chair of the Steering Committee for the National Cancer Institute sponsored ASCUS/LSIL Triage Study (ALTS) and Secretary of the American Society of Colposcopy and Cervical Pathology. I want to express my thanks for providing me the opportunity to present a clinical perspective on the issues related to human papillomavirus and cervical health as I see it in 2004.

Cervical cancer prevention: Where are we in 2004?

I had the privilege of sharing information of cervical cancer screening and human papillomavirus at a 1999 hearing of the House Subcommittee on Health and the Environment. Since that time there has been a "sea change" in cervical cancer screening recommendations and in management of women with abnormal Pap tests. As a result, women in the US and, to some extent, worldwide, will benefit by improved recommendations that focus on detection of the cause of cervical cancer, HPV, and not solely on often subjective cervical cellular changes. However, it must be remembered that the Pap test has successfully decreased cervical cancer incidence approximately 1% per year over the past 26 years. Cervical cancers are now uncommon, the annual incidence per million women ranging from 8 to 14 for squamous cell cancers and from 0.7 to 2.7 for cervical adenocarcinoma. In 1949, the year that Pap smear screening was introduced in the US the 2004 equivalent of 50,000 cases of cervical cancer occurred. Instead, the Pap and subsequent treatment of successfully identified cervical cancer precursors has reduced this rate to 12,200 and is steadily declining yearly. Although cervical cancer has not yet been entirely eliminated in the US, it is surely not an epidemic as some would lead all to believe. However, the potential to nearly eliminate cervical cancer is on the near horizon. For that to happen, we, as educators, as policy makers, and as caregivers must work together, with our only interest being in the well-being of all women. This requires a solid commitment to appropriate education of our youth, to provision of resources that provide access for the best up-to-date cervical cancer screening for all women in the US and for provision of HPV vaccines for all children when they become available. We must not forget that the majority of women who get cervical cancer are those who have either never has a Pap test, or have had one or more Paps but have not had them at recommended intervals.

Commitment to appropriate education of our youth

HPV is the most common sexually transmitted disease in America. Seventy-five to 80 percent of sexually active Americans will be infected with HPV at some point in their lives – meaning that anyone who has ever had sexual relations has a high chance of being exposed to this virus. HPV is sexually transmitted and depending upon the location of HPV induced lesions can be transmitted despite consistent condom use. HPV is asymptomatic and as with most viruses, there is no direct treatment of the virus yet available. However, the immune system most commonly suppresses or eliminates HPV, with the infection usually becoming undetectable within 6 months to 2 years. In rare instances, persistent infection with certain types of HPV can cause cervical cancer. HPV must be present for cervical cancer to develop, however, it is critical to remember that the converse is not true – infection with HPV does NOT mean that a woman will eventually get cervical cancer. Only a small proportion of women infected with HPV will get cervical cancer – for cervical cancer is an uncommon consequence of HPV infection. However, many will use these statistics related to transmissibility and the connection between HPV and cervical cancer to promote abstinence until marriage on the basis of fear. Others will point to the high rate of spontaneous suppression of HPV as reassurance that the almost ubiquitous infection rate of HPV does not justify over-reaction and the fact that most studies show decreased rates of genital warts and cervical cancer amongst women whose partner(s) consistently use condoms. Unfortunately, fear messages based upon overstating the risk of HPV and understating the protection provided by condoms threatens to undermine the tremendous progress made to lower teen pregnancy and STD rates.

What should the educational messages be? There is no question that the more partners one has and the earlier that one begins sexual activity, the higher the risk for infection with any of the sexually transmitted diseases. It is also true that diligent condom use does not consistently prevent HPV transmission, despite decreased rates of genital warts and cervical cancer noted with such use in most studies. So what should education be for our children if we are to best prepare them for their years as adults? Should we teach them that the only sure way of preventing all STDs is to abstain from intercourse until marriage and not discuss protective measures just because not all are definitively prevented? Or should we be realistic and pragmatic, taking into account the reality of people's lives. We are not just discussing the education of children but the preparation of our children to be adults. The median age for marriage in the US continues to rise for both men and women. In 1970 the median age for first marriage was 20.8 years for women and 23.2 years for men. By 2000 these ages had risen to 25.1 years for women and 26.8 years for men. The median age of puberty is 13. Throughout history, virginity (for women) until marriage has been secured primarily by either very early marriage of women soon after puberty, or by sequestering women in strictly controlled separation of the sexes until marriage. That these approaches do not exist in most of the US, nor would they ever be acceptable to a free society, is not arguable. As the "Family Life Education Act of 2001" (H.R. 3469) so correctly stated "Comprehensive sexuality education programs respect the diversity of values and beliefs represented in the community and will compliment and augment the sexuality education children receive from their families". Can we realistically promote abstinence-only in the majority of adults until their late 20s? Sex education must teach both the positives of abstinence until marriage and educate how best to minimize risk for the majority who will undoubtedly at some point choose otherwise. Short of abstinence, condoms remain the best protection against a range of sexually transmitted diseases, including HIV. There is no place in government legislation for regulation of educational or medical policy that falls far outside the arena of the majority of medical and educational research and thought. What government can do is provide funds that make sure that the best messages are taught that encourage young people to delay the onset intercourse and at the same time prepare them with the tools needed to best protect themselves and their partner from sexually transmitted diseases once they do become sexually active. That is the only realistic protection. In my view, the language of the Family Life Education Act, if not distorted to favor one viewpoint over another, provides that balance. The Act lists the following as requirements for a program of family life education:

(1). Is age appropriate and medically accurate

(2). Does not teach or promote religion

(3). Teaches that abstinence is the only sure way to avoid pregnancy or sexually transmitted diseases

(4). Stresses the value of abstinence while not ignoring those young people who have had, or are having sexual intercourse

(5). Provides information about the health benefits and side effects of all contraceptives and barrier methods as a means to prevent pregnancy

(6). Provides information about the health benefits and side effects of all contraceptives and barrier methods as a means to reduce the risk of contracting sexually transmitted diseases, including HIV/AIDS

(7). Encourages family communication about sexuality between parent and child

(8). Teaches young people the skills to make responsible decisions about sexuality, including how to avoid unwanted verbal, physical and sexual advances and how not to make unwanted verbal, physical and sexual advances

(9). Teaches young people how alcohol and drug use can effect responsible decision making.

However, it is imperative that the language of this Act not be distorted to favor one approach over another. While the decision to teach sex education and the content of such education is left to the states and to the individual school districts, the influence of the federal government via funding provided for such programs undeniably influences these prerogatives. Funding for abstinence only education has increased 3000% since the 1996 federal entitlement program sponsoring abstinence-only messages. Promoting an imbalance in sexual education by exclusive funding of abstinence-only education puts the population at-risk for serious consequences secondary to lack of preparation for the inevitable time that one will become sexually active. Additionally, fear messages implicit in statements that over-emphasize medical risks may place healthy sexual relationships hostage to fear. In the 2004 State of the Union address the President proposed "a grassroots campaign to help inform families about these medical risks...We will double federal funding for abstinence programs, so schools can teach this fact of life: Abstinence for young people is the only certain way to avoid sexually transmitted diseases." The president's new budget includes an additional $270 million for programs to encourage teens to abstain from sex. If, in contrast, the new budget included this amount for comprehensive sex education rather than one with an abstinence-only approach, the interests of all Americans, rather than only a special interest group, would be furthered.

Since the late 1980s, both the political context surrounding sexuality education and actual teaching approaches have changed considerably. That abstinence-only education is becoming more common as a result of increased federal funding for abstinence-only programs is undeniable, and despite the Family Education Act pronouncement that family life education "not teach or promote religion", there is no question that some religions have been in the forefront of promoting abstinence only education. Whereas only 2% of sex education classes in the US taught "abstinence only' messages in 1988, 23% did so in 1999. These programs often exclude basic information related to puberty and reproduction, in addition to providing little information on pregnancy and STD prevention other than by abstinence. This approach has been promoted by the federal government despite evidence to the contrary that abstinence only programs show little success in delaying onset of sexual activity until marriage but do contribute to inadequate preparation to avoid pregnancy and STDs when they do become active. That rules and regulations are increasingly interfering with what teachers think should be taught is apparent from data that 90% of teachers believe that students should be taught about contraception but 25% are barred by regulations from doing so.

Most of the trusted medical institutions in the US support comprehensive sex education. This includes the American Medical Association, the American Academy of Pediatrics, the American College of Obstetrics and Gynecology, the American Public Health Association and the American Nurses Association. Additionally, the majority of parents want their children to have comprehensive sex education. I urge you as influential members of the Congress to make decisions regarding sex education that are supported by the majority of Americans and by knowledgeable, respected institutions.

Commitment to providing the best available screening

Cervical cancer is nearly entirely preventable because the cancer occurs on a skin surface that is easily accessible for evaluation, risk of presence of the precancer phase is detectable by the Pap test and by HPV testing and the natural history of progression from precancer to cancer is one that is usually quite long over many years to decades. That cervical cancer should be preventable in most circumstances makes every cervical cancer even more tragic. Only an all-out commitment by private and public payers to provide the best screening available for all women can reduce the burden of this tragedy.

Promoting access to the best cervical screening

The majority of cervical cancers continue to occur in women receiving either no, or inadequate, cervical screening. Therefore, education, outreach and access for all women to equal protection from cervical cancer will provide the maximum benefit in reduction of cervical cancer incidence and mortality. Cervical cancer not infrequently strikes women of late child-bearing age, disrupting families and society much more than many other cancers that occur with highest frequency in the elderly. Wise investment by government in a program of cervical cancer prevention is, therefore, both morally right and economically sound. It is likely that women fail to get adequate cervical screening as a result of a complex milieu of cultural, societal and educational factors. A substantial commitment to understanding the reasons for failure to attend screening is necessary in order to overcome these barriers.

Education about the necessity for the presence of HPV in the etiology of cervical cancer and the commonness of this virus must be balanced with reassurance that attendance at recommended screening provides protection from serious outcome for most. Education must extend to the health care provider as well, for outreach and recruitment to responsible preventative care is doomed to failure without a well-informed and empathetic health services sector. Education must include discussion of the sexually transmitted nature of HPV and the relationship of true Pap test abnormalities with an STD, and must be done without prejudice and with great care, compassion, and reassurance.

A More Efficient Screening System

When I last spoke to a Congressional Subcommittee on this subject I emphasized a number of points that must occur before a more efficient screening system would come to fruition. Many of the limitations to the system that I spoke of then have subsequently been corrected by new national screening and management guidelines issued by the American Cancer Society (ACS), the American College of Obstetrics and Gynecology (ACOG), and the American Society for Colposcopy and Cervical Pathology (ASCCP). These include the optimal age to begin screening, the optimal interval for screening, provision of the best technologies for improved screening, and provision of the most objective and efficient management of women with equivocal Paps.

1). *Optimal age to begin screening*: In order to provide the safest and yet cost-efficient coverage, it was imperative to redirect a large concentration of our cervical cancer screening resources to populations at greatest risk and least likely to be traumatized unnecessarily by medical intervention. New national guidelines accomplished this feat by recommending that cervical cytology screening not begin until age 21 or within 3 years of first intercourse, whichever comes first. These parameters replaced previous guidelines that called for first Pap test at age 18, or at the time of first intercourse. This does not negate the importance of continued medical interaction with young people who have begun sexual activity but do not yet need cervical screening, for it remains very important to test young sexually active women for other STDs and to provide contraceptive services. However, as we learned more about the high-prevalence of transient HPV infections in very young women and the long natural history required for the development of serious cervical disease it became increasingly clear that the previous recommendation to begin Pap screening no latter than age 18 was inefficient and wasted resources better spent on cervical cancer screening of older women at greater risk of having persistent precancer requiring treatment.

(2). *Optimal screening interval*: Annual Pap tests have been the standard in the US for over 50 years, this frequency driven by concerns over false-negative Paps, medicolegal liability and the improbability of being able to accurately predict which women are really low risk on the basis of mostly non-verifiable sexual history factors. These concerns served as the major impediment to implementation of prolonged screening intervals. However, the advent of new technologies that improve the sensitivity and efficiency of detection of cervical disease has fostered guidelines that promote longer screening intervals on the basis of decreased risk for missed cervical precancer and cancer. The new technologies of greatest benefit are liquid-based thin-layer cytology and HPV testing. The 2002 American Cancer Society cervical screening guidelines, in recognition of the improved sensitivity of liquid-based Paps, recommended that women up to age 30 have cervical screening only every 2 years if liquid-based, in contrast to annually if a conventional dry Pap smear. Decreasing the number of screens in a woman's life is advantageous if the risk of missing serious disease is not increased because it becomes less likely that transient unimportant HPV changes will be detected. For women after the age of 30 the opportunity for extending screening intervals is given in both the ACS and the ACOG guidelines, which recommend Pap testing every 2 to 3 years for women of this age having 3 consecutive normal Paps, or every three years for women having a single screen that was negative for high-risk HPV and normal on a Pap. The age of 30 was selected as the beginning age for combined screening with HPV testing and the Pap test because women over the age of 30 are less likely to have transient HPV and more at-risk for HPV-induced precancer. The 3-year interval recommended by ACS, ACOG and the recently published "interim guidance" on the use of this "super screen" was based on the nearly 100% negative predictive value of combined testing for precancer and cancer. Additionally, women negative for high-risk HPV are not at-risk for cervical cancer over the next few years, providing a longer period of reassurance than cytology alone. This extended period of protection is even more important amongst women attending government-funded clinics, because regular attendance for recommended cervical screening is often less guaranteed in this setting. Investment in providing the best protection for women at all economic levels is likely to provide substantial return.

These new technologies and guidelines on their use now provide the opportunity to make a significant impact on both the loss of life and on the inefficiency of the cervical cytology screening program if we have the will and the foresight to integrate the best that these technologies provide. If we do not, the present impasse in further reduction in cervical cancer may remain. Much not only depends upon the willingness of third-party payers to cover appropriately effective emerging technologies, but also upon a full understanding by clinicians

Provision of Vaccines for all Children

Cervical cancer will nearly be eliminated during the lifetime of many attending this meeting. Its demise will come on the heels of the improvements in screening and management we have discussed today, and on the availability in the near future of vaccines against HPVs 16 and 18. If introduced worldwide, vaccination against HPV 16 alone could prevent over 50% of the nearly one-quarter million deaths that occur annually from cervical cancer. A quadravalent vaccine including types 6, 11, 16 and 18 could theoretically prevent 90% of genital warts and 75% of cervical cancers. The potential is not only in reduction of morbidity from genital warts and cervical cancer, and mortality from the latter, but in the possibility that physical, psychological, and financial costs associated with screening, follow-up, and treatment should be significantly decreased. Two different categories of vaccines are presently under development or testing: prophylactic and therapeutic. Prophylactic vaccines are directed to preventing infection from occurring, whereas therapeutic vaccines are designed to either eliminate HPV infections in patients already infected with HPV, or to kill high-grade precancer and invasive cancer cells. Prophylactic HPV vaccines will need to be administered before infection in order to elicit neutralizing antibodies that would either inhibit attachment or entry. Because HPV is easily and frequently transmitted soon after sexual debut, the target population for prophylactic HPV vaccination will necessarily be children that have not attained the age of sexual maturity. Recent studies offer promise that prophylactic HPV vaccines against these types may be 100% effective in preventing both infection with the types included in the vaccine and the precancer that such types may induce.

Again, thank you for the opportunity to address these issues. The war against HPV and cervical cancer will be won. All we have to do is hold the course steady by appropriately educating our youth, providing the best protective cervical screening available for all women, and providing HPV vaccines to all children once these vaccines become available. I will be pleased to answer any questions that you may have.

Mr. SOUDER. Thank you.

Dr. Meeker.

Dr. MEEKER. Thank you.

My name is Meg Meeker, and I am a physician of child and adolescent medicine. I have been practicing adolescent medicine in Michigan for about 20 years. So I represent a population of patients very dear to my heart, that is the children in America.

I am grateful to have the opportunity to speak to you on behalf of my own patients and the 35 million teenagers across the United States. For about 20 years I have taken care of thousands of teens, I have authored two books on teen health issues, and currently speak across the country on teen health issues. I am a fellow of the American Academy of Pediatrics and certified by the American Board of Pediatrics.

Ladies and gentlemen, the epidemic of sexually transmitted diseases among our youth in the United States today is sobering and poorly recognized by the public at large. This year, in 2004, 10 million teenagers and young adults under the age of 25 will contract a new sexually transmitted disease. That translates into approximately 8,000 teenagers in the United States every day contracting a new sexually transmitted disease. Human papillomavirus, as you are hearing, outnumbers all other sexually transmitted infections among our youth and costs our country billions of dollars yearly because it wreaks havoc in the genital tracks of, may I say it again, teen girls and very young women.

We are here to discuss prevention of HPV infections and cervical cancer. If I might for a moment, let me permit you behind closed doors that physicians like myself see every single day. Fifteen years ago I rarely saw abnormal Pap smears in young girls; 10 years I personally witnessed a dramatic rise in the frequency of abnormal Pap smears among my own patient population of young teenage girls, many of those as young as 13; and 4 years ago I had to break the news to one of my young patients, we will call her Amy, just before her 14th birthday that, no, she didn't have full-blown cervical cancer, she had the milder form of severe dysplasia, but needed cervical surgery nonetheless. She had her surgery, 3 months afterwards returned to my practice with signs of very serious depression. The morbidity, not just the mortality, but the morbidity of this disease among young women is tremendous.

Cervical cancer is a young women's disease and deserves our strongest efforts at real and aggressive prevention, not just medical management of the cure, that giving an increased number of Pap smears to young girls will afford. That is very important, but that is medical management of a disease, it is not a primary strategy of prevention of the cervical cancer. So what can we do to truly prevent human papillomavirus infections and cervical cancer in our young women in America?

We could more aggressively train our children to use condoms during sexual intercourse. There are, however, serious drawbacks to this approach. The scientific data, and may I say from the National Institutes of Health condom effectiveness report shows that there is insufficient evidence of any risk reduction for sexual transmission of human papillomavirus even with 100 percent condom use, which I might add, among youth doesn't happen. The primary reason for this, and no one has discussed this, is that HPV is not transmitted like HIV, which is transmitted through bodily fluids; it is transmitted from skin to skin. And even the best condom available out there only covers a certain portion of the skin. So unless we make condoms a lot larger, it is very difficult, with condoms alone, to prevent the transmission of the cervical cancer-causing agent human papillomavirus.

Second, we could increase screening for cervical cancer. While increased screening is very important, and I might add does not take place in the most at-risk population, and that is children, whom I represent, and I am one of the few pediatricians who does gynecology in my practice, I might add, while that is very important, it is a secondary, not a primary strategy for prevention of the disease. At the time of screening, many women may have already become infected and show signs of dysplasia or even more advanced cancer. Screening detects HPV infections, it does not prevent them from occurring. The only way to prevent infections and subsequent sequela in our young girls is to teach them the only way to avoid infection, as Dr. Gerberding's report shows from the CDC, is to abstain from sexual activity during the teen years, the high-risk years.

Distinguished Members of Congress, we are indeed living in schizophrenic times. Every day our children are bombarded with sexual messages from the entertainment industries and multimillion dollar corporations aggressively marketing sex to them from the age of about 8 years old on. I believe, personally, that these messages have a profound effect on their sexual behavior. Teens have begun sexual activity at younger and younger ages, and have dramatically increased the number of sexual partners in recent years. They come to their physician's offices and then we, and I speak for the thousands of doctors who, across the country, work fervently to deflect the damage done to their young bodies, just to their bodies from sexual activity. Daily we "mop up the messes," if you will, of too much sex too soon.

We have become overwhelmed and discouraged because the bottom line is that sexual activity among our youth is out of control. The best medical data on sexually transmitted infections in teens teaches us that there is two successful ways to drive down the STD epidemic of teens in our country: One, delay the onset of sexual debut and two, drive down the numbers of sexual partners.

If we commit to help our young women accomplish these two goals, then we offer the best medical care available to prevent cervical cancer. We physicians cannot fight the uphill battle of rising HPV infections in younger women and out-of-control teen sexual activity alone; we need your help in sending clear and loud messages to our communities and to our youth that sexual activity in teenagers, with or without condoms, is very high-risk behavior.

Thank you very much, Mr. Chairman.

[The prepared statement of Dr. Meeker follows:]

Address to Congressional Committee
Margaret J. Meeker, M.D., F.A.A.P
March 11, 2004

As a pediatrician practicing child and adolescent medicine in a suburban Michigan community, I am grateful to have the opportunity to speak to you on behalf of my own patients and the millions of teens across the U.S. For twenty years, I have cared for thousand of teens; I have authored two books on teen health issues and currently speak across the country on teen health issues. I am a Fellow of the American Academy of Pediatrics and certified by the American Board of Pediatrics.

Ladies and gentlemen, the epidemic of sexually transmitted diseases among our youth in the U.S today is sobering and poorly recognized by the public at large. This year, 10 million teens and young adults under age 25 will contract a new sexually transmitted infection. *Today*, 8,000 children under the age of 18, will contract a new STD. Human papillomavirus, as you are hearing, outnumbers all other sexually transmitted infections among our youth and costs our country billions of dollars yearly because it wreaks havoc in the genital tracts of teen girls and young women.

We are here to discuss prevention of HPV infections and cervical cancer. If I may, permit me to show you what I (and many other physician colleagues with whom I have collaborated) have seen change during the course of my short medical career.

Fifteen years ago, I rarely saw abnormal Pap smears in teen girls. Ten years ago, I personally witnessed a dramatic rise in the frequency of abnormal Pap smears among my patient population of young teenage girls – some as young as thirteen. And four years ago, I had to break the news to one of my young patients, Amy, just before her fourteenth birthday that she had very serious dysplasia of her cervix and required surgery to remove the precancerous tissue. She had her surgery and three months afterward, returned to me with signs of very serious depression. Amy could have been my daughter, your grandchild, or perhaps your niece. Cervical cancer is a young woman's disease and deserves our strongest efforts at real and aggressive prevention because it has devastating effects on the physical and psychological health of our young girls.

So what can we do to prevent HPV infections and cervical cancer in our young girls?

We could more aggressively train our children to use condoms during sexual intercourse. There are, however, serious drawbacks to this approach. The scientific data shows us that "there is insufficient evidence of any risk reduction for sexual transmission of human papillomavirus infection even with 100% condom use" (1). The primary reason for this is that HPV is transmitted from skin to skin contact and condoms cover only a small portion of the skin.

Second, we could increase screening for cervical cancer. While better screening is very important, it is a secondary, not primary strategy for cervical cancer prevention. At the time of screening, many women may have already become infected and show signs of dysplasia or even more advanced cancer. Screening detects HPV infections, but it does not prevent them from occurring.

The only way to *prevent* infections and subsequent sequelae in our young girls and young women is to teach them that the only way to avoid infection, as Dr. Gerberding's report shows, is to abstain from sexual activity during the teen years.

Distinguished members of Congress, we are indeed living in schizophrenic times. Every day, our children are bombarded with sexual messages from the entertainment industries and from multimillion-dollar corporations aggressively marketing sex to them. I believe these messages have a profound effect on their sexual behavior. Teens have begun sexual activity at younger and younger ages and have dramatically increased the number of sexual partners in recent years. They come to their physician's offices and then we – and I speak for thousands of doctors across the country- work fervently to deflect the damage done to their young bodies from sexual activity. Daily, we "mop up the messes" of too much sexual activity, too soon. We have become overwhelmed and discouraged because their sexual activity is out of control.

The best medical data on sexually transmitted infections in teens teaches us that there are two ways to *successfully* drive down these infections in our youth: one- delay the onset of sexual activity, and two- decrease the number of sexual partners (2). The scientific evidence shows that if teens delay their sexual debut, statistically, the number of lifetime sexual partners they have decreases. Thus, their exposure to sexually transmitted infections like HPV goes down.

If we commit to help our young women accomplish these two goals, then we offer the *best medical care* available to prevent cervical cancer. Ladies and gentlemen, we physicians cannot fight the uphill battle of rising HPV infections and out of control teen sexual activity alone. We need your help in sending clear and loud messages to our communities and to our youth that sexual activity in teens- with or without condoms- is *very* high-risk behavior.

1. Workshop Summary: Scientific Evidence on Condom Effectiveness for Sexually Transmitted Disease (STD) Prevention. July 20, 2001. National Institute of Allergy and Infectious Diseases, National Institutes of Health, Department of Health and Human Services. Available at: http://www.niaid.nih.gov/dmid/stds/condomreport.pdf

2. Centers for Disease Control and Prevention. (1991, January4.) Premarital Sexual Experience Among Adolescent Women- United States, 1970-1988. *Morbidity and Mortality Weekly Report*, 39 (51), 929-932.

3. Institute of Medicine. (1997). *The Hidden Epidemic – Confronting Sexually Transmitted Disease* (edited by Thomas R. Eng and William T. Butler). Washington, DC: National Academy Press.

Mr. SOUDER. Thank you.

Dr. Zenilman, you will be our cleanup hitter.

Dr. ZENILMAN. With a name starting in Z, I am used to being at the end.

Mr. SOUDER. I can imagine. Except for those rare days when they reversed the order, those wonderful days.

Dr. ZENILMAN. Good afternoon. Thank you for having me. My name is Jonathan Zenilman. I am professor of medicine at the Johns Hopkins University School of Medicine and chief of infectious diseases at Johns Hopkins Bayview Medical Center. My area of research and clinical expertise for the past 18 years has been in sexually transmitted infections. I am also the president of the American STD Association, representing 450 academic and public health researchers in this area; and also I am a practicing physician and take care of patients with reproductive tract infections at the Baltimore City Health Department and in my own academic practice at Bayview Medical Center.

More important, I am the proud father of three teenagers, one of whom, Aliza Zenilman, with her friend, Mandy Millman, is here with us today in the second row sitting behind me. I thank the committee for extending your warm welcome to her and her friend today.

I address this committee as a private individual, a physician, as a public health practitioner, and as a father who gives patients the advice that I give my own children.

We are hearing and have heard today that HPV infection is almost always asymptomatic and is extremely common. I will therefore limit my comments to highlight issues which have not been already addressed by the previous witnesses.

Some strains, as you know, of HPV are associated with the development of cancer. Recent studies we have performed in a Hopkins suburban clinic in Baltimore, supported by the CDC Sentinel Surveillance Grant previously mentioned, found that the proportion of women infected with high-risk HPV types is 14 percent higher in persons of color and persons with HIV or those at risk for other reproductive tract infections. Extrapolating from these and other data, I would estimate that approximately 1 in 6 to 7 individuals sitting in this room is currently infected with a high-risk HPV type. Let me say, however, and emphasize that Pap smears, which have already been previously testified to as the major control strategy, are actually a screening test for a cancer that is caused by a sexually transmitted viral infection.

In terms of primary prevention of HPV and other STDs, we try to give our adolescents and young adults a moral compass that will help them in making informed choices regarding their sexual health. A British colleague of mine once said, “The most effective contraceptive is ambition,” which requires us as a Nation to provide an environment of educational and economic opportunity, as well as positive recreational outlets for our young people.

Effective prevention of risky sexual behavior and their consequences, teenage pregnancy and sexually transmitted infections, requires two critical components: one, accurate based science-based information on reproductive health and prevention of infection and pregnancy, and two, a social peer and family environment that promotes responsible decisionmaking, allowing teens to make an informed choice. Unfortunately, many teenagers do not have both of those criteria.

Delaying sexual intercourse is a public health message that I and all reproductive health professionals support, in tandem with counseling on responsible sexual behavior. An abstinence-only approach which excludes safer sex messages and includes messages that emphasize intercourse only within the context of marriage, is therefore clearly out of touch with the realities and practices of the vast majority of Americans. We are performing a disservice by focusing only an abstinence-only approach.

Condoms are highly effective in preventing sexually transmitted infections, including genital herpes and HIV infection. In the latter case, condom use is life-saving. In communities where condom use has been universally adopted and supported, dramatic and striking decreases in overall STD and HIV infection rates have been observed.

As a parent, I want public policies that are reality-based and provide the resources necessary for my children, along with my patients, to protect themselves. I want them to have access to medically accurate sexuality education. I want to see support for research efforts to develop and make vaccines and other prevention interventions.

Unfortunately, the debate on human sexuality, sexual behavior, and STDs is all too often framed in an absolutist stark context in which only simplistic solutions are framed to address inherently complex behavioral and social questions. This is not a new phenomenon. More than 60 years ago, Dr. Thomas Turner was a colonel in the U.S. Army during World War II and was in charge of venereal disease control effort for 14 million servicemen and women. He was later to serve as dean of the Johns Hopkins Medical School and died in 2002 at the age of 100. I had the privilege of getting to know Dr. Turner in the late years of his life.

As a sidebar, if you are a venereologist, you may live to be a long age.

During World War II, Dr. Turner and the Army were faced with the same dilemma we now see facing as this Nation develops policies and practices. As only he could, he described the difficulty in providing expedient and simplistic approaches. "If a soldier remained continent, he would not acquire venereal disease. Many did remain continent, but no one in his right mind would expect this of a high percentage of men in their most vigorous and disorganized years. The first paradox, therefore, was preaching continence as an official doctrine, while simultaneously providing instructions and facilities for prevention of disease during and after sexual intercourse. We were repeatedly impaled on the horns of this dilemma. Some worthy folk urged a firm stand on a high moral plane; otherwise accused us of crass hypocrisy."

Dr. Turner held steadfast in pursuing a pragmatic solution, and I implore you to follow Dr. Turner's lead in approaching today's STD problem. Thank you.

[The prepared statement of Dr. Zenilman follows:]

JOHNS HOPKINS
UNIVERSITY
Johns Hopkins Bayview Medical Center
Division of Infectious Diseases
4940 Eastern Ave
Baltimore, MD 21224

Jonathan Zenilman, M.D.
Professor of Medicine
(410) 550-0501 / FAX (410) 550-1169
E-mail: jzenilma@jhmi.edu

Testimony of:

Jonathan M. Zenilman, MD
Professor of Medicine
Johns Hopkins University School of Medicine &
Chief Infectious Division
Johns Hopkins Bayview Medical Center

House Government Reform Committee
Subcommittee on Criminal Justice, Drug Policy and Human Resources
March 11, 2004

JOHNS HOPKINS
U N I V E R S I T Y
Johns Hopkins Bayview Medical Center
Division of Infectious Diseases
4940 Eastern Ave
Baltimore, MD 21224

Jonathan Zenilman, M.D.
Professor of Medicine
(410) 550-0501 / FAX (410) 550-1169
E-mail: jzenilma@jhmi.edu

Testimony of Dr. Jonathan Zenilman

House Government Reform Committee
Subcommittee on Criminal Justice, Drug Policy and Human Resources
March 11, 2004

Good morning, Mr. Chairman, members of the committee. My name is Jonathan Zenilman. I am Professor of Medicine at The Johns Hopkins University School of Medicine, and Chief of the Infectious Diseases Service at the Johns Hopkins Bayview Medical Center. My area of research and clinical expertise for the past 18 years is in sexually transmitted infections. I am also the President of the American STD Association, which represents 450 academic and public health researchers in the area of sexually transmitted infections. I am also a practicing physician, and take care of patients with reproductive tract infections at the Baltimore City Health Department and in my own academic practice at Bayview Medical Center.

More important, I am the proud father of three teenagers, one of whom, Aliza Zenilman, is with us this morning. I thank Congressmen Cummings, Souder, and the Committee for extending their warm welcome to her today.

I address this committee as a private individual, a physician, who counsels patients and their partners about HPV and other sexually transmitted infections; as a public health practitioner; and as a father who gives patients the advice that I give my own children.

We are hearing today that HPV infection is almost always asymptomatic, and is extremely common. In adolescents and young adults alone there are an estimated 9-10 million persons with chronic infections and 4.6 million *new* cases per year.

Some strains of HPV are associated with the development of cervical cancer. HPV strains are classified by number. Strains 16, 18, 31, 45 and about a dozen others are associated with cervical cancer-and are often called "high-risk types". Recent studies we have performed in a Hopkins suburban clinic Baltimore, the proportion of women infected with high risk types of HPV is 14%, and it is higher in persons of color, in persons with HIV or those at risk for other reproductive tract infections. In fact, extrapolating from the National and local data, I would estimate that at least 1 in 6 adults in this hearing room are presently infected with HPV, and 75-80% of persons will have been exposed and infected at some time during their life. New data also suggests, that nearly 90% of persons infected spontaneously clear (or self-cure) the virus.

Cervical cancer is the most important adverse outcome of HPV infection. Let me emphasize that Pap smears are actually a screening test for a cancer that is caused by a sexually transmitted viral infection. Since it takes an average of 10 years or more for cancer to develop, the Pap smear screening program, in combination with recently implemented additional testing for the virus itself, is extremely effective in preventing cancer. The implementation of Pap smear screening has been a resounding public health victory, as evidenced by a continual decrease in cervical cancer rates. The current most effective means of preventing cervical cancer is to ensure that American women have universal access to Pap smear screening and to the subsequent treatment of identified cervical abnormalities.

Last year, researchers published results from a large clinical trial demonstrating that a vaccine was highly effective in preventing infection with HPV-16, one of the major viruses that cause cervical cancer. Trials are currently underway testing the vaccine against the viruses many subtypes. Based on these very promising data, we expect that a vaccine would be available for distribution to the general public in about 5 years.

In terms of primary prevention of HPV and other sexually transmitted infections, we try to give our adolescents and young adults a moral compass that will help them in making informed decisions regarding their sexual health. A British colleague of mine once said, "the most effective contraceptive is ambition," which requires us as a nation to provide an environment of educational and economic opportunity, as well as positive recreational outlets for our young people".

Effective prevention of risky sexual behavior and their consequences, teenage pregnancy and sexually transmitted infections, requires 2 critical components:

- Accurate, science-based information on reproductive health and prevention of infection and pregnancy.
- A social, peer and family environment that promotes responsible decision-making, allowing teens to make an informed choice.

Despite progress in the past few years, the average age of first intercourse for American teenagers is still a bit under 16, which means that half of American teenagers are initiating sexual intercourse while still at a very young age. This is the group at highest risk for sexually transmitted infections. Over 90% of Americans have had sexual intercourse by the time they are 25.

Delaying sexual intercourse is a public health message that I and all reproductive health professionals support -- in tandem with counseling on responsible sexual behavior. An abstinence-only approach which excludes safer sex messages, and includes messages that emphasize intercourse only within the context of marriage is therefore clearly out of touch with the realities and practices of the vast majority of Americans. We are performing a disservice by focusing only on an abstinence-only approach.

In order to reduce the burden of STDs, a clear, two-pronged approach is required, and supported by over 60 years of public health experience and research. First, abstinence is the best way to protect against human papillomavirus (HPV) and other sexually transmitted diseases. The second is that when you become sexually active, use effective contraception and condoms.

Condoms are highly effective in preventing sexually transmitted infections, including genital herpes and HIV infection. In the latter case, condom use is lifesaving. In communities where condom use has been universally adopted and supported, dramatic and striking decreases in overall STD and HIV infection rates have been observed.

Current proposals to provide questionable warning labels and to undermine public confidence in condoms will not reduce the number of persons engaging in risky sexual behavior, and they will clearly not reduce the prevalence of HPV nor of other sexually transmitted infections.

Much has been made of the recent NIH report on condom efficacy. That report noted that "the scientific evidence currently available is not sufficient to recommend condoms as a primary prevention strategy for the prevention of genital HPV infection."' However, this statement has been widely misinterpreted. It does not say that condoms are ineffective, and in fact, there are promising data to suggest that they are.

The same report noted that there is evidence that condom use may actually reduce the risk of cervical cancer. Possible explanations for the protective effect of condoms against cancer may be that condom use reduces the quantity of HPV transmitted and the likelihood of re-exposure to HPV, as well as exposure to a co-factor for cervical cancer, such as chlamydia or genital herpes, which have been identified as potential co-factors for cervical cancer development.

As a parent, I want public policies that are reality-based and provide the resources necessary for my children, along with my patients to protect themselves. I want them to have access to medically accurate sexuality education. I want to see support for research efforts to develop and make vaccines and other prevention interventions.

Unfortunately, the debate on human sexuality, sexual behavior and sexually transmitted infections is all too often framed in an absolutist, stark context, in which only simplistic solutions are framed to address inherently complex behavioral and social questions. This is not a new phenomenon.

More than 60 years ago, Dr. Thomas Turner was a Colonel in the US Army during World War II, and was in charge of the venereal disease control effort for 14 million servicemen and women. He was to serve as the Dean of The Johns Hopkins University School of Medicine in the 1950s and 1960s, and died in 2002 at the age of 100. I had the privilege of getting to know Dr. Turner in the late years of his life.

During World War II, Dr. Turner and the Army were faced with the same dilemma we now seem faced with as the nation develops policies and practices designed to prevent and control STDs. As only he could, he described the difficulty in providing expedient and simplistic approaches in almost poetic terms.

I quote:

...If a soldier remained continent he would not acquire venereal disease; many did remain continent, but no one in his right mind would expect this of a high percentage of men in their most vigorous and disorganized years....

.....The first paradox, therefore, was preaching continence as an official doctrine while simultaneously providing instructions and facilities for prevention of disease during and after sexual intercourse. We were repeatedly impaled on the horns of this dilemma. Some worthy folk urged a firm stand on a high moral plane; others accused us of crass hypocrisy....

Dr. Turner held steadfast in pursuing a pragmatic solution, and I implore you to follow Dr Turner's lead in approaching today's STD problem.

Thank you for allowing me to testify today.

Mr. SOUDER. One of the things I wanted to clear up at the beginning, I understood from our earlier panel, and I thought I heard at least alluded to by several of you, that up to 80 percent of Americans would get HPV sometime during their lifetime. Does everybody agree with that?

[Panel members indicate in the affirmative.]

Mr. SOUDER. Then why I was confused, Dr. Cox, is you said we shouldn't be alarmists. Eighty percent is a pretty high number.

Dr. COX. Well, I didn't say that we shouldn't be alarmed. What I was saying is that we shouldn't overstate the risk.

Mr. SOUDER. But 80 percent? So you are not talking about overstating the risk of people getting HPV.

Dr. COX. Overstating the risk of what you get from HPV.

Mr. SOUDER. The cancer part.

Dr. COX. Right. That is correct.

Mr. SOUDER. But not invasive procedures?

Dr. COX. I think we all have the same goals, and I would agree with Dr. Meeker here, that we all want to try to encourage young people to delay intercourse as long as they possibly can, and give them the health reasons for that. There is no question that is a real positive. We all foster that. The only difference amongst the four or five of us up at this table is the fact that some of us believe that only abstinence should be taught in school, and that would protect individuals from starting intercourse too early, and others of us feel that you have to be more balanced.

Mr. SOUDER. I don't believe that. I believe that is an inaccurate statement, for the record. You have broader disagreements than that, and I am going to explore some of those disagreements.

Dr. COX. OK.

Mr. SOUDER. I agree that is one of the differences of opinions.

First, some have claimed that you can provide medically accurate labels on condoms, and that this would discourage condom use. Do you believe that condom use would be less if things were accurately labeled?

Dr. Coburn, do you believe if we put a label on that gave accurate information, which, by the way, could be argued by putting accurate information as a doctor, any of you want to do this, we face this problem. Let me ask a general labeling question. You were both a doctor and a legislator, and on the Energy and Commerce Health Committee. When we said that certain things that address diseases or health problems, when they run advertising, they have to have warnings on TV, and that they have to accurately address what the product does, what was the discussion about let us don't accurately label versus they might not use that drug? How does this process work, and how do we balance that as legislators? And you both being a legislator and a doctor, could you talk about how we sort this through? Does accurate labeling discourage usage? And what if somebody could have used that medication, but we said it might have side benefits, so they don't use the medication?

Dr. COBURN. Well, let me preface it first. Anybody that is going to be sexually active in our society today who is going to be sexually active, ought to wear a condom. OK? Period. Because it will reduce the risk. The difference is saying that we don't want to tell people the truth because if we give them too much information they might make a bad choice undermines the whole basis under which we run our society. And if you carry that a little further, the logical conclusion is that if you tell everybody to wear a condom and don't tell them anything, then why would they ever come get a Pap smear, because a condom protects them? So you can't be on both sides of the logical argument.

The fact is we need as a policy, a national policy, that we ought to be truthful about the risks of STDs. We shouldn't be alarmists, but we should be truthful, and we should trust our children to make good choices, and we ought to have leadership. And what we don't have in this country today is leadership on this issue. You have not heard the surgeon general talk about the No. 1 STD in this country and the fact that it relates to at least 1.350 million procedures every year, that it costs at least $3 billion, and that we could make a difference on. And it is not about condoms or non-condoms; it is not about abstinence versus non-abstinence. The fact is that we ought to teach our kids to give them the best medical advice, and then if they choose to not use that best medical advice, if they use a device that will help lower their risk, then it ought to be labeled accurately.

And I would take exception. I am head of the President's Advisory Commission on HIV/AIDS. We have not lowered HIV infection in this country. We have as many or more new HIV infections in this country as we had 10 years ago. We have failed miserably. We have spent billions of dollars on this message. We have a higher rate of STDs today than we have ever had; we have a higher rate of HIV infection than we have had; we are spending more to treat. So we have sent the message, and if we applied the same thing to cigarette smokers, well, our society is going to smoke cigarettes and we can't change the culture, leadership is about changing the culture, because it will pay us big dividends both in health and social and emotional aspects of how we interrelate to each other.

So I think we ought to see a label that is accurate. It shouldn't be inflammatory, it should just be scientifically accurate, and there shouldn't be anything wrong with it. But it ought to be accurate not just about HPV, it ought to be accurate about chlamydia, because the studies on chlamydia aren't very good, when we are wanting to protect young women from chlamydia.

Mr. SOUDER. Is there anybody here who opposes more accurate labeling on the condoms?

Dr. COX. My basic concern about labeling the condom as not being an adequate protection from HPV is just you have to cram everything on a condom label in such a small area. I am very concerned about the mixed messages that individuals might get because HPV sounds like HIV, like HSV, like HBV. All these other STDs sound similar, so I am concerned that there might be decreased use on that basis. I would rather see a label that said something like properly used condoms significantly protect against some, but not all, STDs. I just get concerned about the message when you try to put one single STD on there, and how it might be mixed up with others.

Mr. SOUDER. Do you believe that other warnings that we have on other medicines and medications also can discourage usage, and would you favor not labeling them because people might not use them?

Dr. COX. Personally, I don't quite make the connection between those issues, but, yes, I know some people don't take medicines because they worry about the warnings we put out on medicines.

Mr. SOUDER. So would you recommend we label them less accurately?

Dr. COX. No, I am not recommending that at all. I am just saying that I am concerned about the mixed messages individuals may get not his.

Mr. SOUDER. But, see, the double standard, and this is what bothers some of us. We are not arguing about whether we should fund Pap smears, we are not arguing about whether we shouldn't do more treatment questions, look at at-risk populations. We have a specific piece of legislation that says accurate labeling, and there are several parts of this that we are going to pursue, but, first, most of the Democratic Members who were here earlier seem to support accurate labeling. Now, we can argue what is accurate, but that in the accurate labeling problem here is why we should have warnings. And as Dr. Coburn just mentioned the Surgeon General not speaking about this, what some of us are wondering, and this is our challenge, is are people not speaking up about this problem because they have other agendas? Are they blocking warning labels here, where we seem to be putting warning labels on all kinds of things, because they have other agendas and they are uncomfortable with what seems to be the most effective things?

For example, we have heard multiple times, I know I have raised other types of issues, but in smoking we don't give Dr. Zenilman used the word "inherently simplistic messages." Our messages against smoking are inherently simplistic, and the billboards that we see up are very simplistic. Let me just say flat out the data under "Just Say No" were more effective than they were when we gave more inherently complicated messages. We can argue whether there were other things going on, but the plain fact of the matter is inherently simplistic messages move a certain percentage of the population and that, in fact other patterns, also to take the quote from Dr. Turner, at that time the military was also providing cigarettes to people because they believed people couldn't have their behavior changed.

In fact, behavior changed. And if there is something like high-risk sexual behavior, that is causing the amount of problems that we have in the United States, whether it is HPV, HIV and other things, why wouldn't our primary aggressive prevention strategy be abstention. And then acknowledge, as Dr. Coburn just did, look, if you are going to engage in high-risk behavior, make sure it is absolutely clear that it is high-risk behavior, it shouldn't be followed. But if you do, here is what you have to do, and then if you have done that high-risk behavior, we need to treat you and take care of you.

I don't understand where the resistance is to acknowledge that it is aggressively high-risk behavior and needs to be reversed. I don't understand the resistance to this. To just say, oh, well, it is happening; therefore, we have to not be aggressive in our response. We are aggressive on date rape. It is happening all the time; it is probably increasing. But we don't not speak out against date rape. We have sexual harassment as a huge problem in our society, possibly increasing, but we don't not speak out against it because it seems to be something many people do. I don't understand the fatalism that I am hearing.

Dr. ZENILMAN. You asked, actually, quite a complex question, so I will try to distill it down.

I don't think we can compare date rape or sexual harassment to consensual sexual intercourse between teenagers or young adults.

Mr. SOUDER. But the consequences of teen pregnancy, out of wedlock, not finishing school, teen suicides, lack of stability in marriage over long-term, kids having multiple higher rates of different problems, sexually transmitted diseases. How can you say that there aren't those extreme consequences to out-of-wedlock pregnancy in our society, and sexual activity, which is directly related to that?

Dr. ZENILMAN. In reference to the specific, I think that is why this is actually an inherently complex issue. First of all, in the 1940's, the Army did not recognize that cigarettes were a problem. The military and the VA have taken cigarettes out of at least on-site consumption or purchase, which was actually a direct issue.

I would argue that this is a much more complex behavioral issue than cigarette smoking. And, furthermore, I am in agreement with you. I am in agreement with the other members of the panel that our major objective should be to delay onset of sexual intercourse. I think you have heard unanimity from all of the witnesses on this specific issue.

Mr. SOUDER. That should be our primary prevention strategy?

Dr. ZENILMAN. I think that should be the major focus.

Mr. SOUDER. It should be the major focus, the primary preventions strategy?

Dr. ZENILMAN. It should be the major goal in adolescent sexual health. But on the other hand, and you may call it fatalistic, I may call it realistic, recognizing that most people, the vast majority of Americans are not going to follow that advice. So, therefore, in the context of a public health reality, our objective is to minimize the risk to individuals who are engaging in sexual behavior.

Now, I would also argue that I don't like the context of intercourse in teenagers having consensual intercourse or adults having sexual intercourse is not the same as a date rape or sexual harassment. The latter has a lot more of the consequences that you mentioned previously.

Mr. SOUDER. I don't think this data backs that statement up. I believe they are awful and I have worked with them, but you are not going to argue here that out-of-wedlock pregnancy and related things are less damaging overall to a life's career than somebody who has been sexually harassed, which, by the way, may also occur in the teen pregnancy and the out-of-wedlock or non-married sexual activity.

Dr. ZENILMAN. A consensual adult who is actually having sexual relations and is properly informed will be contracepting.

Mr. SOUDER. This isn't really a debate, and I am sorry I got us off into that. We have a substantial disagreement.

Let me go next to the female physicians on our panel. Some have downplayed the threat of HPV infection by suggesting routine tests and, if necessary, treatment can prevent the development of cervical cancer. Can you describe the treatment that a woman would undergo for abnormal cell changes? Dr. Bush, maybe you can start with this, because you referred to this high number. Is cervical cancer or HPV related dysplasia easily treated? And what are some of the side effects of the treatment?

Dr. BUSH. Basically, we encourage women, once they have initiated sexual activity, to begin getting routine annual Pap smears. The reason we are screening is because HPV is the leading cause of cervical cancer, and it can be detected with the Pap smear. So as someone said, HPV causes cervical cancer and it is a preventable disease.

When the women has an abnormal Pap smear, they can be graded into high grade or in low grade or atypia. When a low-grade atypia is found, we may simply repeat the Pap smear because a significant number will spontaneously, because of their immune system, get rid of it. But with persistence, and that is the problem, 10 to 12 percent of people will have persistent infection and it will not go away, and that is associated with the high incidence of cervical cancer. If it is a high-grade lesion, which goes from moderate to severe dysplasia to carcinoma incite two, they are more likely to progress to cancer, and often it does not take 10 to 15 years. As Dr. Coburn mentioned someone in his practice, I could mention someone in my practice who actually initiated sex after age 16, and at 19, very recently, I had to do a leap procedure because of persistent infection.

What happens is we do a colposcopy, which takes a microscope, looks at the cells, we biopsy and take a chunk of the tissue, send it to the lab, let them tell us if the Pap smear was accurate or how far it has; sometimes it is less, sometimes more. With persistent of the infection confirmed by the biopsy results, then you have to remove those cells so that they do not progress. Removing means cryosurgery to kill them, it means an electrical surgical loop procedure to remove the cells, it may mean colonization, which is an outpatient surgical procedure surgical procedure, and it does cause pain; you have to give anesthesia, analgesia for the removal of that tissue, it means that you put the lady at risk whether she becomes pregnant, when she becomes pregnant in the future, not only the risk of premature delivery, but also perhaps stenotic cervix, that she would have to have cesarian section, that her cervix hadn't opened.

To make a long answer short, there is significant morbidity that is associated with an abnormal Pap smear. Persistence of the infection does progress to cervical cancer, and we are talking about 10 to 12 percent of people that have persistence.

Mr. SOUDER. Dr. Meeker, the New York Times, you heard us refer in the first panel when you were here, to this study that we have been kicking around among the members, that a majority of high school teens are virgins, according to the latest CDC data. This is a reversal from a decade ago. As a pediatrician, do you think abstinence is a realistic approach to trying to stop STDs among kids?

Dr. MEEKER. Well, I know it is, because I want to remind everybody that the epidemic of diseases that we are seeing amongst our youth now weren't here 40, 50, 60, 70 years ago, even as recently as 30 years ago. And I would ask have we fundamentally, as human beings, changed? No. I mean, our physiology is the same. What has changed is the direct marketing to our younger and younger children sexually promiscuous advertisements and so on and so forth.

What also has changed is the increase in the number of sexual partners that teenagers have and the earlier onset of sexual activity, and that is what has increased the number of STDs. So children, teenagers, the majority of teenagers will take their cues from significant adults in their life. The Ad Health study shows that. If it is communicated to teenagers, expectations about sexual activity from an authority figure in their life, teenager or a parent, the majority of teenagers will follow that and they will abstain from sexual activity.

I think there are some very significant and very serious misunderstandings about abstinence-only education, if I might. There is a sense that those promoting abstinence-only education are trying to withhold information. That is absolutely not true. What we are trying to do is just teach kids what the very real risks are to condom use. No one in this panel would tell a kid not to use a condom, and we are all willing to say that there is a role in condom use, but our money needs to be and our efforts need to be in teaching kids about abstinence. Everybody here is saying that we need to communicate messages to our kids that will change their behavior, so some say we need to encourage them to use condoms more frequently and better, or our other alternative is to teach them not to be sexually active. Either way, all of us are asking our kids to change their behavior.

We know how well teaching teens about condoms has worked; we have the data. And the data shows us that condom use has increased; young kids will use condoms the first, second, third time, but after that, as their age increases, condom use decreases. So we know what the data shows, and that basically asking them to change their behavior toward increased condom use has not worked. And in the midst of increased condom use, the STD rates, HPV too, have risen. So now I will say why not try the second approach? Why do we not then say what we need to do is put our time and our energy and our money into programs that will teach kids to delay the onset of sexual activity, which is abstinence?

Dr. COX. Chairman Souder, I might add there is a study that was just released this week out of England, where they went to a full-blown condom message, and what they have is a disaster on their hand as they go back and measure, in terms of increased teen pregnancies, increased STDs, and increased onset of early sexual debut. And what they are doing, the government in England now is reassessing whether that program is right, because what they did was actually increased sexual activity. And I am not saying that all condom messages do that, and I would not say that, but the British have decided that maybe they went down the road the wrong way, because they actually have marked increases in all the bad outcomes associated with early sexual activity through a government that was designed to do just exactly the opposite of it.

Mr. SOUDER. Dr. Zenilman, because one of the things we are arguing here are outcomes, and you did a study, you were the lead author, in 1995. And if I can quote from this, I would like to hear your comments on it. That 15 percent of the men who were always condom users had incident sexually transmitted diseases, compared with 15.3 percent of those who never used condoms, 23.5 percent of the women who were always users in incident sexually transmitted diseases, compared to 26.8 percent of never users. This study did not determine if subjects were infected with HPV, it should be pointed out.

In your study there was no significant statistical difference between men and women who always used condoms and those who never used condoms. So how do you explain that study? I would be interested.

Dr. ZENILMAN. Sure. I would be happy to. The title of the study was the validity of self-reported condom use, and the question that was asked was can we use sexually transmitted diseases as a biological marker of condom use. And there is subsequent data to support our hypothesis from other areas, that if you are actually asking somebody within a clinic environment, where the messages are to use condoms all the time, and you are seeing them, that we understand that a certain proportion of people will over-estimate their condom use. In a sense, there is an incentive to say that they use when they did not. So the question in that study was actually not on the efficacy of condom use, but, rather, do patients really tell the truth about their condom use and are there ways that we can develop methods from a behavioral standpoint or from a biological measure to measure that more accurately. I stated actually in the text of the discussion of that article that was really the specific objective of the study and what our hypothesis was.

Mr. SOUDER. So the fact that there were no significant difference between usage of condoms and not, you assumed that your people were lying.

Dr. ZENILMAN. That is correct.

Mr. SOUDER. How did you confirm that they were lying?

Dr. ZENILMAN. Well, embedded in this study there were a large number of partnerships. We never had enough data to actually publish this as a formal manuscript, but if we asked partners of men who said that they used condoms, the men said they used condoms 100 percent of the time. We had a certain number of female partners in that study and we actually looked at the same question and how they responded to the question, and there was no correlation.

Mr. SOUDER. How did you know they weren't lying?

Dr. ZENILMAN. Somebody is.

Now, on a subsequent issue, actually, we do have some more recent biological markers which we are analyzing from that same study.

Mr. SOUDER. Because whenever you get into sexual activity questions, for example, some believe that the number of people who say they are sexually active in certain periods of time in American history will be exaggerated; in other times, when there is a public message that stresses more abstinence, the number of people who say they are abstaining is exaggerated. The problem with this is to make claims based on data where you don't know whether your subjects are lying seems to be a rather tenuous proposition.

Dr. ZENILMAN. Well, with all due respect, sir, that actual paper had been through several series of peer review by journals and had been presented at a number of national meetings and has been validated in subsequent studies. I would be happy to share that with you.

Mr. SOUDER. I wasn't even necessarily referring to your paper, because if your assumption is correct that there is a certain percentage lying, if you agree that a certain percentage lie depending on other variables in the society on whether they are abstaining or not abstaining, this whole question of scientifically saying effectiveness is in fact somewhat challengeable, to say the least, because you can't establish who is and who isn't, and, therefore, the scientific argument that it is effective is fairly shaky.

Dr. ZENILMAN. I think that was a specific objective of the NIH committee which was mentioned. And as I am sure you are well aware, there was a subsequent research meeting which actually established a number of research priorities for the NIH and other HHS agencies to investigate this specific issue. I mean, that is recognized as a research question.

Mr. SOUDER. Dr. Coburn, do you have any comments on this?

Dr. COBURN. I would just say we are seeing the same thing in HIV right now. There are studies out there where people say they tell their partners but don't; and then there are those that say they always use condoms but don't. So the data is skewed based on the lack of truthfulness based on the question that is asked. There is a prejudice when you ask the question, because right now, today, in today's climate, it is important for people who are HIV-infected to always use a condom, it works 86 percent of the time. Well, if they are not, but the standard in the society is to use it, you are going to get an answer that they use it, even though what we know when we have people actually inside the groups that are participating and actually participating in that behavior, what we see is a very different story. And that is why we are seeing, in the gay community, a rise in new infections, because they are not using condoms anymore, because we have done great research in terms of the successful control of the disease for a great many people.

So I think all data is hard to get, and I think this study is important in terms of telling us not about whether there is a comparison of sexually transmitted diseases with condoms or without. It is important in terms of saying it is hard to get truthfulness in some of this, and I think it is true.

I would also say Dr. Cox has been responsible, to a great extent, for our change in how we handle cervical cancer, especially abnormal Paps. This has changed over 5 to 6 years. We are not as aggressive as we used to be because of some of the research that has come on that, and I think that needs to be said, because that knowledge of HPV in terms of low-risk, we aren't as aggressive as we were in the past, and we don't have to be because of some of the research that they have put forth.

Mr. SOUDER. Well, we have had you here for a long time. Let me finish this way. And we will go in reverse order, so you get the first chance. Most of you have come as far as the others, but we will have you start. And I will let you make any comments you want after having heard what each of you said in this panel and what you have heard at the hearing today.

Dr. Zenilman.

Dr. ZENILMAN. So it is a general open?

Mr. SOUDER. Yes. Open mic time.

Dr. ZENILMAN. Right. First of all, I want to thank you and the committee for inviting us. I think really, from what I have heard, there is less disagreement than actually may be innately obvious, because I think the basic messages are there and I think we are in agreement on. I think it is specifically how it is framed. And I think if we could take a little bit of the acrimony out of this, we may be able to be more able to craft a message which is consistent with what everybody wants.

Mr. SOUDER. Thank you.

Dr. Meeker.

Dr. MEEKER. Thank you. I totally agree. I think that, obviously, when you talk about sexual activity and sexual behavior, it is pretty easy for me, because I am talking about kids, and everybody is innately protective of kids, so I am very glad I am not an internist and talking about sexual behavior of 25-year-old women. That is your job. But I think that it is a very emotional topic and one of the great difficulties for us, and I do agree that we are in much more agreement than we believe, is that with the talk and the discussion about the very seriousness of HPV infections and cervical cancer is completely shifting the way we need to approach and rethink condom use.

Heretofore, I believe the general public has believed, and many physicians like me have believed, that condoms are a panacea. And the reason we thought that was pretty well founded, because condoms do work better, to use non-medical language, with HIV than they do with HPV. That is just the way it is. And we felt very secure and safe in just teaching people just use condoms, use condoms, different colors, different flavors, different whatever; anything we needed to do. But this is a new day, and now it is time to attend to the needs of our young women.

Cervical cancer is a young woman's disease. I am a pediatrician here talking about STDs. Isn't that sad? And so we need to dramatically shift our paradigm in how we think and approach sexually transmitted diseases. And I don't hate condoms, but I know that I took an oath 20-some years ago to provide the best medical care that I can to my patients, and as far as cervical cancer that I see in my young women, it is unabashedly to teach them to delay sexual activity as long as possible and to reduce the number of partners; and that is where I will go down fighting for that in years to come, because that is what the young girls in my practice need to hear, and I think the medical community is agreed on that.

We need some serious Federal money and energy in that. We have given it to the HIV/AIDS community, which is wonderful; we are making great strides. Now it is time to turn to our young women and say we will teach you very aggressively to hold off on sexual activity as long as possible. And we really need to be willing to step forward into new territory in that way.

And I thank you for the opportunity to be here.

Mr. SOUDER. Thank you.

Dr. Cox, you have come the farthest.

Dr. COX. And have to go back the farthest tonight, yes, and be back in the clinic tomorrow morning.

I think in most ways we are in agreement. I think, as I said when I started out this discussion earlier, we all agree that delaying intercourse as long as possible is in everybody's benefit, and that is the primary message that should be taught in our sex education classes. I feel very strongly, though, that we need comprehensive sex education that includes all the messages, including those of how to best protect one's self when you do become sexually active; and that they need to be realistic messages. Young people need to be taught that condoms are not 100 percent effective and that they don't work as well for HPV as they do for HIV. But I think that to eliminate or at least diminish the potential of their use would be quite detrimental and might increase the risk of HIV.

I disagree on one statement that was just made, that cervical cancer is a young woman's disease. Cervical cancer is really non-existent, or almost so, below the age of 21. The serious statistics in the last few years have not shown any cervical cancers per 100,000 women in women 21 or below, but 21 to 24 there is 1.7 per 100,000 women that get cervical cancer. And of course, the rates go up and start to plateau off in the forties. I guess we can still call that young women in the forties. But I would agree, though, that the risk of getting cervical cancer is an issue that is increased by having intercourse and getting exposed to high-risk HPV in very young women and teens, and that is where the risk is; it is not that there are great risks of cervical cancer then, but certainly that exposure then puts them at greater risk than if they had gotten exposed to the virus later in life. And we need to make sure that our young women know that.

And if anybody wants to go to the briefing on HPV that I am going to do right after this, I am certainly going to stress the issues in terms of education of our children, that they can't be totally protected by condoms against HPV, and that this virus is most risky when they are at that age. We would like very much to get motivation to delay intercourse, but we also want to make sure that, as we prepare our children to be adults, that they have at least the tools, when they become adults, to protect themselves.

Mr. SOUDER. Can I ask you a technical question? Pardon my ignorance. Does the cervical cancer through HPV, does it incubate a number of years? In other words, could you be exposed to it when you are young and then have it show up?

Dr. COX. Most HPV does, if it is going to express itself, goes through some cellular expression within a couple of years of exposure, but some perhaps may lay in what we call a non-express or latent phase for a number of years and then immunity decreases. And they haven't cleared the virus, which most do, but if it goes a number of years and they haven't, it then may express itself. But I think probably most get some expression early on. And when you get a high-grade lesion in a young women, typically those high-grade pre-cancers will be present for many, many years before they attain the capability of being invasive. So the reason that cervical cytology has diminished the risk and the rate of cervical cancer so dramatically is the capability of picking up those high-grade changes before they become invasive cancer, and treating them.

Mr. SOUDER. If you have the pre-cancer lesions and so on, does that make it more likely that you could be exposed from further sexual activity with different partners later in your life? Is there any kind of reoccurrence vulnerability that develops?

Dr. COX. It is interesting. Most of the studies that have looked at women as they age have shown that with increasing number of partners, individuals appear to become immune to increasing number of types, so that getting exposed to HPV again, they may become less likely to be HPV positive. Of course, increasing number of partners also increases the risks that they may have a viral type that isn't cleared and may eventually get cervical cancer.

But I am not sure I totally answered your question.

Mr. SOUDER. I wouldn't totally understand it if you totally answered it anyway. I was just trying to get a basic understanding. Thank you.

Dr. Bush.

Dr. BUSH. I was just going to piggy-back on that response. The Medical Institute for Sexual Health has published a monogram on condoms, and in it it talks about the cumulative effect of repeated infections, and that does put you at risk for cervical cancer.

What I was going to originally say was that I have been in women's health for 35-plus years, and when I first started, principally dealing with childbirth, when we talked about the use of condoms, it was always derided as the least effective form of contraception. And that is mostly what condoms were used for. And, of course, 100 percent effective was your hormonal contraceptives, and so condoms were considered 85 percent effective for prevention of pregnancy, and we considered that worthless.

It is interesting to me now we say condoms are 85 percent effective for prevention of HIV and we call it highly effective. So that is kind of confusing. I don't know if the 35 years made the difference or what, but that is interesting.

I also wanted to add that when a woman gets infected with HPV, then the persistence of infection is the thing that gives her the increased risk. We don't know which woman is going to get rid of the infection with her immune status and which one is going to persist. So it is like when I am counseling a woman to use the best method to prevent an infection, prevent an infection, then not knowing her immune status, I am going to give her information that will put her at the greatest health-promoting method, and that would be to abstain from sex, to delay sex, to limit her partners, because I feel like I am giving her the best recommendation, to modify her behavior, that will promote the best for her long-term. I too am the mother of children, and this is what I tell my kids, so I feel like it would be unethical for me to tell my patients anything less than the best.

The YRBS study that was put out by the CDC showed that 50 percent of young people are now reporting that they are abstaining from sex, so I feel like the best method to delay sexual activity is having an effect. And I am encouraged by the fact that in the study, when they broke it out with ethnic minorities, the group that showed the greatest progress toward abstinence, increasing their rates of abstinence, were African-American youth. So I feel like the message is being put out there, is being heard, and I would like to see us put as much effort, as much money, as much resources into promoting the method that will give you the best health, that will be primary prevention, as opposed to a second tier, which is the condom.

Mr. SOUDER. Thank you.

Dr. Coburn.

Dr. COBURN. Well, thank you for having this hearing. I think it is important. I still am skeptical that the FDA and the CDC will come up to the bar that they need to. They have made statements; it is my hope that they will do that.

I was just kind of wondering and thinking out loud what if every one of our children aged 12 years and older was taught about HPV and what the consequences would be. What would the behavior change be if they were actually taught in school here is a virus, here is how you get it, here is what is going to happen. I will tell you what would happen: the vast majority of them would delay the onset of sexual activity. And what we are talking about when we talk about abstinence is a realistic look at what are the consequences if you have a behavior other than that. And we are afraid to tell our children the truth, as far as the Government is concerned, and it is time that changed. Our children are worth more than that. We ought to invest in them. We ought to trust them that the majority of the time they are going to make good decisions. They are not going to make bad decisions all the time. And then we ought to support them at the time when they make a bad decision.

The other thing is that Congress ought to continue to support HPV vaccine research, but it needs to be a broad multivalent vaccine. Going after one or two types is halfway, and if we put money into that instead of a good solution to it, a good secondary treatment option rather than prevention, I think we will have failed. So I think oversight in terms of what the CDC and the FDA are doing in terms of vaccines are very important, because if we just go after HPV–16, what we are going to see is the other viruses rise in terms of prevalence, if we haven't decreased the age of onset and the number of partners.

So I thank you for holding this hearing. Prevention is the best message for our youth, and the best message with that is knowledge associated with sexually transmitted disease and an attitude of abstinence. We use that method on every other area where they are at risk; there is no reason that good leadership couldn't use that method on this.

Mr. SOUDER. Well, thank you very much. We will put your full statements in the record. If you have anything else to add, we may have a few written questions for you before we close the hearing record.

With that, the subcommittee stands adjourned.

[Whereupon, at 2:43 p.m., the subcommittee was adjourned, to reconvene at the call of the Chair.]

[Additional information submitted for the hearing record follows:]

Thank you for the opportunity to testify on the human papillomavirus (HPV) and cervical cancer. My name is Dr. Richard Schlegel, and I am the Professor and Chair of the Department of Pathology at the Georgetown University Medical Center.

Worldwide cervical cancer remains one of the primary causes of cancer deaths in women, resulting in more than 250,000 deaths per year. Eighty percent of these deaths occur in developing countries where screening and treatment are absent or seriously deficient. It has been confirmed that cervical cancer derives from HPV infected cells. In other words, HPV is a necessary precursor of cervical cancer. Presently, there are methods available to generate a vaccine against this virus. In fact, I was involved in the research that led to the first generation vaccine. However, the first generation vaccine involves the production of virus-like particles (VLPs) and this method is very expensive and the vaccine that is produced must be stored in a frozen state. This creates tremendous hurdles to successful delivery of the vaccine to developing countries where refrigeration is not always available.

I have been working on the advancement of a new second-generation HPV vaccine that has proven to be highly effective in animal trials. The vaccine can be produced inexpensively in bacteria and is much simpler to purify than the prior formulation. Moreover, the vaccine can be converted to a stable powder, which can be shipped and stored at room temperature. Thus, the new HPV vaccine offers several important advantages over the first generation vaccine, particularly with regard to distributing this prophylactic vaccine to the developing world where it is critically needed.

The cost of the current vaccine is $100 per shot, and each patient needs a series of 3 shots to be effectively immunized. However, the second-generation vaccine would cost much less, in the range of $10 per shot with a total cost of $30 per patient. The savings realized in treatment alone would be enormous. Not to mention the savings that would result from fewer women having to be treated for cervical cancer. It is my understanding that in the U.S. about $6 billion per year is spent in detecting and treating cervical cancer. Of course a dollar amount could never be put on the human suffering avoided and lives saved as a result of this vaccine.

As members of the Subcommittee know, bringing a drug or vaccine to market involves four phases: animal trials, phase 1-3 clinical trials, and commercial production and distribution. On this second-generation vaccine, animal trials are complete and were highly successful. Phase I trials are being funded through a Rapid Award from the National Institutes of Health (NIH). Approximately twenty patients will be in this small trial. The phase II trials would involve about 500 human patients and cost approximately $1.5 million. Typically, this phase is funded by a pharmaceutical company which would then move to commercial production. However, I have been told by a leading expert in the field of vaccine development that pharmaceutical manufacturers have three criteria in determining whether to fund phase two trials. They are:

1) The product is at least as effective as currently available products;

2) There is a clear advantage for the new product over those currently on the market;

3) The product must earn $750 million profit beyond its production costs.

While this vaccine clearly meets the first two criteria, the pharmaceutical industry does not foresee earning $750 million beyond production costs for this vaccine. From a societal view, this is myopic. A cost effective, stable HPV vaccine would save the lives of nearly 250,000 women, which is priceless. On the financial side, however, the elimination of cervical cancer by a vaccine would cut health care costs enormously and yield a great benefit here and in developing countries.

I believe very strongly in this vaccine and its potential. I come to you because I hope you can help us find a way to overcome the lack of support for this new initiative. Indeed, I think this vaccine brings to light a broader policy issue. There must be a way that the government can intervene, as it has done in the case of so-called "orphan drugs", to insure that medications like this one are not stymied because the normal business model does not fit. Too much is at stake not to tackle the challenge.

I appreciate very much your consideration of my testimony and may be contacted to answer any questions you have regarding the research and progress on this second generation vaccine.

To Whom It May Concern:

Thank you for your service and commitment to improving women's healthcare and preventing the unnecessary spread of Cervical Caner and Human Papillomavirus. I hope my personal testimony and experience will be of aid to you as you thoughtfully listen to the advice of experts and deliberate their suggestions.

I am a 21 year old college student. I attended Grayslake Community High School in IL, the student population was about 1650, when I graduated. During my high school years I was a varsity cheerleader, varsity tennis player and I dated the Homecoming King for two years (I was the Prom Queen). I "hung-out" with students that were sexually active both at early ages and with many different partners. I had friends that got pregnant as young as fifteen, had abortions, and contracted various sexually transmitted diseases. I also had a large number of close-friends that were and are virgins as I am.

I was the president of Students Against Destructive Decisions (SADD) for three years and I was a teen trainer for the American Lung Cancer Association with the: Teens Against Tobacco Usage (TATU) program. Just last fall I became certified by the state of Virginia to teach abstinence education.

The message I have from suburbia Illinois is that the two things sexually active teens are worried about are: 1) am I pregnant and 2) did I contract an STD. Condoms, until the outbreak of HPV, generally protected them from both. Those that refrained from sexual intercourse often did so because they did not want to risk either of those two concerns. Yet, the safe sex message being taught in the public schools is that condoms protect, for the most part, from both. When in reality condoms do not protect from HPV.

On the message of Safe Sex vs Abstinence: Teens are clearly told regardless of rhetoric that they will eventually have sex outside of a monogamous relationship and that when they engage in sexual behavior to do it safely (ie use a condom). The truth, according to your third panel, is that there can be "safe sex" from HIV and gonorrhea when wearing a condom but that there is no safe sex from HPV. That message is not given to the general public. Abstinence Education as Dr. Weldon mentioned, often has less results if it is not an ongoing education. Also, as mentioned by panelist Dr. Meeker, the minimum goal should be—abstinence while the girls are young because HPV is more easily contracted while the female body is still developing.

Although, I am a virgin and will be one until I am married, I do not expect that everyone or even most people will make the same personal decision. However, when helping young people decide their position, especially, those educated by our collectively funded public schools; it is robbery to not fully teach them about the dangers and realities of HPV.

Advice

1. Label condoms correctly and focusing funds on HPV education and PAP procedures. If you recall, the second concern of those sexually active is: contracting a STD. Thus,

educating them on HPV might cause young people to refrain from sexual activity (which would buy time to develop cures).

2. The concern that abstinence education does not work is fool-hearted because it has not been tried. It is impossible to measure the effectiveness of a program of this nature if there is not a clear message, hope for success, and clear expectations communicated for years. Currently, teens are told by the actions of society, particularly the government and some community leaders that they *will* be promiscuous, the question is just *when*. Why, when teen are expected to engage in sexual relations, should they not do what is expected of them? They have no standard to live up to. Nothing to strive for.
3. For what it is worth, I would request serious consideration of a clear message about the truths of HPV and let young people conclude as they will. Precautionary messages will help bring about prevention, not absolutely but in a much larger number than communicating constant doom.

Thank you for your time, service, and consideration,

Jane A. Grisham

Testimony of
Senator Connie Lawson, Indiana General Assembly
For Women In Government

Before the House Subcommittee on
Criminal Justice, Drug Policy and Human Resources
United States House of Representatives
Washington, DC

February 5, 2004

Mr. Chairman and Members of the Subcommittee,

My name is Connie Lawson and I am a second-term State Senator from Indiana. I am pleased to offer this testimony today on behalf of Women In Government. Women In Government is a bi-partisan, non-profit, educational association of elected and appointed women in state government. I currently serve on our Board of Directors and am also on our organization's Cervical Cancer Task Force.

Given that cervical cancer is one of the most preventable types of cancer due to early detection techniques, no American women should die of this disease. Thus, Women In Government has chosen eliminating cervical cancer over the next ten years as one of our organization's top priorities. In 2003, we formed a Cervical Cancer Task Force to address this issue and in January 2004, we launched a new campaign called the "Challenge to Eliminate Cervical Cancer." The campaign challenges state legislatures across the country to pass our members' bills and resolutions calling for improved public education about cervical cancer and HPV and broadened access to the most advanced screening tests – regardless of women's socioeconomic status. Already, members of our organization have introduced or plan to introduce legislation or resolutions in approximately 10 states.

My testimony today addresses the subject of HPV, which studies show is the cause of virtually all cervical cancers, and the important role that HPV testing in cervical cancer screening can play in helping to eliminate this deadly disease.

It is important to note that cervical cancer rates have decreased significantly over the last 60 years, due to widespread screening using the traditional Pap smear. However, according to the American Cancer Society, over 10,500 women will be diagnosed with and approximately 3,900 women will die of cervical cancer this year. This cancer, however, is nearly 100 percent preventable. It is a slow-developing disease that can usually be treated before abnormal cells develop into cancer. So, why are thousands of women still dying? Two key barriers have blocked our way.

First, cervical cancer disproportionately affects minority women and those with lower incomes, because they are less likely to have access to routine screening. Hispanic women, for example, are twice as likely to be diagnosed with cervical cancer as Caucasian women. Approximately half of all cervical cancer cases are in women who have *never* been screened, and 10 percent are in women who haven't been screened in the last five years. Thus, despite the high level of preventive care offered in this country, we must do more to extend life-saving technology to all age-appropriate women.

Second, in women who *are* screened periodically, studies show that the Pap smear's ability to identify women with cervical cancer or its early signs ranges between only 51 percent and 85 percent. Now, however, research shows that a test for HPV is much more effective at identifying women needing early intervention to stop the disease. A recent study of over 11,000 women showed that its sensitivity was over 97 percent. The test is now approved by the U.S. Food and Drug Administration for women 30 and older, for use along with the Pap smear, and is recognized in the screening guidelines of several leading medical groups. These organizations include the American College of Obstetricians and Gynecologists, the American Cancer Society and the Association of Reproductive Health Professionals.

But having advanced technology is only the first step toward eliminating cervical cancer. Every woman – no matter what her socioeconomic status -- must be *informed* about and *have access to* routine cervical cancer screening using the most up-to-date techniques. Education about cervical cancer and HPV is especially important because the more women know about their healthcare and the tests available to them, and what results of those tests mean, the more empowered they can be to take an active role in ensuring their own good health.

To help accomplish these objectives, and as part of Women In Government's "Challenge to Eliminate Cervical Cancer campaign," I have recently introduced a resolution in Indiana. The resolution calls on our legislative council to direct the appropriate committee to review the data regarding cervical cancer and HPV and evaluate current methods of public education and access to regular cervical cancer screening and options for increasing screening accuracy.

I look forward to working with my colleagues in the Indiana legislature to pass this resolution and then helping Women In Government benefit from my experience so that they too can advance this issue throughout the states.

While Women In Government members are tackling this important issue in our own states, I urge the Congress to similarly take action on improving cervical cancer education and screening programs at the federal level. I appeal to the Congress to make better screening tests available to *all* women – including underserved women.

Only by working on this issue at both the state and federal levels can we reach the attainable goal of finally eliminating the threat of cervical cancer for the women of America.

Thank you for the opportunity to provide this testimony.

Testimony of
Walter Kinney, M.D.

Before the House Subcommittee on
Criminal Justice, Drug Policy and Human Resources
United States House of Representatives
Washington, DC

March 11, 2004

Mr. Chairman and Members of the Subcommittee,

Thank you for the opportunity to explain the important and growing role of testing women for human papillomavirus (HPV) in cervical cancer screening programs in the United States.

My name is Dr. Walter Kinney. I am a gynecologic oncologist, which means that I am responsible for the care of women with genital cancers, including cervical cancer. I am an Associate Clinical Professor of Obstetrics and Gynecology at the University of California at Davis, and I practice in Sacramento at the Kaiser Permanente facility here. My testimony today reflects my own opinions (rather than those of my employer) which were formed from my experience in my current position as well as from years of clinical research in the area of cervical cancer. I have authored or co-authored 20 studies published in peer-reviewed medical journals on cervical cancer, HPV and HPV testing, and have helped to develop the categories in the current Bethesda system, by which Pap smears are diagnosed. I have also participated in the development of the current guidelines for cervical cancer prevention from the American Cancer Society, and the American Society of Colpcoscopy and Cervical Pathology. I am presently in the process of developing a set of standards for response to abnormal Pap smears at the request of the American College of Obstetrics and Gynecology.

There is now consensus in the medical community that infection with "high risk" types of human papillomavirus (HPV) must be present for a woman to develop cervical cancer. Research shows that determining a woman's HPV status helps identify her risk of having or developing cervical cancer or precancer – thus allowing her to either be monitored closely and treated early, or to safely avoid frequent, repeat examinations. In contrast, if we rely on Pap smears alone, even frequent testing is associated with a significant potential for false negative results – thus raising the possibility that cervical disease will develop undetected into invasive cancer. I believe the ability to accurately assess this risk can significantly help to improve the effectiveness and efficiency of cervical cancer screening programs in the U.S.

As you may well be aware, HPV is a highly prevalent virus: The cumulative lifetime risk of having ever carried HPV is 80-90 percent for adults who have been sexually active. HPV can be present in some people's mouths or under their fingernails. Carriage therefore does not require sexual intercourse. For the vast majority of women HPV is suppressed by the immune system without their awareness and without ever causing them any harm. As a consequence it is not a "disease", in that the vast majority of women who carry it are not adversely affected by it in any way. Transient carriage of HPV is normal, and should be not be stigmatized. It does not mean infidelity or promiscuity, nor should it be associated with gonorrhea or syphilis in the minds of patients. Stigmatizing HPV erroneously in this fashion means that women will not want to be tested, and that we are at risk of losing the potential benefit of better cervical cancer prevention that HPV testing can provide.

HPV does not directly lead to cancer. Rather, long term carriage of HPV enables abnormal cervical cells to reproduce unchecked by the body's natural defenses – sometimes leading to cervical disease or cancer. Most women will suppress HPV before significant cell changes occur. Only persistent carriage of HPV – usually lasting more than decade – can lead to cervical cancer.

The traditional method of cervical cancer prevention has been the annual Pap smear. In this test, cells are scraped from the cervix and then examined under a microscope. The Pap smear has several flaws. First, it is not a "sensitive" test, which means it often fails to identify women who have early signs of cervical disease. An evaluation in 1999 by the Agency for Health Care Policy and Research found that, on average, Pap testing is only 51 percent accurate at identifying women with moderate or high-grade cervical lesions. A Kaiser Permanente study published in the journal *Cancer* in 2000 showed that 28 percent of women diagnosed with invasive cervical cancer had had only normal Pap results in the preceding 3 years. The American Cancer Society reports that 40 percent of women with cervical cancer had normal Pap results within the previous five years. Newer "liquid-based" Pap tests – which flush cervical cells clear of debris so they can be viewed more clearly on the slide – have been shown to increase the sensitivity of the Pap. However, the fact remains that that Pap is a subjective test, dependent upon individual interpretation and judgment, regardless of how the slide is prepared.

Another problem with Pap smears is that they often produce ambiguous results. Five to seven percent of the 50 million Pap smears performed in the U.S. each year produce inconclusive results known as ASC-US (atypical squamous cells of undetermined significance). Few of these women actually have cellular changes that require treatment, yet most have traditionally undergone unnecessary additional testing and procedures, which can be anxiety-producing, uncomfortable and inconvenient for women, while also increasing healthcare costs. Finally, adding to the uncertainty around Pap smears, their results are difficult to reproduce, because different individuals may interpret the same slide differently. In a major study by the National Cancer Institute (NCI), fewer than 50 percent of high-grade precancerous lesions diagnosed by Pap smear at referring universities had the diagnosis confirmed upon later review.

In contrast, studies show that HPV testing has a higher sensitivity than the Pap smear for identifying women with early signs of cervical disease or cancer, which translates into a higher negative predictive value (the ability to rule out disease). A study of over 11,000 women published recently in the leading medical journal, *The Lancet*, showed that the sensitivity for HPV testing was 97.1 percent, compared to 76.6 percent for the Pap test. Additionally, studies show that the negative predictive value of HPV testing in conjunction with a Pap smear in women aged 30 and over ranges between 99.93 percent and 100.0 percent for high-grade cervical disease or cancer – higher than the Pap alone.

So what does all of this mean? Because of its high sensitivity and negative predictive value, HPV testing adds more certainty to cervical cancer screening. HPV testing already is the standard of care for follow-up evaluation of women with ASC-US Pap results, having been shown conclusively to offer a better assessment than repeating the Pap or performing a more invasive procedure called colposcopy. This approach has been validated by a major NCI study and confirmed in consensus guidelines published in the *Journal of the American Medical Association* in 2002.

Recently, in 2003, the U.S. Food and Drug Administration also approved the Hybrid Capture II high-risk HPV DNA test for routine screening in conjunction with a Pap smear for women aged 30 and older. Studies suggest that women who test negative on both the HPV and Pap tests can be very reassured that they are not at current risk, and can be safely screened less frequently than those who are HPV positive. In fact, one round of negative HPV and normal Pap test results can provide reassurance equal to or better than three normal consecutive annual Paps. Additionally, research shows that using HPV testing in such a manner can save more lives and reduce healthcare costs to a greater degree than traditional Pap smear-only programs.

Thus, the American College of Obstetricians and Gynecologists (ACOG) and the American Cancer Society (ACS) have recently updated their screening guidelines to include HPV testing in combination with a Pap smear every three years for women aged 30 and over. Both groups offered this as a viable alternative to more frequent testing using just the Pap.

Use of HPV testing in routine cervical cancer screening is increasing and numerous insurance companies already reimburse for it. In January of this year, Kaiser Permanente's Northern California region announced that it would offer and recommend HPV testing in addition to a Pap smear to all women 30 and over. Under this protocol, those women who opt for HPV testing along with their Pap smear will still have routine gynecologic exams. However, if their HPV and Pap tests are both normal, they will not be re-screened for another three years – in accordance with the ACOG and ACS guidelines. Women who are positive for HPV but have normal Pap results will be re-screened every year, also in accordance with the new guidelines. Those who are HPV positive and have abnormal Pap results will be referred to colposcopy. The goal is to provide screening with the best tests, by focusing resources on the women who truly need them.

For a program such as this to succeed, I believe that education of clinicians and women is essential. Physicians must understand how to factor a woman's HPV status into their screening recommendations. They must also know how to sensitively communicate information about HPV and a woman's HPV test results in order to reduce anxiety. Conversely, women must understand that less-frequent screening does not mean that annual gynecologic examinations no longer are needed. Additionally, women must understand the meaning of an HPV test result so that this information can be empowering rather than anxiety-provoking.

In summary, with proper education of healthcare professionals and women, I believe that HPV testing offers tremendous opportunities to improve cervical cancer screening for American women, while reducing healthcare costs by enabling resources to be focused on those women who need them most.

Thank you for the opportunity to comment on this matter.

Walter Kinney M.D.

Testimony of Christine Baze Guay

House Subcommittee on Criminal Justice, Drug Policy and Human Resources
U.S. House of Representatives
Washington, DC
March 11, 2004

To the Chairman and Members of the Subcommittee:

I would like to thank the subcommittee for the opportunity to provide written testimony about a topic that is so personal and important to me. As a cervical cancer survivor, I believe I can share some insight into the devastation that diagnosis and treatment of this disease can bring to an individual's life.

My name is Christine Baze Guay. I am a 35-year-old musician living outside of Boston. When I was diagnosed with cervical cancer in April of 2000, I knew very little about the disease or about HPV, the virus that causes it. Now I know this is a cancer that can be prevented and I have chosen to use my voice and my experience to help other women avoid it. As you evaluate the issue of HPV, I urge you to consider that, for a woman, understanding HPV, knowing her HPV status and not being embarrassed to talk about it with her doctor, can help ensure that she never goes through what I went through.

My story begins with music. I started playing the piano at age four and never stopped. A classical pianist for 20 years, my identity was wrapped in the music I performed. It allowed me to have a voice, share emotion, and connect with people – it was what made me feel like myself. It wasn't until grad school that I considered singing and playing the piano together, and it wasn't until years later that I would discover the joy of writing my own material. The evolution was magical. Before I knew it, I had my own band, steady gigs, a large following, and was said to be "the next big thing that comes out of Boston."

But all that changed when I woke up one day in January of 2000 and saw blood. Lots of it. I called my gynecologist, he said not to worry, that women spot between cycles. I said I've never spotted, and this was a LOT of blood. Once in the office, I was assured that I was "stressed" and that nothing was wrong. I was to return in two months for my annual exam, and not worry about it. So I did just that. I went on playing my music and dreaming of being a rock star.

Then I went in for my annual exam in March, and my pap test came back abnormal. I had never had an abnormal pap, and I had been going for my annual tests faithfully since I was 18 years old, so I was confused and concerned. I returned to the office for a colposcopy, and my doctor explained that he was seeing dysplasia - cell changes - and that they would need to be removed. He took a biopsy and told me about a procedure called "LEEP." He asked me to come back in a week to review the results of the biopsy and schedule the procedure. When I asked him what this all meant, he explained that, if left untreated, the dysplastic cells could turn into cancer of the cervix. I said "cancer?"

He then assured me that I did not have cancer, that I had normal paps every year (including the year before), that this type of cancer is slow growing, but that we needed to get the cells out of my body before they did turn cancerous.

The day of my follow-up appointment I got a phone call at 8:15AM. It was a woman confirming an appointment I did not have with a doctor I did not know. When I questioned her, she said my gynecologist had set it up for me and asked me if I had spoken to him. I said I had not, but was scheduled to meet with him later that morning to review the results of my colposcopy. I asked her if she was calling about my LEEP procedure. When she hesitated, I insisted on knowing who this doctor was and what this appointment was for. She finally said, "I'm so sorry Christine. Dr. Duska is a gynecologic oncologist and I am calling from the North Shore Cancer Center."

I looked at my husband and said "I have cancer."

It's weird how life can change dramatically in one moment in time. That phone call was my moment, and from that came a whirlwind of terror and sadness that is hard to put into words. I was diagnosed with invasive cervical cancer with extensive lymphatic invasion. Ten days after my diagnosis I had a radical hysterectomy. A month after that I had another surgery move my ovaries out of the radiation "frying zone." A week after that I started five weeks of daily pelvic radiation, concurrent with four rounds of chemotherapy, followed by three rounds of internal radiation. At 31 years old, I was physically depleted and emotionally devastated.

Most people are aware of the physical impact cancer and treatment can have on a person – it becomes apparent to everyone around you. What is less obvious is the emotional impact. After my treatment ended, the depression that followed was stifling. I felt like I had no idea of who I was, what was to become of me, my life, or what was I supposed to do.

I finally realized that I was indeed depressed, and I needed to attack the depression the same way I attacked the cancer. I started taking an anti-depressant, went to individual therapy, joined a cancer group and then a "young" cancer group. I started doing yoga, reiki, and acupuncture. We bought a house and I painted every inch. We got a puppy and she became my lifeline. Eventually it worked. I felt like I was getting my life back. But the music was nowhere to be found. It had stopped the day I was diagnosed, and I had yet to find the passion again. The one thing that always made me feel like me was gone – and I didn't think I was going to get it back.

Then I saw the movie "Harold and Maude," and became completely inspired by Maude's enthusiasm for life and every experience that comes with it. The soundtrack by Cat Stevens rang in my head, and when I heard the song, "Trouble," something clicked and I realized it was the song of the last year and a half of my life. I ran to my piano and started playing and singing that song. I felt it. I cried. It was the day the music returned to my life.

Now I am almost four years in remission, and I have decided to use my voice, my music, and my story to help educate other women about cervical cancer and what can be done to prevent it. I started a non-profit organization called popsmear.org and I organize benefit concerts around the country to raise awareness and money for the fight against cervical cancer. As a survivor, I do not want anyone to have to endure what I had to. And they don't have to.

My cancer was undetected for years. The standard pap test has a very high false negative rate, and women can be told they are "normal" when they are not. Despite my yearly visits, it wasn't until my doctor's office started using more modern technology (a liquid-based pap test), that my cancer was found. In addition, we know now the cause of cervical cancer – HPV – and there is an FDA-approved test that can determine who is at increased risk. All women need to understand the role of HPV and that cervical cancer IS preventable. It is crucial for women to have the information necessary to advocate for themselves, and that all women have access to these technologies that can save lives. Women also need the ability to talk about HPV with their doctor without feeling self-conscious or judged.

I am the lucky one – I did not lose my life to this disease. But, I can never have children. My digestive system and vagina are continuously reacting and changing as a result of radiation damage. I also live with the fear that it will return, and that I will not be so lucky. Cancer has changed my life dramatically. However, I am choosing to do something about it and advocate on behalf of all women. I'm just a musician, but I believe that I can make a difference. I believe that cervical cancer can be eliminated if people are educated about HPV and have access to the latest technologies. This is a cancer that we have the answer to - we need to use it.

I thank you for this opportunity and your consideration on this issue.

ACOG Statement to the Committee on Government Reform
Subcommittee on Criminal Justice, Drug Policy and Human Resources

Prevention of the Human Papillomavirus and Cervical Cancer
United States House of Representatives

March 11, 2004

The American College of Obstetricians and Gynecologists (ACOG), on behalf of its 46,000 partners in women's health care, is pleased to offer this statement to the House Committee on Government Reform, Subcommittee on Criminal Justice, Drug Policy and Human Resources. We thank Chairman Souder, Ranking Member Cummings, and the entire subcommittee for their leadership to address prevention efforts to reduce the incidence of cervical cancer.

ACOG Fellows care for and treat women of all ages. We believe that improving women's health is a vital investment, and that a strong commitment to preventive health care helps preserve the reproductive health and lives of all women.

As physicians dedicated to improving women's health care, ACOG is committed to decreasing the rate of cervical cancer and preventing those Human Papillomavirus (HPV) infections that lead to it. We believe Congress' highest priority in reaching this goal should be to expand underserved women's access to Pap test examinations. Although Pap testing does not lower the incidence of the genital HPV infection, it detects cellular changes caused by the virus, changes which can then be treated, when necessary, before they progress to cervical cancer.

What is HPV?

HPV is the name of a group of viruses with more than 100 different strains, of which approximately 30 are sexually transmitted. Only a small fraction of women with HPV are at high risk for cervical cancer. Certain types of HPV cause warts on the hands or feet, while some genital strains cause visible genital warts. Only a small number of strains, which do not leave warts, eventually lead to cervical cancer.

THE AMERICAN COLLEGE OF OBSTETRICIANS AND GYNECOLOGISTS • WOMEN'S HEALTH CARE PHYSICIANS
409 12TH STREET SW WASHINGTON DC 20024-2188
MAILING ADDRESS: PO BOX 96920 WASHINGTON DC 20090-6920
Phone: 202/638-5577
Internet: http://www.acog.org

Timely Screening is Critical

Cervical cancer is treatable and curable with regular exams. The cervicovaginal smear, or Pap test, is one of the few tests available that detects the presence of a premalignant lesion allowing for the prevention of cancer, and its success rate in reducing deaths from cervical cancer is proven. According to statistics, the availability and use of the Pap test reduced deaths from cervical cancer by over 60 percent between the years 1950 to 1980. The American Cancer Society estimates that in 2004, about 10,520 cases of invasive cervical cancer will be diagnosed in the United States, and about 3,900 women will die from the disease.

It is most important to note that, according to the National Cancer Institute, about half of women with newly diagnosed cervical cancer have never had a Pap test, and another 10 percent have not had a test in the past five years. This makes increasing access to Pap testing among underserved women a high priority.

Access to Screening

Despite improved screening rates due to the federally funded National Breast and Cervical Cancer Early Detection Program (NBCCEDP), access to care is still problematic for some women; race, educational level, and age tend to predict access. African-American women have higher death rates from cervical cancer, and women with less than a high school education are less likely to have testing than women with more education. Cervical cancer has a peak incidence between the ages of 40 and 55, yet women in this age group are less likely to have been screened with cervical cytology testing than are younger women.

Recent advances in our knowledge of the development of cervical cancer as well as technological changes in cancer screening have led ACOG to revise our guidelines regarding cervical cytology testing. Human Papillomavirus infections are common in young women, but in most, the immune system is effective in fighting the virus and preventing precancerous changes from occurring.

Because most HPV infections resolve spontaneously and cervical cancer is exceedingly rare in adolescents, ACOG now recommends that cervical cancer screening begin approximately 3 years after first sexual intercourse—but no later than age 21 years. Women younger than 30 years of age should have a Pap test each year. Women who are 30 or older, who are at low risk, and who have had 3 consecutive negative Pap tests may be screened every 2-3 years. Women who are 30 or older may also choose to have an HPV test at the time of their Pap test. If they receive negative results on both tests, they should be rescreened no sooner than 3 years. ACOG strongly encourages regular gynecologic visits as a part of preventive health care.

Again, we thank the Committee for addressing this important issue. As of 2002, the Centers for Disease Control and Prevention, through the NBCCEDP, have provided breast and cervical cancer screening services to more than 1.5 million underserved women. We hope Congress and the Administration will continue to eradicate cervical cancer through timely screening, and by focusing efforts on expanding access to reproductive health care to all women.

Additions to the Record by the Subcommittee

Table of Contents

(1) Follow-Up Questions to CDC, NIH and FDA

(2) Congressional Correspondence with Federal Agencies Regarding HPV

(3) Federal HPV Prevention Law

(4) HPV Facts

(5) Congressional Research Service Memorandum on HPV

(6) CDC HPV Prevention Report

(7) American Cancer Society Detail Guide on Cervical Cancer

(8) NIH Consensus Statement on Cervical Cancer

(9) NIH Workshop Executive Summary on Condom Effectiveness

(10) NCI Letter to House Subcommittee on Health and Environment

(11) Medical Institute for Sexual Health HPV Prevention Report

(12) Studies on HPV

(13) Background on Virginity Pledge Study

(14) Congressional Women's Caucus Letter of Support for HPV Education Law

(15) ACOG's Opposition to HPV Education Law

(16) American Cancer Society

(17) Government Spending on "Safe" Sex and Abstinence

(18) UK "Comprehensive" Sex Education Outcomes

(19) HPV and Gay and Lesbian Health

(20) Miscellaneous Documents

1. Follow-Up Questions to CDC, NIH and FDA

ONE HUNDRED EIGHTH CONGRESS

Congress of the United States

House of Representatives

COMMITTEE ON GOVERNMENT REFORM

2157 RAYBURN HOUSE OFFICE BUILDING

WASHINGTON, DC 20515–6143

MAJORITY (202) 225–5074
FACSIMILE (202) 225–3974
MINORITY (202) 225–5051
TTY (202) 225–6852

www.house.gov/reform

March 18, 2004

Honorable Tommy G. Thompson
Secretary
Department of Health and Human Services
200 Independence Avenue, S.W.
Washington, D.C. 20201

Dear Secretary Thompson,

Thank you for your leadership in protecting the health of all Americans. I particularly would like to thank you for the January 2004 report "Prevention of Genital Human Papillomavirus Infection" issued by the Centers for Disease Control and Prevention (CDC).

The Subcommittee held a hearing on March 11 to discuss this report and other issues related to HPV and cervical cancer.

Please find attached additional questions related to these topics directed to the CDC, National Institutes for Health (NIH) and the Food and Drug Administration (FDA) by the Subcommittee for publication in the hearing record.

Thank you again.

Sincerely,

Mark E. Souder
Chairman,
Subcommittee on Criminal Justice,
Drug Policy and Human Resources

Enclosures

CDC

1. According to the CDC's testimony, about 20 million Americans at any given point in time are currently infected with HPV, about 5.5 million people become newly infected with the virus each year, 10,520 women will be diagnosed with cervical cancer this year and 3,900 women will die from it. (a) How many women undergo invasive procedures each year to assess the status of their abnormal pap smears secondary to HPV? (b) How many women in total undergo invasive surgery to treat conditions, including cervical cancer, related to HPV infection annually? (c) Has there been an increase in abnormal PAP tests over the past thirty years? (d) Has there been an increase in the number of women undergoing invasive treatment related to HPV-infected over the past thirty years? (e) How many men undergo treatment for HPV-related conditions each year?

2. Since the enactment Public Law 106-354, the Breast and Cervical Cancer Prevention and Treatment Act of 2000, has the percentage of women treated who were identified under the CDC's testing programs for breast and cervical cancer increased, decreased or remained the same?

3. Effective screening has been credited for the significant decline in cervical cancer deaths in the U.S. (a) What percentage of at-risk women is not receiving cervical cancer screening as recommended? (b) Which test is more reliable to identify women at risk for cervical cancer, the PAP smear or HPV DNA screening? (c) Does the CDC cervical cancer screening program provide HPV DNA diagnostic testing? (d) Women at risk for cervical cancer can be identified with PAP and HPV DNA testing. How can those at risk for other HPV cancers, including men, be screened or identified?

4. When Dr. Gerberding was appointed director of the CDC on July 3, 2002, she stated, "We must evaluate programs and messages that have shown success. For example, the country of Uganda has reduced its HIV infection rate. Its comprehensive program includes a strong emphasis on abstinence, marital fidelity and responsible sexual behavior. Abstinence and monogamy, along with the avoidance of risky behaviors, are the first line of defense against HIV/AIDS." The January 2004 CDC HPV prevention report that advocates abstinence, monogamy and risk avoidance echoes this statement by Dr. Gerberding.

Please provide the overall CDC funding amounts for efforts to prevent HIV, STDs and unwanted pregnancy that specifically promote (a) abstinence; (b) monogamy, (c) partner reduction; and (d) "safer" sex, including condoms and contraception?

5. A vaccine for hepatitis B has been available for two decades, yet since 1999 the incidence of acute hepatitis B has increased among males 20 and older and among females over the age of 40. Based on these trends and the fact that more than 20 million

Americans are already infected with HPV, if an effective HPV vaccine became available within the next decade, how long would it be before a significant decrease in HPV prevalence would occur in the United States?

6. Over the past decade, CDC has sought to address issues involving stigma associated with HIV and some behaviors linked to HIV transmission. Popular culture-- including television, movies, magazines, and music-- has glamorized drug abuse, promiscuity and casual sex. Peer pressure also contributes to adolescents experimenting with sex and drugs. As a result, healthy behaviors, including abstinence, and youngsters who have chosen to practice these behaviors have been stigmatized. (1) Does the CDC recognize the stigma associated with abstinence and virginity that pressures many adolescents to engage in sexual activity and other risky behaviors? (2) What efforts, if any, is CDC sponsoring to address this stigma against virginity and abstinence?

7. The January 2004 CDC HPV prevention report states, "There is evidence that indicates that the use of condoms may reduce the risk of cervical cancer." During questioning at the Subcommittee hearing, Dr. Thompson stated that only two studies showed a reduction in cervical cancer risk associated with condom use. Are two studies that show such an association between condom use and reduced cervical cancer risk sufficient to make claims that condom use reduces cervical cancer risk?

8. In November 2002, a meta-analysis of "the best available data describing the relationship between condoms and HPV-related conditions" from the previous two decades was published in the journal *Sexually Transmitted Diseases*. The meta-analysis concluded: "There was no consistent evidence of a protective effect of condom use on HPV DNA detection, and in some studies, condom use was associated with a slightly increased risk for these lesions." (a) Would the studies cited in this meta-analysis be sufficient to make claims that condom use increases risk for HPV-related lesions? (b) What might be the cause for the association between condom use and increased risk for lesions?

NIH

1. An April 1996 National Institutes of Health Consensus Development Conference Statement on Cervical Cancer concluded, "Primary prevention of HPV infection will require (1) directing education efforts toward adolescents and health care providers regarding the strong causal link between acquisition of HPV as a sexually transmitted disease and development of cervical cancer and its precursors, (2) encouraging delayed onset of sexual intercourse, (3) developing an effective prophylactic vaccine, and (4) developing effective vaginal microbicides. The data on the use of barrier methods of contraception to prevent the spread of HPV is controversial but does not support this as an effective method of prevention."

Since April 1996, what is the total amount NIH has spent on research and other efforts to develop effective (a) HPV or cervical cancer vaccines; (b) microbicides; and (c) behavioral change interventions that delay the onset of sexual activity?

2. There are at least 18 strands of HPV that can cause cancer according to data published in the February 6, 2003 issue of The New England Journal of Medicine. (a) Of the HPV vaccine candidates currently undergoing trials, do any protect against all high risk strains of HPV infection? (b) If a vaccine does not protect against all high risk strands of HPV, is it then possible for a woman to become infected with a strain of HPV to which the vaccine does not provide immunity and thereby still develop cervical cancer?

3. A study published last year in the Journal of the National Cancer Institute found that an HPV vaccine now in development may not effectively protect women against infection during ovulation. What impact would this shortcoming potentially have on the overall effectiveness of HPV vaccination?

4. Would an HPV vaccine provide effective protection against persistent infection for someone who may already have been exposed to HPV?

5. HPV has been detected in some prostate tumors. Is there sufficient evidence to suggest that HPV infection may be associated with the development of prostate cancer?

6. HPV is associated with a number of cancers. What other viruses are associated with the development of cancer?

FDA

1. In December 2000, Public Law 106-554 was signed by President Clinton, directing the FDA to "reexamine existing condoms labels... to determine whether the labels are medically accurate regarding the overall effectiveness or lack of effectiveness in preventing sexually transmitted diseases, including HPV." On February 12, 2004, the Subcommittee requested that the FDA provide "a detailed summary of all actions taken to enact this law since it was signed on December 21, 2000," including "meeting dates, meeting participants, and number of full time employees assigned to implementing this law." The FDA response dated March 10, 2004 did not provide the specific details the Subcommittee requested. The Subcommittee again would request a detailed summary of all actions taken to enact this law since it was signed on December 21, 2000, including specific meeting dates, meeting participants, the topics discussed at each meeting and the number of full time employees assigned to implementing this law.

2. In July 2003, the FDA warned Berlex Laboratories, a unit of German drug maker Schering, that an advertisement for Yasmin birth control pills was misleading because it, in part, overstated the product's effectiveness. How long did it take the FDA to review these claims and to make this determination that the company was providing misleading claims of effectiveness?

3. Is there any published scientific data available indicating that labels providing "medically accurate regarding the overall effectiveness or lack of effectiveness" of condoms in preventing HPV and other STDs would discourage condom use?

4. Does the labeling on any other contraceptives notify consumers that a product does not prevent STDs?

5. "Microbicides" have been suggested as potential protection against HPV and other STDs. (a) What microbicides currently are available? (b) Please explain the effectiveness or lack of effectiveness of existing microbicides in protecting against HPV, HIV/AIDS and other STDs? (c) The spermicide Nonoxynol-9 (N-9) has been promoted for the prevention of pregnancy and STDs. For nearly 15 years, a growing number of studies have actually demonstrated an increased risk for HIV infection associated with N-9 use. Now researchers report in the March 2004 issue of the medical journal Obstetrics and Gynecology that the chances of becoming pregnant over a six-month period may be as high as 22 percent for women who rely on N-9 for contraception. The Subcommittee wrote to the FDA on April 9, 2003 and stated "N-9 was originally intended for use as a spermicide for contraception, yet in this regard, there are no data to indicate that condoms with N-9 are any more effective than condoms that do not contain N-9. The availability of condoms laced with N-9, therefore, provide no benefit over what is otherwise available for contraception but do cause increased risks for HIV infection. This danger with no

known beneficial offset calls into question the overall safety and effectiveness of such products and thereby the FDA approval for production and sale." With the growing evidence that N-9 use is not effective and may be dangerous, will the FDA consider pulling N-9 products from commercial availability until its safety and effectiveness can be proven?

6. FDA requires products to undergo clinical trials to demonstrate safety and effectiveness before they are marketed for their stated purpose(s). In the FDA testimony delivered to the Subcommittee, it is stated that "our current guidance recommends that the package insert for condoms contain the following statement: If used properly, latex condoms will help to reduce the risk of transmission of HIV infection (AIDS) and many other sexually transmitted diseases, including chlamydia infections, genital herpes, genital warts, gonorrhea, hepatitis B, and syphilis." The FDA testimony further states, "scientific studies on STDs characterized by genital ulcers, e.g., genital herpes and syphilis, are inconclusive as to whether the risks of these diseases is lowered for condom users." In 2001, a report entitled "Scientific Evidence on Condom Effectiveness for Sexually Transmitted Disease (STD) Prevention" prepared by the FDA with the National Institute of Allergy and Infectious Diseases of the National Institutes of Health, the Centers for Disease Control and Prevention and the U.S. Agency for International Development evaluated the published data on latex condoms and STD prevention. In the report, the panel "concluded that there was no evidence that condom use reduced the risk of HPV infection" and "The Panel agreed that the published epidemiologic data were insufficient to draw meaningful conclusions about the effectiveness of the latex male condom to reduce the risk of transmission of genital ulcer diseases (genital herpes, syphilis and chancroid)." In fact the, panel found that there was only sufficient data to demonstrate that condom use could reduce "HIV transmission in both men and women who engage in vaginal intercourse" and "indicated that the latex male condom could reduce the risk of gonorrhea for men."

There seems to be some confusion about the overall possible effectiveness of condoms for preventing STDs. (a) When did condoms undergo FDA approved clinical trials to determine effectiveness in preventing the transmission of STDs? (b) Did clinical trials of condoms specifically examine the effectiveness of condoms against HPV or cervical cancer?

Department of Health and Human Services
Follow-up Questions and Answers on
HPV and Cervical Cancer Hearing
March 11, 2004
Subcommittee on Criminal Justice, Drug Policy and Human Resources
Committee on Government Reform
U.S. House of Representatives

CDC Questions

Question 1: According to the CDC's testimony, about 20 million Americans at any given point in time are currently infected with HPV, about 5.5 million people become newly infected with the virus each year, 10,520 women will be diagnosed with cervical cancer this year and 3,900 women will die from it.
(a) How many women undergo invasive procedures each year to assess the status of their abnormal pap smears secondary to HPV?
(b) How many women in total undergo invasive surgery to treat conditions, including cervical cancer, related to HPV infection annually?
(c) Has there been an increase in abnormal PAP tests over the past thirty years?
(d) Has there been an increase in the number of women undergoing invasive treatment related to HPV-infected over the past thirty years?
(e) How many men undergo treatment for HPV-related conditions each year?

Response: Data are not available to answer all of these questions. However, by evaluating two recent studies that assessed the burden of HPV-related conditions in the United States, *(HW Chesson, JM Blandford, TL Gift, G Tao, KL Irwin. The estimated direct medical costs of sexually transmitted diseases among American youth, 2000. Perspect Sexual Reprod Health 2004;36:11-19 and H Weinstock, S Berman, W Cates. Sexually transmitted diseases in American youth: Incidence and Prevalence Estimates, 2000. Perspect Sexual Reprod Health 2004;36:6-10),* we can derive some estimates. About 2.1 million women undergo colposcopy, a procedure in which the cervix is viewed with a microscope and special lighting to see whether the cells have undergone any changes. About 1.9 million women each year are diagnosed and treated for cervical intraepithelial neoplasia (CIN), (also called cervical dysplasia) CIN is classified as I, II or III depending on its severity. The more severe forms, CIN II and CIN III can become cancer, but this is rare if the woman receives adequate treatment. Treatments include removing the abnormal cells through special procedures using lasers, freezing, or cauterizing the areas with the abnormal cells. The only HPV-related condition for which men commonly receive treatment are anal or genital warts. Using estimates provided in the articles, about 250,000 cases of anal or genital warts occur in men each year, and about 75%, or 187,500 men are treated. Treatments include topical ointments, or removal by laser, freezing, or surgery.

Question 2: Since the enactment Public Law 106-354, the Breast and Cervical Cancer Prevention and Treatment Act of 2000, has the percentage of women treated who were identified under the CDC's testing programs for breast and cervical cancer increased, decreased or remained the same?

Response:

- The number of patients being referred for treatment has not changed over time.
- Prior to the enactment of the Treatment act, approximately 96% of the women diagnosed with cancer through the program initiated therapy – however, this was no easy task, and unfortunately took away valuable time and resources that could have been used to get more women screened (Battelle Study). With respect to treatment following the Act, CMS may be better suited to answer this question.

Question 3: Effective screening has been credited for the significant decline in cervical cancer deaths in the U.S. (a) What percentage of at-risk women is not receiving cervical cancer screening as recommended? (b) Which test is more reliable to identify women at risk for cervical cancer, the PAP smear or HPV DNA screening? (c) Does the CDC cervical cancer screening program provide HPV DNA diagnostic testing? (d) Women at risk for cervical cancer can be identified with PAP and HPV DNA testing. How can those at risk for other HPV cancers, including men, be screened or identified?

Response:

(a) According to BRFSS and NHIS, an estimated 15% of women 18-65 have never been screened for cervical cancer, and between 20-30% have not had screening within the past 2-3 years.

(b) CDC's decisions regarding the use of any new technology are based on analysis and re-analysis of the best evidence available. *Pap* Test*:* The Pap test is widely accepted and in part responsible for greatly reducing deaths from cervical cancer in America. The Pap test is still the gold standard for determining the current cervical cancer risk. Only a few women with abnormal PAP tests will ever develop cervical cancer.

(c) For current absolute risk of cervical cancer the Pap test is more reliable than the HPV test. The CDC administered screening program tests for current risk, as future risk is speculative. The Breast and Cervical Cancer Program provides HPV DNA screening if certain abnormal PAP test results are found. (For ASC-US Pap results, and for surveillance for LSIL results at 1 year if colposcopy results is negative.)

(d) CDC is not currently aware of any screening for the other cancers, and there is no proven method of adequately screening men for HPV.

Question 4: When Dr. Gerberding was appointed director of the CDC on July 3, 2002, she stated, "We must evaluate programs and messages that have shown success. For example, the country of Uganda has reduced its HIV infection rate. Its comprehensive program includes a strong emphasis on abstinence, marital fidelity and responsible sexual behavior. Abstinence and monogamy, along with the avoidance of risky behaviors, are the first line of defense against HIV/AIDS." The January 2004 CDC HPV prevention report that advocates abstinence, monogamy and risk avoidance echoes this statement by Dr. Gerberding.

Please provide the overall CDC funding amounts for efforts to prevent HIV, STDs and unwanted pregnancy that specifically promote (a) abstinence; (b) monogamy, (c) partner reduction; and (d) "safer" sex, including condoms and contraception?

Response: CDC's HIV/STD and pregnancy prevention efforts compose a comprehensive program that, like the Ugandan approach, includes messages encouraging abstinence, delaying sexual debut, monogamy, partner reduction, and risk reduction, including correct and consistent condom use for sexually active persons with multiple partners. These messages are part of the comprehensive programs funded by CDC through state and local health departments, education departments, and community-based organizations. It is not possible to identify specific expenditures for the categories listed above as these messages are delivered as part of overall prevention programs. In FY 2003, $319 million was distributed to health departments for HIV prevention services; $57 million was provided directly to CBOs for HIV prevention activities; and $107.1 to state and local health departments for STD prevention and control

CDC is supporting specific research related to abstinence among young people. For example, *Parents Matter* is a community-based study evaluating the effectiveness of two programs designed to reduce sexual risk behavior among young people through effective parent-child communication. This is a five-year research project. Funding for the project totals $4.5 million dollars. One of the first publications being prepared from the study examines predictors of parental abstinence communication since communication about abstinence and delaying sexual activity is an important part of keeping youth free from HIVand other STDs and preventing unwanted pregnancy.

CDC also supports *Project Connect*, an integrated multi-level intervention, which is designed to work with parents, providers, schools and communities to create environments for adolescents that prevent STD, including HIV, and teen pregnancy. As such, outcome goals include delay in sexual initiation and return to abstinence among sexually active adolescents. These goals will be met through improved relationships and communication in families, increased connection to health care services, and school environments that support and encourage healthy behavior. The study is being implemented and evaluated in middle schools and high schools in the Los Angeles Unified School District. Project Connect is an eight year study (2 years of development, 5 years of intervention and evaluation, 1 year analysis and report writing) and is currently in its 2nd year. The total costs are expected to be $9.5 million.

In addition, in FY 2003 CDC funded state and national organizations to promote science-based strategies including abstinence to prevent teen pregnancy, HIV & STD ($532, 906); and regional training centers to assist providers in integrating adolescent reproductive health and HIV/STD through dissemination of information on teen pregnancy trends and issues and best practices in teen pregnancy prevention including abstinence ($450,000). In addition, CDC funds a series of research projects that seek to find the best methods for delaying the onset on sexual activity, increasing the effective use of contraceptives, and decreasing numbers of partners.

With regard to school health, in FY 2004, CDC is currently funded for $46.7M for HIV programs. This number has remained level for the last decade. CDC recognizes that the only certain way to prevent HIV, sexually transmitted diseases, and unplanned pregnancy is to *not* engage in sexual intercourse. CDC is committed to helping to increase the percentage of young people who have chosen not to engage in intercourse. In the context of such serious health threats, CDC funds state and large urban school districts and non-governmental organizations to support their efforts to prevent HIV infection among youth. State and local education agencies choose the curricula and programs that are suitable for their communities. CDC requires that all CDC-funded HIV prevention and health education policies, programs, materials, and presentations used at the local level be locally determined and consistent with community values. In the 2001 *Journal of School Health*, it was reported that 91.5% of middle/ junior high schools and 96.1% of high schools used abstinence as the most effective method to avoid pregnancy, HIV or other STDS (1). CDC is committed to tracking how the programs are being delivered (2).

Additionally in FY 2003, CDC funded $2.3 million to 12 state education agencies and two national organizations to help adolescents avoid early sexual debut and to avoid or reduce unintended pregnancies, infection from STDs, and HIV/AIDS infection.
The twelve states and one territory are CO, KS, LA, MI, MN, NM, NV, RI, NC, WA, WI, WY, and Palau. These organizations are focusing on abstinence only and/or abstinence as a critical component of broader approaches. They include faith-based agencies, HIV community planning groups, community agencies that serve young people, parents, families, juvenile justice agencies, and organizations that are focusing on reducing sexual risks for HIV, other STDs, and pregnancy among young people.

Question 5: A vaccine for hepatitis B has been available for two decades, yet since 1999 the incidence of acute hepatitis B has increased among males 20 and older and among females over the age of 40. Based on these trends and the fact that more than 20 million Americans are already infected with HPV, if an effective HPV vaccine became available within the next decade, how long would it be before a significant decrease in HPV prevalence would occur in the United States?

Response: Acceptance rates by high-risk adults for hepatitis B vaccine have been high when vaccine is offered in the setting in which these adults are receiving care or evaluation, such as health care institutions or STD clinics. There is not a national program for hepatitis B vaccination of adults, and overall vaccine coverage among adults is low. In contrast, the incidence of hepatitis B has declined dramatically among children and adolescents for whom national programs for universal immunization are in place. Hepatitis B vaccination impacts (including other countries that started vaccinating widely before the U.S. did) may provide some information on changes in the epidemiology of infection and disease; however, one must use caution in comparing the two infections and drawing conclusions on HPV vaccination potential directly from the HBV story, as HBV and HPV do not have exactly the same modes of transmission nor the same risk factors for infection and disease. The physiology of infection clearances for HBV and HPV are also not comparable.

Prevention of HBV infection through adolescent immunization may provide a useful model for the prevention of HPV infection. While HBV is acquired during adolescence, infection rates are lower than those found among young adults. This information became the driving force behind establishment of an adolescent immunization visit at 11-12 years of age to provide hepatitis B and other vaccines needed to protect teenagers from disease. In addition, vaccination is recommended for all adolescents (11-18 years) not previously vaccinated against hepatitis B. This adolescent immunization strategy has achieved modestly successful rates of vaccination coverage (about 60%) since they were first published in 1996, and immunization rates continue to increase. The adolescent immunization visit could provide the platform for the use of vaccines against HPV infection.

If an effective HPV vaccine were available, decreases might be realized in the incidence of pre-malignant cervical changes earlier than decreases in cervical cancer rates, which would predict subsequent decreases in cervical cancer deaths. Additionally, we do not know if HPV vaccine will have an impact on existing pre-cancerous lesions or early cancers. If these regress, do not progress or progress slower after vaccination, one would see further decreases in cervical cancer deaths at a later date.

Question 6: Over the past decade, CDC has sought to address issues involving stigma associated with HIV and some behaviors linked to HIV transmission. Popular culture-- including television, movies, magazines, and music-- has glamorized drug abuse, promiscuity and casual sex. Peer pressure also contributes to adolescents experimenting with sex and drugs. As a result, healthy behaviors, including abstinence, and youngsters who have chosen to practice these behaviors have been stigmatized. (1) Does the CDC recognize the stigma associated with abstinence and virginity that pressures many adolescents to engage in sexual activity and other risky behaviors? (2) What efforts, if any, is CDC sponsoring to address this stigma against virginity and abstinence?

Response: CDC's comprehensive school health efforts include messages about abstinence (even for young people who have already had sex) and delaying sexual debut. Our programs support these two strategies among young people, and send young people an affirming message that abstinence and delay are healthy, positive choices. For example, CDC's Division of Adolescent and School Health has developed **Guidelines**

for Effective School Health Education to Prevent the Spread of AIDS (see http://www.cdc.gov/nccdphp/dash/sexualbehaviors/guidelines/guidelines.htm) that include the following goals:

School systems should make programs available that will enable and encourage young people who have not engaged in sexual intercourse and who have not used illicit drugs to continue to

- Abstain from sexual intercourse until they are ready to establish a mutually monogamous relationship within the context of marriage;
- Refrain from using or injecting illicit drugs.

For young people who have engaged in sexual intercourse or who have injected illicit drugs, school programs should enable and encourage them to–

- Stop engaging in sexual intercourse until they are ready to establish a mutually monogamous relationship within the context of marriage;
- To stop using or injecting illicit drugs.

Question 7: The January 2004 CDC HPV prevention report states, "There is evidence that indicates that the use of condoms may reduce the risk of cervical cancer." During questioning at the Subcommittee hearing, Dr. Thompson stated that only two studies showed a reduction in cervical cancer risk associated with condom use. Are two studies that show such an association between condom use and reduced cervical cancer risk sufficient to make claims that condom use reduces cervical cancer risk?

Response: Dr. Thompson did not state that only two studies showed a reduction in cervical cancer risk. He stated that among the studies showing reduction of cervical cancer risk, two had results that were statistically significant. His testimony in this regard was based on CDC's Report to Congress entitled "Prevention of Genital HPV Infection". That report describes nine studies that evaluated women with cervical cancer. Seven of the nine found a reduction in risk of cancer in women using condoms. Among these seven studies, the magnitude of risk reduction ranged from 20-80%; two of the seven studies showed statistically significant risk reduction. Statistical significance refers to the likelihood that study findings could be due to chance and not to the amount of risk reduction or the quality of the study design. Conclusions about risk typically are based on the findings of the whole body of clinical studies, including consideration of the adequacy of study design and direction of potential bias, and also on biologic plausibility. The NIH Workshop Summary: Scientific Evidence on Condom Effectiveness for STD Prevention concluded that "study findings did suggest that condom use might afford some protection in reducing the risk of HPV-associated diseases, including genital warts in men and cervical neoplasia in women." A meta-analysis published in November 2002 in the journal Sexually Transmitted Diseases concluded that available data "suggest that…condoms may protect against genital warts, CIN II or II and invasive cervical cancer."

Question 8: In November 2002, a meta-analysis of "the best available data describing the relationship between condoms and HPV-related conditions" from the previous two decades was published in the journal *Sexually Transmitted Diseases*. The meta-analysis concluded: "There was no consistent evidence of a protective effect of condom use on HPV DNA detection, and in some studies, condom use was associated with a slightly increased risk for these lesions." (a) Would the studies cited in this meta-analysis be sufficient to make claims that condom use increases risk for HPV-related lesions? (b) What might be the cause for the association between condom use and increased risk for lesions?

Response:

(a) The published meta-analysis considered six studies of condoms and HPV DNA detection in women. Of these six, three showed risk reduction and the amount of risk reduction ranged from 10-80%. Three other studies showed no risk reduction (e.g. women who used condoms had a higher risk for HPV infection). However, as the authors point out, none of these studies were designed specifically to look at condoms and HPV, and it is difficult to draw conclusions. The CDC Report to Congress reports a similar but more recent systematic literature review that also shows inconsistent findings and concludes the effect of condom use on HPV infection is unknown.

(b) Since there is no apparent biologic reason why condom use would increase risk of HPV infection, a likely explanation is that the study design might not have been adequate to correctly assess condom use and HPV infection. All studies of HPV infection have serious methodologic limitations that hamper their interpretation. These limitations can lead to an incorrect estimate of the association between condom use and HPV infection, most likely an underestimate (or even finding a harmful effect). If people tend to use condoms with riskier partners or over-report condom use, or if consistent condom users are lumped together with inconsistent users in the analysis, or if women were already infected with HPV prior to condom use, this can bias the results toward showing that condoms have no or little protective effect, or even a harmful effect.

FDA QUESTIONS

Question 1: In December 2000, Public Law 106-554 was signed by President Clinton, directing the FDA to "reexamine existing condoms labels…to determine whether the labels are medically accurate regarding the overall effectiveness or lack of effectiveness in preventing sexually transmitted diseases, including HPV." On February 12, 2004, the Subcommittee requested that the FDA provide "a detailed summary of all actions taken to enact this law since it was signed on December 21, 2000," including "meeting dates, meeting participants, and number of full time employees assigned to implementing this law." The FDA response dated March 10, 2004 did not provide the specific details the Subcommittee requested. The Subcommittee again would request a detailed summary of all actions taken to enact this law since it was signed on December 21, 2000, including specific meeting dates, meeting participants, the topics discussed at each meeting and the number of full time employees assigned to implementing this law.

Response: FDA has taken its responsibility to comply with PL 106-554 very seriously. The statute was enacted in December 2000, and in April 2001, after consultation with Agency legal counsel regarding the interpretation of the condom labeling review provision, we began to develop an implementation plan to fulfill our obligations. In the three years that have elapsed since then, the Agency has carried out this plan, which included a survey of the current labeling on marketed condoms, a review of the Agency's current labeling guidance as well as policies that led up to it, and comprehensive and systematic review of the published literature and other clinical considerations. This last element of the plan was both helped and complicated by developments that unfolded after PL 106-554 was enacted. These events included the summary report from the interagency workshop that was issued in June 2001, new findings regarding the risks of HIV transmission associated with use of nonoxynol-9 (a spermicide contained in the lubricant of some condoms), and – most recently – CDC's *Report to Congress: Genital HPV Infection*. The body of literature addressed by these departmental initiatives encompasses the results from several hundred studies, and the process of reviewing them and systematically evaluating their contributions to our overall understanding of condom protection against various STDs has been a laborious effort.

Our activities to comply with PL 106-554 also included consultations with colleagues in both NIH and CDC, participation in a second workshop on condom study methodology (December 2002), coordination on an Agency policy regarding nonoxynol-9 (N-9), monitoring of and response to *ad hoc* inquiries and new actions taken by condom manufacturers, and development of a detailed concept paper that is the blueprint for the Agency's planned regulatory response. FDA's efforts to implement this statute have involved input from Agency clinicians and epidemiologists, regulatory and compliance staff, legal counsel, and management of the Center for Devices and Radiological Health. Because of the involvement of individuals from various FDA components and levels on this effort over the past three years, and because these employees have worked on PL 106-554 in addition to many other assignments and projects, it is difficult to identify precisely the number of employees who have worked on implementation of PL 106-554, and such a number would not provide a meaningful picture of the Agency's work on this specific initiative. As requested, however, we have tried to give a more complete picture of the history of our work in the enclosed outline of meetings and work initiatives associated with implementing the new statute. This outline includes only formal meetings that could be retrospectively identified and does not include numerous informal consultations among agency staff.

As indicated in the Agency's testimony at the March 11th hearing, the review of the medical literature is complete and the Agency is now in the process of writing up the results of that review and developing a new guidance document that will propose revised language for condom labeling. FDA is also developing a proposed rule to amend the condom classification to designate this guidance document as a special control for condoms. We expect to issue these proposals for public comment later this year.

Question 2: In July 2003, the FDA warned Berlex Laboratories, a unit of German drug maker Schering, that an advertisement for Yasmin birth control pills was misleading because it, in part, overstated the product's effectiveness. How long did it take the FDA to review these claims and to make this determination that the company was providing misleading claims of effectiveness?

Response: FDA became aware of the Berlex Laboratories advertisement for Yasmin birth control pills on May 16, 2003, and issued the referenced warning letter on July 10, 2003. However, it should be noted that the review involved in sending this company a warning letter is not directly comparable to the agency's ongoing review of condom labeling. The former situation involved examining comparative effectiveness statements made in a single advertisement for a particular product. FDA examined information already submitted to it by that product's manufacturer as part of the drug approval process and based its letter on the absence in those materials of information sufficient to meet the specific regulatory standard applicable to this type of comparative drug claim. FDA's review of condom labeling, by contrast, involves examination of existing product labeling for an entire class of products, in light of current scientific knowledge, to determine objectively whether that labeling is medically accurate with respect to overall effectiveness against a diverse range of STDs. As indicated in our prior testimony, this evaluation has required FDA to undertake an extensive independent review of current literature and other information.

Question 3: Is there any published scientific data available indicating that labels providing "medically accurate regarding the overall effectiveness or lack of effectiveness" of condoms in preventing HPV and other STDs would discourage condom use?

Response: Although FDA certainly would be concerned if labeling in some way discouraged use of a condom when its use would be appropriate, studies to evaluate such responses are, in essence, human behavior trials. We are not aware of such studies.

Question 4: Does the labeling on any other contraceptives notify consumers that a product does not prevent STDs?

Response: Users of intrauterine devices (IUDs), tubal occlusion devices, and natural skin condoms should not expect protection against STDs, and labeling for those products should contain the statement that:

This product is intended to prevent pregnancy. It does not protect against HIV infection and other sexually transmitted diseases.

Similarly, all prescription contraceptive products, including all hormonal contraceptive products (birth control pills, vaginal rings, and patches) are required to bear a labeling statement that they do not protect against STDs including HIV (AIDS). Labeling for the two approved drugs for emergency contraception state the same. FDA has proposed that over-the-counter (OTC) vaginal contraceptives containing N-9 also bear labeling indicating that they do not protect against AIDS and other sexually transmitted diseases, 68 FR 2254.

Question 5: "Microbicides" have been suggested as potential protection against HPV and other STDs. (a) What microbicides currently are available? (b) Please explain the effectiveness or lack of effectiveness of existing microbicides in protecting against HPV, HIV/AIDS and other STDs?(c) The spermicide Nonoxynol-9 (N-9) has been promoted for the prevention of pregnancy and STDs. For nearly 15 years, a growing number of studies have actually demonstrated an increased risk for HIV infection associated with N-9 use. Now researchers report in the March 2004 issue of the medical journal Obstetrics and Gynecology that the chances of becoming pregnant over a six-month period may be as high as 22 percent for women who rely on N-9 for contraception. The Subcommittee wrote to the FDA on April 9, 2003 and stated "N-9 was originally intended for use as a spermicide for contraception, yet in this regard, there are no data to indicate that condoms with N-9 are any more effective than condoms that do not contain N-9. The availability of condoms laced with N-9, therefore, provide no benefit over what is otherwise available for contraception but do cause increased risks for HIV infection. This danger with no known beneficial offset calls into question the overall safety and effectiveness of such products and thereby the FDA approval for production and sale." With the growing evidence that N-9 use is not effective and may be dangerous, will the FDA consider pulling N-9 products from commercial availability until its safety and effectiveness can be proven?

Response: There are no prescription or OTC microbicides approved for prevention of HPV, HIV/AIDs or other STDs.

The spermicide N-9 is a non-ionic surfactant that works as a vaginal contraceptive by damaging the cell membrane of sperm. It has been shown in certain in vitro studies to damage the cell wall of certain STD pathogens and to have activity against certain bacterial and viral STD pathogens, including HIV. Because N-9 kills the AIDS virus (HIV) and other STD pathogens in vitro, it has been suggested, over the years, that the drug might help prevent or reduce the risk of transmission of the AIDS virus and other STDs in humans. However, labeling for N-9 vaginal contraceptive products and lubricants containing N-9 has never stated or suggested this. Although information available to the general public may create the misperception that N-9 might help decrease the risk of becoming infected with the AIDS virus and other STDs, more recently, a number of studies have demonstrated that N-9 does not protect against the AIDS virus (HIV) or other STDs. However, only a few recent studies have suggested that there may be a greater risk of HIV infection associated with frequent N-9 use. These studies used a very high-risk population of commercial sex workers as subjects. FDA is working to address this risk information in light of the intended use of N-9 products as contraceptives.

As you note, the March 2004 medical journal Obstetrics and Gynecology published spermicide efficacy studies involving N-9 vaginal spermicides, which showed that the probability of pregnancy during typical use for spermicides containing N-9 was between 10-22 (this means that per year, 10-22 women out of 100 will become pregnant). N-9 spermicides may be just as effective as other non-hormonal birth control methods; 14-15 women will become pregnant using the male latex condom, 20-32 women will become pregnant using the diaphragm or cervical cap, 19-27 women will become pregnant using natural family planning, etc. The typical use pregnancy rates were obtained from the literature - R.A. Hatcher, J. Trussell, F. Stewart et al., Contraceptive Technology, 17th revised edition (1998) and 18th edition (in press), and data adapted from clinical trial product information submitted to FDA and NIH.

The N-9 efficacy studies described above are for stand-alone vaginal contraceptives containing N-9, such as films, suppositories, foams and gels. These studies show that N-9 is effective in preventing pregnancy when used correctly. FDA has decided to allow these products to remain on the marketplace, but will require manufacturers to label their products with warnings that advise consumers that N-9-containing OTC vaginal contraceptive drug products do not protect against the AIDS virus and other STDs and that frequent use by women at risk for HIV may increase their risk of getting HIV from infected partners. FDA published a proposed rule requiring these warnings for OTC vaginal contraceptives on January 16, 2003, 68 FR 2254. FDA has also published a call for data notice on December 13, 2003 (68 FR 75585) for vaginal lubricants and moisturizers, some of which contain N-9. These are drugs that were not previously reviewed by FDA when the OTC drug review process began. The review will determine if these ingredients are generally recognized as safe and effective for their labeled uses.

Condoms containing N-9 are not under the purview of FDA's proposed rule of 1/16/03. Condoms are medical devices. N-9, a drug, is added to the lubricant system of some condoms in order to provide a spermicidal effect in the event of condom breakage or slippage where there might be semen spillage in the vagina. In 1981, data supporting the addition of N-9 to the condom lubricant system included results from post-coital testing showing a great reduction in sperm motility. FDA believed that confirmatory contraceptive studies – which would need to be unusually large to show an expected small added effect – were unnecessarily burdensome.

FDA believes that a significant portion of the market for condoms with N-9 consists of heterosexual couples at low HIV risk who use this product for contraceptive protection. We believe that this is a reasonably safe use of a condom with N-9, and the data do not support removal of this product from the market for these low risk populations. The studies that suggested an increased risk of HIV transmission associated with frequent use of N-9 tested the use of stand-alone spermicides by women, not the use of condoms with N-9 in the lubricant. Given that condoms themselves are an effective barrier to transmission of HIV, and that N-9 does not compromise these barrier properties, it is not clear how those study findings relate to condoms with N-9. However, the Agency is currently reviewing labeling of condoms with N-9 to make sure that information regarding appropriate use of this product is properly presented to the consumer in light of new information about the potential risks of N-9.

Question 6: FDA requires products to undergo clinical trials to demonstrate safety and effectiveness before they are marketed for their stated purpose(s). In the FDA testimony delivered to the Subcommittee, it is stated that "our current guidance recommends that the package insert for condoms contain the following statement: If used properly, latex condoms will help to reduce the risk of transmission of HIV infection (AIDS) and many other sexually transmitted diseases, including chlamydia infections, genital herpes, genital warts, gonorrhea, hepatitis B, and syphilis." The FDA testimony further states, "scientific studies on STDs characterized by genital ulcers, e.g., genital herpes and syphilis, are inconclusive as to whether the risks of these diseases is lowered for condom users." In 2001, a report entitled "Scientific Evidence on Condom Effectiveness for Sexually Transmitted Disease (STD) Prevention" prepared by the FDA with the National Institute of Allergy and Infectious Diseases of the National Institutes of Health, the Centers for Disease Control and Prevention and the U.S. Agency for International Development evaluated the published data on latex condoms and STD prevention. In the report, the panel "concluded that there was no evidence that condom use reduced the risk of HPV infection" and "The Panel agreed that the published epidemiologic data were insufficient to draw meaningful conclusions about the effectiveness of the latex male condom to reduce the risk of transmission of genital ulcer diseases (genital herpes, syphilis and chancroid)." In fact the, panel found that there was only sufficient data to demonstrate that condom use could reduce "HIV transmission in both men and women who engage in vaginal intercourse"

and "indicated that the latex male condom could reduce the risk of gonorrhea for men."

There seems to be some confusion about the overall possible effectiveness of condoms for preventing STDs. (a) When did condoms undergo FDA approved clinical trials to determine effectiveness in preventing the transmission of STDs? (b) Did clinical trials of condoms specifically examine the effectiveness of condoms against HPV or cervical cancer?

Response: Latex condoms were devices marketed prior to May 28, 1976, the enactment date of the Medical Device Amendments. Like all other pre-amendments devices, condoms were classified under the Federal Food, Drug, and Cosmetic Act after consideration by an expert panel of the information available at that time about their safety and effectiveness.

In the specific case of condoms, the panel's recommendations were based not on clinical trials but on the extensive experience with, and widespread use of, condoms for many years, through which the device's safety and effectiveness were considered to be well documented. Based on the panel's recommendations and after consideration of public comment, by a regulation finalized in 1980, FDA classified condoms used for both contraceptive and prophylactic purposes (defined by the regulation as "preventing transmission of venereal diseases") into Class II. 21 C.F.R. 884.5300. (Condoms containing N-9 in the lubricant were also placed in Class II, in 1982, under 21 C.F.R. 884.5310.)

Because condoms are class II devices, manufacturers seeking to introduce new condoms to the market use the 510(k) premarket notification pathway. In such submissions to the agency, manufacturers must demonstrate that the new condom is substantially equivalent to a legally marketed predicate device -- a condom already on the market. Usually, a sponsor's demonstration of substantial equivalence does not require new clinical studies.

In the years since their initial classification, FDA has followed the development of new information related to the safety and effectiveness of condoms. As mentioned in our testimony, FDA has introduced several labeling changes, including regulations regarding expiration dating and latex allergy warnings and guidance documents addressing other aspects of labeling, including STD prevention. These changes reflect our ongoing monitoring of the safety and effectiveness of condoms for their dual purpose of contraception and protection against STDs.

As you know, FDA participated in the 2000 interagency workshop on condom effectiveness against STDs as well as a more comprehensive review of the literature. We reviewed the Condom Fact Sheet and STD Fact Sheets currently available on PHS websites. In our ongoing implementation of PL 106-554, we are also considering the new CDC Report to Congress on Genital HPV Infection, as well as other clinical considerations. The CDC report highlights many of the important clinical studies of the association of condom use and the clinical course of HPV infection and clinical sequelae. As you heard during testimony at the March 11th hearing, we believe – and CDC concurs – that condom use provides a risk reduction for the clinical sequelae of HPV, including genital warts and cervical cancer. As stated in the Agency testimony, we are reexamining condom labeling under PL 106-554 and propose any changes needed to ensure that such labeling neither overstates nor understates expected STD risk reduction.

NIH QUESTIONS

Question 1: Since April 1996, what is the total amount NIH has spent on research and other efforts to defelop effective (a.) HPV or cervical cancer vaccines; (b) microbicides; and (c) behavioral change interventions that delay the onset of sexual activity?

Response: The NIH continues to support research efforts in the areas of HPV/cervical cancer vaccines, microbicides, and behavioral change interventions that delay the onset of sexual activity, and in FY 2001 to FY 2003 the NIH supported the following:

(a) HPV/cervical cancer vaccines (NIH Totals)

FY 2001 Actual $12.4M
FY 2002 Actual $9.8M
FY 2003 Actual $14.9M

HPV and Cervical Cancer Vaccines (NCI Only)

FY 1996 - $ 2,391,818
FY 1997 - $ 3,757,143
FY 1998 - $ 7,413,227
FY 1999 - $ 8,028,804
FY 2000 - $10,153,834
FY 2001 - $14,077,133
FY 2002 - $ 9,851,591
FY 2003 - $18,755,467

Total Research Funding for HPV Research (in millions) (NCI Only)

FY 1996 - $27.3
FY 1997 - $34.1
FY 1998 - $34.2
FY 1999 - $37.8
FY 2000 - $39.7
FY 2001 - $46.3

FY 2002 - $44.3
FY 2003 - $56.4

Total Research Funding for Cervical Cancer Research (in millions) (NCI Only)

FY 1996 - $51.6
FY 1997 - $55.8
FY 1998 - $55.2
FY 1999 - $66.3
FY 2000 - $67.0
FY 2001 - $72.6
FY 2002 - $67.6
FY 2003 - $79.0

(b) microbicides

Topical Mircrobicides (NIH Totals)
FY 2001 Actual $47.0M
FY 2002 Actual $55.8M
FY 2003 Actual $57.9M

***Note: None for NCI**

(c) behavioral interventions

Behavioral change interventions that delay the onset of sexual activity (NIH Totals)

FY 2001 Actual $12.4M
FY 2002 Actual $14.5M
FY 2003 Actual $17.3M

***Note: None for NCI**

Question 2: There are at least 18 strands of HPV that can cause cancer according to data published in the February 6, 2003 issue of The New England Journal of Medicine.

(a) Of the HPV vaccine candidates currently undergoing trials, do any protect against all high risk strains of HPV infection?

Response: The current vaccines being tested protect against two types of HPV that are oncogenic: type 16, which accounts for 50 percent of all cervical cancers worldwide, and type 18, which accounts for an additional 10-20 percent.

(b) If a vaccine does not protect against all high risk strands of HPV, is it then possible for a woman to become infected with a strain of HPV to which the vaccine does not provide immunity and thereby still develop cervical cancer?

Response: Because current vaccines will protect against between 60-70 percent of cervical cancers, it is possible that a vaccinated women could get cervical cancer from one of the other oncogenic types of HPV. In the future, there may be vaccines developed to protect against these additional types. Therefore, it is important that a woman continue to be screened for cervical cancer, even if she has been vaccinated.

Question 3: A study published last year in the Journal of the National Cancer Institute found that an HPV vaccine now in development may not effectively protect women against infection during ovulation. What impact would this shortcoming potentially have on the overall effectiveness of HPV vaccination?

Response: We know that in the short-term (one to two years) the vaccine's effectiveness is near 100 percent against persistent HPV and is not affected by a woman's cyclical hormone changes. The ongoing trials are designed to help answer the remaining question as to whether cyclical fluctuations affect duration of the vaccine's protection, and if booster vaccinations will be needed.

Question 4: Would an HPV vaccine provide effective protection against persistent infection for someone who may already have been exposed to HPV?

Response: There are no human data to suggest that a vaccine can treat an existing infection. Animal studies suggest that it cannot, and this is another question being addressed in the current NCI vaccine trial.

Question 5: HPV has been detected in some prostate tumors. Is there sufficient evidence to suggest that HPV infection may be associated with the development of prostate cancer?

Response: HPV is such a potent carcinogenic agent in the anogenital region that it has been suggested as a potential factor in the development of cancer in many tissues, including the prostate. Despite its proven association with virtually all cervical cancer and fractions of vaginal, vulvar, penile, and anal cancer, there is to date no persuasive evidence of HPV's role in prostate cancer. In addition, false positive detection of HPV DNA has been a historical problem, which might account for some early reports of an association of HPV with neoplasia of the prostate, colon, ovary, and bladder.

Question 6: HPV is associated with a number of cancers. What other viruses are associated with the development of cancer?

Response: HPV is associated with cervical cancer, anogenital cancers, and possibly oral and esophageal cancers. Epstein-Barr Virus (EBV) is associated with nasopharangeal carcinoma, Burkitt's lymphoma, and possibly other lymphomas. Hepatitis B and Hepatitis C Virus are associated with liver cancer. Human Herpes Virus 8 (HHV-8; also known as KSHV, or Kaposi's sarcoma-associated herpesvirus) is associated with Kaposi's Sarcoma. HTLV-I (human T-lymphotropic virus type I) is associated with adult T-cell leukemia (ATL). In an indirect manner, Human Immunedeficiency Virus (HIV) suppresses the immune system and provides a permissive environment for cancers to develop.

2. Congressional Correspondence with Federal Agencies Regarding HPV

Congressional Correspondence with Federal Agencies Regarding HPV

Date	Addressee and Agency	Content	Author(s)	Date of Response
October 29, 1999	Dr. Richard Klausner, NCI	Request for a conference to develop consensus statement on condom effectiveness	Representative Coburn	November 16, 1999 from Dr. Klausner, NCI
March 30, 2001	Dr. Anthony Fauci, NIAID	Request for consensus statement on condom effectiveness	Chairman Souder with Rep. Weldon	April 17, 2001 from Marc Smolonsky, NIH OD
March 30, 2001	Dr. Judith Wasserheit, CDC	Requests an update on the status of the enactment of P.L. 106-554	Chairman Souder with Reps. Weldon, Myrick and Pitts	May 9, 2001 from Dr. Jeffrey Koplan, CDC
May 24, 2001	Dr. Jeffrey Koplan, CDC	Response to May 9, 2001 letter requesting an update on the status of P.L. 106-554	Chairman Souder with Rep. Weldon	No response
March 5, 2002	Dr. Jeffrey Koplan, CDC	Requests an update on the status of the enactment of P.L. 106-554	Chairman Souder with Reps. Weldon, C. Smith and Pitts	May 17, 2002 from Dr. David Fleming, CDC
November 19, 2003	Dr. Julie Gerberding, CDC	Expresses disappointment with enactment of P.L. 106-554	Chairman Souder	December 18, 2003 from Dr. Julie Gerberding, CDC
September 7, 2000	Dr. Jane Henney, FDA	Requests a review of condom labeling regarding HPV	Representative Coburn	October 20, 2000 from Ms. Melinda Plaisier, FDA

August 23, 2001	Dr. Bernard Schwetz, FDA	Requests an update on the status of condom relabeling required by P.L. 106-554	Chairman Souder	November 20, 2001 from Ms. Melinda Plaisier, FDA
February 12, 2004	Dr. Mark McClellan, FDA	Requests an update on the status of condom relabeling required by P.L. 106-554	Chairman Souder	March 10, 2004 from Mr. Amit Sachdev, FDA
August 19, 2003	Ms. Dana Corrigan, HHS OIG	Requests a review to determine if federal agencies are complying with P.L. 106-554	Chairman Souder (with original request from former Rep. Coburn)	September 29, 2003 from Ms. Dana Corrigan, OIG
July 18, 2001	Secretary Thompson, HHS	Expresses dissatisfaction with enactment of P.L. 106-554 by CDC and FDA	Former Rep. Coburn	No response
May 15, 2002	Secretary Thompson, HHS	Expresses dissatisfaction with enactment of P.L. 106-554 by CDC and FDA; requests update on status of law	Chairman Tauzin with Rep. Pitts	September 10, 2003 from Secretary Thompson, HHS
November 21, 2003	Ambassador Tobias, State Department	Outlines intentions of HPV provision of P.L. 108-025	Rep. J. Davis	No response to date
March 4, 2004	Ambassador Tobias, State Department	Requests correction of erroneous HPV statements in President's Global AIDS Plan	Chairman Souder	No response to date

TOM A. COBURN, M.D
2D DISTRICT, OKLAHOMA

COMMITTEE ON COMMERCE
SUBCOMMITTEES:
HEALTH AND ENVIRONMENT
ENERGY AND POWER

Congress of the United States
House of Representatives
Washington, DC 20515–3602

215 STATE STREET, SUITE 815
MUSKOGEE, OK 74401
(918) 687-2533
(918) 682-8503 (FAX)

120 S. MISSOURI, ROOM 105
CLAREMORE, OK 74017
(918) 341-9336
(918) 341-9437 (FAX)

34 "A" STREET N.E., ROOM 202
MIAMI, OK 74354
(918) 542-5337
(918) 542-5367 (FAX)

RECEIVED
1999 NOV -2 P 2: 48
NIH EXECUTIVE SECRETARIAT

October 29, 1999

The Honorable Richard D. Klausner, M.D.
Director
National Cancer Institute
National Institutes of Health
9000 Rockville Pike
Bethesda, MD 20892

Dear Dr. Klausner,

Thank you for arranging the October 25th meeting between representatives of the NCI, NIH and FDA with Dr. Tom Fitch to formulate a consensus statement regarding the scientific data relating to the ineffectiveness of condoms in preventing the transmission of the human papillomavirus (HPV). I appreciate your responsiveness to my request in such a timely manner.

I was disappointed that some of the participants in this meeting had not read several of the major studies regarding the ineffectiveness of condoms in preventing HPV transmission. On short notice, Dr. Fitch pulled himself away from his practice in San Antonio, Texas, and made himself available to develop a consensus statement based upon all of the available data. Without a full review of all of the relevant studies by all of the participants, it was impossible to develop a consensus that reflected the available scientific findings.

I would suggest that since the group failed to reach a consensus, we schedule another meeting in the near future comprised of an expert panel that has had the opportunity to review all of the relevant data. I would once again request that Dr. Fitch be included along with several other experts with whom I have consulted on this issue.

Please do not hesitate to contact me or Roland Foster of my staff to discuss the arrangement and composition of this panel at your convenience. I can be reached at (202) 225-2701.

Thank you again for your assistance.

Sincerely,

Tom

Tom A. Coburn, M.D.
Member of Congress

173930

429 CANNON HOUSE OFFICE BUILDING
WASHINGTON, DC 20515
(202) 225-2701 Fax: (202) 225-3038

PRINTED ON RECYCLED PAPER

E-mail: rep.coburn@mail.house.gov
Web site: www.house.gov/coburn

DEPARTMENT OF HEALTH & HUMAN SERVICES

Public Health Service

National Institutes of Health
National Cancer Institute
Bethesda, Maryland 20892

NOV 16 1999

The Honorable Tom Coburn
House of Representatives
Washington, DC 20515

Dear Dr. Coburn:

I am pleased to respond to your letter of October 29 regarding our efforts to determine the effectiveness of condoms in preventing infection with human papillomavirus (HPV). We very much appreciate the willingness of Dr. Tom Fitch to participate, on short notice, in a meeting with staff from the National Cancer Institute, the National Institute of Allergy and Infectious Diseases (NIAID), and the Food and Drug Administration to begin to address this question. In what may have been a pure stroke of luck, Dr. Fitch told me that the cancellation of a previous commitment meant that he was able to travel to Bethesda with minimal disruption to his patient care responsibilities.

Dr. Penny Hitchcock presented the goals of the meeting at its outset: 1) reach common ground on HPV infection and condoms as independent issues; 2) reach agreement on what criteria should be used to identify papers for review; 3) finalize the list of papers; and 4) reach agreement on a timeline. From your letter, it appears as though there may have been a misunderstanding as to the expectation about reaching consensus at the meeting itself. Certainly, we would all agree that this is an important public health issue that warrants careful consideration. Our initial meeting was the first step in this process, and I agree that another meeting with broad representation would be appropriate.

Based on our telephone conversation, I am pleased that we both agree on the need for more communication on the nature, extent, and definitiveness of the evidence currently available to us regarding the efficacy of condoms. Concerning HPV infection, and HPV associated diseases, none of us feel that the literature leads to clear conclusions that condom use strongly protects against HPV infection. On the other hand, the quality of the data and studies available to us do not, to everyone's satisfaction, rule out some level of protection.

Clearly, the available data do not lend themselves to a straightforward, simple answer. Among the participants at the meeting of October 25, there were different interpretations of the data, with some concluding that the studies to date provide sufficient information, while others found the studies to be lacking in design, methodology, or clarity with respect to the question at hand. Such differences of opinion are not unusual in the research community, and this is one of the challenges we face in trying to draw conclusions from disparate published data.

Page 2 - The Honorable Tom Coburn

Given these complexities, I have spoken with Dr. Fauci, Director of NIAID, about moving forward with a larger, more inclusive meeting. He has agreed that Dr. Hitchcock would be the appropriate individual to lead this effort. We envision broad representation from other Federal agencies, the inclusion of health professionals such as Dr. Fitch and his colleagues, and others, including behavioral researchers. This meeting would also focus more broadly on all sexually transmitted diseases rather than limiting its focus on HPV transmission. We appreciate your confidence in the National Institutes of Health to lead this effort.

Sincerely,

Richard D. Klausner, M.D.
Director
National Cancer Institute

ONE HUNDRED SEVENTH CONGRESS

Congress of the United States

House of Representatives

COMMITTEE ON GOVERNMENT REFORM

2157 RAYBURN HOUSE OFFICE BUILDING
WASHINGTON, DC 20515–6143

FACSIMILE (202) 225–3974
MAJORITY (202) 225–5074
MINORITY (202) 225–5051
TTY (202) 225–6852

www.house.gov/reform

March 30, 2001

Anthony S. Fauci, M.D.
Director
National Institute of Allergy and Infectious Diseases
National Institutes of Health
Building 31, Room 7A-03C
Bethesda, MD 20892-2520

Dear Dr. Fauci,

As you know, nearly 13,800 new cases of invasive cervical cancer were diagnosed last year and this year alone about 4,600 women will die from the disease. Tens of thousands of other women will be diagnosed and treated for pre-cancerous conditions which researchers believe are about 4 times more common than invasive cervical cancer. Virtually all cervical cancer is linked to the human papillomavirus (HPV). With at least 24 million Americans carrying the virus and 5.5 million new infections occurring each year, HPV is the most common sexually transmitted disease.

Dr. Richard D. Klausner, Director of the National Cancer Institute (NCI) at the National Institutes of Health (NIH) stated in a in a February 19, 1999 letter to then-Commerce Committee Chairman Tom Bliley that "condoms are ineffective against HPV" and that "additional research efforts by NCI on the effectiveness of condoms in preventing HPV transmission are not warranted." This statement echoes the conclusions of both the NIH and the American Cancer Society. According to the NIH Consensus Development Conference Statement on Cervical Cancer from April 1- 3, 1996, "the data on the use of barrier methods of contraceptives to prevent the spread of HPV… does not support this as an effective method of prevention." The American Cancer Society found "research shows that condoms cannot protect against infection with HPV."

Public Law 106-554 mandates that the Centers for Disease Control (CDC) and its grantees and contractors begin stating "medically accurate information regarding the effectiveness or lack of effectiveness of condoms in preventing" HPV infection. Last June, while Congress was debating this extremely important public health measure designed to protect women's health, the Sexually Transmitted Diseases office of NIAID's Division of Microbiology and Infectious Diseases convened a meeting entitled "Scientific

Evidence on Condom Effectiveness and STD Prevention" with the intent of preparing a paper on this topic based upon the available science. Nearly ten months later, this document has still not been released.

Recently the Physicians Consortium filed a Freedom of Information Act (FOIA) request with NIAID to obtain documents associated with the development of this paper. We are writing to request all of the documents that the Physicians Consortium requested in its FOIA. We understand that NIAID has set a deadline to complete the paper within the next two weeks. We would, therefore, also request a final copy of the paper along with all of the scientific studies that were reviewed to reach the conclusions contained therein.

Thank you for your prompt attention to this matter.

Sincerely,

Mark E. Souder
Chairman
Subcommittee on Criminal Justice,
Drug Policy and Human Resources
Committee on Government Reform

Dave Weldon, M.D.
Member of Congress

Enclosure: Physicians Consortium FOIA letter

CC: The Honorable Tommy G. Thompson
Secretary
Department of Health and Human Services

The Physicians Consortium

Harrisburg office: 1240 North Mountain Road,
Harrisburg PA, 17112 (612) 827-9552

Mr. Paul Marshall
FOIA Coordinator
Office of Policy Analysis
NIAID
Building 31, Room 7A-52
31 Center Drive MSC 2520
Bethesda, MD 20892-2520

March 27, 2001

Dear Mr. Marshall:

RE: FOIA REQUEST

This FOIA is divided into two parts: A FOIA request for certain documents with an immediate effective date and a FOIA request for additional documents with an effective date of Wednesday, April 4, 2001.

On June 12th and 13th, 2000, a meeting titled "Scientific Evidence on Condom Effectiveness and STD Prevention" was held at the Hyatt Dulles in Herndon, Virginia. Penny Hitchcock, former Chief of the STD branch of NIAID, was responsible until recently for coordinating the preparation of a paper yet to be released.

Under FOIA, the Physicians Consortium requests the following

FOIA with an immediate effective date:

1. The initial draft version prepared after the June meeting and the draft version released to the external review panel on or about March 15, 2001. Please e-mail these documents to diggsthis@aol.com and hwallismd@worldnet.att.net. If the initial draft is not in a format that can be e-mailed, then fax it to (719) 548-5941.

FOIA with an effective date of April 4, 2001:

The Physicians Consortium wishes to be sensitive to the ongoing efforts to finalize the paper. Therefore, the effective date for the additional documents requested under this FOIA is April 4, 2001. While expediency in receiving documents under this FOIA is important to us, much more important is that the final paper be medically accurate, scientifically complete and sound and void of a bias intended to support existing public health doctrines.

The documents to be included under the second part of this FOIA are:

2. Any and all draft versions of the report as it has evolved, excluding the specific draft versions covered in point 1 (above), but including any draft versions developed after the version released to the external review panel on or about March 15, 2001.
3. The audio transcript of the June 12th and 13th meeting.
4. Any and all documents (including, but not limited to, memoranda, scientific papers, reports and others) distributed to participants at the June 12th and 13th meeting. This would include documents that originated from NIAID and other federal agencies as well as documents that originated from outside participants to the meeting.
5. Any and all comments, either by mail, e-mail, facsimile, or in any other form, relating to the preparation of the report and to each draft version. This should include correspondence within NIAID and to/from NIH, FDA, CDC, U.S. Agency for International Development, other federal agencies not listed, and all non-governmental individuals and organizations.
6. Any and all internal documents and memoranda relating to Penny Hitchcock's involvement with the project, the delay of the paper, and the decision whereby Dr. Hitchcock was removed or removed herself from the project. This request should include any and all memoranda from NIH or affiliated agencies to Dr. Hitchcock and from Dr. Hitchcock to HIH or affiliated agencies relating to the preparation, content or delay of the paper. Included in this request would be any correspondence related to the paper sent by Dr. Hitchcock to NIH and affiliated agencies in the month prior to her disassociation with the project and since.

All documents on file or produced before April 4, the effective date of this FOIA, should be subject to this FOIA.

The Physicians Consortium, in addition to representing approximately 2,000 physicians providing medical services to tens of thousands of patients, is a not-for-profit public interest group which intends to disseminate the requested information to members of Congress, appropriate news media, and the American public at large. Thus, the Physicians Consortium requests a fee waver of all applicable search charges related to this FOIA request, pursuant to 5USC§552(a)(4)(A)(iii); Larson v. Central Intelligence Agency, 843 F.2d 1482 (D.C. Cir. 1988); Judicial Watch Inc. v. United States Department of Commerce, No. 95-0133 (D.D.C. May 16, 1995). Disclosure of this information is in the public interest because it is likely to contribute significantly to the public understanding of the activities of NIAID and NIH.

We understand that certain copying charges may be charged for this request. Please notify us if such charges reach $200.

If you have any questions regarding this FOIA request, please do not hesitate to call us.

Sincerely,

Hal Wallis, M.D

Cc: Secretary Tommy Thompson, Department of Health and Human Services
Rep. Dan Burton, Chairman, House Committee on Government Reform
Rep. Mark Souder, Chairman Criminal Justice, Drug Policy and Human Resources Subcommittee, House Committee on Government Reform
Marc Wheat, House Committee on Commerce
Rep. Ernest Istook, Jr.

ONE HUNDRED SEVENTH CONGRESS

Congress of the United States

House of Representatives

COMMITTEE ON GOVERNMENT REFORM

2157 RAYBURN HOUSE OFFICE BUILDING

WASHINGTON, DC 20515–6143

FACSIMILE (202) 225–3974
MAJORITY (202) 225–5074
MINORITY (202) 225–5051
TTY (202) 225–6852

www.house.gov/reform

March 30, 2001

Judith N. Wasserheit. M.D., M.P.H.
Director
Sexually Transmitted Diseases Prevention Division
National Center for HIV, Sexually Transmitted Diseases and Tuberculosis Prevention
Centers for Disease Control and Prevention
1600 Clifton Road, N.E.
Atlanta, GA 30333

Dear Dr. Wasserheit,

As you know, nearly 13,800 new cases of invasive cervical cancer were diagnosed last year and this year alone about 4,600 women will die from the disease. Tens of thousands of other women will be diagnosed and treated for pre-cancerous conditions which researchers believe are about 4 times more common than invasive cervical cancer. Virtually all cervical cancer is linked to the human papillomavirus (HPV). With at least 24 million Americans carrying the virus and 5.5 million new infections occurring each year, HPV is the most common sexually transmitted disease.

Over the past two years, Congress has made cervical cancer treatment and prevention a priority. The Breast and Cervical Cancer Treatment Act (P.L. 106-354) was approved and signed into law October 2000, will provide medical assistance for breast and cervical cancer-related treatment services to low-income women who have already been screened for cancer under CDC's early detection program. Likewise, in December Congress passed and the President signed legislation to address the prevention of HPV infection (P.L.106-554). Both of these laws were approved overwhelmingly and are extremely important steps towards eliminating cervical cancer and saving women's lives.

Despite its prevalence, very few Americans are aware of HPV. Only one in five American women are aware of the link between cervical cancer and HPV according to a 2000 survey conducted by the National Cervical Cancer Public Education Campaign. According to a report in the November 2000 journal Obstetrics and Gynecology, an astounding 87 percent of high school students have not heard of HPV.

Obviously if we are to prevent HPV infection and the invasive and non-invasive conditions it can cause, more must be done to raise the public's awareness about the virus and the medically accurate facts regarding its transmission and possible consequences. The HPV prevention provisions of P.L. 106-554 lay the groundwork to meet these goals.

This law specifically requires the CDC to:

- Determine the prevalence of HPV in the United States;
- Develop and distribute educational materials to the public and health care professionals regarding HPV prevention, modes of transmission, the link between HPV and cervical cancer and the lack of effectiveness of condoms in preventing HPV and the importance of regular Pap smears;
- Ensure that all educational and prevention materials prepared for the public by the federal government and its grantees regarding HPV and other sexually transmitted diseases contain medically accurate information regarding the effectiveness or lack of effectiveness of condoms in preventing HPV infection.

As you know, a progress report must be made to the Congress by the end of this year, however because of this law's importance to protecting women's health, we are very interested in knowing what actions the CDC-- and particularly your division-- has taken over the past 4 months to enact these requirements. Furthermore, with the development of new testing technologies to identify infection with particular strains of HPV, what action is the CDC considering in making diagnosis with HPV-16 or other high risk strains a reportable condition. Such surveillance data is extremely important to public health authorities and to us as policy makers.

Thank you for your prompt attention to this inquiry. We look forward to a timely written response and working with you to ensure that this law is promptly and properly enacted to protect the health and lives of women.

Sincerely,

Mark E. Souder
Chairman
Subcommittee on Criminal Justice,
Drug Policy and Human Resources
Committee on Government Reform

Dave Weldon, M.D.
Member of Congress

Sue Myrick
Member of Congress

Joseph Pitts
Member of Congress

CC: Honorable Tommy G. Thompson
Secretary
Department of Health and Human Services

DEPARTMENT OF HEALTH & HUMAN SERVICES

Public Health Service

Centers for Disease Control
and Prevention (CDC)
Atlanta GA 30333

MAY 9 2001

The Honorable Mark E. Souder
United States House of Representatives
Washington, D.C. 20515-6143

Dear Mr. Souder:

I am responding to your letter to Dr. Judith N. Wasserheit, Director, Division of STD Prevention, concerning the Centers for Disease Control and Prevention's (CDC) progress toward the prevention and treatment of human papillomavirus (HPV)16, and making HPV 16 and other high-risk HPV types reportable.

As you know, the provisions of P.L. 106-554 authorize surveillance and educational activities critical to understanding the epidemiology and impact of HPV, as well as better informing healthcare providers, public health professionals, and the public about HPV prevention. Below is a summary of activities CDC is undertaking to address the HPV provision of P.L. 106-554.

- Continuation of a longitudinal study of the incidence of HPV infection in adolescent females, aged 12-19 years, in Atlanta, Georgia. Results of this study may contribute important information on the determinants of progression from HPV infection to development of precancerous cells.
- Performance of additional HPV prevalence and epidemiology surveillance in nationally representative samples using CDC's National Health and Nutrition Examination Survey. This project will provide specific information on HPV 16.
- Establishment of six to eight sentinel surveillance sites to monitor the prevalence of high-risk HPV types in women.
- Implementation of formative research and a patient survey to develop and pilot health messages for HPV patients and their partners.
- Performance of a provider survey of knowledge, attitudes, and practices regarding HPV diagnoses and treatment. This survey will assess perceptions, practices, barriers, and facilitators regarding HPV risk assessment, testing, treatment, counseling, and partner services.

Page 2 - The Honorable Mark E. Souder

With respect to making infection with high-risk HPV types a reportable condition, each state determines which conditions or diseases are reportable within their state. In this regard, in April 1999, CDC, in collaboration with the American Cancer Society, convened a panel of internationally recognized experts to provide recommendations for HPV prevention activities and research in the United States. This expert panel specifically recommended against establishing routine reporting for genital HPV infection at this time. The panel indicated that such action would be premature due to critical gaps in knowledge about HPV epidemiology, lack of widespread availability and experience with HPV tests, current inability to distinguish the more than 90 percent of HPV-infected women who will eliminate the infection without problems from the small minority who will develop precancerous cervical changes, and the absence of effective therapy. CDC will continue to work closely with states and other partners to expand the knowledge base and best practices for HPV prevention. A copy of the panel's report is enclosed.

We appreciate your commitment to the prevention and treatment of cervical cancer and look forward to furthering HPV prevention and control in the United States. A copy of this letter is being sent to The Honorable Sue Myrick, The Honorable Dave Weldon, M.D., and The Honorable Joseph Pitts who cosigned your letter.

Sincerely,

Jeffrey P. Koplan

Jeffrey P. Koplan, M.D., M.P.H.
Director

Enclosure

ONE HUNDRED SEVENTH CONGRESS

Congress of the United States

House of Representatives

COMMITTEE ON GOVERNMENT REFORM

2157 RAYBURN HOUSE OFFICE BUILDING

WASHINGTON, DC 20515–6143

FACSIMILE (202) 225–3974
MAJORITY (202) 225–5074
MINORITY (202) 225–5051
TTY (202) 225–6852

www.house.gov/reform

May 24, 2001

Jeffrey P. Koplan, M.D., M.P.H.
Director,
Centers for Disease Control and Prevention
1600 Clifton Rd.
Atlanta, GA 30333

Dear Dr. Koplan,

Thank you for your May 9 letter responding to our correspondence of March 30 addressed to Dr. Judith Wasserheit regarding the Human Papillomavirus Education and Prevention provisions contained within Public Law 106-554.

We were very disappointed with your response. In our initial inquiry, we specifically asked what actions the CDC has taken over the past four-- now five-- months to enact the requirements of this law. Instead of an update of actions taken, we were provided an incomplete summarization of certain requirements of the law.

We would ask again (1) What actions has the CDC taken since December to implement this vitally important law that protects women's health? Please include with your response any and all internal memos or other documents pertaining to this law.

Noticeably absent in your summary of the law is a provision that requires the CDC, other federal agencies and all contractors, grantees and subgrantees of the Department of Health and Human Services to "contain medically accurate information regarding the effectiveness or lack of effectiveness of condoms in preventing" HPV and other STDs. Specifically the law states:

`(c) HPV Education and Prevention-

`(1) IN GENERAL- The Secretary shall prepare and distribute educational materials for health care providers and the public that include information on HPV. Such materials shall address--

`(A) modes of transmission;

`(B) consequences of infection, including the link between HPV and cervical cancer;

`(C) the available scientific evidence on the effectiveness or lack of effectiveness of condoms in preventing infection with HPV; and

`(D) the importance of regular Pap smears, and other diagnostics for early intervention and prevention of cervical cancer purposes in preventing cervical cancer.

`(2) MEDICALLY ACCURATE INFORMATION- Educational material under paragraph (1), and all other relevant educational and prevention materials prepared and printed from this date forward for the public and health care providers by the Secretary (including materials prepared through the Food and Drug Administration, the Centers for Disease Control and Prevention, and the Health Resources and Services Administration), or by contractors, grantees, or subgrantees thereof, that are specifically designed to address STDs including HPV shall contain medically accurate information regarding the effectiveness or lack of effectiveness of condoms in preventing the STD the materials are designed to address."

This law took effect December 21, 2000 and states very clearly that all educational and prevention materials printed from that date forward by the CDC and others must contain medically accurate information regarding the effectiveness or lack of effectiveness of condoms against STDs. Yet a CDC Fact Sheet entitled "Condoms and Their Use in Preventing HIV and Other STDs" updated on January 31, 2001 reads:

"The correct and consistent use of latex condoms during sexual intercourse- vaginal, anal, or oral-can greatly reduce a person' s risk of acquiring or transmitting most STDs, including HIV infection, gonorrhea, chlamydia, trichomonas, human papilloma virus infection (HPV), and hepatitis B."

As you know, this statement is <u>not</u> "medically accurate," as specifically required by federal law.

Dr. Richard D. Klausner, Director of the National Cancer Institute has told Congress that "condoms are ineffective against HPV." Like wise, a 1996 National Institutes of Health Consensus Development Conference Statement on Cervical Cancer found that the scientific data on the use of barrier methods of contraception such as condoms "does not support this as an effective method of prevention" of HPV. The American Cancer Society concurs, stating "research shows that condoms cannot protect against infection with HPV." And a draft of a soon-to-be released paper on condom effectiveness, prepared by the National Institute of Allergy and Infectious Disease with CDC participation, concludes "that there was no evidence that condom use reduced the risk of HPV infection."

Yet these conclusions determined from published scientific data are not reflected in the statement printed in the CDC Fact Sheet. We are gravely concerned by both the failure to comply with the statute and the potential impact of providing scientifically inaccurate information which may endanger the health-- and in some cases, the lives-- of women.

(2) Please provide an explanation of why this provision of the law and these scientific facts were overlooked.

We would also like to know (3) what is the CDC doing to inform its contractors, grantees and subgrantees about the ineffectiveness of condoms in preventing HPV infection and the legal requirement to provide such medically accurate information? (4) What penalties are typically levied against organizations that receive federal funds and do not comply with federal legal requirements? Would such organizations be required to return federal funds or possibly be prohibited from receiving federal funds in the future? (5) Please also provide a complete listing, including addresses, of all CDC contractors, grantees and subgrantees receiving any federal funds for HIV/STD education and prevention.

Finally, a recent report in the "STD Advisor" stated that a CDC advisory committee plans to reinforce condom messages in an upcoming "MMWR Report and Recommendations" publication. (4) Could you please explain the intent of the CDC in releasing this report at this time? (5) Will this report reflect the conclusions of the NIAID, NCI and the published scientific data regarding the lack of effectiveness of condoms in preventing HPV infection as legally required?

Thank you for your prompt attention to this inquiry. We look forward to working with you to ensure that this law is properly enacted to protect the health and lives of women.

Sincerely,

Mark E. Souder
Chairman
Subcommittee on Criminal Justice,
Drug Policy and Human Resources

Dave Weldon, M.D.
Member of Congress

CC: Honorable Tommy Thompson
Secretary
Department of Health and Human Services

ONE HUNDRED SEVENTH CONGRESS

Congress of the United States

House of Representatives

COMMITTEE ON GOVERNMENT REFORM

2157 RAYBURN HOUSE OFFICE BUILDING
WASHINGTON, DC 20515-6143

MAJORITY (202) 225-5074
FACSIMILE (202) 225-3974
MINORITY (202) 225-5051
TTY (202) 225-6852

www.house.gov/reform

March 5, 2002

Dr. Jeffrey P. Koplan, MD MPH
Director
Centers for Disease Control and Prevention
1600 Clifton Road
Atlanta, GA 30333

Dear Dr. Koplan,

The Centers for Disease Control and Prevention (CDC) and the Association of Schools of Public Health recently provided a $940,000 grant to Planned Parenthood of Southwest and Central Florida and the University of South Florida to conduct a study to determine how people react when they are diagnosed with human papillomavirus (HPV) infection. The data from this research is intended to develop an educational message to prevent HPV infection and cervical cancer.

This study was required by Public Law 106-554. Specifically the law states:

"(1) IN GENERAL. The Secretary, acting through the Centers for Disease Control and Prevention, shall conduct prevention research on HPV, including—

"(A) behavioral and other research on the impact of HPV-related diagnosis on individuals;

"(B) formative research to assist with the development of educational messages and information for the public, for patients, and for their partners about HPV;

"(C) surveys of physician and public knowledge, attitudes, and practices about genital HPV infection; and

"(D) upon the completion of and based on the findings under subparagraphs (A) through (C), develop and disseminate educational materials for the public and health care providers regarding HPV and its impact and prevention."

Because the results of this study will impact the educational materials that will be developed and disseminated to the public regarding HPV infection and cervical cancer, it is essential that the research and the data obtained be scientifically pure and not skewed by political motivations. In this regard, we find it baffling that a Planned Parenthood affiliate would be chosen to conduct this study. As you know, Planned Parenthood aggressively opposed the law requiring this HPV study and has for some time promoted a political agenda that has misled the public about the lack of condom effectiveness in preventing HPV infection. Clearly, a far more objective organization could have been selected to conduct this study.

Could you please provide the Planned Parenthood of Southwest and Central Florida and the University of South Florida proposal that was submitted for this study along with answers to the following questions:

(1) Is the CDC sponsoring any organizations or researchers other than Planned Parenthood affiliates to conduct research on this topic?
(2) As you know, the Planned Parenthood study will include only the agency's own clients and therefore will not represent a broad cross-section of women. It is fair to assume that Planned Parenthood clients are likely to have different attitudes and values than women who seek health services from family doctors or health care providers that do not promote or perform abortions. If only Planned Parenthood clients are being interviewed for this research, the opinions of the vast majority of American women will be omitted from consideration and analysis and the research will be unfairly and unscientifically skewed. What efforts are you making to determine the attitudes of women who are not Planned Parenthood clients about HPV?
(3) What specific questions will be asked of study participants?

Could you also provide recent educational materials from the Planned Parenthood of Southwest and Central Florida that address HPV and condoms? As you know, since December 21, 2000, federal law requires all educational and prevention materials printed by the CDC and its partners to contain medically accurate information regarding the effectiveness or lack of effectiveness of condoms against STDs. We would like to verify that an organization conducting research for the CDC is both complying with the law and providing medically accurate information to the public.

Could you also provide an update as to what actions the CDC has taken since December 2000 to educate health care providers, CDC grantees and partners, the media and the public about HPV, its link to cervical cancer and the lack of effectiveness of condoms in preventing HPV infection as mandated by Public Law 106-554?

Finally, have any efforts been made to evaluate whether CDC partners are complying with the federal requirement that all educational and prevention materials "contain medically accurate information regarding the effectiveness or lack of effectiveness of condoms in preventing the STD the materials are designed to address?"

Thank you for your attention to this matter. We look forward to a prompt reply.

Sincerely,

Mark E. Souder
Chairman
Subcommittee on Criminal Justice,
Drug Policy and Human Resources

Dave Weldon, M.D.
Member of Congress

Chris Smith
Member of Congress

Joe Pitts
Member of Congress

DEPARTMENT OF HEALTH & HUMAN SERVICES

Public Health Service

Centers for Disease Control
and Prevention (CDC)
Atlanta GA 30333

MAY 17 2002

JUN 4 2002

The Honorable Mark E. Souder
House of Representatives
Washington, D.C. 20515-6143

Dear Mr. Souder:

This is in response to your letter to Dr. Jeffrey P. Koplan, former Director of the Centers for Disease Control and Prevention (CDC), requesting information on funding provided by CDC to support a study to assess the impact on women when diagnosed with human papillomavirus (HPV) infection. Please excuse the delay of this response.

CDC is conducting formative research on the psychological impact of HPV diagnosis on women at five sites around the nation. These sites were competitively selected, and included are the University of South Florida (USF), the University of Oklahoma, the University of South Carolina, the Los Angeles County Department of Health Services, and the Washington State Department of Health. Each of these research sites will collaborate with a number of clinical sites, which include primary care centers, public health clinics, women's health centers, HIV care clinics, community health centers, family medicine clinics, university health centers, family planning clinics, Indian Health Service clinics, sexually transmitted disease (STD) clinics, and a Veterans Administration women's clinic. USF is the only research site with plans to recruit participants from Planned Parenthood clinics. Each of the sites involved in this study contributes important data on women from various segments of the population. Aggregating data across the sites will provide a representative picture of the impact of HPV diagnosis and American women's attitudes toward HPV.

In fiscal year (FY) 2001, CDC provided $295,161 to USF to conduct the first of 3 years of such formative research. The research plan at USF requires laboratory testing of specimens obtained via Papanicolaou (Pap) smears from 1,000 women. This is expected to yield a sample of approximately 100 HPV-positive women who are willing to be interviewed regarding the psychosocial impact of their HPV diagnosis. Due to the short time frame of the study and the number of women to be screened, it is necessary to collaborate with clinics where Pap smears are routinely obtained from large numbers of women. Thus, USF proposes to collaborate with its Student Health Center and Planned Parenthood of Southwest and Central Florida.

Regarding your request for the USF study protocol, the research protocol is currently pending review and approval by the CDC Institutional Review Board and cannot be considered a final research plan. Once the plan is finalized, I will forward it to you under separate cover. In response to your request for Planned Parenthood of Southwest and Central Florida's materials on HPV and condoms, CDC does not provide funding for these materials. Please contact Ms. Barbara Zdavecky, President and CEO of Planned Parenthood of Southwest and Central Florida, at telephone (941) 365-3913 if you wish to obtain these materials.

CDC is also conducting formative research to develop a provider survey that will assess knowledge, attitudes, and practices regarding HPV diagnosis and treatment. This survey will also assess perceptions, practice barriers, and facilitators regarding HPV risk assessment, testing, treatment, counseling, and partner services. All of the findings, from formative and survey research, will underpin the development and dissemination of educational materials and health messages.

Finally, in reference to efforts to evaluate whether CDC partners are complying with the requirements of Public Law 106-554 regarding the content of educational materials, CDC has taken the following steps:

- Informed grantees, subgrantees, contractors, and a wide range of public health partners about the requirements of the law, especially those requirements regarding the content of educational materials.

- Communicated the requirements of Public Law 106-554 through conference calls with the National Coalition of STD Directors and the National Alliance of State and Territorial AIDS Directors.

- Collaborated with the National Institutes of Health to develop a fact sheet with educational messages reflecting the latest science in STD prevention. This fact sheet is currently undergoing clearance.

Should CDC become aware of any inconsistencies in the implementation of the requirements of Public Law 106-554 by any CDC grantee, we will notify the organization and provide technical assistance and guidance to assist in correcting the information.

We appreciate your continued commitment to the prevention and treatment of HPV and cervical cancer. An identical letter is being sent to Representatives Dave Weldon, M.D., Chris Smith, and Joe Pitts who cosigned your letter.

Sincerely,

David Fleming

David W. Fleming, M.D.
Acting Director

ONE HUNDRED EIGHTH CONGRESS

Congress of the United States

House of Representatives

COMMITTEE ON GOVERNMENT REFORM
2157 RAYBURN HOUSE OFFICE BUILDING
WASHINGTON, DC 20515–6143

MAJORITY (202) 225-5074
FACSIMILE (202) 225-3974
MINORITY (202) 225-5051
TTY (202) 225-6852

www.house.gov/reform

November 19, 2003

Julie L. Gerberding, M.D., M.P.H.
Director
Centers for Disease Control and Prevention
1600 Clifton Road, N.E.
Atlanta, GA 30333

Dear Dr. Gerberding,

Thank you for making your staff available on November 17 to discuss the Center for Disease Control and Prevention's implementation of Public Law 106-554. The Congressional staff delegation at this meeting included representatives from the Senate Health, Education, Labor and Pensions Committee, the House Energy and Commerce Committee, the Republican Study Committee, the office of Congressman Dave Weldon. M.D. of the House Appropriations Committee, and the House Subcommittee on Criminal Justice, Drug Policy and Human Resources.

As you know, this law directs the CDC to undertake a number of activities to educate the public about human papillomavirus (HPV), including its health consequences and how infection can be prevented. The conversation between CDC and Congressional staff focused on the legal requirements under this Act directing CDC to develop a report by December 21, 2003 recommending "the best strategies to prevent future [HPV] infections, based on the available science."

It is very disappointing to learn that CDC has not taken appropriate actions to ensure compliance with the law and will miss the legal deadline for releasing these very important and much needed prevention recommendations.

Consider that in the United States, approximately 20 million people are currently infected with genital HPV and more than 5 million new infections occur annually. Experts agree that nearly all cases of cervical cancer are directly associated with HPV infection. HPV is also associated with more than one million pre-cancerous lesions. An estimated 13,000 new cases of invasive cervical cancer are diagnosed annually in the

U.S. and tens of thousands of other women will be treated for HPV related pre-cancerous conditions. Cervical cancer kills nearly 5,000 women every year in the U.S.; by way of comparison, AIDS kills about 3,800 women every year. Yet few Americans have ever even heard of HPV and most are unaware of its risks or how to protect themselves from infection.

The commitment of CDC made by Dr. Ed Thompson, Deputy Director for Public Health Services, and the CDC staff that the agency will release HPV prevention recommendations in January is very much appreciated. With January designated as Cervical Cancer Awareness Month, the release at this time, while statutorily overdue, would be very appropriate.

Specifically, Dr. Thompson and CDC staff committed to:

(1) issuing HPV prevention recommendations based on available science no later than the third week of January;

(2) including Dr. Tom Coburn, a practicing obstetrician/family physician who cares for patients affected by HPV and the author of the federal HPV law, or his designee in the development of these recommendations; and

(3) providing routine progress updates to staff, including drafts of the recommendations.

We also strongly encourage CDC to focus on data that has been peer reviewed and published in scientific journals and to refrain from issuing theoretical, hypothetical or unproven bases for protection.

In addition to the HPV prevention report, Public Law 106-554 requires CDC to undertake a number of other activities related to HPV education and research. We look forward to frequent progress updates on the status of these efforts.

Thank you, and Dr. Thompson, for CDC's commitment to beginning efforts to educate the public about the dangers of HPV and how to protect against HPV infection.

Sincerely,

Mark E. Souder
Chairman
Subcommittee on Criminal Justice,
Drug Policy and Human Resources

cc: Honorable Tommy Thompson
Secretary
Department of Health and Human Services

Honorable Judd Gregg
Chairman
Senate Committee on Health, Education, Labor and Pensions

Honorable Billy Tauzin
Chairman
House Energy and Commerce Committee

Honorable Michael Bilirakis
Chairman
House Subcommittee on Health

Honorable Dave Weldon, M.D.
Member of Congress
House Appropriations Committee

Honorable Sue Myrick
Chair
Republican Study Committee

Honorable Tom Coburn, M.D.

DEPARTMENT OF HEALTH & HUMAN SERVICES | Public Health Service

Centers for Disease Control
and Prevention (CDC)
Atlanta GA 30333

DEC 1 8 2003

The Honorable Mark E. Souder
House of Representatives
Washington, D.C. 20515-6143

Dear Mr. Souder:

Thank you for your letter regarding Congressional, Department of Health and Human Services (HHS), and Centers for Disease Control and Prevention (CDC) staff discussions surrounding implementation of PL 106-554. I appreciate your deep interest in ensuring that the public is properly educated about human papillomavirus (HPV) as well as your personal interest in CDC's response to certain requirements related to HPV in PL 106-554.

I am pleased that staff were able to more fully discuss the implementation of the PL 106-554 during the November 17 meeting. We understand well the need to provide strategies for prevention with respect to HPV. As always, any strategies we present will be based on the best available science. Additionally, we are committed to further advancing the field by continuing our research and surveillance activities in this critical area and by working collaboratively with public- and private- sector agencies and external experts.

Your letter lists a number of matters that were discussed at the meeting. We are committed to meeting, to the best of our ability, your expectations, and the requirements of the law by providing by the third week in January "a detailed summary of the significant findings and problems and the best strategies to prevent future [HPV] infections based on available science." As for involving Dr. Coburn and providing drafts of the report to Congress, I would like to suggest that you and/or your staff meet with Dr. Ed Thompson, CDC's Deputy Director for Public Health Services in the near future to discuss specifically the best way to address these matters. And I would reiterate my requests from earlier in the year, that, at your convenience, you and I meet to discuss your concerns.

I certainly want to keep you updated on our progress with the implementation of the requirements of PL 106-554, and I look forward to future discussions with you.

Sincerely,

Julie Louise Gerberding

Julie Louise Gerberding, M.D., M.P.H.
Director

TOM A. COBURN, M.D.
2D DISTRICT, OKLAHOMA

COMMITTEE ON COMMERCE

SUBCOMMITTEES:
HEALTH AND ENVIRONMENT
ENERGY AND POWER

Congress of the United States
House of Representatives
Washington, DC 20515–3602

215 STATE STREET, SUITE 615
MUSKOGEE, OK 74401
(918) 687-2533
(918) 682-8503 (FAX)

120 S. MISSOURI, ROOM 105
CLAREMORE, OK 74017
(918) 341-9336
(918) 341-9437 (FAX)

34 "A" STREET N.E., ROOM 202
MIAMI, OK 74354
(918) 542-5337
(918) 542-5367 (FAX)

September 7, 2000

The Honorable Jane E. Henney, M.D.
Commissioner
Food and Drug Administration
Parklawn Building
5600 Fishers Lane
Rockville, MD 20857

Dear Dr. Henney,

As a practicing physician who has cared for countless women who have become infected with human papillomavirus (HPV) despite their belief that they were having "safe sex" by using a condom, I am gravely concerned that unless the Food and Drug Administration reconsiders the existing label for condom packages more young women will become victims of this horrible virus that can cause cancer and death.

As you know, HPV is the cause of virtually all cervical cancer. The virus is present in 99.7 percent of all cervical cancers according to a study published last year in the Journal of Pathology. HPV has also been linked to oral cancer and cancer of the vagina, prostate, penis and anus, as well as genital warts. Many of those infected, however, have no visible symptoms. While not everyone infected will develop cancer, every year 15,000 cases of cervical cancer are diagnosed and 5,000 women die from the disease. Hundreds of thousands of other women will be diagnosed and treated for pre-cancerous conditions which some researchers estimate are about four times more common than invasive cervical cancer. And despite the fact that it is the most common sexually transmitted virus in the United States, over three-fourths of the respondents in a recent poll have never heard of HPV.

Dr. Richard Klauser, Director of the National Cancer Institute (NCI), has stated "condoms are ineffective against HPV" and the American Cancer Association has concurred, acknowledging that "research shows that condoms ("rubbers") cannot protect against infection with HPV." According to Dr. Klausner, the evidence that condoms do not protect against HPV is so definitive that "additional research efforts by NCI on the effectiveness of condoms in preventing HPV transmission is not warranted."

The labeling on condoms— approved by the FDA— is extremely misleading. "If used properly, latex condoms are effective against pregnancy, AIDS and other STD's" according to the label on LifeStyles condoms. Trojan and TrustEx state that "latex condoms will help reduce the risk of transmission of HIV infection (AIDS) and many other sexually transmitted diseases." A LifeStyles Condom press release issued in July even went as far as to state that

429 CANNON HOUSE OFFICE BUILDING
WASHINGTON, DC 20515
(202) 225-2701 Fax: (202) 225-3038

E-mail: rep.coburn@mail.house.gov
Web site: www.house.gov/coburn

"the proper and consistent use of latex condoms is the most effective way to prevent the spread of such diseases, including HIV, AIDS and HPV (human papaloma virus)." These claims are absolutely untrue in regard to HPV.

Ironically, all latex condoms are required to contain a warning that they contain rubber latex which may cause allergic reactions. The most recent data show that only 15 people died from latex allergies during a four year period. This is a significant contrast to the 5,000 women who die a year from cervical cancer of which nearly all is associated with HPV.

Interestingly enough, the labeling on birth control pills addresses cervical cancer and states the ineffectiveness of oral contraceptives in preventing STDs. While HPV is not sited per se, both genital warts and cervical cancer are addressed in the packaging of birth control pills. "Oral contraceptives do not protect against transmission of HIV (AIDS) and other sexually transmitted diseases such sexually transmitted diseases such chlamydia, genital herpes, genital warts, gonorrhea, hepatitis B, and syphilis," according to the labeling of ORTHO-CYCLEN and ORTHO TRI-CYCLEN. Furthermore, "some studies have found an increase in the incidence of cancer of the cervix in women who use oral contraceptives. However, this findings may be related to factors other than the use of oral contraceptives."

It bewilders me that birth control pills, which are commonly understood to prevent only pregnancy and not STDs, would address these health concerns while condom labels not only fail to address HPV and cervical cancer, but provide misleading information about their effectiveness.

In light of this information, I would like to know:

1) If the FDA intends to revise condoms labels to more accurately reflect the scientific facts about their ineffectiveness against HPV and the correlation between HPV and cervical cancer. If not, please provide an explanation as to why the agency feels this information should be withheld from consumers.

2) What liability do you expect that the condom manufacturers, the FDA or any other government agencies have assumed due to the fact that this information on HPV has been available for some time but yet withheld and, instead, misleading information about condom effectiveness has been prescribed on condom packaging.

Thank you for your attention to this matter. I look forward to a prompt reply. If you have any questions, please do not hesitate to contact me.

Sincerely,

Tom A. Coburn, M.D.
Vice Chair
Commerce Subcommittee on Health & Environment

Enclosures

Food and Drug Administration
Rockville MD 20857

OCT 20 2000

The Honorable Tom A. Coburn
Vice Chairman
Subcommittee on Health and Environment
Committee on Commerce
House of Representatives
Washington, D.C. 20515

Dear Mr. Vice Chairman:

Thank you for your letter of September 7, 2000, expressing your concerns about the effectiveness of condoms in preventing transmission of sexually-transmitted diseases (STDs), particularly the human papillomavirus (HPV), and the labeling of condoms in this respect. Your questions will be restated followed by our response.

1. **If the FDA intends to revise condom labels to more accurately reflect the scientific facts about their ineffectiveness against HPV and the correlation between HPV and cervical cancer. If not, please provide an explanation as to why the agency feels this information should be withheld from consumers.**

The Food and Drug Administration (FDA or the Agency) is in the process of taking a comprehensive look at condom labeling, including the primary display panel, the back panel, the package insert, and the individual foil pack.

As we understand it, almost a year after Dr. Richard Klausner, Director, National Cancer Institute (NCI), sent a letter dated February 19, 1999, to Chairman Bliley, House Committee on Commerce (which you quoted in your letter), Drs. Anthony Fauci, Director, National Institute of Allergy and Infectious Diseases (NIAID), and Klausner responded to a separate request from your office. This response led to the agreement to hold a conference that would examine the available data on condom effectiveness for STD protection. A steering committee, made up of representatives from NIAID, NCI, the National Institute for Child Health and Human Development, the Centers for Disease

Control and Prevention, FDA, and the United States Agency for International Development, planned the meeting. The Public Health Service conference, entitled "Scientific Evidence on Condom Effectiveness and STD Prevention," took place on June 12-14, 2000. The conference panel reviewed more than 100 published studies and heard from a variety of experts in the field. Presentations and deliberations highlighted some difficulties with understanding condom effectiveness. In particular, although studies show that condoms provide significant protection against some STDs (including and especially HIV/AIDS), currently-available data do not clearly answer the question of whether or to what extent condoms protect against transmission of HPV. A summary of the June workshop is being prepared by the National Institutes of Health and should be available shortly. Our review of condom labeling will address this and many other questions.

2. **What liability do you expect that the condom manufacturers, the FDA or any other government agencies have assumed due to the fact that this information on HPV has been available for some time but yet withheld and, instead, misleading information about condom effectiveness has been prescribed on condom packaging.**

FDA has not assumed any such liability. We have no information about the liability assumed by condom manufacturers or other government agencies.

Thanks again for your interest in this matter. If you have further questions, please let us know.

Sincerely,

Melinda K. Plaisier
Associate Commissioner
for Legislation

ONE HUNDRED SEVENTH CONGRESS

Congress of the United States

House of Representatives

COMMITTEE ON GOVERNMENT REFORM

2157 RAYBURN HOUSE OFFICE BUILDING

WASHINGTON, DC 20515–6143

MAJORITY (202) 225–5074
FACSIMILE (202) 225–3974
MINORITY (202) 225–5051
TTY (202) 225–6852

www.house.gov/reform

August 23, 2001

Bernard A. Schwetz, D.V.M., Ph.D.
Acting Principal Deputy Commissioner
Food and Drug Administration
5600 Fishers Lane
Rockville MD 20857-0001

Dear Dr. Schwetz,

I look forward to working with you in protecting the health of all Americans and improving the safety of food, drugs and medical devices.

Public Law 106–554 requires the Food and Drug Administration (FDA) to "reexamine existing condom labels" and "determine whether the labels are medically accurate regarding the overall effectiveness or lack of effectiveness of condoms in preventing sexually transmitted diseases, including HPV."

As you know, the National Institutes of Health along with the U.S. Agency for International Development, the Centers for Disease Control and Prevention and the FDA released last month a report entitled "Scientific Evidence on Condom Effectiveness for STD Prevention." This report provided the single most comprehensive review of the published scientific data on the effectiveness of condoms in preventing sexually transmitted diseases (STDs). In the executive summary, the document states "for HPV, the Panel concluded that there was **no** [emphasis added] epidemiological evidence that condom use reduced the risk of HPV infection." In addition to HPV, the panel reviewed the effectiveness of condoms in preventing infection with seven other STDs—HIV, gonorrhea, chlamydia, syphilis, chancroid, trichomoniasis, and genital herpes. The report concluded that "the evidence available" on the effectiveness of condoms against these infections "should not be interpreted as proof of the adequacy or inadequacy of the condom to reduce the risk of STDs other than HIV transmission in men and women and gonorrhea in men."

The FDA "Guidance for Industry Uniform Contraceptive Labeling" issued on July 23, 1998 directs manufacturers to include the following statement in consumer labeling regarding transmission of STDs:

"For latex condoms for men:

> "(On the condom wrapper/Principal display panel)
> If used properly, latex condoms will help reduce the risk of HIV infection (AIDS) and many sexually transmitted diseases.
>
> "(Directions For Use)
> If used properly, latex condoms will help reduce the risk of HIV infection (AIDS) and many sexually transmitted diseases, including chlamydia, genital herpes, genital warts, gonorrhea, hepatitis B, and syphilis."

These statements do not reflect the NIH review of the available published data on condom effectiveness, and therefore are not "medically accurate" as mandated by federal law.

Public Law 106–554 also requires that all "educational and prevention materials prepared and printed from this date forward [December 15, 2000] for the public and health care providers by the Secretary (including materials prepared through the Food and Drug Administration, the Centers for Disease Control and Prevention, and the Health Resources and Services Administration), or by contractors, grantees, or subgrantees thereof, that are specifically designed to address STDs including HPV shall contain medically accurate information regarding the effectiveness or lack of effectiveness of condoms in preventing the STD the materials are designed to address."

Could you please provide the Subcommittee with an update as to what specific actions the FDA has taken—or intends to take—to ensure that:

(1) Condom labeling reflects the conclusions of the NIH report; and

(2) FDA educational and prevention materials (including those posted on the FDA website) have been revised to ensure that such materials are "medically accurate" as required by law?

Because Public Law 106–554 requires the FDA to review the medical accuracy of condom labels, please also elaborate at to how the FDA intends to address condoms that contain the spermicide Nonoxynol-9 (N-9).

As you know, studies have indicated since 1989 that use of N-9 may actually increase the risk of HIV infection. In a Dear Colleague letter dated August 4, 2000, Dr. Helene Gayle of the Centers for Disease Control and Prevention (CDC) stated, "given that N-9 has now been proven ineffective against HIV transmission, the possibility of risk, with no benefit, indicates that N-9 should not be recommended as an effective means of HIV prevention."

In contrast, the FDA website states "although it has not been scientifically proven, it is possible that nonoxynol-9 may reduce the risk of transmission of the AIDS virus during intercourse as well. Using a spermicide along with a latex condom is therefore advisable, and is an added precaution in case the condom breaks."

This statement is quite troubling for several reasons. It is, first and foremost, medically inaccurate. It also encourages a behavior that numerous data indicate increase HIV risk. And it also provides advice that admittedly "has not been scientifically proven."

Could you please explain:

(3) Why, and how often, does the FDA provide consumers with recommendations that have "not been scientifically proven?" In other words, are there are other instances in which the FDA recommends the use of a device or drug that has no proven efficacy?

(4) Has the FDA verified that products containing N-9 are safe and effective? If not, does the FDA intend to halt the production, sale or marketing of condoms containing N-9 until such products undergo proper trials to determine if they are safe and effective?

(5) If the FDA does intend to allow the further production of condoms with N-9, what changes in labeling for such products will be required?

Thank you for your prompt attention to this matter. If you have any questions, please contact Roland Foster of the Subcommittee on Criminal Justice, Drug Policy and Human Resources at (202) 225-2577.

Sincerely,

Mark E. Souder
Chairman
Subcommittee on Criminal Justice,
Drug Policy and Human Resources

Enclosure

* The condoms should be made of latex (rubber).
* The package should say that the condoms are to prevent disease.

If the package doesn't say anything about preventing disease, the condoms may not provide the protection you want even though they may be the most expensive ones you can buy.

Novelty condoms, for example, will not be labeled for either disease- or pregnancy-prevention. Condoms that don't cover the entire penis are not labeled for disease prevention and should not be used for this purpose. For proper protection, a condom must unroll to cover the entire penis.

Some condom packages bear the words "DATE MFG." This is the date when the condoms were made, not an expiration date. FDA requires that all condoms to which a spermicide has been added be labeled with the expiration date of the spermicide. New York state requires an expiration date on all condoms sold in that state. To gain access to the New York market, therefore, most of the five domestic manufacturers of condoms will now include this date on all their packages, usually abbreviated "EXP." The condom should not be purchased or used after that date.

Condoms are available in almost all pharmacies; many supermarkets and other stores also carry them. They are also available from vending machines. When purchasing condoms from vending machines, as from any source, be sure they are latex, labeled for disease prevention, and are not outdated. Do not purchase condoms from a vending machine located where it may be subject to extreme temperatures or direct sunlight. Extreme temperatures--especially heat--can make latex brittle or gummy.

Condoms should be stored in a cool, dry place out of direct sunlight. Closets or drawers usually make good storage places. Condoms should not be kept in a pocket, wallet or purse for more than a few hours at a time because they may be exposed to extreme temperatures. Places that may get very hot, such as car glove compartments, are particularly poor storage areas.

When opening a condom, handle the package gently. Don't use teeth, sharp fingernails, scissors, or other sharp instruments as these may damage the condom. And make sure you can see what you're doing!

After you open the package, inspect the condom. If the material sticks to itself or is gummy, the condom is no good. Check the condom top for other obvious damage such as brittleness, tears and holes, but don't unroll the condom to check it because this could damage it.

Spermicides

Spermicides, which kill sperm, are used for birth control either alone or with barrier contraceptives such as the diaphragm or cervical cap. Scientists have observed that, in test tubes, a spermicide called nonoxynol-9 kills organisms that cause STDs. Although it has not been scientifically proven, it is possible that nonoxynol-9 may reduce the risk of transmission of the AIDS virus during intercourse as well. Using a spermicide along with a latex condom is therefore advisable, and is an added precaution in case the condom breaks. Some condoms come with nonoxynol-9 already added. Their packages are required to be labeled with the expiration date of the spermicide, and they should not be used after that date.

Some experts think that even if a condom with spermicide is used, additional spermicide in the form of a jelly, cream or foam should be added. These are sold over the counter in pharmacies and some supermarkets. (Although swallowing small amounts of spermicide has not proven harmful in animal tests, it is not known if this is true for humans. For that reason, and because spermicides have a bitter taste, for oral sex it may be best to use a

DEPARTMENT OF HEALTH & HUMAN SERVICES

Public Health Service

Food and Drug Administration
Rockville MD 20857

NOV 20 2001

The Honorable Mark E. Souder
Chairman
Subcommittee on Criminal Justice,
Drug Policy and Human Resources
Committee on Government Reform
House of Representatives
Washington, DC 20515 - 6148

Dear Mr. Chairman:

Thank you for your letter of August 23, 2001 expressing your concerns about the Food and Drug Administration's (FDA or the Agency) implementation of the section of Public Law 106-554, pertaining to labeling of condoms. We apologize for the delay in responding.

FDA is currently developing an implementation plan for carrying out Public Law 106-554. Our plan will consider the recently released report, **Workshop Summary:** *Scientific Evidence on Condom Effectiveness for Sexually Transmitted Disease (STD) Prevention,* (July 20, 2001), as well as other important findings (including new publications since the workshop was held in June 2000) to determine what modifications to current condom labeling are appropriate. We are also evaluating the appropriate regulatory mechanism for effecting such change.

As you know, Public Law 106-554 also has provisions regarding educational materials on the human papilloma virus (HPV) for health care providers and the public, these are directed at all components of the Department of Health and Human Services. Over the past year, the National Institutes of Health (NIH) and the Centers for Disease Control and Prevention (CDC) have developed new information on condoms and HPV. FDA will be working with public health officials from both agencies to ensure consistent and accurate information about HPV and other STDs and condom use.

Your letter points out that the FDA website still posts an article from a September 1990 issue of FDA Consumer, about condom use. To improve consumer access, FDA posts and maintains all articles from this consumer magazine. A carefully worded disclaimer at the beginning of each article addresses the concern about dated material. Nevertheless, we understand your concerns about the text of one paragraph in that article regarding nonoxynol-9 (N9), a spermicide contained in the lubricant of some condoms. As you may know, Helene Gayle's August 4, 2000, letter to CDC grantees was based on study results presented at the International AIDS Conference in July 2000 (Durban, South Africa). This was a study of commercial sex workers in Africa and southeast Asia who used vaginal preparations containing N9. As described below, FDA is still considering the applicability of this study to a U.S population, in the context of its ongoing review of the safety and effectiveness of over-the-counter (OTC) vaginal spermicides containing N9.

Regarding your questions on FDA's review of and regulatory plans for products containing N9, in 1980, an Advisory Review Panel, consisting of medical and scientific experts, reviewed OTC vaginal contraceptives already on the market and concluded that vaginal spermicides containing N9 were safe and effective for OTC use. In a 1995 proposed rule, the Agency tentatively concurred with the Panel's general recommendations regarding safety but stated that clinical studies were necessary to establish the effectiveness of the spermicide's final formulation when used in humans.

In addition, some specific safety issues relating to local vaginal irritation were raised. Consequently, the Agency requested additional safety and efficacy information to support the marketing of N9, but in the interim, the proposed rule allowed for the continued marketing of OTC vaginal spermicides containing N9. These issues were discussed at the November 22, 1996, Non-prescription Drugs Advisory Committee Meeting at which time the committee concurred with the Agency to allow interim marketing of N9-containing vaginal spermicides, pending results from the proposed rule.

In response to this proposed rule, NIH's National Institute of Child Health and Human Development (NICHD) advised the Agency of its intention to conduct a clinical trial to evaluate the efficacy, safety, and acceptability of different formulations and doses of vaginal spermicides containing N9 available on the market. The NICHD studies were originally projected to be completed in 2001; however, because of the difficulty in recruiting subjects for the trials, the estimated completion

Page 3 - The Honorable Mark E. Souder

time is two to three years from now. FDA will evaluate the results of these trial studies when completed. FDA is also evaluating the published study reports, including the recent study to which you alluded, and other recent medical literature suggesting that N9 is not antimicrobial and does not protect against infection from the AIDS virus and other STDs. Because of the safety concerns raised in these studies, the Agency is considering proposing a new rule to require new labeling warnings for marketed OTC N9-containing vaginal spermicides to alert consumers that these products will not protect against transmission of the AIDS virus or other STDs.

With respect to condoms containing N9 in the lubricant, as noted above, FDA is devising a plan to review the labeling of all condoms, including those containing N9 in the lubricant, and will also make changes there as appropriate. It is important to note that the labeling of condoms with N9 in the lubricant does not make any claims regarding the ability of N9 to provide an increase in protection against STDs.

Thank you again for contacting us concerning this matter. If you have further questions, please let us know.

Sincerely yours,

Jacilyn Dupont for

Melinda K. Plaisier
Associate Commissioner
for Legislation

ONE HUNDRED EIGHTH CONGRESS

Congress of the United States

House of Representatives

COMMITTEE ON GOVERNMENT REFORM

2157 RAYBURN HOUSE OFFICE BUILDING

WASHINGTON, DC 20515–6143

MAJORITY (202) 225–5074
FACSIMILE (202) 225–3974
MINORITY (202) 225–5051
TTY (202) 225–6852

www.house.gov/reform

February 12, 2004

Mark B. McClellan, M.D., Ph.D.
Commissioner
U. S. Food and Drug Administration
5600 Fishers Lane
Rockville MD 20857-0001

Dear Dr. McClellan,

As you know, Public Law 106–554 requires the Food and Drug Administration (FDA) to "reexamine existing condom labels" and "determine whether the labels are medically accurate regarding the overall effectiveness or lack of effectiveness of condoms in preventing sexually transmitted diseases, including HPV."

Experts agree that infection with certain strains of the human papillomavirus (HPV) is the primary cause of nearly all cervical cancer. According to the American Cancer Society, nearly 13,000 women develop invasive cervical cancer annually in the United States and over 4,000 women die of the disease every year. HPV infection is also associated with other cancers and more than one million pre-cancerous lesions. By way of comparison, nearly the same number of women die annually as a result of cervical cancer as do of HIV/AIDS in the United States.

The Centers for Disease Control and Prevention (CDC) estimates 20 million Americans are currently infected with HPV and 5.5 million Americans become infected with HPV every year.

On January 30, 2004, the CDC issued a report to Congress entitled "Prevention of Genital Human Papillomavirus Infection" pursuant to Public Law 106-554 that concluded, "Even consistent and correct use of condoms would not be expected to offer complete protection from HPV infection." According to the CDC, therefore, "The available scientific evidence is not sufficient to recommend condoms as a primary prevention strategy for the prevention of genital HPV infection."

The CDC report should come as no surprise to the FDA as its findings reflect prior conclusions by the National Institutes for Health and the American Cancer Society. A meta-analysis reviewing "the best available data describing the relationship between condoms and HPV-related conditions" from the past two decades published in the November 29, 2002 edition of the journal *Sexually Transmitted Diseases* found, "There was no consistent evidence of a protective effect of condom use on HPV DNA detection, and in some studies, condom use was associated with a slightly increased risk for these lesions."

Three years after Public Law 106-554 was signed by President Clinton, condom labels still do not warn consumers about the lack of protection against HPV infection. The Subcommittee urges FDA to act on the release of CDC's HPV prevention report and immediately relabel condoms to alert consumers that condoms do not provide effective protection against HPV infection.

Please also provide the Subcommittee with the following:

(1) The agency's timetable for relabeling condoms in compliance with Public Law 106-554; and

(2) A detailed summary of all actions taken to enact this law since it was signed on December 21, 2000. Please include meeting dates, meeting participants, and number of full time employees assigned to implementing this law.

Thank you for your attention to this very important subject. I look forward to working with you to ensure the public is receiving medically accurate information from which to make fully informed health decisions based upon scientific data. Please respond to this request prior to the March 11 Subcommittee hearing that will address the federal response to cervical cancer and HPV.

Sincerely,

Mark E. Souder
Chairman,
Subcommittee on Criminal Justice,
Drug Policy and Human Resources

ONE HUNDRED EIGHTH CONGRESS

Congress of the United States

House of Representatives

COMMITTEE ON GOVERNMENT REFORM

2157 RAYBURN HOUSE OFFICE BUILDING

WASHINGTON, DC 20515–6143

MAJORITY (202) 225-5074
FACSIMILE (202) 225-3974
MINORITY (202) 225-5051
TTY (202) 225-6852

www.house.gov/reform

August 19, 2003

Ms. Dara Corrigan
Acting Principal Deputy Inspector General
Office of the Inspector General
Department of Health and Human Services
330 Independence Avenue, S.W.
Washington, D.C. 20201

Dear Ms. Corrigan,

Dr. Tom Coburn, a former member of the U.S. House of Representatives, recently contacted the Subcommittee regarding the failure of the Centers for Disease Control and Prevention (CDC) and the Food and Drug Administration (FDA) to comply with the legal requirements of Public Law 106-554. This law is intended to educate the public about the dangers of human papillomavirus (HPV) and to prevent its spread and its harmful consequences, which include cervical cancer and death. This policy was overwhelmingly supported by Congress and signed into law by President Clinton on December 21, 2000.

I request that the Office of the Inspector General conduct a thorough investigation to determine whether Public Law 106-554 has been faithfully executed and, if not, to make recommendations to ensure that the appropriate agencies immediately comply with the directives and intent of this law. Please also determine if federal agencies and organizations receiving federal funds are complying with P.L. 106-554 by providing medically accurate information about HPV, reflecting the findings of the July 2001 scientific report entitle "Scientific Evidence on Condom Effectiveness for STD Prevention" issued by NIH/CDC/FDA/USAID.

A copy of Dr. Coburn's correspondence outlining the allegations against CDC and FDA is attached.

Thank you for your attention to this serious matter.

Sincerely,

Mark E. Souder
Chairman,
Subcommittee on Criminal Justice,
Drug Policy and Human Resources

Attachment

cc: Honorable Claude A. Allen
Honorable Tom A. Coburn, M.D.

DEPARTMENT OF HEALTH & HUMAN SERVICES

Food and Drug Administration
Rockville MD 20857

MAR 1 0 2004

The Honorable Mark E. Souder
Chairman
Subcommittee on Criminal Justice,
Drug Policy, and Human Resources
Committee on Government Reform
House of Representatives
Washington, D.C. 20515-6143

Dear Chairman Souder:

Thank you for the letter of February 12, 2004, regarding the Food and Drug Administration's (FDA or the Agency) implementation of Public Law (P.L.) 106-554 with respect to the labeling of condoms. FDA has complied with P.L. 106-554 by carefully reexamining existing condom labeling to determine whether the labels are medically accurate regarding the overall effectiveness or lack of effectiveness of condoms in preventing sexually transmitted diseases (STDs), including human papilloma virus (HPV). As directed by this law, the Agency has not confined its examination to labeling addressing HPV transmission, but has examined condom labeling regarding the transmission of other STDs as well.

FDA agrees with the Centers for Disease Control and Prevention's recent report to Congress entitled, "Prevention of Human Papillomavirus Infection." The report indicates that:

> *While available scientific evidence suggests that the effect of condoms in preventing HPV infection is unknown, condom use has been associated with lower rates of the HPV-associated diseases of genital warts and cervical cancer. The available scientific evidence is not sufficient to recommend condoms as a primary prevention strategy for the prevention of genital HPV infection. There is evidence that indicates that the use of condoms may reduce the risk of cervical cancer.*

With respect to your specific concerns, they are repeated below followed by our response:

1. **The Agency's timetable for relabeling condoms in compliance with Public Law 106-544.**

   P.L. 106-554 directs FDA to reexamine condom labeling, not only with respect to their "overall effectiveness" in preventing STDs, but also with respect to their "lack of effectiveness." FDA is working to present a balanced view of condom performance, being careful neither to overstate device effectiveness nor to discourage device usewhere it is appropriate. The Agency is working on developing a proposed rule to be accompanied by draft labeling guidance for public comment later this year.

2. **A detailed summary of all actions taken to enact this law since it was signed on December 21, 2000. Please include meeting dates, meeting participants, and number of full time employees assigned to implementing this law.**

A team of experts from FDA's Center for Devices and Radiological Health (CDRH), as well as staff from the Department of Health and Human Services Office of General Counsel, Food and Drug Division, have worked on this effort since enactment of P.L. 106-554 (see enclosure).

To accomplish this task, the Agency staff has conducted a comprehensive systematic review of the published medical literature on condoms and STDs. Given the enormous scope of this effort, we have just completed this literature review and are now looking at how the results from this review would impact condom labeling.

Based on the review of the literature, CDRH has developed a regulatory plan to provide condom users with a consistent labeling message about STDs and the protection they should expect from condom use. FDA is preparing new guidance on condom labeling to address these issues, with the target of publishing that guidance as a draft for public comment later this year. FDA also anticipates proposing to amend the classification regulations for condoms to designate the labeling guidance as a special control for these devices (an additional measure that will provide assurance of safety and effectiveness).

Thank you again for the opportunity to update the Subcommittee on this important public health issue. Dr. Daniel Schultz, the Director of CDRH's Office of Device Evaluation will be representing FDA at the March 11 hearing before the Subcommittee.

Sincerely,

Amit K. Sachdev
Associate Commissioner
for Legislation

Enclosure

FDA Office Staffs Working to Implement P.L. 106-554

Center for Devices and Radiological Health (CDRH)
Office of the Center Director (OCD)
Office of Device Evaluation (ODE)
Office of Compliance (OC)
Office of Health and Industry Programs (OHIP)
Office of Science and Technology (OST)
Office of Surveillance and Biometrics (OSB)

DHHS Office of General Counsel, Food and Drug Division (OGC)

Condom Meetings

Discussions of changes to condom 510(k) guidance:

Attendees: Relevant staff from FDA

Meetings range from February 2001 through February 2002

CDRH working group meetings to review literature on condom effectiveness for sexually transmitted diseases:

Attendees: Relevant staff from FDA

Meetings range from October 2002 to present

Planning and update CDRH management on progress regarding condom labeling review:

Attendees: Relevant staff from FDA

Meetings range from July 2001 to present

NIH Workshop

Attendees: Relevant staff from FDA

December 2002

WHO Announcement of Findings from COL-1492 Study Re: N9

Attendees: Relevant staff from FDA

July 2001

Meetings with various stakeholders

Attendees: Relevant staff from FDA

Meetings range from March 2001 through March 2003

Condom labeling focus testing and planning

Attendees: Relevant staff from FDA

Meetings range from April 2001 through present

Tom A. Coburn, M.D.
FAMILY PRACTICE
P.O. Box 1760
Muskogee, Oklahoma 74402
(918) 687-8950

August 12, 2003

Ms. Dara Corrigan
Acting Principal Deputy Inspector General
Office of the Inspector General
Department of Health and Human Services
330 Independence Avenue, S.W.
Washington, D.C. 20201

Dear Ms. Corrigan,

Cervical cancer is a largely preventable disease, yet according to the American Cancer Society, an estimated 13,000 new cases of invasive cervical cancer were diagnosed in 2002 and over 4,000 women die of the disease every year. Tens of thousands of others will be treated for related pre-cancerous conditions.

Experts agree that infection with certain strains of the human papillomavirus (HPV) is one of the strongest risk factors for cervical cancer. HPV infection, in fact, is associated with nearly all cervical cancer. HPV has also been linked to other forms of cancer and to genital warts.

HPV is the most common sexually transmitted disease and scientific studies have repeatedly concluded that condoms do not provide effective protection against HPV infection. In 2001, the National Institutes of Health along with the U.S. Agency for International Development, the Centers for Disease Control and Prevention (CDC) and the Food and Drug Administration (FDA) released a report entitled "Scientific Evidence on Condom Effectiveness for STD Prevention." This report provided the single most comprehensive review of the published scientific data on the effectiveness of condoms in preventing sexually transmitted diseases (STDs). The document states "for HPV, the Panel concluded that there was no epidemiological evidence that condom use reduced the risk of HPV infection."

Because of the widespread prevalence of HPV, a general lack of knowledge about the disease and how to prevent its transmission, the significant numbers of Americans harmed or killed as a result of HPV infection every year, and the failure of the Centers for Disease Control and Prevention (CDC) and the Food and Drug Administration (FDA) to address the epidemic, Congress passed and President Clinton signed Public Law 106-554 in 2000.

This law requires CDC to educate the public about HPV and the lack of effectiveness of condoms in preventing HPV infection. All educational materials produced by CDC and other federal agencies and federal grantees are also required to provide similar medically accurate information about HPV and condoms. The law directs the FDA to "reexamine existing condoms labels... to determine whether the labels are medically accurate regarding the overall effectiveness or lack of effectiveness in preventing sexually transmitted diseases, including HPV." The law also required CDC to conduct HPV research and provide recommendations regarding "the best strategies to prevent future [HPV] infections."

As the author of this law and a practicing physician who has cared for countless patients affected by HPV, I am deeply troubled by the federal bureaucracy's continued failure to address the HPV and to adhere to and abide by the legal requirements of P.L. 106-554.

I sent a letter to the Department of Health and Human Services July 18, 2001 regarding my concerns and requested that the Department take "appropriate actions to properly enact the law." I did not receive a response and it is obvious that actions to properly enact the law have still not been undertaken.

Expressing similar concerns, Congressmen Billy Tauzin, Chairman of the House Energy and Commerce Committee, and Joe Pitts sent a letter to the Department of Health and Human Services in May 2002 requesting an update on the status of the implementation of the law but 15 months later have still not received a response.

An independent review by another Congressional Subcommittee has found that two and a half years after the effective date of the federal HPV prevention and education law, CDC and FDA have largely ignored the law and maintain the indifferent attitude towards the HPV epidemic that prompted the need for this law.

In addition to ignoring much of the law, the areas of the law that CDC has implemented have been done so in a manner that appears to deliberately undermine its intent.

The law is clear that the CDC and other government agencies and partners must provide "medically accurate information regarding the effectiveness or lack of effectiveness of condoms" in preventing HPV and other sexually transmitted diseases (STDs). Yet in a July 2001 "Dear Colleague" letter to its partners, the CDC issued inaccurate information regarding the effectiveness of condoms. The CDC states "epidemiological studies have generally not demonstrated an association between condom use and the risk of HPV infection, but these studies are inconclusive because of limitations in how they were designed. Again, these limitations would generally lead to an underestimation of the protective effect." The inaccurate claim that studies are "inconclusive" is repeated several times in the CDC letter. The CDC letter also provides what is labeled "Theoretical Basis for Protection" that claims "consistent and correct use of latex condoms would be expected to protect against transmission of genital ulcer diseases and HPV in some, but not all, instances." This is medically inaccurate and does not reflect the available clinical science.

The law also states that the "educational material" on HPV required to be printed by this law "and all other relevant educational and prevention materials prepared and printed from this date forward for the public and health care providers by the Secretary (including materials prepared through the Food and Drug Administration, the Centers for Disease Control and Prevention, and the Health Resources and Services Administration), or by contractors, grantees, or subgrantees thereof, that are specifically designed to address STDs including HPV shall contain medically accurate information regarding the effectiveness or lack of effectiveness of condoms in preventing the STD the materials are designed to address." The law provides a clear mandate for all federal agencies and private partners. Yet the CDC's July 2001 letter states that the requirement is limited to only materials "funded by CDC." To the contrary, the law does not apply to only CDC funded materials. It is, rather, a requirement that all organizations receiving federal funding must abide by as a condition of eligibility for federal funding.

The CDC was directed to conduct a number of research activities on HPV. These included investigating the impact of HPV-related diagnosis on individuals, the development of educational messages and information for the public, patients and their partners and determine the public and the medical community's knowledge and awareness about HPV. The CDC has provided a $940,000 grant to Planned Parenthood of Southwest and Central Florida to conduct this study. Planned Parenthood opposed the enactment of this law and has consistently downplayed the impact of HPV infection on women's health and distorted the facts about the lack of effectiveness of condoms in preventing HPV. The selection of such a biased organization is just another indication that CDC is intentionally undermining this law.

The actions and lack of actions taken by the CDC and FDA to undermine this law are both illegal and threaten the health of millions of Americans.

The following chart outlines the provisions of Public Law 106-554 and the status of the each:

Public Law 106-554 Provision	Status
Conduct HPV prevalence and prevention research	CDC has selected Planned Parenthood, which opposed the enactment of the HPV law, to conduct this research.
Progress reports on HPV research to be submitted to Congress before January 2001	Incomplete -- Over one and a half years overdue.
Develop and disseminate educational materials on HPV and its prevention	Incomplete.
Report providing recommendations of the best strategies to prevent HPV infection	Due December 2003.

All educational materials on STDs, HPV and condoms prepared by federal agencies and their partners must provide medically accurate information including the lack of effectiveness of condoms in preventing infection	CDC has issued inaccurate claims based upon a "theoretical" and unproven hypothesis, inconsistent with both the law and scientific data.
Condom labels to be rewritten to be medically accurate to reflect the effectiveness or lack of effectiveness in preventing HPV and other STDs	Incomplete.

I would request that the Office of the Inspector General conduct a thorough investigation to determine why Public Law 106-554 has been both misinterpreted and largely ignored by CDC and FDA and to make recommendations to ensure that these agencies immediately comply with the directives and intent of this law. Please also determine if federal agencies and organizations receiving federal funds are providing medically accurate information about HPV, reflecting the findings of the 2001 scientific report issued by NIH/CDC/FDA/USAID.

Thank you for your assistance with this request. Please do not hesitate to contact me if you have any questions or if I can be of any assistance with this investigation.

Sincerely,

Tom A. Coburn, M.D.
Member of Congress (retired)

cc: Honorable Judd Gregg, U.S. Senate
Honorable Billy Tauzin, Member of Congress
Honorable Joe Pitts, Member of Congress
Honorable David Weldon, MD, Member of Congress
Honorable Mark Souder, Member of Congress
Honorable Sue Myrick, Member of Congress

DEPARTMENT OF HEALTH & HUMAN SERVICES

Office of Inspector General

Washington, D.C. 20201

SEP 29 2003

The Honorable Mark E. Souder
Chairman, Subcommittee on Criminal Justice,
Drug Policy and Human Resources
Committee on Government Reform
House of Representatives
Washington, D.C. 20515

Dear Mr. Souder:

Thank you for your letter of August 19, 2003, which follows up on a request to the subcommittee from Dr. Tom Coburn, a former member of the House of Representatives regarding Public Law 106-554. This law is intended to educate the public about the dangers of human papillomavirus (HPV) and to prevent its spread and harmful effects, which include cervical cancer and death. The Centers for Disease Control (CDC) and the Food and Drug Administration (FDA) are charged with carrying out this law. You requested that the Office of Inspector General (OIG) conduct an investigation to determine whether Public Law 106-554 has been faithfully executed and, if not, to make recommendations to ensure that the appropriate agencies immediately comply with the directives and intent of this law. You also asked if we would determine if Federal agencies and organizations receiving Federal funds are complying with Public Law 106-554 by providing medically accurate information about HPV.

We appreciate your interest in this matter and will consider the questions that you raise as part of our upcoming round of work planning. As such, we would be interested in meeting with you and your staff, as well as staff from CDC and FDA, as we seek to determine what might be an appropriate approach for this office. As you know, we received a similar letter from your former colleague, Dr. Tom Coburn. We have sent a similar letter to Dr. Coburn and offered to meet with him as well.

Additionally, you may be interested to know that among the 2004 work planned by our Office of Evaluation and Inspections (OEI) is a study on the National Breast and Cervical Cancer Early Detection Program. While this study will not focus on the issues that you raise about HPV and Public Law 106-554, it is part of the OIG's effort to begin examining public health issues, including sexually transmitted diseases and related grants, from a management and oversight perspective.

Page 2 – The Honorable Mark E. Souder

If you have any questions, please do not hesitate to contact me or one of your staff may contact George Grob, Deputy Inspector General for Management and Policy at (202) 619-2482.

Sincerely,

Dara Corrigan
Acting Principal Deputy Inspector General

cc: The Honorable Tom A. Coburn, M.D.
Dr. Julie Gerberding, CDC
Dr. Mark McClellan, FDA

Tom A. Coburn, M.D.
FAMILY PRACTICE
P.O. Box 1760
Muskogee, Oklahoma 74402
(918) 682-4318

July 18, 2001

Honorable Tommy G. Thompson
Secretary
U.S. Department of Health and Human Services
200 Independence Avenue, S.W.
Washington, D.C. 20201

Dear Secretary Thompson,

On July 5, the Centers for Disease Control and Prevention (CDC) distributed a "Dear Colleague" letter regarding the implementation of the HPV Education and Prevention Law of 2000 (Public Law 106-554). As the author of this law, I was troubled by the CDC's misinterpretation of the law and the likely health impact that will result from this misinterpretation.

As you know, the National Cancer Institute, the American Cancer Society and numerous published scientific studies have concluded that the human papillomavirus (HPV) is the cause of nearly all cervical cancer and that condoms do not provide effective protection against HPV infection. Despite this science, the CDC has intentionally misled the public about the dangers of HPV and the shortcomings of condoms.

As a practicing physician who sees the ravages of HPV infection every week, and more and more frequently in young women and girls, I am appalled by the CDC's intentional cover-up of the HPV epidemic and the attempt to manipulate the law which I authored.

The CDC "Dear Colleague" letter violates both the spirit and letter of the law in two important areas.

(1) CLINICAL SCIENCE

The law is clear that the CDC and other government agencies and partners must provide "medically accurate information regarding the effectiveness or lack of effectiveness of condoms" in preventing HPV and other sexually transmitted diseases (STDs).

Yet the CDC letter provides inaccurate information regarding the effectiveness of condoms. The CDC states "epidemiological studies have generally not demonstrated an association between condom use and the risk of HPV infection, but these studies are inconclusive because of limitations in how they were designed. Again, these limitations would generally lead to an underestimation of the protective effect." The inaccurate claim that studies are "inconclusive" is repeated several times. The CDC goes on to provide what it labels "Theoretical Basis for Protection" which claims "consistent and correct use of latex condoms would be expected to protect against transmission of genital ulcer diseases and HPV in some, but not all, instances."

The CDC has repeatedly distorted the truth with this "theoretical" rationalization for protection despite the fact that it is contradicted by the clinical science.

In a letter to Congress, Dr. Richard D. Klausner, Director of the National Cancer Institute (NCI), stated that "condoms are ineffective against HPV." The science in this regard is so clear that Dr. Klausner concluded "additional research efforts by NCI on the effectiveness of condoms in preventing HPV transmission are not warranted."

In follow-up, the NCI was asked why the NCI and CDC had reached differing conclusions on the overall effectiveness of condoms in preventing HPV infection. Dr. Douglas Lowy, Deputy Director of NCI's Division of Basic Sciences, explained that "the NCI conclusion that condoms are ineffective against HPV infection is based on the results of several long term studies that have failed to show that barrier contraceptives prevent cervical HPV infection, dysplasia, or cancer." Dr. Lowy provided published studies to substantiate the NCI statements.

A June 2000 workshop co-sponsored by the U.S. Agency for International Development, Food and Drug Administration, CDC, and the National Institutes for Health was held to evaluate the published evidence on latex condoms in regards to their effectiveness against preventing STDs. "For HPV, the Panel concluded that there was no evidence that condom use reduced the risk of HPV infection."

The science and the law are clear, and the CDC has ignored both.

(2) APPLICATION

The law also states that "educational material" on HPV required to be printed by this law "and all other relevant educational and prevention materials prepared and printed from this date forward for the public and health care providers by the Secretary (including materials prepared through the Food and Drug Administration, the Centers for Disease Control and Prevention, and the Health Resources and Services Administration), or by contractors, grantees, or subgrantees thereof, that are specifically designed to address STDs including HPV shall contain medically accurate information regarding the effectiveness or lack of effectiveness of condoms in preventing the STD the materials are designed to address."

The law provides a clear mandate for all federal agencies and private partners. Yet the CDC's letter states that the requirement is limited to only materials "funded by CDC." To the contrary, the law does not apply to only CDC funded materials. It is, rather, a requirement that all organizations receiving federal funding must abide by as a condition of eligibility for federal funding. This was well understood during the drafting of the law and is clear from the actual language of the law.

It is bewildering why the CDC, or any federal agency, would provide funding to any organization that was not providing medically accurate information. It is also extremely disturbing that the CDC would misrepresent the medically accurate truth and intentionally confuse the public. Such actions will only ensure that more and more young women and men become infected and even die as a result of HPV infection.

The CDC seems to have forgotten that it is charged with disease control and "prevention." Millions of Americans already have HPV, most of which are unaware that they infected and have probably never even heard of the virus or its consequences. In addition to cervical cancer, prostate cancer, a leading cause of death in men, is now also believed to be linked to HPV. This year alone, tens of thousands of women will be treated for HPV-related pre-cancerous conditions and nearly 5,000 women in American will die of cervical cancer. Nearly all of these deaths could have been prevented. The emotional toll of this disease is impossible to determine and unless action is taken, the financial toll will be staggering as HPV infects more and more Americans.

I would ask you to take the appropriate actions to properly enact the law and educate the public with the truth about HPV so we can start saving lives.

I have attached a copy of the CDC Dear Colleague letter as well as the actual language of the law. Please do not hesitate to contact me if you have any questions or need additional information.

Sincerely,

Tom

Tom A. Coburn, M.D.
Member of Congress (retired)

Enclosures

cc: Honorable Claude A. Allen, Deputy Secretary, HHS
Honorable David Weldon, MD, Member of Congress
Honorable Mark Souder, Member of Congress
Honorable Billy Tauzin, Member of Congress

DEPARTMENT OF HEALTH & HUMAN SERVICES　　Public Health Service

Centers for Disease Control
and Prevention (CDC)
Atlanta, GA 30333

July 5, 2001

Dear Colleague:

During the 2001 appropriations process, the United States Congress enacted Public Law 106-554, which authorizes surveillance and educational activities critical to understanding the epidemiology and impact of genital human papillomavirus (HPV). The provisions of this law also identify activities important to better informing health care providers, public health professionals, and the public about HPV prevention.

Specifically, the language requires:

- implementation of sentinel surveillance to monitor the prevalence of specific types of HPV;
- prevention research on HPV in areas of the behavioral impact of HPV-related diagnosis;
- formative research to assist in the development of educational messages for providers, patients and their partners, and the public; and
- surveys of physician and public knowledge, attitudes, and practices about genital HPV infection.

Upon completion of the above activities and, based on the findings, the Centers for Disease Control and Prevention (CDC) will develop and disseminate educational materials for health care providers and the public.

This law further requires that all educational and prevention materials prepared after December 21, 2000, by the Department of Health and Human Services, its agencies and their grantees, subgrantees, and contractors that are specifically designed to address sexually transmitted diseases (STDs) including HPV, shall contain "medically accurate information regarding the effectiveness or lack of effectiveness of condoms in preventing the STD the materials are designed to address."

To assist you in preparing those materials, following is a document that provides prevention messages on the effectiveness of condoms in reducing the transmission of specific STDs, as per P.L.106-554. The document also contains background information, including the theoretical basis for protection and related laboratory and epidemiological studies. Please ensure that all educational materials developed after December 21, 2000, and funded by CDC use the appropriate message or messages. A printed copy of this document will also be mailed to you.

The HPV provisions authorized in P.L.106-554 are enclosed. If you have any questions, please don't hesitate to call our Office of Communications at (404) 639-8890.

Sincerely,

Helene D. Gayle

Helene D. Gayle, M.D., M.P.H.
Director, National Center for HIV, STD, and TB Prevention

Genital Ulcer Diseases and Human Papillomavirus

Prevention message for genital ulcer diseases and HPV infections
Genital ulcer diseases and HPV infections can occur in genital areas that are covered or protected by a latex condom. They can also occur in areas that are not covered or protected. Latex condoms, when used consistently and correctly, can reduce the risk of genital herpes, syphilis, chancroid, and HPV infection, only when the infected areas are covered or protected by the condom. In addition, the use of latex condoms has been associated with a reduction in risk of HPV-associated diseases, such as cervical cancer.

Genital ulcer diseases include genital herpes, syphilis, and chancroid. These diseases are transmitted primarily through "skin-to-skin" contact from sores/ulcers or infected skin that looks normal. HPV infections, like genital ulcer diseases, are transmitted through contact with infected genital skin or mucosal surfaces/fluids. Although these infections can occur in genital areas that are covered or protected by the condom, they can also occur in areas that are not.

Theoretical Basis for Protection: Protection against genital ulcer diseases and HPV depends on the site of the sore/ulcer or infection. Latex condoms can only protect against transmission when the ulcers or infections are in genital areas that are covered or protected by the condom. Thus, consistent and correct use of latex condoms would be expected to protect against transmission of genital ulcer diseases and HPV in some, but not all, instances.

Laboratory Studies that determine whether or not organisms can penetrate latex condoms under conditions more stringent than those during intercourse, demonstrate that latex condoms provide an impermeable barrier to organisms considerably smaller than those that cause genital ulcer diseases and HPV infections.

Epidemiological Studies that compare infection rates among condom users and nonusers provide evidence that latex condoms can protect against the transmission of syphilis and genital herpes. However, because some epidemiological studies show little or no protection, the body of evidence is considered inconclusive. Many of the studies are also inconclusive regarding the level of protection because of limitations in design. In general, these limitations would lead to an underestimation of the protective effect. No conclusive studies have specifically addressed the transmission of chancroid and condom use.

Epidemiological studies have generally not demonstrated an association between condom use and the risk of HPV infection, but these studies are inconclusive because of limitations in how they were designed. Again, these limitations would generally lead to an underestimation of the protective effect. Study results do, however, show an association between condom use and risk reduction of HPV-associated diseases, including genital warts, cervical dysplasia and cervical cancer.

For bibliography on condom effectiveness, contact
CDC's National Prevention Information Network
at **(800) 458-5231** or **www.cdcnpin.org**

SEC. 516. (a) HUMAN PAPILLOMAVIRUS. —Part B of title III of the Public Health Services Act (42 U.S.C. 243 et seq.) is amended by inserting before section 318 the following section:

HUMAN PAPILLOMAVIRUS

SEC. 317P. (a) SURVEILLANCE. —

(1) IN GENERAL. —The Secretary, acting through the Centers for Disease Control and Prevention, shall—

(A) enter into cooperative agreements with States and other entities to conduct sentinel surveillance or other special studies that would determine the prevalence in various age groups and populations of specific types of human papillomavirus (referred to in this section as 'HPV') in different sites in various regions of the United States, through collection of special specimens for HPV using a variety of laboratory-based testing and diagnostic tools; and

(B) develop and analyze data from the HPV sentinel surveillance system described in subparagraph (A).

(2) REPORT. —The Secretary shall make a progress report to the Congress with respect to paragraph (1) no later than 1 year after the effective date of this section.

(b) PREVENTION ACTIVITIES; EDUCATION PROGRAM. —

(1) IN GENERAL. —The Secretary, acting through the Centers for Disease Control and Prevention, shall conduct prevention research on HPV, including—

(A) behavioral and other research on the impact of HPV-related diagnosis on individuals;

(B) formative research to assist with the development of educational messages and information for the public, for patients, and for their partners about HPV;

(C) surveys of physician and public knowledge, attitudes, and practices about genital HPV infection; and

(D) upon the completion of and based on the findings under subparagraphs (A) through (C), develop and disseminate educational materials for the public and health care providers regarding HPV and its impact and prevention.

(2) REPORT; FINAL PROPOSAL. —The Secretary shall make a progress report to the Congress with respect to paragraph

(1) not later than 1 year after the effective date of this section, and shall develop a final report not later than 3 years after such effective date, including a detailed summary of the significant findings and problems and the best strategies to prevent future infections, based on available science.

(c) HPV EDUCATION AND PREVENTION. —

(1) IN GENERAL. —The Secretary shall prepare and distribute educational materials for health care providers and the public that include information on HPV. Such materials shall address—

(A) modes of transmission;

(B) consequences of infection, including the link between HPV and cervical cancer;

(C) the available scientific evidence on the effective-ness or lack of effectiveness of condoms in preventing infection with HPV; and

(D) the importance of regular Pap smears, and other diagnostics for early intervention and prevention of cervical cancer purposes in preventing cervical cancer.

(2) MEDICALLY ACCURATE INFORMATION. —Educational material under paragraph (1), and all other relevant educational and prevention materials prepared and printed from this date forward for the public and health care providers by the Secretary (including materials prepared through the Food and Drug Administration, the Centers for Disease Control and Prevention, and the Health Resources and Services Administration), or by contractors, grantees, or subgrantees thereof, that are specifically designed to address STDs including HPV shall contain medically accurate information regarding the effectiveness or lack of effectiveness of condoms in preventing the STD the materials are designed to address. Such requirement only applies to materials mass produced for the public and health care providers, and not to routine communications. ''.

(b) LABELING OF CONDOMS. —The Secretary of Health and Human Services shall reexamine existing condom labels that are authorized pursuant to the Federal Food, Drug, and Cosmetic Act to determine whether the labels are medically accurate regarding the overall effectiveness or lack of effectiveness of condoms in preventing sexually transmitted diseases, including HPV.

MAY-17-2002 13:07

Congress of the United States
Washington, DC 20515

May 15, 2002

Honorable Tommy G. Thompson
Secretary
Department of Health and Human Services
200 Independence Avenue, S.W.
Washington, D.C. 20201

Dear Secretary Thompson:

The Energy and Commerce Committee has consistently made cervical cancer treatment, prevention and awareness a priority. The Breast and Cervical Cancer Treatment Act (P.L. 106-354), which provides medical assistance to low-income women with breast and cervical cancer, was authored by this Committee. Likewise, the Committee developed legislation (P.L.106-554) to address the prevention of human papillomavirus (HPV) infection, the cause of nearly all cervical cancer. Both of these life-saving laws were approved overwhelmingly and are extremely important components in the effort to eliminate cervical cancer and towards saving women's lives.

The Committee is very concerned about the lack of progress that the Centers for Disease Control and Prevention (CDC) and the Food and Drug Administration have made in implementing the HPV prevention law. The Department was required by law to submit a progress report prepared by CDC to Congress before January of this year regarding the prevalence of HPV in various age groups, demographics and regions of the United States. This has not been done. The Committee looks forward to receiving this report soon.

In addition, we would like to know the status of several other aspects of this law. The CDC was directed to conduct a number of research activities on HPV. These included investigating the impact of HIV-related diagnosis on individuals, the development of educational messages and information for the public, patients and their partners and determine the public and the medical community's knowledge and awareness about HPV. The CDC has provided a $940,000 grant to Planned Parenthood of Southwest and Central Florida to conduct this study. The Committee is disturbed by this decision due to fact that Planned Parenthood opposed the enactment of this law and has consistently downplayed the impact of HPV infection on women's health and distorted the facts about the (lack of) effectiveness of condoms in preventing HPV. We would like a detailed explanation as to why the CDC chose such a biased organization to conduct this research. Please also provide a list of other organizations that have received grants to conduct similar research.

P.L. 106-554 requires CDC to educate health care providers, CDC grantees and partners, the media and the public about HPV and the lack of effectiveness of condoms in preventing HPV infection. Please provide an update on what actions the CDC has taken in this regard.

This law also requires all HHS agencies, contractors, grantees, and subgrantees to provide medically accurate information regarding the effectiveness or lack of effectiveness of condoms in preventing STDs, including HPV. There has been evidence that some CDC-supported organizations have failed to comply with this legal requirement. What efforts, if any, have been made to evaluate whether HHS partners are complying?

In addition to these actions by the CDC, the FDA was directed to "reexamine existing condoms labels… to determine whether the labels are medically accurate regarding the overall effectiveness or lack of effectiveness in preventing sexually transmitted diseases, including HPV." Please provide a status report on the relabeling of condoms in this regard, including a timetable for the new labeling.

In addition, a new study, conducted by the International Agency for Research on Cancer of the World Health Organization concluded that that there is a significant connection between the use of birth control pills and cervical cancer. The research found that women infected with HPV who had used birth control pills for five years or more were nearly three times more likely to develop cervical cancer than HPV infected women who had never taken the pill. Women who had taken the pill for 10 years or more were four times more likely to get the disease than those who had never taken it. The Committee believes it is in the best interest of women's health for them to be aware of this potential danger. What efforts is the FDA undertaking to add this risk to the labeling of birth control pills? Is the CDC providing any educational materials to the medical community or the public about this risk?

Thank you for your assistance with this request. The Committee deeply appreciates and applauds your commitment to protecting the health of women and all Americans.

Sincerely,

Billy Tauzin
Chairman
Committee on Energy and Commerce

Joe Pitts
Member of Congress

TOTAL P.03

SENT BY: 9-25- 3 ; 11:00AM ; 51154;# 2/ 5

THE SECRETARY OF HEALTH AND HUMAN SERVICES
WASHINGTON, D.C. 20201

SEP 10 2003

The Honorable W.J. (Billy) Tauzin
Chairman
Committee on Energy and Commerce
House of Representatives
Washington, D.C. 20515

Dear Mr. Chairman:

Thank you for your letter expressing concern about the progress the Centers for Disease Control and Prevention (CDC) and the Food and Drug Administration (FDA) have made in implementing the Breast and Cervical Cancer Treatment Act (Public Law 106-554), which addresses the prevention of human papillomavirus (HPV) infection and related cervical cancer.

As required in the HPV legislation, the Department of Health and Human Services (HHS) directed CDC to prepare a draft progress report relative to the provisions contained within Public Law 106-554. The progress report is enclosed. The most complex provision of this legislation is the requirement that CDC conduct sentinel surveillance to monitor trends in genital HPV infection. To comply with this provision, CDC designed a 3-year study involving 35 clinics. These clinics must consecutively enroll at least 200 eligible women per year for 3 years to provide adequate sample size and ensure scientific rigor. Due to delays in IRB approval, clinics could not begin to enroll participants and initiate data collection until 2003. Once CDC completes the analysis of these data, it will issue a Final Report.

Since the law's enactment, CDC has advised me that it has implemented the following activities:

- initiated sentinel surveillance activities in collaboration with six health departments throughout the country to determine the prevalence in various age groups and populations of specific types of HPV infection in the United States;
- initiated collection of additional HPV prevalence and surveillance information in nationally representative population samples, using CDC's National Health and Nutrition Examination Survey (NHANES) that will provide specific information on HPV-16, one of the most common high-risk types of HPV associated with cervical cancer;
- initiated several formative research activities to assess knowledge and attitudes of the public and HPV-infected individuals about HPV healthcare-seeking and sexual behaviors and HPV information needs;
- completed formative research to develop a provider survey that will assess knowledge, attitudes, and practices regarding HPV diagnoses and treatment and developed a draft provider survey and a sampling plan. A package describing the study is under development and will be submitted shortly to the Office of Management and Budget (OMB). The provider survey will assess perceptions, practice barriers, and facilitators regarding HPV risk assessment, testing, treatment, counseling, and partner services.

Page 2 - The Honorable W.J. (Billy) Tauzin

On December 2, 2002, CDC posted on its website a fact sheet entitled *Male Latex Condoms and Sexually Transmitted Diseases*. The fact sheet is consistent with language provided in Public Law 106-554 to contain medically accurate information regarding the effectiveness or lack of effectiveness of condoms in preventing sexually transmitted diseases. CDC has also developed a set of disease-specific fact sheets that meet the same criteria. These individual fact sheets are currently in the clearance process, and will soon be distributed, and will also be available on CDC's website.

In response to your concerns about the funding of Planned Parenthood of Southwest and Central Florida, CDC funded the University of South Florida (USF) and four other sites to conduct formative research on the psychological impact of HPV diagnosis on women. This research will yield information on knowledge and awareness of HPV, the psychosocial impact of an HPV diagnosis, and will guide the development of counseling and educational messages for women with HPV. These sites were competitively selected and include the University of Oklahoma, the University of South Carolina, the Los Angeles County Department of Health Services, and the Washington State Department of Health, in addition to USF. Each of these research sites will collaborate with a number of clinical sites including primary care centers, public health clinics, women's health centers, HIV care clinics, community health centers, family medicine clinics, university health centers, family planning clinics, Indian Health Service clinics, sexually transmitted disease (STD) clinics, and a Veterans Administration women's clinic. USF is the only research site with plans to recruit participants from Planned Parenthood clinics. Each of the sites involved in this study will contribute important data on women from various segments of the population. Aggregating data across the sites will provide a representative picture of the impact of HPV diagnosis and American women's attitudes toward HPV.

Although USF requested approximately $940,000 in fiscal year 2001, CDC was only able to provide $295,161 to USF to conduct the first of three years of the formative research. In the second year (FY 2002), USF received $295,153, and in the third year (FY 2003) $430,195. The third-year funding represents an increase over the previous two years because USF was able to expand the study to include local STD and community clinics, thus increasing the valuable diversity in the study population. USF provided $25,000 per clinic to the two Planned Parenthood clinics during each year of the study, allowing the clinics to hire a recruiter for this study. The employee's job responsibilities are limited to study recruitment. The research conducted at USF has yielded laboratory testing of specimens obtained via Papanicolaou (Pap) smears from over 1,000 women. This screening yielded 52 women with HPV who were interviewed regarding the psychosocial impact of their HPV diagnosis. Information from these women has been used to develop a quantitative survey instrument, which is being pilot-tested in multiple geographic areas for use in the next phase of the HPV formative research. Both the qualitative interviews and the results from the quantitative survey will be used to develop educational messages for women who have high-risk HPV.

Page 3 - The Honorable W.J. (Billy) Tauzin

Due to the short timeframe of the study and the number of women to be screened, CDC indicated it is necessary to collaborate with clinics where Pap smears are routinely obtained from large numbers of women. Thus, USF continues to collaborate with its Student Health Center and Planned Parenthood of Southwest and Central Florida. In addition, in year three, USF will begin collaborating with other partners, including a local STD clinic and a local community clinic.

We are enclosing a copy of the USF protocol, *An Assessment of the Social, Emotional, Physical and Behavioral Impacts of an HPV-Related Diagnosis*, for your information.

In reference to efforts to evaluate whether CDC partners are complying with the requirement of Public Law 106-554 regarding the content of educational materials, CDC advises me that is has taken the following steps:

- informed grantees, subgrantees, contractors, and a wide range of public health partners about the requirements of the law, especially those requirements regarding the content of educational materials;
- communicated the requirements of Public Law 106-554 through conference calls with the National Coalition of STD Directors and the National Alliance of State and Territorial AIDS Directors.

Should HHS become aware of any inconsistencies in the implementation of the requirements of Public Law 106-554 by any CDC grantee, we will have CDC notify the organization and provide technical assistance and guidance to assist in correcting the information.

Since the legislation was enacted, FDA has met with condom manufacturers and other parts of the public health service to identify relevant information on the effectiveness of condoms against STDs, including HPV infection. In that same timeframe, several new studies and reports on condom effectiveness have also become available. FDA is currently reviewing the relevant data and expects to complete that review this fall. If the agency's review supports the need for a change in condom labeling, FDA will work with manufacturers to make appropriate changes. Moreover, if the FDA review supports it, changes in condom labeling will be proposed.

CDC is aware of the International Agency for Research on Cancer's (IARC) study mentioned in your letter. The agency has determined that the IARC findings obtained from research in selected developing countries are not consistent with research carried out in the United States and do not warrant informing the American medical community or the public at large. The World Health Organization (WHO) has determined the IARC findings are not sufficient to change current WHO guidelines. CDC will continue to carefully review the evidence and promptly respond to any new data that may indicate the need to modify current recommendations to the medical community or the American public.

Page 4 - The Honorable W.J. (Billy) Tauzin

Please call me if you have any further thoughts or questions. I look forward to working with you on this issue. I will also provide this response to Representative Joseph Pitts who co-signed your letter.

Sincerely,

Tommy G. Thompson

Enclosures

JO ANN DAVIS
FIRST DISTRICT, VIRGINIA

COMMITTEES:
ARMED SERVICES

INTERNATIONAL RELATIONS

GOVERNMENT REFORM
CHAIRWOMAN, CIVIL SERVICE AND AGENCY REORGANIZATION SUBCOMMITTEE

www.house.gov/joanndavis

Congress of the United States
House of Representatives
Washington, DC 20515–4601

WASHINGTON OFFICE:
1123 LONGWORTH HOUSE OFFICE BUILDING
WASHINGTON, DC 20515
TELEPHONE: (202) 225–4261

DISTRICT OFFICES:
4904-B GEORGE WASHINGTON MEMORIAL HWY.
YORKTOWN, VA 23692
(757) 874–6687

4500 PLANK ROAD, SUITE 105-A
FREDERICKSBURG, VA 22407
(540) 548–1086

1623 TAPPAHANNOCK BOULEVARD
P.O. BOX 3106
TAPPAHANNOCK, VA 22560
(804) 443–0668

November 21, 2003

Ambassador Randall Tobias
Office of the Global AIDS Coordinator
Department of State
2201 C Street, NW
Suite 1004
Washington, D.C. 20520

Dear Ambassador Tobias:

Public Law 108-025 requires a report to be submitted to Congress that shall include "an analysis of the prevalence of human papilloma virus (HPV) in sub-Saharan Africa and the impact that condom usage has upon the spread of HPV in sub-Saharan Africa." As the author of this provision-passed unanimously in the House International Relations Committee-I wanted to share my thoughts and expectations in regards to this important provision.

Scientific studies have concluded that HPV is the cause of nearly all cervical cancer. HPV is also associated with more than one million precancerous lesions of varying severity. According to the National Cervical Cancer Coalition, cervical cancer rates are highest in sub-Saharan Africa and Central America. Eighty percent of the world's cervical cancer cases, in fact, are in Africa, Asia and South America. Each year about 470,000 new cases are reported, with about 225,000 deaths occurring as a result of cervical cancer. In sub-Saharan Africa, cervical cancer is the leading cancer death in women. Many of those infected with HPV are co-infected with HIV.

While the focus of P.L. 108-025 is treating and preventing HIV/AIDS, tuberculosis and malaria, HPV poses a significant health threat to millions around the world, most of whom are women. It is vitally important that our efforts to curb and treat HIV do not ignore those affected by HPV and do not have the unintended consequence of facilitating the spread of HPV to unsuspecting victims.

Many of the women in the countries that are to be assisted by the President's global AIDS initiative have little access to health care services that are vitally important to women's health, including regular Pap testing and treatment for HPV-related abnormalities. It is essential, therefore, that women in these nations be given medically accurate information that allows them to protect themselves against HPV infection and cervical cancer.

Studies have concluded that condoms do not provide effective protection to prevent HPV infection. A June 2000 workshop co-sponsored by the U.S. Agency for International

Tobias, Randal
November 21, 2003
Page 2

Development, Food and Drug Administration, Centers for Disease Control and Prevention, and National Institutes for Health was held to evaluate the published evidence on latex condoms in regards to their effectiveness against preventing STDs. "For HPV, the Panel concluded that there was no evidence that condom use reduced the risk of HPV infection." In a 1999 statement to Congress, Dr. Richard D. Klausner, then-Director of the National Cancer Institute (NCI), stated that "condoms are ineffective against HPV." Dr. Douglas Lowy, Deputy Director of NCI's Division of Basic Sciences, explained that "the NCI conclusion that condoms are ineffective against HPV infection is based on the results of several long term studies that have failed to show that barrier contraceptives prevent cervical HPV infection, dysplasia, or cancer."

To date, global HIV prevention efforts have focused almost exclusively on condom promotion. The reliance on the promotion of condoms ignores the scientific fact that condoms do not prevent transmission of HPV and thereby help facilitate the spread of the virus among those who mistakenly believe condoms are protective. HIV does not exist in a vacuum and it is unfair to continue to ignore the unique threats posed, especially to women and girls, by HPV.

As the U.S. undertakes the global HIV prevention and AIDS treatment initiative, we must monitor the impact our efforts have upon the spread of HPV to ensure we are not unintentionally harming the health of women we are intending to help by contributing to the spread of HPV. It would be a cruel and tragic irony if our efforts to alleviate the suffering from AIDS resulted in increased deaths from cervical cancer.

The intent of the HPV study mandated by P.L. 108-025 is, therefore, to gain a better understanding of the size, scope and impact of the HPV epidemic in the sub-Saharan Africa to ensure that social marketing and promotion of condoms does not contribute to the spread of HPV.

I would expect that a number of studies would be necessary to complete this directive.

First, HPV prevalence testing would be necessary from a cross section of ages and populations including girls, married women, pregnant women and prostitutes in each of the countries studied. Prevalence studies should also determine risk factors for infection including number of primary and secondary sexual partners, age of sexual debut, condom use, and commercial sex work. Perhaps this research could be conducted with ongoing HIV prevalence studies to streamline efforts. The subjects of these tests should consent to testing, be notified of positive or abnormal test results and be referred to treatment, if necessary.

For the second part of this directive regarding condom use and HPV rates, I would also expect a number of studies to be conducted. One should examine whether those with abnormal Pap test or diagnosed with HPV used condoms. Another should be a long term study to examine the correlation between condom promotion and availability and HPV rates. A study of condom users over a period of time would be the most useful to determine whether these subjects become infected with HPV as well as other STDs including HIV and chlamydia.

These studies should not be limited to female subjects, as HPV has also been connected with other forms of cancer, affecting both men and women.

I would suggest consulting with the Medical Institute for Sexual Health and the Institute for Youth Development on this research. Additional funding for the studies could be provided by the National Institutes of Health.

Because invasive cervical cancer with HIV infection is one clinical case definition for AIDS, I strongly encourage the Administration to include HPV testing, Pap testing and treatment for HPV related conditions as components of the Administration's global AIDS initiative. I would also encourage the Administration to require that all U.S. funded condom promotion efforts require those distributing condoms provide medically accurate information to the recipients that condom can not effectively prevent HPV infection.

Congratulations on your selection and confirmation as the first Global AIDS Coordinator. My thoughts and prayers will be with you and the President as you undertake this great mission. Please do not hesitate to contact me or Melissa Smith in my office at 202-225-4261 if I can be of any assistance.

With kind regards, I remain

Sincerely,

Jo Ann Davis
Member of Congress

ONE HUNDRED EIGHTH CONGRESS

Congress of the United States

House of Representatives

COMMITTEE ON GOVERNMENT REFORM

2157 RAYBURN HOUSE OFFICE BUILDING

WASHINGTON, DC 20515–6143

MAJORITY (202) 225-5074
FACSIMILE (202) 225-3974
MINORITY (202) 225-5051
TTY (202) 225-6852

www.house.gov/reform

March 4, 2004

Ambassador Randall L. Tobias
U.S. Global AIDS Coordinator
Department of State
2201 C Street, NW
Suite 1004
Washington, DC 20520

Dear Ambassador Tobias:

Thank you for your leadership implementing the President's global HIV/AIDS initiative.

"The President's Emergency Plan for AIDS Relief: U.S. Five Year Global HIV/AIDS Strategy" recently delivered to Congress provides a well considered blue print for addressing the HIV/AIDS pandemic and represents the single largest humanitarian effort focused on a specific disease by any nation in history. I look forward to working with you to ensure the success of this noble endeavor in both preventing the further spread of HIV and providing care to those who are impacted by the disease.

While the focus of Public Law 108-25, which authorized the President's global AIDS initiative, is treating and preventing HIV/AIDS, tuberculosis and malaria, it also addresses another serious infectious disease, human papillomavirus (HPV). HPV poses a significant health threat to millions of women around the world because it is the cause of nearly all cervical cancers. It is vitally important that in our efforts to curb and treat HIV, we do not ignore those affected by HPV.

According to the National Cervical Cancer Coalition, cervical cancer rates are highest in sub-Saharan Africa and Central America. Eighty percent of the world's cervical cancer cases, in fact, are in Africa, Asia and South America. Each year about 470,000 new cases are reported, with about 225,000 deaths occurring as a result of cervical cancer. In sub-Saharan Africa, cervical cancer is the leading cancer death among women. Many of those infected with HPV are co-infected with HIV.

Because of the importance of properly addressing HPV, I want to bring to your attention an error contained within "The President's Emergency Plan for AIDS Relief: U.S. Five Year Global HIV/AIDS Strategy." On page 80 of the document in "Appendix B: Human Papilloma Virus in sub-Saharan Africa and the Impact of Condom Use on Its Spread," the report states "correct and consistent use of condoms can be expected to decrease (though not eliminate) the risk of transmitting HPV." The source cited for this claim is "'Workshop Summary: Scientific Evidence on Condom Effectiveness for Sexually Transmitted Disease (STD) Prevention,' the National Institute of Allergy and Infectious Diseases (NIAID), June 12-13, 2000." A closer read of this NIAID workshop states "For HPV, the Panel concluded that there was no epidemiological evidence that condom use reduced the risk of HPV infection." This finding can be found on page ii of the document's "Executive Summary." On page 26 of the report, it re-iterates that "There was no evidence that condom use reduced the risk of HPV infection."

This conclusion of NIAID echoes the assessments reached by the National Cancer Institute (NCI), the American Cancer Society, the Centers for Disease Control and Prevention (CDC), and a published meta-analysis of the best data published over the past two decades.

In a letter to the U.S. House Commerce Committee dated February 19, 1999, NCI director Dr. Richard D. Klausner stated "Condoms are ineffective against HPV because the virus is prevalent not only in the mucosal tissue (genitalia) but also on dry skin of the surrounding abdomen and groin, and it can migrate from those areas into the vagina and the cervix. Additional research efforts by NCI on the effectiveness of condoms in preventing HPV transmission are not warranted." In a separate letter to the U.S. House Commerce Committee dated April 8, 1999, Dr. Douglas Lowy, NCI Deputy Director of Basic sciences, stated "The NCI conclusion that condoms are ineffective against HPV infection is based on the results of several long term studies that have failed to show that barrier contraceptives prevent cervical HPV infection, dysplasia, or cancer."

The American Cancer Society's "Detailed Guide: Cervical Cancer" dated October 21, 2003 states "Recent studies show that condoms ('rubbers') do not protect well against HPV infection. This is because HPV can be passed from person to person by skin-to-skin contact with any HPV-infected area of the body, such as skin of the genital or anal area not covered by the condom. The absence of visible warts cannot be used to decide whether caution is needed, because HPV can be passed to another person even when there are no visible warts or other symptoms."

In November 2002, a meta-analysis of "the best available data describing the relationship between condoms and HPV-related conditions" from the previous two decades was published in the journal *Sexually Transmitted Diseases*. The meta-analysis concluded: "There was no consistent evidence of a protective effect of condom use on HPV DNA detection, and in some studies, condom use was associated with a slightly increased risk for these lesions. ... Complete protection from genital HPV infection may be impossible because infections may occur at ... sites not covered by the condom."

On January 30, 2004, the CDC released "Report to Congress: Prevention of Human Papillomavirus Infection" that found "the available scientific evidence is not sufficient to recommend condoms as a primary prevention strategy for the prevention of genital HPV infection."

The findings of the CDC, NIAID, NCI, American Cancer Society and the most comprehensive meta-analysis of published scientific data contradict the statement on page 80 published in "The President's Emergency Plan for AIDS Relief: U.S. Five Year Global HIV/AIDS Strategy."

The United States Leadership Against HIV/AIDS, Tuberculosis, and Malaria Act of 2003, Public Law 108-25, requires "an analysis of the prevalence of Human Papilloma Virus (HPV) in sub-Saharan Africa and the impact that condom usage has upon the spread of HPV in sub-Saharan Africa." I, therefore, request a correction to this document and an updated analysis to reflect the available science on HPV.

The "U.S. Five Year Global HIV/AIDS Strategy" also states "additional HPV epidemiological research in developing countries is needed to develop more effective HPV and cervical cancer prevention strategies."

I welcome efforts to conduct additional research on HPV and expanding access to HPV/cervical testing and treatment in developing countries. It is, however, unnecessary to develop a new strategy on HPV prevention as the CDC "Report to Congress: Prevention of Human Papillomavirus Infection" took three years to research and develop.

The CDC HPV prevention strategy states, "Because genital HPV infection is most common in men and women who have had multiple sex partners, abstaining from sexual activity (i.e. refraining from any genital contact with another individual) is the surest way to prevent infection. For those who choose to be sexually active, a monogamous relationship with an uninfected partner is the strategy most likely to prevent future genital HPV infections. For those who choose to be sexually active but who are not in a monogamous relationship, reducing the number of sexual partners and choosing a partner less likely to be infected may reduce the risk of genital HPV infection."

The CDC's HPV prevention recommendations are fully consistent with the President's HIV prevention strategy that emphasizes abstinence and being faithful. These recommendations, therefore, could be incorporated into global HIV prevention programs. This is particularly important for women in countries with little access to important health care services, such as regular Pap testing and treatment for HPV-related abnormalities. It is essential for these women to be given medically accurate information that empowers them to protect themselves against HPV infection and cervical cancer.

HIV, after all, does not exist in a vacuum and it is unfair to ignore the unique threats posed, especially to women and girls, by HPV.

The Subcommittee will hold a hearing on HPV March 11. I would invite your staff to attend to learn more, along with me, about HPV.

Thank you again for your leadership. I look forward to working with you on this important endeavor.

Sincerely,

Mark E. Souder
Chairman
Subcommittee on Criminal Justice,
Drug Policy and Human Resources

3. Federal HPV Prevention Law

The HPV Provisions of Public Law 106-554

The Consolidated Appropriations Act of 2001 was approved by Congress on December 15, 2000 and was signed by President Clinton on December 21, 2000, becoming Public Law 106-554. The following are the provisions relating to HPV education and prevention contained within this law:

Sec. 516. (a) Human Papillomavirus.--Part B of title III of the Public Health Services Act (42 U.S.C. 243 et seq.) is amended by inserting before section 318 the following section:

``human papillomavirus

``Sec. 317P. (a) Surveillance.--

``(1) In general.--The Secretary, acting through the Centers for Disease Control and Prevention, shall--

``(A) enter into cooperative agreements with States and other entities to conduct sentinel surveillance or other special studies that would determine the prevalence in various age groups and populations of specific types of human papillomavirus (referred to in this section as `HPV') in different sites in various regions of the United States, through collection of special specimens for HPV using a variety of laboratory-based testing and diagnostic tools; and

``(B) develop and analyze data from the HPV sentinel surveillance system described in subparagraph (A).

``(2) Report.--The Secretary shall make a progress report to the Congress with respect to paragraph (1) no later than 1 year after the effective date of this section.

``(b) Prevention Activities; Education Program.--

``(1) In general.--The Secretary, acting through the Centers for Disease Control and Prevention, shall conduct prevention research on HPV, including--

``(A) behavioral and other research on the impact of HPV-related diagnosis on individuals;

``(B) formative research to assist with the development of educational messages and information for the public, for patients, and for their partners about HPV;

``(C) surveys of physician and public knowledge, attitudes, and practices about genital HPV infection; and

``(D) upon the completion of and based on the findings under subparagraphs (A) through (C), develop and disseminate educational materials for the public and health care providers regarding HPV and its impact and prevention.

``(2) Report; final proposal.--The Secretary shall make a progress report to the Congress with respect to paragraph (1) not later than 1 year after the effective date of this section, and shall develop a final report not later than 3 years after such effective date, including a detailed summary of the significant findings and problems and the best strategies to prevent future infections, based on available science.

``(c) HPV Education and Prevention.--

``(1) In general.--The Secretary shall prepare and distribute educational materials for health care providers and the public that include information on HPV. Such materials shall address--

``(A) modes of transmission;

``(B) consequences of infection, including the link between HPV and cervical cancer;

``(C) the available scientific evidence on the effectiveness or lack of effectiveness of condoms in preventing infection with HPV; and

``(D) the importance of regular Pap smears, and other diagnostics for early intervention and prevention of cervical cancer purposes in preventing cervical cancer.

``(2) Medically accurate information.--Educational material under paragraph (1), and all other relevant educational and prevention materials prepared and printed from this date forward for the public and health care providers by the Secretary (including materials prepared through the Food and Drug Administration, the Centers for Disease Control and Prevention, and the Health Resources and Services Administration), or by contractors, grantees, or subgrantees thereof, that are specifically designed to address STDs including HPV shall contain medically accurate information regarding the effectiveness or lack of effectiveness of condoms in preventing the STD the materials are designed to address. Such requirement only applies to materials mass produced for the public and health care providers, and not to routine communications.".

(b) labeling of condoms.--The Secretary of Health and Human Services shall reexamine existing condom labels that are authorized pursuant to the Federal Food, Drug, and Cosmetic Act to determine whether the labels are medically accurate regarding the overall effectiveness or lack of effectiveness of condoms in preventing sexually transmitted diseases, including HPV.

Status of HPV-related Provisions of Public Law 106-554

Public Law 106-554 Provision	Status
CDC directed to conduct HPV prevalence and prevention research	Ongoing; Final reports expected in early 2005.
CDC to deliver progress report to Congress by December 21, 2001	Delivered September 12, 2003, nearly three years late.
CDC to develop and disseminate educational materials on HPV and its prevention for the public and health care providers	CDC estimates that educational materials for the public will be completed in December 2004 and those for health care providers will be completed in May 2005.
CDC to issue recommendations of the best strategies to prevent HPV infection by December 21, 2003.	Delivered January 30, 2004.
All educational materials on STDs, HPV and condoms prepared by federal agencies and their partners must provide medically accurate information including the lack of effectiveness of condoms in preventing infection	On July 5, 2001, CDC issued inaccurate claims about condom effectiveness against HPV infection based upon a theoretical and unproven hypothesis, inconsistent with both the law and scientific data; Websites and other educational materials by government agencies and government partners continue to omit these requirements.
Condom labels to be reviewed and rewritten by FDA to ensure that such labels are medically accurate and reflect the effectiveness or lack of effectiveness in preventing HPV and other STDs.	Incomplete.

4. HPV Facts

HPV Fact Sheet

What is HPV?

There are more than 100 different strains of HPV, or human papillomavirus, and over 30 of those strains are transmitted through sex. HPV infection is recognized as the primary cause of cervical cancer. The virus is present in 99.7 percent of all cervical cancers according to a study published in the Journal of Pathology. HPV is also associated with more than one million pre-cancerous lesions, oral cancer, cancer of the vagina, penis, anus, head and neck, as well as genital warts. In addition, HPV has been detected in some prostate tumors. An infected mother may transmit HPV to her newborn with affected children facing prolonged, difficult treatment for respiratory papillomatosis. Genital warts have been reported in children, although such lesions are rare.

How widespread is HPV and cervical cancer?

In 2001, cervical cancer was estimated to be the 12th most commonly new diagnosed cancer among women in the U.S. About 24 million Americans are currently infected with HPV according to the National Cancer Institute and an estimated 5.5 million Americans become infected with HPV every year. On March 8, 2004, researchers from the Colorado Health Sciences Center reported that more than 30 percent of women in a recent study were found to be infected with a strain of HPV linked to cervical and anal cancer. In comparison, 18.7 percent of men carried HPV-16, one of 10 high-risk strains of the virus.

While not everyone infected with HPV will develop cervical cancer, an estimated 13,000 new cases of invasive cervical cancer are diagnosed annually in the United States and over 4,000 women die of the disease every year. According to the American Cancer Society, non-invasive cervical cancer may be 4 times as widespread as the invasive type. By comparison, nearly the same number of women die annually in the U.S. as a result of HIV/AIDS as cervical cancer. In addition, over 1,350,000 women will have invasive procedures each year just to assess the status of their abnormal pap smears secondary to HPV.

HPV infection accounts for over half of all the new sexually transmitted diseases that occur every year among young Americans aged 15- 24 according to a study published in the January/February 2004 edition of Allan Guttmacher Institute's *Perspectives on Sexual and Reproductive Health*. Of the 9.1 million new STDs acquired by this age group in 2000, HPV accounted for 4.6 million. In comparison, HIV accounted for 15,000.

The rate of cervical cancer cases in African-American women (11.4 per 1,000) is higher than the rate in white women (7.1 per 1,000), and African-American women are about 33 percent more likely to die from it.

Do condoms prevent the transmission of HPV?

No. Studies have repeatedly concluded that condoms do not provide effective protection against HPV infection.

In January 2004, the CDC issued a report to Congress entitled, "Prevention of Genital Human Papillomavirus." The report found:

> "Because genital HPV infection is most common in men and women who have had multiple sex partners, abstaining from sexual activity (i.e. refraining from any genital contact with another individual) is the surest way to prevent infection. For those who choose to be sexually active, a monogamous relationship with an uninfected partner is the strategy most likely to prevent future genital HPV infections. For those who choose to be sexually active but who are not in a monogamous relationship, reducing the number of sexual partners and choosing a partner less likely to be infected may reduce the risk of genital HPV infection. …
>
> "The available scientific evidence is not sufficient to recommend condoms as a primary prevention strategy for the prevention of genital HPV infection."

The CDC's findings echo the scientific consensus, including that of a 2001 report entitled "Scientific Evidence on Condom Effectiveness for Sexually Transmitted Disease (STD) Prevention" prepared by the National Institute of Allergy and Infectious Diseases of the National Institutes of Health in consultation with the FDA, the Centers for Disease Control and Prevention and the U.S. Agency for International Development which evaluated the published data on latex condoms and STD prevention and "concluded that there was no evidence that condom use reduced the risk of HPV infection."

In a February 19, 1999 letter to the House Commerce Committee, Dr. Richard D. Klausner, then-Director of the National Cancer Institute (NCI), stated that "condoms are ineffective against HPV." The science in this regard is so clear that Dr. Klausner concluded "additional research efforts by NCI on the effectiveness of condoms in preventing HPV transmission are not warranted."

According to the American Cancer Society, "research shows that condoms cannot protect against infection with HPV. This is because HPV can be passed from person to person with any skin-to-skin contact with any HPV-infected area of the body, such as skin of the genital or anal area not covered by the condom. The absence of visible warts cannot be used to decide whether caution is warranted, since HPV can be passed on to another person even when there are no visible warts or other symptoms. HPV can be present for years with no symptoms."

Furthermore, risk factors for HPV infection include early sexual debut, multiple sexual partners, and partners with multiple sexual partners. Those who are misled into believing condoms will protect them against HPV infection may, as a result, engage in these behaviors that increase their risk for HPV infection and cervical cancer.

The CDC has stated "there is evidence that indicates that the use of condoms may reduce the risk of cervical cancer." How can this be true if condoms do not prevent infection with the virus that causes cervical cancer?

The CDC statement that condoms "may" reduce the risk of cervical cancer is inconclusive at best and contradicted by most scientific studies. The January 2003 CDC report entitled "Prevention of Genital Human Papillomavirus Infection" finds only "three studies on genital HPV infection and condom use showed a protective effect, but most studies on genital HPV infection and condom use did <u>not</u> show a protective effect" (emphasis added).

The National Cancer Institute has refuted this CDC claim. Dr. Douglas Lowy, Deputy Director of NCI's Division of Basic Sciences, explained that "the NCI conclusion that condoms are ineffective against HPV infection is based on the results of several long term studies that have failed to show that barrier contraceptives prevent cervical HPV infection, dysplasia, or cancer" in an April 8, 1999 letter to Congressman Michael Bilirakis, Chairman of the Commerce Committee's Subcommittee on Health and the Environment.

Absence of cervical cancer does not mean that a woman with HPV will not require treatment. Many women who are infected with HPV, but do not yet have cervical cancer, will require invasive treatment for pre-cancerous lesions. Over 1,350,000 women will have invasive procedures each year just to assess the status of their abnormal pap smears secondary to HPV. Many of these will be at increased risk for infertility, premature delivery or other HPV-related conditions.

Furthermore both men and women infected with HPV but without cancer can still spread the virus to others who may develop cancer.

Aren't regular Pap tests and treatment sufficient to prevent HPV infection from threatening women's health?

Regular Pap screening or HPV DNA testing for women are both extremely important to diagnose, monitor and, if necessary, treat HPV infection and related precancers and cancerous conditions of the cervix. However, similar screening tests do not exist for many of the other conditions caused by HPV infection. Likewise, there is no test to identify HPV infection in men.

And while treatment can prevent the progression of cervical disease or death from cervical cancer, treatment does not eradicate HPV or prevent it from causing future health problems. Furthermore, treatment can often be invasive, unpleasant, and costly and not preclude the necessity for additional treatments.

Cervical cancer is treated using surgery, radiation and chemotherapy; sometimes two or more methods are used. The most common types of surgery include cryosurgery, laser surgery, cone biopsy, simple hysterectomy, radical hysterectomy and pelvis lymph node dissection, and pelvic exenteration. Radiation therapy may involve external radiation or internal radiation (radioactive materials implanted in the tumor).

Treatment for cervical dysplasia—a premalignant or precancerous change in the cells of the cervix that may progress to cancer—include surgery, cone biopsy, cryosurgery, laser surgery, and electrosurgery.

The direct medical cost of treating a patient with cervical cancer is $9,200 to $13,360, while surgery to remove a precancerous lesion is $1,100 to $4,360. The financial burden of HPV in the U.S. has been estimated to range from $1.6 billion to $6 billion annually, making HPV one of the most costly sexually transmitted diseases after HIV/AIDS, according to a December 1999 CDC report

Screening and treatment are the key strategies for disease management but the best protection against cervical cancer and HPV related diseases remains prevention of HPV infection.

Doesn't HPV infection usually resolve itself and, therefore, not pose a significant health problem?

It is true that most women with HPV infection do not develop cervical cancer and the body's own immune system usually eradicates the virus. However, tens of thousands of those who do become infected must be treated every year for HPV-related health conditions and over 4,000 women die annually from cervical cancer. HPV infection cannot be "cured" medically. No HPV vaccine currently exists, and even if the body clears HPV naturally, infection can be re-established over and over again if there is repeated exposure.

Why have so few Americans ever heard of this pervasive disease that kills thousands of women every year?

Despite the fact that HPV is the most common sexually transmitted disease in the United States and the second most costly, over three-fourths of respondents in a recent poll have never heard of HPV.

The CDC, the federal agency charged with disease prevention, currently provides no guidance to states on how to curtail the spread of HPV and insufficient leadership to health care providers on how to counsel or even recognize those infected.

Public Law 106-554, passed by Congress and signed by President Clinton in 2000, directed CDC to issue a report not later than December 21, 2003 detailing the "best strategies to prevent future [HPV] infections, based on the available science." In January 2004, the CDC issued a report to Congress entitled, "Prevention of Genital Human Papillomavirus." The report found:

> "Because genital HPV infection is most common in men and women who have had multiple sex partners, abstaining from sexual activity (i.e. refraining from any genital contact with another individual) is the surest way to prevent infection. For those who choose to be sexually active, a monogamous relationship with an uninfected partner is the strategy most likely to prevent future genital HPV infections. For those who choose to be sexually active but who are not in a monogamous relationship, reducing the number of sexual partners and choosing a partner less likely to be infected may reduce the risk of genital HPV infection. … The available scientific evidence is not sufficient to recommend condoms as a primary prevention strategy for the prevention of genital HPV infection."

Public Law 106-554 also directs the FDA to "reexamine existing condoms labels… to determine whether the labels are medically accurate regarding the overall effectiveness or lack of effectiveness in preventing sexually transmitted diseases, including HPV." In the three years since the enactment of this law, FDA has not acted to make condom manufacturers comply with this statutory requirement.

The American College of Obstetricians and Gynecologists (ACOG) has claimed that educating the public that condoms do not protect against HPV infection "will simply increase the likelihood that people will fail to use condoms, and put men and women at unnecessary risk." Is this true?

By this same logic, it is then also possible that by inaccurately claiming condoms do prevent cervical cancer, at risk women will develop a false sense of security and be less likely to receive cervical cancer screening or treatment.

There is, however, no evidence to substantiate the claim that providing medically accurate information will reduce condom use. A June 13, 2000 letter from the U.S. Consumer Product Safety Commission to the Congressional Research Service stated that "based on our data compiled over more than 25 years and the experience of our staff, there is no scientific or anecdotal evidence" that indicates that requiring informational labels on products "actually contributed to decreased use of such products."

Updated March 10, 2004

5. Congressional Research Service Memorandum on HPV

Congressional Research Service

Memorandum November 17, 2003

TO: House Subcommittee on Criminal Justice, Drug Policy and Human Resources
Attention: Roland Foster

FROM: Judith A. Johnson
Specialist in Life Sciences
Domestic Social Policy Division

SUBJECT: **Human Papillomavirus**

In order to provide the information you requested on human papillomavirus (HPV), I contacted the following four organizations: the Centers for Disease Control and Prevention (CDC), the National Institutes of Health (NIH), the American College of Obstetricians and Gynecologists (ACOG), and the Partnership for Prevention. Copies of the responses I received from CDC and the Partnership for Prevention are attached; NIH replied that they do not have the type of information you are seeking (copy of email response is attached). ACOG has not yet responded. I also looked at reports on the Kaiser Family Foundation website on the topic of HPV and Sexually Transmitted Diseases prepared by Kaiser and the American Social Health Association. Copies of these reports are also attached. In response to your request, I am providing below a consolidation of the information obtained on HPV, primarily from CDC, on the overall size, cost, and impact of HPV in the United States. Most of the information was taken verbatim from CDC documents.

1. The overall prevalence and incidence of HPV in the United States.

According to information provided on the CDC website, an estimated 20 million Americans are currently infected with HPV (prevalence) and an estimated 5.5 million Americans become infected with HPV each year (incidence).[1] An estimated 75% of the reproductive age population has been infected with sexually transmitted HPV and an estimated 15% of Americans ages 15 to 49 are currently infected. A U.S. study published in 1998 found that an average of 14% of female college students became infected with genital HPV each year. About 43% of the women in the 1998 study were infected with HPV

[1] All statistics in this Section 1 were found in the following document: *Tracking the Hidden Epidemics 2000 – Trends in STDs in the United States: A Closer Look at HPV Infection.* See: [http://www.cdc.gov/nchstp/od/news/RevBrochure1pdfcloselookhpv.htm].

during the 3-year study period. Although less data are available on HPV among men, levels of current infection in men appear to be similar to those in women.

HIV-positive individuals have a higher prevalence of HPV infection and precancerous lesions on the cervix and anus than HIV-negative individuals. A San Francisco study of gay and bisexual men found that 60% of HIV-negative men had HPV and almost all HIV-positive men with severely compromised immune systems were infected with HPV. Similarly, a six-city study among high risk and HIV-infected women found that 26% of HIV-negative women were infected with HPV but 70% of HIV-positive women with severely comprised immune systems were infected with HPV.

2. A detailed description of all HPV-related medical conditions and how each is treated.

Of the more than 100 HPV viruses that have been identified, about 30 can infect the genital area and are spread (almost always) through sexual contact.[2] Some are considered "high-risk" types and may cause abnormal Pap smears and cancer of the cervix, anus, and penis. Others are "low-risk," and they may cause mild Pap smear abnormalities and genital warts. However, most HPV infections are subclinical: they have no signs or symptoms. Therefore, most infected persons are completely unaware they are infected and can transmit the virus to a sex partner. Genital warts are extremely common and can appear within several weeks, several months or even years after sexual contact with an infected person. Therefore, it is often difficult for patients to determine when they became infected and which sexual partner was the source of the infection.

Visible genital warts can be removed, but no treatment is better than another and no single treatment is ideal for all cases. In most patients treatment can induce wart-free periods. If left untreated, visible genital warts may resolve on their own, remain unchanged, or increase in size or number. Determining whether treatment of genital warts will reduce transmission is difficult because laboratory markers of infectivity have not been established and because some clinical studies have found HPV DNA in genital tissue following treatment. Currently available therapies for genital warts may reduce, but probably do not eradicate, infectivity. Whether the reduction in viral DNA that results from current treatment regimens impacts future transmission remains unclear. The natural history of genital warts is generally benign; the types of HPV that usually cause external genital warts are not associated with cancer. No evidence indicates that either the presence of genital warts or their treatment is associated with the development of cervical cancer.[3] Recurrence of genital warts within the first several months after treatment is common and usually indicates recurrence rather than reinfection.

Treatment of external genital warts can either be administered in the doctor's office (cryotherapy, surgical removal, electrocautery, laser surgery, podophyllin resin, trichloroacetic acid, bichloroacetic acid, interferon injection) or applied at home by the

---

[2] Genital HPV Infection. See: [http://www.cdc.gov/nchstp/dstd/Fact_Sheets/FactsHPV.htm].

[3] Visible genital warts usually are caused by HPV types 6 or 11. Other HPV types that cause flat, nearly invisible abnormal growths (as compared with types 6 and 11) in the anogenital region (e.g., types 16, 18, 31, 33, 35, 39, 45, 51, 52, 56, 58, 59, 68, and 69) have been strongly associated with cancer in both men and women. See: [http://cis.nci.nih.gov/fact/3_20.htm].

patient (podofilox cream, imiquimod cream). Treatment of internal genital warts (cervix, vagina, urinary tract, anus, rectum, mouth) usually occurs in the doctor's office.[4]

Subclinical HPV infection is even more common than genital warts and there is currently no treatment available. Most HPV infections appear to be temporary and are probably cleared up by the body's immune system. One 1998 study in college students showed that in 91% of women with new HPV infections, HPV became undetectable within 2 years.[5] However, reactivation or reinfection with HPV is always possible.

The single most important risk factor for cervical cancer–regardless of whether warts are present or not–is persistent cervical infection with certain types of HPV. HPV type 16 accounts for more than 50% of cervical cancers and high-grade dysplasia (abnormal cell growth), and HPV 16 along with types 18, 31, and 45 account for about 80% of cervical cancers.[6] Regular screening with a cervical Pap test is an effective low cost screening test for the prevention of invasive cervical cancer.[7] Cervical cancer is treated using surgery, radiation and chemotherapy; sometimes two or more methods are used. The most common types of surgery include cryosurgery, laser surgery, cone biopsy, simple hysterectomy, radical hysterectomy and pelvic lymph node dissection, and pelvic exenteration (radical hysterectomy and bladder, vagina, rectum, and part of colon may be removed as well). Radiation therapy may involve external radiation or internal radiation (radioactive materials implanted in the tumor). Chemotherapy uses drugs to stop the growth of cancer cells, either by killing the cells or by stopping the cells from dividing. When taken by mouth or injected into a vein or muscle, the drugs enter the bloodstream and can reach cancer cells throughout the body. The type and stage of the cervical cancer being treated determines which chemotherapy drug is used and the method of administration.[8]

Cervical dysplasia is a premalignant or precancerous change in the cells of the cervix which may progress to cancer without treatment. Mild dysplasia (also called low-grade squamous intraepithelial lesions or low-grade SILs) is a common condition, especially in young women, and a majority of cases return to normal over several months to a few years. Sometimes, mild dysplasia can progress to moderate or severe dysplasia, also called high-grade SILs. High-grade SILs are not cancer, but they may eventually lead to cancer and are treated by a doctor when they are detected. Treatments for cervical dysplasia include surgery, cone biopsy, cryosurgery, laser surgery, and electrosurgery.[9]

---

[4] For more detailed information, see: *Sexually Transmitted Diseases Treatment Guidelines 2002-Human Papillomavirus Infection* at [http://www.cdc.gov/std/treatment/6-2002TG.htm]

[5] The polymerase chain reaction (PCR) and another technique (Southern blot hybridization) were used to detect HPV in cell samples from the cervix and vagina. Gloria Y. F. Ho, et al., Natural History of Cervicovaginal Papillomavirus Infection in Young Women, *The New England Journal of Medicine*, vol. 338, Feb. 12, 1998, pp. 423-428.

[6] Ibid.

[7] For more detailed information, see: *Cervical Cancer and Pap Test Information* at [http://www.cdc.gov/cancer/nbccedp/info-cc.htm]

[8] More detailed information on cervical cancer treatment can be found at [http://www.nci.nih.gov/cancerinfo/pdq/treatment/cervical/patient/] for patients, and [http://www.nci.nih.gov/cancerinfo/pdq/treatment/cervical/healthprofessional] for physicians.

[9] Guidelines for the treatment of cervical dysplasia can be found at :

(continued...)

3. The overall annual cost for testing and treatment of HPV-related medical conditions.

In the United States, HPV is associated with about 80% of the 12,000 cases and 4,100 deaths due to cervical cancer each year.[10] HPV is also associated with more than one million precancerous lesions of varying severity. The direct medical cost of treating a patient with cervical cancer is $9,200 to $13,360, while surgery to remove a precancerous lesion is $1,100 to $4,360.[11] The financial burden of HPV in the U.S. has been estimated to be from $1.6 billion to $6 billion annually, making HPV one of the most costly sexually transmitted diseases (STDs) after HIV infection.[12]

4. The annual number of HPV-related diagnoses requiring invasive medical procedures.

Almost all of the invasive medical procedures for HPV are linked to cervical cancer. In the United States, HPVs are associated with about 80% of the 12,000 cases and 4,100 deaths due to cervical cancer each year. They are also associated with more than one million precancerous lesions of varying severity.[13]

5. A ranking of all sexually transmitted diseases, including HPV, in order by: cost for testing and treatment; prevalence; and, associated deaths, including HPV-related cervical cancer deaths.

---

[9] (...continued)
[http://www.guidelines.gov/summary/summary.aspx?doc_id=3286&nbr=2512&string=cervical+AND+cancer].

[10] A. Jemel et al., Cancer Statistics, 2003, *CA – A Cancer Journal for Clinicians*, vol. 53, Jan./Feb. 2003.

[11] Preventing Emerging Infectious Diseases: A Strategy for the 21st Century, Box 2: Economic Costs for Patient Care from Infectious Diseases, United States visited at [www.cdc.gov/ncidod/emergplan/box02.htm]. Also, an article in the January 2003 issue of *Emerging Infectious Disease* examined the cost-effectiveness of an HPV vaccine and calculated many of the resultant costs of screening and treatment. See attached and online at: [http://www.cdc.gov/ncidod/EID/vol9no1/02-0168.htm].

[12] CDC, Prevention of Genital HPV Infection and Sequelae: Report of an External Consultants' Meeting, Atlanta, GA: CDC, National Center for HIV, STD and TB Prevention; Dec. 1999.

[13] See Box 2, p. 2 in: CDC. Preventing Emerging Infectious Diseases: A Strategy for the 21st Century, at [http://www.cdc.gov/ncidod/emergplan/box02.htm]; and Cancer Statistics, 2003.

Table 1. Cost of Sexually Transmitted Diseases, 1994

STD	Cost (in millions)
Sexually transmitted HIV	$4,683
Pelvic Inflammatory disease	4,148
HPV	3,827
Chlamydia	2,013
Gonorrhea	1,051
Cervical cancer	737
Herpes simplex	237
Hepatitis B	156
Syphilis	106
Chancroid	1

Source: Institute of Medicine, The Hidden Epidemic: Confronting Sexually Transmitted Diseases, 1997.

Table 2. Prevalence of Sexually Transmitted Diseases

STD	Prevalence
Herpes	45,000,000
HPV	20,000,000
Chlamydia	2,000,000
Hepatitis B	417,000
Gonorrhea	n/a
Syphilis	n/a
Trichomoniasis	n/a
Bacterial vaginosis	n/a

Source: Tracking the Hidden Epidemics 2000 – Trends in STDs in the United States. [http://www.cdc.gov/nchstp/dstd/Stats_Trends/Trends2000.pdf]

According to CDC, there has not been a recent study summarizing in a comparable manner all deaths from STDs. In 2002, there were approximately 9,000 AIDS deaths among those who were infected through sexual transmission of HIV. Other deaths due to AIDS that year were associated with other sources of transmission.[14] **Table 3** below provides data from 1992 regarding deaths among women.

---

[14] The most current HIV/AIDS surveillance report with these data can be found at: [http://www.cdc.gov/hiv/stats/hasrlink.HTM].

Table 3. Mortality Related to Sexually Transmitted Diseases in U.S. Women, 1992

STD	Deaths
Cervical cancer	5,210
HIV	2,665
Hepatitis B and Hepatitis C	960
Syphilis	99
Pelvic inflammatory disease	220
Ectopic pregnancy	18
Gonorrhea	43
Other	4
Total	**9,179**

Source: American Journal of Public Health, vol. 87(6), June 1997, pp. 938-944.

6. A description of all HPV specific prevention and education programs supported by the Centers for Disease Control and Prevention or other federal agencies.

CDC provided me with a copy of a August 2003 Report to Congress entitled "Human Papillomavirus: Surveillance and Prevention Research," which was prepared by CDC in response to the Public Health Service Act Section 317P. This report describes activities undertaken to date to address the requirements of that section. However, there are additional programs at CDC that address cervical cancer.

I trust this information will be useful to your office. If you have any further questions, please do not hesitate to call (202-707-7077).

Attachment

6. CDC HPV Prevention Report

REPORT TO CONGRESS

Prevention of Genital Human Papillomavirus Infection

Centers for Disease Control and Prevention

Department of Health and Human Services

Julie Louise Gerberding, M.D., M.P.H.
Director
Centers for Disease Control and Prevention
January 2004

Table of Contents

Executive Summary	**Pages 3-5**
Introduction	**Pages 6-7**
Epidemiology of Genital HPV Infection	
Incidence and Prevalence of Genital HPV Infection	**Pages 8-10**
Prevalence of Sequelae of Genital HPV Infection	**Page 10**
Natural History of Genital HPV Infection	**Pages 10-11**
Transmission and Prevention of Genital HPV Infection	
Transmission	**Pages 11-12**
Prevention of Genital HPV Infection	**Pages 12**
Reducing Duration of Infectiousness	**Pages 12-13**
Reducing Efficiency of Transmission	**Page 13**
Condoms	**Pages 13-16**
Microbicides	**Page 16**
Reduction of Sexual Behavior Risk	**Pages 16**
Vaccines	**Pages 16-17**
Prevention of Cervical Cancer	**Pages 17-18**
Summary of Strategies to Prevent Genital HPV Infection	**Pages 18-19**
References	**Pages 20-35**

Prevention of Genital Human Papillomavirus Infection

Executive Summary

This report describes key aspects of the epidemiology of genital HPV infection and its transmission, and summarizes the best strategies to prevent infections with genital HPV as well as the HPV-associated diseases of genital warts and cervical cancer.

Genital infection with human papillomavirus (HPV) is very common in sexually active men and women and can sometimes have serious health consequences. About 20 million Americans are currently infected, and about 5.5 million people become newly infected each year. The virus can infect the genital skin and the linings of the vagina, cervix, rectum, and urethra. Most infections cause no clinical problems and go away on their own without treatment. Some infections lead to genital warts in men and women, and abnormal Papanicolaou (Pap) tests in women. Treatments are directed to abnormal cells associated with HPV rather than the virus itself; currently there is no curative treatment for HPV infection.

Of greatest importance, persistent infection with certain types of HPV is a leading cause of cervical cancer. Progression from cervical cancer precursor lesions to invasive cancer is a slow process, estimated to take 10–15 years. Cervical cancer is an uncommon consequence of HPV infection in women, especially if they are screened for cancer regularly with Pap tests and have appropriate follow-up of abnormalities. The purpose of screening with the Pap test is to detect cervical abnormalities that can be treated, thereby preventing progression to invasive cervical cancer, and also to detect invasive cervical cancer at a very early stage. If detected early and managed promptly, survival rates for cervical cancer are over 90%. In the past 40 years, widespread cervical cancer screening using the Pap test and treatment of precancerous cervical abnormalities have resulted in a dramatic decrease in the incidence and mortality due to cervical cancer in the United States. However, each year in the United States, an estimated 12,200 women develop cervical cancer and 4,100 women die from it. Of women in the United States who develop cervical cancer, about half have never had a Pap test.

Because genital HPV infection is most common in men and women who have had multiple sex partners, abstaining from sexual activity (i.e. refraining from any genital contact with another individual) is the surest way to prevent infection. For those who choose to be sexually active, a monogamous relationship with an uninfected partner is the strategy most likely to prevent future genital HPV infections. For those who choose to be sexually active but who are not in a monogamous relationship, reducing the number of sexual partners and choosing a partner less likely to be infected may reduce the risk of genital HPV infection.

All published epidemiologic studies of HPV have methodologic limitations that make the effect of condoms in the prevention of HPV infection unknown. While a few studies on genital HPV and condom use showed a protective effect, most studies on genital HPV infection and condom use did not show a protective effect. Recognizing that the optimal study design to ensure valid measurements can be problematic, it remains important that further research be done to help determine the efficacy of condoms in preventing HPV infection.

Nevertheless, available studies suggest that condoms reduce the risk of the clinically important outcomes of genital warts and cervical cancer. One possible explanation for the protective effect of condoms against warts and cancer is that condom use could reduce the quantity of HPV transmitted or decrease the likelihood of re-exposure, thereby decreasing the chance of developing clinical disease. An alternative explanation is that condom use may reduce exposure to a co-factor for cervical cancer, such as chlamydia or genital herpes, thereby reducing the chance of cervical cancer.

The available scientific evidence is not sufficient to recommend condoms as a primary prevention strategy for the prevention of genital HPV infection. There is evidence that indicates that the use of condoms may reduce the risk of cervical cancer.

Regarding other possible prevention approaches, no data indicate that treatment of clinical lesions or use of microbicides will prevent transmission of infection, although HPV vaccines are likely to become available in the next few years and may become an important prevention tool.

Summary of Strategies to Prevent Genital HPV Infection

Based on currently available science, the following recommendations summarize the strategies most likely to be effective in preventing future infections with genital HPV infection and cervical cancer.

Individual Strategies

- The surest way to eliminate the risk for future genital HPV infections is to refrain from any genital contact with another individual.
- For those who choose to be sexually active, a long-term, mutually monogamous relationship with an uninfected partner is the strategy most likely to prevent future genital HPV infections. However, it is difficult to determine whether a partner who has been sexually active in the past is currently infected.
- For those choosing to be sexually active and who are not in long-term mutually monogamous relationships, reducing the number of sexual partners and choosing a partner less likely to be infected may reduce the risk of genital HPV infection. Partners less likely to be infected include those who have had no or few prior sex partners.
- While available scientific evidence suggests that the effect of condoms in preventing HPV infection is unknown, condom use has been associated with lower rates of the HPV-associated diseases of genital warts and cervical cancer. The available scientific evidence is not sufficient to recommend condoms as a primary prevention strategy for

the prevention of genital HPV infection. There is evidence that indicates that the use of condoms may reduce the risk of cervical cancer.

- Regular cervical cancer screening for all sexually active women and treatment of precancerous lesions remains the key strategy to prevent cervical cancer.

- In the future, receiving a safe and effective HPV vaccine to help prevent genital HPV infection as well as the HPV-associated diseases of genital warts and cervical cancer would be an important prevention measure. However, an effective HPV vaccine would not replace other prevention strategies.

Public Health Strategies

Public health agencies should:

- Promote increased cervical cancer screening among never and rarely-screened women and appropriate follow-up of those with abnormal Pap tests.

- Work with public and private partners to increase awareness about prevention of genital HPV infection and cervical cancer among health care providers and in the general public.

- Collaborate with private industry to promote and accelerate the development of a safe and effective HPV vaccine.

- Continue epidemiologic, laboratory, and behavioral research on genital HPV infection, including studies of the prevalence of HPV in the United States, research on the attitudes and concerns of women diagnosed with HPV infection (e.g., concerns about cancer or about transmission), and surveys of provider knowledge and practices regarding HPV.

Introduction

Human papillomaviruses (HPV) are members of the Papillomaviridae family of DNA viruses. Because HPV cannot be cultured easily in the laboratory, HPV infection is most commonly diagnosed by detecting HPV DNA. Differences in sequences of DNA are used to determine different HPV types. More than 100 HPV types have been identified, over 30 of which infect the genital area. Genital HPV infections are estimated to be the most common sexually transmitted infection in the United States, with an estimated 5.5 million persons becoming newly infected every year (1). Although the majority of infections cause no symptoms and are self-limited, genital HPV is of public health concern because persistent infection with certain types can cause cervical cancer in women.

Genital HPV infections are categorized according to their association with cervical cancer. Infections with low-risk types, primarily types 6 and 11, can cause benign or low-grade cervical cell changes and genital warts, but are not associated with cervical cancer. Infection with high-risk types, primarily types 16, 18, 31, and 45, can cause low-grade cervical cell abnormalities, high-grade cervical cell abnormalities that are precursors to cancer, and genital cancers. Most genital infections with either high-risk or low-risk HPV types go away on their own, without clinical consequences. Currently, one HPV DNA test is FDA-approved for use in women for cervical cancer screening; no HPV test is available for men.

The sequela of genital HPV infection with greatest public health importance is cervical cancer. Cervical cancer is relatively uncommon in the United States because widespread cervical Papanicolaou (Pap) testing can detect precancerous lesions before they develop into cancer. However, in many developing countries where cervical cancer screening activities are limited, cervical cancer is the most common cancer in women. Based on multiple lines of evidence, both the International Agency for Research on Cancer and the National Institutes of Health (NIH) have concluded that high-risk genital HPV infections act as carcinogens in the development of cervical cancer (2;3). While infection with high-risk types appears to be "necessary" for the development of cervical cancer, it is not "sufficient" because cancer does not develop in the vast majority of women with HPV infection (2;3). Other co-factors appear to be necessary for the development of cervical cancer (described in *Natural History of Genital HPV Infection*, page 10). HPV infection is also associated with anogenital cancers at other sites including the vulva, vagina, penis and anus. Each of these is substantially less common than cervical cancer, with the exception of anal cancer in homosexual men (4-8). The association of genital types of HPV with non-genital cancer is less well established, but studies support a possible role in a subset of head and neck (9) and esophageal (10) cancers. In each of these non-genital cancers, there are clearly cancers arising independent of HPV, a situation quite different from cancer of the cervix. While a few studies suggest a possible association of HPV with cancer of the prostate (11), the findings are not consistent and the most recent studies do not indicate that HPV is associated with these cancers (12;13).

Because of the public health importance of cervical cancer, this report focuses on the prevention of genital HPV infection and its sequelae in heterosexual men and women. The report describes key aspects of the epidemiology of genital HPV infection and its transmission, and summarizes the best strategies to prevent infections with genital HPV as well as the HPV-associated diseases of genital warts and cervical cancer.

Epidemiology of Genital HPV Infection

Incidence and Prevalence of Genital HPV Infection

Accurately assessing the extent of genital HPV infection in the U.S. population has been difficult for many reasons. Data on prevalence and incidence of HPV infection are limited because there is no routine screening for HPV infection, and it is often unclear whether a newly diagnosed infection is recently acquired or longstanding. Neither HPV infection nor genital warts are routinely reported to state health departments for the following reasons: (a) no standard justification for recommending STD case reporting (e.g., patient care measures such as curative treatment for patients and their sex partners, or monitoring ongoing prevention programs) exists for genital HPV infection or warts, (b) most infections clear spontaneously, and (c) case reporting would create a large burden for providers, health departments and laboratories given the high prevalence of infection (14).

Cases of cervical cancer are routinely reported to cancer registries such as the National Cancer Institute Surveillance, Epidemiology, and End Results (SEER) program, and Centers for Disease Control and Prevention (CDC)-supported state cancer registries. However, because cervical cancer is a rare and late manifestation of HPV infection, cancer surveillance provides limited information on the burden and current trends of HPV infections. CDC is conducting a survey of the general U.S. population and a survey of women attending different types of clinics to improve measures of the prevalence of genital HPV. Results for the U.S. population survey will be available in late 2005, and, for the clinic based survey, in 2007. Data from these studies will be useful in evaluating the impact of future prevention strategies on HPV prevalence.

Because of the above issues, the magnitude of genital HPV infection is derived from extrapolations of epidemiologic studies. Studies that detect HPV DNA measure current infection, and studies that detect HPV antibodies using blood tests provide approximations of lifetime infection. Overall, in the United States, an estimated 20 million people (15% of the population) are currently infected with HPV, 50–75% of which is with high-risk types, and about 5.5 million people are infected every year (1). It has been estimated that at least 50% of sexually active men and women acquire genital HPV infection at some point in their lives; a recent estimate suggests that 80% of women will have acquired genital HPV by age 50 (15;16). An estimated 9.2 million sexually active adolescents and young adults 15 to 24 years of age are currently infected with HPV (17).

Prevalence studies in the United States have primarily included convenience samples of women attending managed care, STD, or university clinics. Studies have found that the prevalence of HPV infection is lowest in women who have never had sexual intercourse (18-21). Genital HPV infection is especially common among sexually active young women (less than 25 years of age), with prevalence decreasing with older age (22-30). While results vary by population studied, and sampling and detection methods used, overall they indicate that prevalence of genital HPV infection in sexually active young women in the United States ranges from 17–84% (22-29); most studies have reported a prevalence greater than 30% (22;23;25-27). In a study conducted in Portland, Oregon, 32% of young women ages 16 to 24 years had genital HPV DNA detected versus only 4% of women ages older than 45 years (24). The higher rates in younger women appear to be related to transmission of new infection during the early years of sexual activity, with infection clearing over time in most women (28;31). By far, the most common infections are with the high-risk types. Infection with multiple types of HPV occurs in approximately 5–30% of infected women (23;32-34). HPV infection is most likely to be detected in women who have cervical cancer precursors; in one study, over 85% of women with cervical cancer precursors had detectable HPV DNA (34).

These findings are supported by studies of incident (new) genital HPV infections, which can more accurately determine rates, as well as behavioral risk factors for infection. Studies of HPV incidence have been conducted in a variety of settings with variable follow-up periods. Incidence of HPV infection in college women studied for two to three years was 32–43% (21;28). Other studies assessing populations of women using routine gynecological or family planning services found incidences of 11–32% in one year, and 44–55% in three years (29;31;33;35;36). The incidence of high-risk types, such as HPV-16, is higher than the incidence of low-risk types (28;29;31). For example, in one study, the incidence in one year was 32% for high-risk HPV types compared with 18% for low-risk HPV types (29).

The risk factors consistently associated with HPV infection in women are young age (age less than 25 years) and sexual behavior, specifically number of sex partners, as described below (*Transmission and Prevention of Genital HPV,* page 11). Other risk factors identified include early age of first sexual intercourse, and male partner sexual behavior. Less consistently identified risk factors include smoking, oral contraceptive use, nutritional factors, and lack of circumcision of male partners (20). Many of the identified risk factors are likely markers for unmeasured sexual behavior (21;25;37-39). In addition, immune suppression is associated with HPV detection. Studies in women with HIV infection, undergoing dialysis, or after kidney transplant, demonstrate that HPV detection is particularly common with immune suppression (17;40-43).

The prevalence of genital HPV infection in men is more difficult to assess because it is not clear which are the optimal anatomic sites or specimens to test. Most published studies have been conducted outside the United States, in men attending STD or university clinics, or among male partners of women with HPV infection. HPV DNA can be detected at various anogenital sites, including the penis, urethra, scrotum, or anus, as well as in urine and semen (44-56). In heterosexual men, infection is most commonly detected on the penis (54-57). A recent study that evaluated HPV DNA in the distal penis (urethra, glans, coronal sulcus, foreskin) documented higher prevalence of infection in uncircumcised men than in circumcised men (19.6% vs. 5.5%) (46). Prevalence of genital HPV infection in heterosexual men in the populations studied ranges from 16–45%; detection is highly dependent on the anatomic sites or specimens tested (e.g., urine, semen) (45;46;49;52). Risk factors for HPV detection in men include greater lifetime number of sex partners, number of recent sex partners, being uncircumcised, or current genital warts (45;46;52). The relationship of young age with HPV detection is not as consistent in men as in women (45;49;52).

HPV serologic (blood) tests that detect antibodies to the outer proteins of HPV have been useful in assessing previous HPV infection. They complement the studies that are based on HPV DNA detection because HPV DNA is not persistently detectable in most infected people. However, these tests likely underestimate the true extent of previous infection because only 50–70% of persons with detectable HPV DNA develop antibodies (58-60). A recently completed study of the U.S. population conducted by CDC showed that 18% of women and 7% of men aged 12 to 49 had antibodies to HPV-16 (61). The strongest predictors of antibody positivity in both women and men were various measures of past sexual activity, including lifetime number of partners. Antibody prevalence is substantially higher in populations with greater sexual activity. For example, a study of patients attending a U.S. STD clinic found HPV-16 antibody prevalence rates of 55% in women and 33% in men (62).

Prevalence of Sequelae of Genital HPV Infection
Estimates for genital warts are relatively imprecise; however, limited data suggest that each year in the U.S. as many as 100 per 100,000 persons develop genital warts (63), and 1.4 million currently have genital warts (about one percent of the sexually active U.S. population) (64). Rarely, genital HPV infection with low-risk types may be transmitted from mother to baby during delivery resulting in respiratory tract warts in the baby, an illness known as recurrent respiratory papillomatosis (RRP). Estimates of the incidence rate for RRP are also relatively imprecise, but range from 0.4 to 1.1 cases per 100,000 children (65).

Rates of cervical cancer have fallen by approximately 75% since the introduction of Pap testing programs. Cervical cancer incidence in the U.S. is currently estimated to be 8.3 per 100,000 women, with approximately 12,200 new cases and 4,100 deaths occurring annually (66).

Natural History of Genital HPV Infection
Most HPV infections are transient and asymptomatic, causing no clinical problems. Studies have shown that 70% of new HPV infections clear within one year, and as many as 91% clear within two years (28;33;67;68). The median duration of new infections is typically eight months (28;67). HPV-16 is more likely to persist than other HPV types (28); however, most HPV-16 infections become undetectable within two years (28). Factors associated with persistence include older age, high-risk HPV types, infection with multiple HPV types, and immune suppression (69;70). The gradual development of an effective immune response is thought to be the likely mechanism for HPV DNA clearance.

HPV infection that persists is the most important risk factor for cervical cancer precursors and invasive cervical cancer (15;67;69-71). A recent study found that the risk for developing cervical cancer precursors was 14 times higher for women who had at least three positive tests for high-risk HPV compared with that for women who had negative tests (68). However, most women with persistent HPV infection do not develop low-grade cervical cell abnormalities, cervical cancer precursors or cervical cancer (28;31;68;72).

Skin and mucosal changes caused by genital HPV infection --both genital warts and cervical cell abnormalities-- often go away without treatment, probably as a result of the development of an effective immunologic response. Rates of spontaneous clearance and progression to cancer without treatment vary for low-grade and high-grade cervical cell abnormalities. Low-grade cervical cell abnormalities usually clear spontaneously (60% of cases) and rarely progress to cancer (1%), while high-grade cervical cell abnormalities have lower rates of spontaneous clearance (30–40%) and much higher rates of progression to cancer without treatment (greater than 12%) (73).

In addition to persistent infection with high-risk types of genital HPV, other co-factors appear to be necessary for the development of cervical cancer (74). Factors such as long-term use of oral contraceptives, a high number of live births, and immune suppression have been found in some studies to be associated with cervical cancer (74-81). In addition, recent studies have demonstrated that co-infection with *Chlamydia trachomatis* or herpes simplex virus type-2 (HSV-2), the cause of genital herpes, may increase the risk of both cervical cancer precursors and cervical cancer (81;82).

Transmission and Prevention of Genital HPV Infection

Transmission

Genital HPV infection is primarily transmitted by genital contact, usually through sexual intercourse (20;83). In virtually all studies of HPV prevalence and incidence, the most consistent predictors of infection have been various measures of sexual activity, most importantly, the number of sex partners (28;31;64;84). Among women, the risk of acquiring a genital HPV infection increases with increasing number of lifetime male sex partners (25;26;84-87). Similar to infection with other STD, having sex with a new partner may be a stronger risk factor than having sex with a steady partner (21;31). With each new partner, an adolescent female substantially increases her risk of acquiring genital HPV (31). The source of transmission is usually from persons who are asymptomatic and do not realize they are infected (64). Among women who report no previous sexual intercourse, 0–8% have HPV infection supporting the premise that the major route of transmission is sexual (18-21).

Although less well-examined, another variable that increases a woman's risk of HPV infection is the sexual activity of her partner. A study of adolescent females found that those with a partner who had multiple sex partners were at increased risk of HPV infection (31). A study of college students in Seattle found that those with male sex partners with at least one prior partner had a five-fold increased risk of infection compared to those whose male partners had no prior partners. Women whose male partners had an unknown number of prior sex partners had an even higher (eight-fold) risk for acquiring HPV infection (21). This study also reported that women who had known a sex partner at least eight months before initiating a sexual relationship were less likely to acquire genital HPV infection. It was hypothesized that this was due to a greater chance of spontaneous clearance of infection in men who might have been infected with HPV in a previous sexual relationship (21).

Other types of genital contact in the absence of penetrative intercourse (oral-genital, manual-genital, and genital-genital contact) leading to HPV transmission have been described, but these routes of transmission are less common than sexual intercourse (21;88-90). For example, a recent study of college-aged women in Seattle reported a two-year genital HPV incidence rate of 39% among sexually active women and 8% among women who had not engaged in penetrative vaginal intercourse. Almost all of the infections in women who had not engaged in sexual intercourse appeared to be related to genital contact other than penetrative intercourse (21). This study also found minimal evidence of HPV transmission through oral sex (either transmitted from the genital area to the mouth or the mouth to the genital area) (21). Genital HPV infection also may be transmitted by non-sexual routes, but this is extremely uncommon. Non-sexual routes of genital HPV transmission include transmission from a mother to a newborn baby, which is rare (91;92), and transmission by inanimate objects such as environmental surfaces and clothing, which has been hypothesized but has never been documented (93-96).

Prevention of Genital HPV Infection

Prevention of genital HPV infection is important to reduce the prevalence of genital warts and abnormal Pap tests, as well as cervical cancer. Cervical cancer screening programs have been highly effective in reducing rates of cervical cancer in the United States (97;98); decreasing the incidence of genital HPV infection should also reduce rates of cervical cancer(16).

In general, for a given sexually transmitted disease, the number of new infections transmitted to a susceptible population is a function of three variables: duration of infectiousness, efficiency (likelihood) of transmission of infection, and number of new sex partners a person has while infected (99). In the absence of measures to reduce susceptibility in the population (such as the use of effective vaccines), strategies addressing each of these variables can reduce transmission of infection. Such strategies include reducing the duration of infectiousness by treatment, decreasing the efficiency of transmission by measures aimed at reducing infectivity (e.g., condoms, microbicides), and reducing the number of sex partners. The following is a summary of what is currently known about the value of each of these approaches for preventing genital HPV infection.

Reducing Duration of Infectiousness

The most common approach to reducing infectiousness of an STD is treatment. In contrast to bacterial STD for which transmission can be prevented through curative treatment, there is only limited evidence that treatment of HPV-associated lesions is useful to prevent HPV transmission. There is no effective systemic therapy for genital HPV, as exists for bacterial and some other viral STD. Treatments are directed to lesions associated with HPV, and HPV infections in the absence of detectable disease are not treated. Current treatment options for both genital warts and cervical cancer precursors include various local approaches that remove the lesion (e.g., cryotherapy, electrocautery, laser therapy, surgical excision). Genital warts are also treated with topical pharmacologic agents (100). Treatment of genital warts and cervical cancer precursors might reduce infectiousness (100). Although this premise is difficult to test directly because assays for infectivity do not exist, it is supported by several observations. First, in some studies larger amounts of HPV DNA have been found in high-grade than in low-grade cervical lesions (101). Second, after clearance of genital warts after treatment with immune stimulating drugs (e.g. imiquimod), the amount of HPV DNA in the skin can be reduced (102). Third, clearance of HPV DNA can occur after standard therapy for cervical high-grade lesions (103-111). However, clinically normal skin and mucosa near HPV-associated lesions often contain HPV (112;113). This reservoir is thought to explain the typical recurrence rates of 10–20% after treatment of cervical lesions (114;115) and 20–50% after treatment of genital warts (100). It might also help explain the fact that treatment of partners does not influence recurrence rates of genital warts (116). Thus, based on the limited existing data, currently available therapies for HPV-related lesions may reduce but probably do not eliminate infectiousness; the impact of the reduction in viral concentration which occurs with treatment remains unclear.

Reducing Efficiency of Transmission

Efficiency of transmission, or the likelihood that an infection will be transmitted from an infected person to an uninfected person, can be affected by several variables, such as immunity. However, for STD, the most common approach is the use of physical barriers such as condoms. In the future, other methods that may decrease the likelihood that an infection will be transmitted could include chemical barriers, such as microbicides or a combination of chemical and physical approaches.

Condoms

Evidence for the effectiveness of the male latex condom to prevent various STD among heterosexual men and women was the subject of a recent NIH report (117). The report concluded that for the majority of STD, published data were not adequate to definitively assess the effectiveness of condoms to prevent STD. The review also concluded that most epidemiologic studies that evaluated condom use had significant methodologic problems. For HPV specifically, the NIH report concluded that most of the reviewed studies did not obtain sufficient information on condom use to allow careful evaluation of the association between condom use and HPV infection or disease. The report also concluded that there was no epidemiologic evidence that condom use reduced the risk of HPV infection, but that condom use might afford some protection in reducing the risk of HPV-associated diseases, including warts in men and cervical neoplasia (cervical cancer precursors and invasive cancer) in women (117). More recently, an even more detailed review of the published literature on condoms and HPV infection and its sequelae came to similar conclusions as the NIH report and elaborated on the many methodologic issues affecting studies of condoms for HPV prevention (118). In addition, several other recent studies reported that, for women and men, use of male condoms reduces the risk of genital herpes and chlamydia, both of which may be co-factors for the development of cervical cancer (81;82;119-124). Below is a summary of current scientific evidence on the effectiveness of male condoms for prevention of genital HPV.

As described above, available clinical and epidemiologic data indicate that genital HPV infection is transmitted by contact with infected skin or mucosa. Laboratory studies have demonstrated that latex condoms provide an essentially impermeable barrier to particles the size of HPV (125;126). Studies of HPV infection in men demonstrate that most HPV infections (both HPV DNA and HPV-associated lesions) are located on parts of the penis that would be covered by a condom (48;54-57;63;127-129). However, even consistent and correct use of condoms would not be expected to offer complete protection from HPV infection because infections also may occur on sites not covered or protected by a condom. In men, HPV infection can occur on the scrotum, groin area, base of the penis, and anus (54-57). In women, HPV infection can occur on the outside of the vulva, which can come into contact with the genital skin of a man using a condom

Published studies that have assessed the effectiveness of male condoms to prevent HPV infection or any STD other than HIV are limited by multiple methodologic issues (117;118). In general, these limitations are likely to underestimate condom effectiveness (130-132). Studies with optimal designs would collect information on consistent and correct condom use and would be able to determine whether HPV infection preceded or followed condom use. In addition, several recent studies have demonstrated that many individuals use condoms in situations of perceived STD risk (e.g., with sex partners known to have STD or who have other partners), thereby complicating valid comparisons with those not using condoms, who often have lower sexual risks (133;134). Furthermore, valid estimates of condom effectiveness can be obtained only when users and nonusers have similar levels of exposure to infected partners as illustrated in a recent study of gonorrhea and chlamydia (123). This study showed a protective effect for condoms among persons whose sex partners were known to be infected, but not among those whose partners were not known to be infected. Data on whether partners have HPV infection has not been available for most studies of condoms and HPV infection.

Studying the relationship between condom use and HPV infection is particularly difficult compared to other STD. In contrast to viral STD such as HIV and genital herpes for which highly accurate blood tests allow conclusive determination of infection, accurate blood tests for genital HPV infection do not exist at present. The detectability of HPV DNA in a given individual varies over time (68;135); therefore, determining if a person is infected or if an infection is new or pre-existing is very difficult. Finally, it is also difficult to study outcomes that take many years to develop (e.g., high-grade cervical cell abnormalities, invasive cervical cancer). The optimal study design to ensure valid measurements is a randomized, controlled trial. However, because randomization (assigning some individuals to use condoms and assigning others not to use condoms) can be problematic and potentially unethical (118), this study design is rarely used.

We evaluated 46 peer-reviewed publications in English available after January 1966 that included information on the association between condom use and HPV infection or a sequelae (e.g., genital warts, HPV-associated lesions including cervical cancer precursors, or invasive cervical cancer) (21;26;28;30;31;39;46;48;49;52;84;86;87;136-168). We excluded publications that evaluated HIV-infected persons or used only HPV blood tests. These studies represent a variety of geographic areas and populations. Of the 46 studies, 23 evaluated condom use and prevalent or incident HPV infection by detection of HPV DNA, and 25 evaluated sequelae of infection. The studies of sequelae included five that measured clinical findings of warts or HPV-suggestive lesions on the external genital skin, 10 that measured low- or combined low-grade and high-grade cervical cell abnormalities, six that evaluated high-grade cervical cell abnormalities, and nine that evaluated cervical cancer, six of which were studies of invasive cervical cancer. In most studies, condom use was generally defined broadly, as "ever versus never" or "use versus non-use"; in some studies the definition of condom use was not specified. Only 14 studies measured consistent condom use, and none measured correct use. Forty studies were cross-sectional (so the temporal relationship between condom use and HPV outcome could not be easily determined); two studies were randomized.

Of the 23 studies that measured HPV infection, 18 were conducted in women only, four in men only, and one in both women and men. Estimates of the level of risk reduction varied broadly. Three studies in women reported a protective effect of condoms which was statistically significant (151;152;153). None of the studies measured exposure to infected partners.

Of the 10 studies that measured either low-grade cervical cell abnormalities, or combined low-grade and high-grade cervical cell abnormalities, one study found a statistically significant reduction in cervical cell abnormalities.

Of the five studies that measured external genital HPV-associated lesions, three evaluated women (all genital warts), three evaluated men (one with genital warts and two with HPV suggestive lesions of the penis), and one evaluated both women and men (48;139;142;145;164) Of the three studies in women, one found a statistically significant reduction (30%) in genital warts (164) and one found a reduction in risk that was not statistically significant (142). All three studies in men found statistically significant protection with levels ranging from 30–70% (48;145;164).

Of the six studies that measured cervical cancer precursors (including carcinoma in situ), two studies found a reduction of risk which was statistically significant (136;137;146;154;158;166). Nine studies evaluated women with cervical cancer, six of which were invasive cervical cancer (138;140;143;149;155;156;159;162;166). Of the nine studies, seven found a reduction in risk of cancer in women using condoms, two of which were statistically significant. The reduction in risk ranged from 20–80%.

Three studies evaluated the effect of condoms on clearance of HPV DNA or HPV-associated lesions; all of these studies found a benefit of condom use for both men and women (145;167;168). Two of these studies were the first studies of condoms and HPV infection to be conducted as randomized controlled trials, an approach which can substantially reduce bias. In the randomized studies, monogamous couples were randomized to condom use or nonuse; females with a male partner that used condoms had significantly higher rates of clearance of both HPV infection (53% vs. 35%), and cervical cell changes (23% vs. 4%) than the females whose male partner did not use condoms (168). Also, men in the study had significantly faster regression of genital lesions consistent with HPV infection (167).

Available studies suggest that condoms reduce the risk of the clinically important outcomes of genital warts and cervical cancer. One possible explanation for the protective effect of condoms against warts and cancer is that condom use could reduce the quantity of HPV transmitted or decrease the likelihood of re-exposure, thereby decreasing the chance of developing clinical disease (14;118;168). An alternative explanation is that condom use may reduce exposure to a co-factor for cervical cancer, such as chlamydia or genital herpes, thereby reducing the chance of cervical cancer (81;82;119-122;124;169).

However, all published epidemiologic studies have significant methodologic limitations which make the effect of condoms in prevention of HPV infection unknown. As noted on page 14, three studies on genital HPV and condom use showed a protective effect, but most studies on genital HPV infection and condom use did not show a protective effect.

Given these observations, as well as the facts that laboratory studies show that latex condoms provide a barrier to HPV and that most genital HPV in men is located on areas of the skin covered by a condom, the cumulative body of available scientific evidence suggests that condoms may provide some protection in preventing transmission of HPV infections but that protection is partial at best. The available scientific evidence is not sufficient to recommend condoms as a primary prevention strategy for the prevention of genital HPV infection. There is evidence that indicates that the use of condoms may reduce the risk of cervical cancer.

Microbicides
Evaluation of the ability of microbicides to prevent genital HPV infection has been hampered by the difficulties with in vitro cultivation of HPV (14). Recent laboratory work suggests that some compounds may inhibit HPV (170-174). There are also some reports of a potential effect of microbicides in the prevention of cervical cancer (143;156;159;172;175). Future microbicides may be effective in preventing HPV, as well as other sexually transmitted infections. Clinical studies of some of the compounds found to have an effect on HPV in the laboratory are underway.

Reduction of Sexual Behavior Risk
Because of the important role sexual contact plays in the transmission of genital HPV infection and because of limited evidence that other prevention approaches are highly effective, the most effective personal prevention approach is to avoid contact with genital HPV infection by limiting the number and type of sexual partners. The studies that demonstrate genital HPV transmission by sexual intercourse and other genital contact support the premise that abstaining from all genital contact, including non-penetrative contact, is the most effective approach to preventing infection (21;88;90;176). However, no studies have evaluated the effectiveness of programs which promote limiting the number of partners in preventing genital HPV infection. For individuals who choose to be sexually active, data from studies of both HPV incidence and prevalence support the notion that long-term monogamy with a single partner is likely to be the next most effective approach to prevent infection.

The choice of partner is likely to be important in the success of this approach because approximately 20% of women with only one lifetime sex partner have HPV infection (25;177). Knowing if a man is infected with HPV is difficult because most infected men are asymptomatic (64). Furthermore, testing men to find out if they are infected is impractical because of uncertain sensitivity of HPV testing in men and the lack of a test which has been approved for this purpose. The most important factors that decrease the likelihood that a man is infected with genital HPV include his having had a limited number of prior sex partners (45;52), possibly having a longer period of time since his last partner (allowing prior infections to spontaneously resolve) (21), and being circumcised (46;52). The most important factor that may decrease the likelihood that a woman is infected with genital HPV include her having had a limited number of prior sex partners (21;28). In addition, characteristics which may increase the chance that a partner is infected with genital HPV include the presence of genital warts, an abnormal Pap test in women, and immune suppression (64). However, determining a partner's sexual history or assuring their monogamy in a long-term relationship is sometimes difficult, a problem that could reduce the effectiveness of partner selection approaches to prevention.

Vaccines
In contrast to other prevention approaches, vaccines can reduce susceptibility in uninfected partners by stimulating the immune system. A variety of HPV vaccines are under investigation which may provide immunity to a combination of high-risk or high- and low-risk HPV types

(178). The goals of HPV vaccines are to prevent HPV-associated sequelae including genital warts, cervical cancer precursors, and cervical cancer by preventing HPV infection altogether or by reducing the chance of persistent infection if infection does occur. A recently completed economic model concluded that vaccination for HPV, in combination with continued cervical cancer screening, would be a cost effective health intervention (179). In addition, a recent study projected that an effective vaccine could prevent 1,300 deaths annually from cervical cancer if all 12-year-old girls currently living in the United States were vaccinated (180). Although an effective HPV vaccine would be a major advance in approaches to HPV prevention, it would not replace other prevention strategies such as cervical cancer screening or protective sexual behaviors since vaccines would not work for all genital HPV types and would likely not be 100% effective.

HPV vaccines have shown encouraging success in clinical trials (181). Recently, a vaccine for HPV-16 given to adolescent girls demonstrated 91% efficacy in preventing HPV-16 infection and essentially complete protection (100% efficacy) in preventing persistent HPV-16 infection. Although there were only a few cases, the vaccine also appears promising in the prevention of cervical cancer precursors (181). Studies of other formulations of HPV-16 vaccines as well as vaccines with multiple HPV types are underway and are likely to provide an important new approach for genital HPV prevention within the next several years. Surveys of young women who are potential candidates for an HPV vaccine indicate that they have positive attitudes about receiving a vaccine (182).

Prevention of Cervical Cancer

Decades ago, cervical cancer was one of the most common and deadly cancers in women in the United States (97;183). In the past 40 years, widespread cervical cancer screening using the Pap test, and treatment of precancerous cervical abnormalities have resulted in a dramatic decrease in the incidence and mortality due to cervical cancer in the United States (97;183). The purpose of screening with the Pap test is to detect cervical abnormalities that can be treated, thereby preventing progression to invasive cervical cancer, and also to detect invasive cervical cancer at a very early stage. Progression from cervical cancer precursor lesions to invasive cancer is a slow process, estimated to take 10–15 years (16). If detected early and managed promptly, survival rates for cervical cancer are over 90%. In 2003, an estimated 12,200 women in the U.S. will develop cervical cancer and an estimated 4100 women will die from the disease (66). Approximately half of the cases will occur in women who have never been screened, and an additional 10% will occur in women not screened within the past 5 years (2). A recent national survey indicated that cervical cancer screening is not adequate among some women in the U.S; approximately 18% of women have not had a Pap test in the last 3 years (184). The most important factors associated with inadequate cervical cancer screening include absence of a usual source of health care, lack of health insurance, and immigration to the U.S. in the last 10 years. Other factors included older age, low income, low level of education, presence of chronic disabilities, and Asian and American Indian/Alaska Native race/ethnicity (184). Death rates from cervical cancer in the U.S. are higher among foreign-born women than women born in the U.S. (185).

New technologies including liquid-based cytology and testing for high-risk HPV types may offer potential advantages over conventional Pap testing. The American Cancer Society and other organizations have incorporated these technologies into new guidelines for cervical cancer screening (115;186;187). However, the largest gain in reducing the burden of cervical cancer incidence and deaths could best be achieved by increasing screening rates among women who have never or rarely been screened (186).

Summary of Strategies to Prevent Genital HPV Infection

Based on currently available science, the following recommendations summarize the strategies most likely to be effective in preventing future infections with genital HPV infection and cervical cancer.

Individual Strategies

- The surest way to eliminate the risk for future genital HPV infections is to refrain from any genital contact with another individual.

- For those who choose to be sexually active, a long-term, mutually monogamous relationship with an uninfected partner is the strategy most likely to prevent future genital HPV infections. However, it is difficult to determine whether a partner who has been sexually active in the past is currently infected.

- For those choosing to be sexually active and who are not in long-term mutually monogamous relationships, reducing the number of sexual partners and choosing a partner less likely to be infected may reduce the risk of genital HPV infection. Partners less likely to be infected include those who have had no or few prior sex partners.

- While available scientific evidence suggests that the effect of condoms in preventing HPV infection is unknown, condom use has been associated with lower rates of the HPV-associated diseases of genital warts and cervical cancer. The available scientific evidence is not sufficient to recommend condoms as a primary prevention strategy for the prevention of genital HPV infection, but it does indicate that the use of condoms may reduce the risk of cervical cancer.

- Regular cervical cancer screening for all sexually active women and treatment of precancerous lesions remains the key strategy to prevent cervical cancer.

- In the future, receiving a safe and effective HPV vaccine to help prevent genital HPV infection as well as the HPV-associated diseases of genital warts and cervical cancer would be an important prevention measure. However, an effective HPV vaccine would not replace other prevention strategies.

Public Health Strategies

Public health agencies should:

- Promote increased cervical cancer screening among never and rarely-screened women and appropriate follow-up of those with abnormal Pap tests.

- Work with public and private partners to increase awareness about prevention of genital HPV infection and cervical cancer among health care providers and in the general public.

- Collaborate with private industry to promote and accelerate the development of a safe and effective HPV vaccine.

- Continue epidemiologic, laboratory, and behavioral research on genital HPV infection, including studies of the prevalence of HPV in the United States, research on the attitudes and concerns of women diagnosed with HPV infection (e.g., concerns about cancer or about transmission), and surveys of provider knowledge and practices regarding HPV.

Reference List

(1) Cates W, Jr. Estimates of the incidence and prevalence of sexually transmitted diseases in the United States. American Social Health Association Panel. Sexually Transmitted Diseases 1999; 26(4:Suppl):Suppl-7.

(2) NIH Consensus Statement Online 1996 April 1-3 [October 28, 2003]. pp 1-38.

(3) World Health Organization. IARC Monograph on the Evaluation of Carcinogenic Risks to Humans: Human Papillomaviruses. [64]. 1995. Lyons, IARC.

(4) Daling JR, Weiss NS, Klopfenstein LL, Cochran LE, Chow WH, Daifuku R. Correlates of homosexual behavior and the incidence of anal cancer. JAMA 1982; 247(14):1988-1990.

(5) Daling JR, Weiss NS, Hislop TG, Maden C, Coates RJ, Sherman KJ et al. Sexual practices, sexually transmitted diseases, and the incidence of anal cancer. New England Journal of Medicine 1987; 317(16):973-977.

(6) Holly EA, Whittemore AS, Aston DA, Ahn DK, Nickoloff BJ, Kristiansen JJ. Anal cancer incidence: genital warts, anal fissure or fistula, hemorrhoids, and smoking. Journal of the National Cancer Institute 1989; 81(22):1726-1731.

(7) Koblin BA, Hessol NA, Zauber AG, Taylor PE, Buchbinder SP, Katz MH et al. Increased incidence of cancer among homosexual men, New York City and San Francisco, 1978-1990. American Journal of Epidemiology 1996; 144(10):916-923.

(8) Ries L, Kosery C, Hankey B, MillerB, Clegg L, Edwards B. SEER Cancer Statistics Review 1973-1996. Bethesda, MD: National Cancer Institute, 1999.

(9) Herrero R, Castellsague X, Pawlita M, Lissowska J, Kee F, Balaram P et al. Human papillomavirus and oral cancer: the International Agency for Research on Cancer multicenter study. Journal of the National Cancer Institute 2003; 95(23):1772-1783.

(10) Syrjanen KJ. HPV infections and oesophageal cancer. Journal of Clinical Pathology 2002; 55(10):721-728.

(11) Cuzick J. Human papillomavirus infection of the prostate. Cancer Surveys 1995; 23:91-95.

(12) Adami HO, Kuper H, Andersson SO, Bergstrom R, Dillner J. Prostate cancer risk and serologic evidence of human papilloma virus infection: a population-based case-control study. Cancer Epidemiology, Biomarkers & Prevention 2003; 12(9):872-875.

(13) Rosenblatt KA, Carter JJ, Iwasaki LM, Galloway DA, Stanford JL. Serologic evidence of human papillomavirus 16 and 18 infections and risk of prostate cancer. Cancer Epidemiology, Biomarkers & Prevention 2003; 12(8):763-768.

(14) Division of STD Prevention. Prevention of Genital HPV Infection and Sequelae: Report of an External Consultants' Meeting. 1999. Atlanta, GA., Department of Health and Human Services, Atlanta: Centers for Disease Control and Prevention (CDC).

(15) Koutsky LA, Galloway DA, Holmes KK. Epidemiology of genital human papillomavirus infection. Epidemiologic Reviews 1988; 10:122-163.

(16) Myers ER, McCrory DC, Nanda K, Bastian L, Matchar DB. Mathematical model for the natural history of human papillomavirus infection and cervical carcinogenesis. American Journal of Epidemiology 2000; 151(12):1158-1171.

(17) Weinstock H, Berman S, cates W. Sexually Transmitted Infections in American Youth: Incidence and Prevalence Estimates, 2000. Perspectives on Sexual and Reproductive Health. In press.

(18) Fairley CK, Chen S, Tabrizi SN, Leeton K, Quinn MA, Garland SM. The absence of genital human papillomavirus DNA in virginal women. International Journal of STD & AIDS 1992; 3(6):414-417.

(19) Rylander E, Ruusuvaara L, Almstromer MW, Evander M, Wadell G. The absence of vaginal human papillomavirus 16 DNA in women who have not experienced sexual intercourse. Obstetrics & Gynecology 1994; 83(5:Pt 1):1-7.

(20) Koutsky LA, Kiviat NB. Genital human papillomavirus. In: Holmes KK, Sparling PF, Mardh PA et al, editors. Sexually Transmitted Diseases. New York: McGraw-Hill, 1999: 347-359.

(21) Winer RL, Lee SK, Hughes JP, Adam DE, Kiviat NB, Koutsky LA. Genital human papillomavirus infection: incidence and risk factors in a cohort of female university students. American Journal of Epidemiology 2003; 157(3):218-226.

(22) Baken LA, Koutsky LA, Kuypers J, Kosorok MR, Lee SK, Kiviat NB et al. Genital human papillomavirus infection among male and female sex partners: prevalence and type-specific concordance. Journal of Infectious Diseases 1995; 171(2):429-432.

(23) Bauer HM, Ting Y, Greer CE, Chambers JC, Tashiro CJ, Chimera J et al. Genital human papillomavirus infection in female university students as determined by a PCR-based method. JAMA 1991; 265(4):472-477.

(24) Bauer HM, Hildesheim A, Schiffman MH, Glass AG, Rush BB, Scott DR et al. Determinants of genital human papillomavirus infection in low-risk women in Portland, Oregon. Sexually Transmitted Diseases 1993; 20(5):274-278.

(25) Ley C, Bauer HM, Reingold A, Schiffman MH, Chambers JC, Tashiro CJ et al. Determinants of genital human papillomavirus infection in young women. Journal of the National Cancer Institute 1991; 83(14):997-1003.

(26) Peyton CL, Gravitt PE, Hunt WC, Hundley RS, Zhao M, Apple RJ et al. Determinants of genital human papillomavirus detection in a US population. Journal of Infectious Diseases 2001; 183(11):1554-1564.

(27) Wheeler CM, Parmenter CA, Hunt WC, Becker TM, Greer CE, Hildesheim A et al. Determinants of genital human papillomavirus infection among cytologically normal women attending the University of New Mexico student health center. Sexually Transmitted Diseases 1993; 20(5):286-289.

(28) Ho GY, Bierman R, Beardsley L, Chang CJ, Burk RD. Natural history of cervicovaginal papillomavirus infection in young women. New England Journal of Medicine 1998; 338(7):423-428.

(29) Giuliano AR, Harris R, Sedjo RL, Baldwin S, Roe D, Papenfuss MR et al. Incidence, prevalence, and clearance of type-specific human papillomavirus infections: The Young Women's Health Study. Journal of Infectious Diseases 2002; 186(4):462-469.

(30) Burk RD, Kelly P, Feldman J, Bromberg J, Vermund SH, DeHovitz JA et al. Declining prevalence of cervicovaginal human papillomavirus infection with age is independent of other risk factors. Sexually Transmitted Diseases 1996; 23(4):333-341.

(31) Moscicki AB, Hills N, Shiboski S, Powell K, Jay N, Hanson E et al. Risks for incident human papillomavirus infection and low-grade squamous intraepithelial lesion development in young females. JAMA 2001; 285(23):2995-3002.

(32) Rousseau MC, Pereira JS, Prado JC, Villa LL, Rohan TE, Franco EL. Cervical coinfection with human papillomavirus (HPV) types as a predictor of acquisition and persistence of HPV infection. Journal of Infectious Diseases 2001; 184(12):1508-1517.

(33) Franco EL, Villa LL, Sobrinho JP, Prado JM, Rousseau MC, Desy M et al. Epidemiology of acquisition and clearance of cervical human papillomavirus infection in women from a high-risk area for cervical cancer. Journal of Infectious Diseases 1999; 180(5):1415-1423.

(34) Herrero R, Hildesheim A, Bratti C, Sherman ME, Hutchinson M, Morales J et al. Population-based study of human papillomavirus infection and cervical neoplasia in rural Costa Rica. Journal of the National Cancer Institute 2000; 92(6):464-474.

(35) Sellors JW, Karwalajtys TL, Kaczorowski J, Mahony JB, Lytwyn A, Chong S et al. Incidence, clearance and predictors of human papillomavirus infection in women.[comment]. CMAJ Canadian Medical Association Journal 2003; 168(4):421-425.

(36) Woodman CB, Collins S, Winter H, Bailey A, Ellis J, Prior P et al. Natural history of cervical human papillomavirus infection in young women: a longitudinal cohort study. Lancet 2001; 357(9271):1831-1836.

(37) Franco EL, Duarte-Franco E, Ferenczy A. Cervical cancer: epidemiology, prevention and the role of human papillomavirus infection. CMAJ Canadian Medical Association Journal 2001; 164(7):1017-1025.

(38) Fairley CK, Chen S, Ugoni A, Tabrizi SN, Forbes A, Garland SM. Human papillomavirus infection and its relationship to recent and distant sexual partners. Obstetrics & Gynecology 1994; 84(5):755-759.

(39) Davidson M, Schnitzer PG, Bulkow LR, Parkinson AJ, Schloss ML, Fitzgerald MA et al. The prevalence of cervical infection with human papillomaviruses and cervical dysplasia in Alaska Native women. Journal of Infectious Diseases 1994; 169(4):792-800.

(40) Fairley CK, Chen S, Tabrizi SN, McNeil J, Becker G, Walker R et al. Prevalence of HPV DNA in cervical specimens in women with renal transplants: a comparison with dialysis-dependent patients and patients with renal impairment. Nephrology Dialysis Transplantation 1994; 9(4):416-420.

(41) Moscicki AB, Ellenberg JH, Vermund SH, Holland CA, Darragh T, Crowley-Nowick PA et al. Prevalence of and risks for cervical human papillomavirus infection and squamous intraepithelial lesions in adolescent girls: impact of infection with human immunodeficiency virus. Archives of Pediatrics & Adolescent Medicine 2000; 154(2):127-134.

(42) Jamieson DJ, Duerr A, Burk R, Klein RS, Paramsothy P, Schuman P et al. Characterization of genital human papillomavirus infection in women who have or who are at risk of having HIV infection. American Journal of Obstetrics & Gynecology 2002; 186(1):21-27.

(43) Sun XW, Kuhn L, Ellerbrock TV, Chiasson MA, Bush TJ, Wright TC, Jr. Human papillomavirus infection in women infected with the human immunodeficiency virus. New England Journal of Medicine 1997; 337(19):1343-1349.

(44) Aynaud O, Poveda JD, Huynh B, Guillemotonia A, Barrasso R. Frequency of herpes simplex virus, cytomegalovirus and human papillomavirus DNA in semen. International Journal of STD & AIDS 2002; 13(8):547-550.

(45) Baldwin SB, Wallace DR, Papenfuss MR, Abrahamsen M, Vaught LC, Kornegay JR et al. Human papillomavirus infection in men attending a sexually transmitted disease clinic. Journal of Infectious Diseases 2003; 187(7):1064-1070.

(46) Castellsague X, Bosch FX, Munoz N, Meijer CJ, Shah KV, de Sanjose S et al. Male circumcision, penile human papillomavirus infection, and cervical cancer in female partners. New England Journal of Medicine 2002; 346(15):1105-1112.

(47) Fife KH, Coplan PM, Jansen KU, DiCello AC, Brown DR, Rojas C et al. Poor sensitivity of polymerase chain reaction assays of genital skin swabs and urine to detect HPV 6 and 11 DNA in men. Sexually Transmitted Diseases 2003; 30(3):246-248.

(48) Hippelainen M, Syrjanen S, Hippelainen M, Koskela H, Pulkkinen J, Saarikoski S et al. Prevalence and risk factors of genital human papillomavirus (HPV) infections in healthy males: a study on Finnish conscripts. Sexually Transmitted Diseases 1993; 20(6):321-328.

(49) Lazcano-Ponce E, Herrero R, Munoz N, Hernandez-Avila M, Salmeron J, Leyva A et al. High prevalence of human papillomavirus infection in Mexican males: comparative study of penile-urethral swabs and urine samples. Sexually Transmitted Diseases 2001; 28(5):277-280.

(50) Olatunbosun O, Deneer H, Pierson R. Human papillomavirus DNA detection in sperm using polymerase chain reaction. Obstetrics & Gynecology 2001; 97(3):357-360.

(51) Rintala MA, Pollanen PP, Nikkanen VP, Grenman SE, Syrjanen SM. Human papillomavirus DNA is found in the vas deferens. Journal of Infectious Diseases 2002; 185(11):1664-1667.

(52) Svare EI, Kjaer SK, Worm AM, Osterlind A, Meijer CJ, van den Brule AJ. Risk factors for genital HPV DNA in men resemble those found in women: a study of male attendees at a Danish STD clinic. Sexually Transmitted Infections 2002; 78(3):215-218.

(53) Wikstrom A, Popescu C, Forslund O. Asymptomatic penile HPV infection: a prospective study. International Journal of STD & AIDS 2000; 11(2):80-84.

(54) Van Doornum GJ, Prins M, Juffermans LH, Hooykaas C, van den Hoek JA, Coutinho RA et al. Regional distribution and incidence of human papillomavirus infections among heterosexual men and women with multiple sexual partners: a prospective study. Genitourinary Medicine 1994; 70(4):240-246.

(55) Weaver BA, Feng Q, Holmes KK, Kiviat N, Lee S, Meyer C et al. Evaluation of Genital Sites and Sampling Techniques for HPV DNA Detection in Men. Journal of Infectious Diseases. In press.

(56) Perez J, Trigg B, Wheeler C. Detection of Genital Human Papillomavirus (HPV) in Men Using Different Sampling Strategies. [Abstract P 090] International Papillomavirus Conference, October 4-9, 2002, Paris, France.

(57) Weaver B, Feng Q, Kiviat N, Holmes K, Lee S, Meyer C et al. Evaluation of genital sampling techniques for HPV DNA detection. [Abstract O019] International Papillomavirus Conference October 4-9, 2002. Paris, France.

(58) Carter JJ, Koutsky LA, Hughes JP, Lee SK, Kuypers J, Kiviat N et al. Comparison of human papillomavirus types 16, 18, and 6 capsid antibody responses following incident infection. Journal of Infectious Diseases 2000; 181(6):1911-1919.

(59) Wideroff L, Schiffman M, Haderer P, Armstrong A, Greer CE, Manos MM et al. Seroreactivity to human papillomavirus types 16, 18, 31, and 45 virus-like particles in a case-control study of cervical squamous intraepithelial lesions. Journal of Infectious Diseases 1999; 180(5):1424-1428.

(60) Wideroff L, Schiffman MH, Hoover R, Tarone RE, Nonnenmacher B, Hubbert N et al. Epidemiologic determinants of seroreactivity to human papillomavirus (HPV) type 16 virus-like particles in cervical HPV-16 DNA-positive and-negative women. Journal of Infectious Diseases 1996; 174(5):937-943.

(61) Stone KM, Karem KL, Sternberg MR, McQuillan GM, Poon AD, Unger ER et al. Seroprevalence of Human Papillomavirus Type 16 Infection in the United States. Journal of Infectious Diseases 2002; 186.

(62) Slavinsky J, III, Kissinger P, Burger L, Boley A, DiCarlo RP, Hagensee ME. Seroepidemiology of low and high oncogenic risk types of human papillomavirus in a predominantly male cohort of STD clinic patients. International Journal of STD & AIDS 2001; 12(8):516-523.

(63) Chuang TY, Perry HO, Kurland LT, Ilstrup DM. Condyloma acuminatum in Rochester, Minn., 1950-1978. I. Epidemiology and clinical features. Archives of Dermatology 1984; 120(4):469-475.

(64) Koutsky L. Epidemiology of genital human papillomavirus infection. American Journal of Medicine 1997; 102(5A):3-8.

(65) Armstrong LR, Preston EJ, Reichert M, Phillips DL, Nisenbaum R, Todd NW et al. Incidence and prevalence of recurrent respiratory papillomatosis among children in Atlanta and Seattle. Clinical Infectious Diseases 2000; 31(1):107-109.

(66) ACS. Cancer Facts and Figures 2003.

(67) Molano M, Van den BA, Plummer M, Weiderpass E, Posso H, Arslan A et al. Determinants of clearance of human papillomavirus infections in Colombian women with normal cytology: a population-based, 5-year follow-up study. American Journal of Epidemiology 2003; 158(5):486-494.

(68) Moscicki AB, Shiboski S, Broering J, Powell K, Clayton L, Jay N et al. The natural history of human papillomavirus infection as measured by repeated DNA testing in adolescent and young women. Journal of Pediatrics 1998; 132(2):277-284.

(69) Ho GY, Burk RD, Klein S, Kadish AS, Chang CJ, Palan P et al. Persistent genital human papillomavirus infection as a risk factor for persistent cervical dysplasia. Journal of the National Cancer Institute 1995; 87(18):1365-1371.

(70) Hildesheim A, Schiffman MH, Gravitt PE, Glass AG, Greer CE, Zhang T et al. Persistence of type-specific human papillomavirus infection among cytologically normal women. Journal of Infectious Diseases 1994; 169(2):235-240.

(71) Schlecht NF, Platt RW, Duarte-Franco E, Costa MC, Sobrinho JP, Prado JC et al. Human papillomavirus infection and time to progression and regression of cervical intraepithelial neoplasia. Journal of the National Cancer Institute 2003; 95(17):1336-1343.

(72) Koutsky LA, Holmes KK, Critchlow CW, Stevens CE, Paavonen J, Beckmann AM et al. A cohort study of the risk of cervical intraepithelial neoplasia grade 2 or 3 in relation to papillomavirus infection. New England Journal of Medicine 1992; 327(18):1272-1278.

(73) Ostor AG. Natural history of cervical intraepithelial neoplasia: a critical review. International Journal of Gynecological Pathology 1993; 12(2):186-192.

(74) Munoz N. Human papillomavirus and cancer: the epidemiological evidence. Journal of Clinical Virology 2000; 19(1-2):1-5.

(75) Munoz N, Bosch FX. Epidemiology of cervical cancer. IARC Scientific Publications 1989;(94):9-39.

(76) Smith JS, Green J, Berrington dG, Appleby P, Peto J, Plummer M et al. Cervical cancer and use of hormonal contraceptives: a systematic review. Lancet 2003; 361(9364):1159-1167.

(77) Castellsague X, Bosch FX, Munoz N. Environmental co-factors in HPV carcinogenesis. Virus Research 2002; 89(2):191-199.

(78) Castellsague X, Munoz N. Chapter 3: Cofactors in human papillomavirus carcinogenesis--role of parity, oral contraceptives, and tobacco smoking. Journal of the National Cancer Institute Monographs 2003;(31):20-28.

(79) Hildesheim A, Herrero R, Castle PE, Wacholder S, Bratti MC, Sherman ME et al. HPV co-factors related to the development of cervical cancer: results from a population-based study in Costa Rica. British Journal of Cancer 2001; 84(9):1219-1226.

(80) Sedjo RL, Fowler BM, Schneider A, Henning SM, Hatch K, Giuliano AR. Folate, vitamin B12, and homocysteine status. findings of no relation between human papillomavirus persistence and cervical dysplasia. Nutrition 2003; 19(6):497-502.

(81) Castle PE, Giuliano AR. Chapter 4: Genital tract infections, cervical inflammation, and antioxidant nutrients--assessing their roles as human papillomavirus cofactors. [Review] [50 refs]. Journal of the National Cancer Institute Monographs 2003;(31):29-34.

(82) Smith JS, Munoz N, Herrero R, Eluf-Neto J, Ngelangel C, Franceschi S et al. Evidence for Chlamydia trachomatis as a human papillomavirus cofactor in the etiology of invasive cervical cancer in Brazil and the Philippines. Journal of Infectious Diseases 2002; 185(3):324-331.

(83) Schiffman M, Kjaer SK. Chapter 2: Natural history of anogenital human papillomavirus infection and neoplasia. Journal of the National Cancer Institute Monographs 2003;(31):14-19.

(84) Karlsson R, Jonsson M, Edlund K, Evander M, Gustavsson A, Boden E et al. Lifetime number of partners as the only independent risk factor for human papillomavirus infection: a population-based study. Sexually Transmitted Diseases 1995; 22(2):119-127.

(85) Castle PE, Shields T, Kirnbauer R, Manos MM, Burk RD, Glass AG et al. Sexual behavior, human papillomavirus type 16 (HPV 16) infection, and HPV 16 seropositivity. Sexually Transmitted Diseases 2002; 29(3):182-187.

(86) Burk RD, Ho GY, Beardsley L, Lempa M, Peters M, Bierman R. Sexual behavior and partner characteristics are the predominant risk factors for genital human papillomavirus infection in young women. Journal of Infectious Diseases 1996; 174(4):679-689.

(87) Jamison JH, Kaplan DW, Hamman R, Eagar R, Beach R, Douglas JM, Jr. Spectrum of genital human papillomavirus infection in a female adolescent population. Sexually Transmitted Diseases 1995; 22(4):236-243.

(88) Coutlee F, Trottier AM, Ghattas G, Leduc R, Toma E, Sanche G et al. Risk factors for oral human papillomavirus in adults infected and not infected with human immunodeficiency virus. Sexually Transmitted Diseases 1997; 24(1):23-31.

(89) Fairley CK, Gay NJ, Forbes A, Abramson M, Garland SM. Hand-genital transmission of genital warts? An analysis of prevalence data. Epidemiology & Infection 1995; 115(1):169-176.

(90) Marrazzo JM, Stine K, Koutsky LA. Genital human papillomavirus infection in women who have sex with women: a review. American Journal of Obstetrics & Gynecology 2000; 183(3):770-774.

(91) Watts DH, Koutsky LA, Holmes KK, Goldman D, Kuypers J, Kiviat NB et al. Low risk of perinatal transmission of human papillomavirus: results from a prospective cohort study. American Journal of Obstetrics & Gynecology 1998; 178(2):365-373.

(92) af G, V, Eklund C, Wang Z, Sapp M, Schiller JT, Dillner J et al. A survey of seroprevalence of human papillomavirus types 16, 18 and 33 among children. International Journal of Cancer 1999; 80(4):489-493.

(93) Ferenczy A, Bergeron C, Richart RM. Human papillomavirus DNA in fomites on objects used for the management of patients with genital human papillomavirus infections. Obstetrics & Gynecology 1989; 74(6):950-954.

(94) Roden RB, Lowy DR, Schiller JT. Papillomavirus is resistant to desiccation. Journal of Infectious Diseases 1997; 176(4):1076-1079.

(95) Bergeron C, Ferenczy A, Richart R. Underwear: contamination by human papillomaviruses. American Journal of Obstetrics & Gynecology 1990; 162(1):25-29.

(96) Ferenczy A, Bergeron C, Richart RM. Carbon dioxide laser energy disperses human papillomavirus deoxyribonucleic acid onto treatment fields. American Journal of Obstetrics & Gynecology 1990; 163(4:Pt 1):t-4.

(97) Eddy DM. Screening for cervical cancer. Annals of Internal Medicine 1990; 113(3):214-226.

(98) Kiviat N, Koutsky L, Paavonen J. Cervical Neoplasia and Other STD-Related Genital Tract Neoplasias. Sexually Transmitted Diseases. 3rd Edition. New York: McGraw-Hill, 1999: 811-832.

(99) Garnett GP, Anderson RM. Sexually transmitted diseases and sexual behavior: insights from mathematical models. Journal of Infectious Diseases 1996; 174:Suppl-61.

(100) Beutner KR, Reitano MV, Richwald GA, Wiley DJ. External genital warts: report of the American Medical Association Consensus Conference. AMA Expert Panel on External Genital Warts. Clinical Infectious Diseases 1998; 27(4):796-806.

(101) Abba MC, Mouron SA, Gomez MA, Dulout FN, Golijow CD. Association of human papillomavirus viral load with HPV16 and high-grade intraepithelial lesion. International Journal of Gynecological Cancer 2003; 13(2):154-158.

(102) Tyring SK, Arany I, Stanley MA, Tomai MA, Miller RL, Smith MH et al. A randomized, controlled, molecular study of condylomata acuminata clearance during treatment with imiquimod. Journal of Infectious Diseases 1998; 178(2):551-555.

(103) Costa S, De Simone P, Venturoli S, Cricca M, Zerbini ML, Musiani M et al. Factors predicting human papillomavirus clearance in cervical intraepithelial neoplasia lesions treated by conization. Gynecologic Oncology 2003; 90(2):358-365.

(104) Elfgren K, Jacobs M, Walboomers JM, Meijer CJ, Dillner J. Rate of human papillomavirus clearance after treatment of cervical intraepithelial neoplasia. Obstetrics & Gynecology 2002; 100(5:Pt 1):t-71.

(105) Bollen LJ, Tjong AHS, van d, V, Mol BW, ten Kate FW, ter Schegget J et al. Prediction of recurrent and residual cervical dysplasia by human papillomavirus detection among patients with abnormal cytology. Gynecologic Oncology 1999; 72(2):199-201.

(106) Bodner K, Bodner-Adler B, Wierrani F, Kimberger O, Denk C, Grunberger W. Is therapeutic conization sufficient to eliminate a high-risk HPV infection of the uterine cervix? A clinicopathological analysis. Anticancer Research 2002; 22(6B):3733-3736.

(107) Jain S, Tseng CJ, Horng SG, Soong YK, Pao CC. Negative predictive value of human papillomavirus test following conization of the cervix uteri. Gynecologic Oncology 2001; 82(1):177-180.

(108) Kjellberg L, Wadell G, Bergman F, Isaksson M, Angstrom T, Dillner J. Regular disappearance of the human papillomavirus genome after conization of cervical dysplasia by carbon dioxide laser. American Journal of Obstetrics & Gynecology 2000; 183(5):1238-1242.

(109) Kucera E, Sliutz G, Czerwenka K, Breitenecker G, Leodolter S, Reinthaller A. Is high-risk human papillomavirus infection associated with cervical intraepithelial neoplasia eliminated after conization by large-loop excision of the transformation zone? European Journal of Obstetrics, Gynecology, & Reproductive Biology 2001; 100(1):72-76.

(110) Nagai Y, Maehama T, Asato T, Kanazawa K. Persistence of human papillomavirus infection after therapeutic conization for CIN 3: is it an alarm for disease recurrence? Gynecologic Oncology 2000; 79(2):294-299.

(111) Lin CT, Tseng CJ, Lai CH, Hsueh S, Huang KG, Huang HJ et al. Value of human papillomavirus deoxyribonucleic acid testing after conization in the prediction of residual disease in the subsequent hysterectomy specimen. American Journal of Obstetrics & Gynecology 2001; 184(5):940-945.

(112) Ferenczy A, Mitao M, Nagai N, Silverstein SJ, Crum CP. Latent papillomavirus and recurring genital warts. New England Journal of Medicine 1985; 313(13):784-788.

(113) Colgan TJ, Percy ME, Suri M, Shier RM, Andrews DF, Lickrish GM. Human papillomavirus infection of morphologically normal cervical epithelium adjacent to squamous dysplasia and invasive carcinoma. Human Pathology 1989; 20(4):316-319.

(114) Mitchell MF, Tortolero-Luna G, Cook E, Whittaker L, Rhodes-Morris H, Silva E. A randomized clinical trial of cryotherapy, laser vaporization, and loop electrosurgical excision for treatment of squamous intraepithelial lesions of the cervix. Obstetrics & Gynecology 1998; 92(5):737-744.

(115) Wright TC, Jr., Cox JT, Massad LS, Twiggs LB, Wilkinson EJ, ASCCP-Sponsored Consensus Conference. 2001 Consensus Guidelines for the management of women with cervical cytological abnormalities. JAMA 2002; 287(16):2120-2129.

(116) Krebs HB, Helmkamp BF. Treatment failure of genital condylomata acuminata in women: role of the male sexual partner. American Journal of Obstetrics & Gynecology 1991; 165(2):337-339.

(117) National Institute of Allergy and Infectious Diseases. Workshop Summary: Scientific Evidence on Condom Effectiveness for Sexually Transmitted Disease (STD) Prevention.: 2001.

(118) Manhart LE, Koutsky LA. Do condoms prevent genital HPV infection, external genital warts, or cervical neoplasia? A meta-analysis. Sexually Transmitted Diseases 2002; 29(11):725-735.

(119) Baeten JM, Nyange PM, Richardson BA, Lavreys L, Chohan B, Martin HL, Jr. et al. Hormonal contraception and risk of sexually transmitted disease acquisition: results from a prospective study. American Journal of Obstetrics & Gynecology 2001; 185(2):380-385.

(120) Radcliffe KW, Ahmad S, Gilleran G, Ross JD. Demographic and behavioural profile of adults infected with chlamydia: a case-control study. Sexually Transmitted Infections 2001; 77(4):265-270.

(121) Wald A, Langenberg D, Kexel E, Izu A, Ashley R, Corey L. [abstract B9E] National STD Prevention Conference, San Diego, CA, March 4-7, 2002. 3-4-0002.

(122) Wald A, Langenberg AG, Link K, Izu AE, Ashley R, Warren T et al. Effect of condoms on reducing the transmission of herpes simplex virus type 2 from men to women. JAMA 2001; 285(24):3100-3106.

(123) Warner L, Newman DR, Austin HA, Kamb ML, Douglas JM, Malotte CK et al. Condom Effectiveness for Reducing Transmission of Gonorrhea and Chlamydia: The Importance of Assessing Partner Infection Status. American Journal of Epidemiology. In press.

(124) Williams KM, Wingood GM, DiClemente RJ, Crosby RA, Hubbard MD, Liau A et al. Prevalence and correlates of Chlamydia trachomatis among sexually active African-American adolescent females. Preventive Medicine 2002; 35(6):593-600.

(125) Lytle CD, Duff JE, Fleharty B, Bidinger RL, Cyr WH, Routson LB. A sensitive method for evaluating condoms as virus barriers. Journal of AOAC International 1997; 80(2):319-324.

(126) Lytle CD, Routson LB, Seaborn GB, Dixon LG, Bushar HF, Cyr WH. An in vitro evaluation of condoms as barriers to a small virus. Sexually Transmitted Diseases 1997; 24(3):161-164.

(127) Kennedy L, Buntine DW, O'Connor D, Frazer IH. Human papillomavirus--a study of male sexual partners. Medical Journal of Australia 1988; 149(6):309-311.

(128) Krebs HB, Schneider V. Human papillomavirus-associated lesions of the penis: colposcopy, cytology, and histology. Obstetrics & Gynecology 1987; 70(3:Pt 1):t-304.

(129) Schultz RE, Miller JW, MacDonald GR, Auman JR, Peterson NR, Ward BE et al. Clinical and molecular evaluation of acetowhite genital lesions in men. Journal of Urology 1990; 143(5):920-923.

(130) Zenilman JM, Weisman CS, Rompalo AM, Ellish N, Upchurch DM, Hook EW, III et al. Condom use to prevent incident STDs: the validity of self-reported condom use. Sexually Transmitted Diseases 1995; 22(1):15-21.

(131) Weir SS, Feldblum PJ. Condom use to prevent incident STDs. Sexually Transmitted Diseases 1996; 23(1):76-77.

(132) Galavotti C, Cabral R, Beeker C. Condom use to prevent incident STDs. Sexually Transmitted Diseases 1996; 23(1):77-79.

(133) Turner CF, Miller HG. Zenilman's anomaly reconsidered: fallible reports, ceteris paribus, and other hypotheses. Sexually Transmitted Diseases 1997; 24(9):522-527.

(134) Peterman TA, Lin LS, Newman DR, Kamb ML, Bolan G, Zenilman J et al. Does measured behavior reflect STD risk? An analysis of data from a randomized controlled behavioral intervention study. Project RESPECT Study Group. Sexually Transmitted Diseases 2000; 27(8):446-451.

(135) Schneider A, Kirchhoff T, Meinhardt G, Gissmann L. Repeated evaluation of human papillomavirus 16 status in cervical swabs of young women with a history of normal Papanicolaou smears. Obstetrics & Gynecology 1992; 79(5:(Pt 1):t-8.

(136) Adam E, Berkova Z, Daxnerova Z, Icenogle J, Reeves WC, Kaufman RH. Papillomavirus detection: demographic and behavioral characteristics influencing the identification of cervical disease. American Journal of Obstetrics & Gynecology 2000; 182(2):257-264.

(137) Becker TM, Wheeler CM, McGough NS, Parmenter CA, Jordan SW, Stidley CA et al. Sexually transmitted diseases and other risk factors for cervical dysplasia among southwestern Hispanic and non-Hispanic white women. JAMA 1994; 271(15):1181-1188.

(138) Donnan SP, Wong FW, Ho SC, Lau EM, Takashi K, Esteve J. Reproductive and sexual risk factors and human papilloma virus infection in cervical cancer among Hong Kong Chinese. International Journal of Epidemiology 1989; 18(1):32-36.

(139) Evans BA, Tasker T, MacRae KD. Risk profiles for genital infection in women. Genitourinary Medicine 1993; 69(4):257-261.

(140) Fasal E, Simmons ME, Kampert JB. Factors associated wih high and low risk of cervical neoplasia. Journal of the National Cancer Institute 1981; 66(4):631-636.

(141) Figueroa JP, Ward E, Luthi TE, Vermund SH, Brathwaite AR, Burk RD. Prevalence of human papillomavirus among STD clinic attenders in Jamaica: association of younger age and increased sexual activity. Sexually Transmitted Diseases 1995; 22(2):114-118.

(142) Fonck K, Kidula N, Kirui P, Ndinya-Achola J, Bwayo J, Claeys P et al. Pattern of sexually transmitted diseases and risk factors among women attending an STD referral clinic in Nairobi, Kenya. Sexually Transmitted Diseases 2000; 27(7):417-423.

(143) Hildesheim A, Brinton LA, Mallin K, Lehman HF, Stolley P, Savitz DA et al. Barrier and spermicidal contraceptive methods and risk of invasive cervical cancer. Epidemiology 1990; 1(4):266-272.

(144) Hillman RJ, Ryait BK, Botcherby M, Taylor-Robinson D. Human papillomavirus DNA in the urogenital tracts of men with gonorrhoea, penile warts or genital dermatoses. Genitourinary Medicine 1993; 69(3):187-192.

(145) Hippelainen MI, Hippelainen M, Saarikoski S, Syrjanen K. Clinical course and prognostic factors of human papillomavirus infections in men. Sexually Transmitted Diseases 1994; 21(5):272-279.

(146) Ho GY, Kadish AS, Burk RD, Basu J, Palan PR, Mikhail M et al. HPV 16 and cigarette smoking as risk factors for high-grade cervical intra-epithelial neoplasia. International Journal of Cancer 1998; 78(3):281-285.

(147) Juarez-Figueroa LA, Wheeler CM, Uribe-Salas FJ, Conde-Glez CJ, Zampilpa-Mejia LG, Garcia-Cisneros S et al. Human papillomavirus: a highly prevalent sexually transmitted disease agent among female sex workers from Mexico City. Sexually Transmitted Diseases 2001; 28(3):125-130.

(148) Kataja V, Syrjanen S, Yliskoski M, Hippelinen M, Vayrynen M, Saarikoski S et al. Risk factors associated with cervical human papillomavirus infections: a case-control study. American Journal of Epidemiology 1993; 138(9):735-745.

(149) Kjaer SK, de Villiers EM, Dahl C, Engholm G, Bock JE, Vestergaard BF et al. Case-control study of risk factors for cervical neoplasia in Denmark. I: Role of the "male factor" in women with one lifetime sexual partner. International Journal of Cancer 1991; 48(1):39-44.

(150) Kjaer SK, van den Brule AJ, Bock JE, Poll PA, Engholm G, Sherman ME et al. Determinants for genital human papillomavirus (HPV) infection in 1000 randomly chosen young Danish women with normal Pap smear: are there different risk profiles for oncogenic and nononcogenic HPV types? Cancer Epidemiology, Biomarkers & Prevention 1997; 6(10):799-805.

(151) Kjaer SK, Svare EI, Worm AM, Walboomers JM, Meijer CJ, van den Brule AJ. Human papillomavirus infection in Danish female sex workers. Decreasing prevalence with age despite continuously high sexual activity. Sexually Transmitted Diseases 2000; 27(8):438-445.

(152) Kotloff KL, Wasserman SS, Russ K, Shapiro S, Daniel R, Brown W et al. Detection of genital human papillomavirus and associated cytological abnormalities among college women. Sexually Transmitted Diseases 1998; 25(5):243-250.

(153) Mayaud P, Gill DK, Weiss HA, Uledi E, Kopwe L, Todd J et al. The interrelation of HIV, cervical human papillomavirus, and neoplasia among antenatal clinic attenders in Tanzania. Sexually Transmitted Infections 2001; 77(4):248-254.

(154) Munoz N, Bosch FX, de Sanjose S, Vergara A, del Moral A, Munoz MT et al. Risk factors for cervical intraepithelial neoplasia grade III/carcinoma in situ in Spain and Colombia. Cancer Epidemiology, Biomarkers & Prevention 1993; 2(5):423-431.

(155) Parazzini F, Negri E, La Vecchia C, Fedele L. Barrier methods of contraception and the risk of cervical neoplasia. Contraception 1989; 40(5):519-530.

(156) Peters RK, Thomas D, Hagan DG, Mack TM, Henderson BE. Risk factors for invasive cervical cancer among Latinas and non-Latinas in Los Angeles County. Journal of the National Cancer Institute 1986; 77(5):1063-1077.

(157) Sellors J, Mahoney JB, Kacqorowski J, et al. Prevalence and predictors of human papillomavirus infection in women in Ontario, Canada. Can Med Assoc J 2000; 163:503-508.

(158) Shlay JC, McGill WL, Masloboeva HA, Douglas JM, Jr. Pap smear screening in an urban STD clinic. Yield of screening and predictors of abnormalities. Sexually Transmitted Diseases 1998; 25(9):468-475.

(159) Slattery ML, Overall JC, Jr., Abbott TM, French TK, Robison LM, Gardner J. Sexual activity, contraception, genital infections, and cervical cancer: support for a sexually transmitted disease hypothesis. American Journal of Epidemiology 1989; 130(2):248-258.

(160) Svare EI, Kjaer SK, Worm AM, Osterlind A, Moi H, Christensen RB et al. Risk factors for HPV infection in women from sexually transmitted disease clinics: comparison between two areas with different cervical cancer incidence. International Journal of Cancer 1998; 75(1):1-8.

(161) Syrjanen K, Vayrynen M, Castren O, Yliskoski M, Mantyjarvi R, Pyrhonen S et al. Sexual behaviour of women with human papillomavirus (HPV) lesions of the uterine cervix. British Journal of Venereal Diseases 1984; 60(4):243-248.

(162) Thomas DB, Ray RM, Pardthaisong T, Chutivongse S, Koetsawang S, Silpisornkosol S et al. Prostitution, condom use, and invasive squamous cell cervical cancer in Thailand. American Journal of Epidemiology 1996; 143(8):779-786.

(163) Wang PD LR. Risk factors for cervical intraepithelial neoplasia in Taiwan. Gynecologic Oncology 1996; 62:10-18.

(164) Wen LM, Estcourt CS, Simpson JM, Mindel A. Risk factors for the acquisition of genital warts: are condoms protective? Sexually Transmitted Infections 1999; 75(5):312-316.

(165) Young TK, McNicol P, Beauvais J. Factors associated with human papillomavirus infection detected by polymerase chain reaction among urban Canadian aboriginal and non-aboriginal women.[comment]. Sexually Transmitted Diseases 1997; 24(5):293-298.

(166) Zondervan KT, Carpenter LM, Painter R, Vessey MP. Oral contraceptives and cervical cancer--further findings from the Oxford Family Planning Association contraceptive study. British Journal of Cancer 1996; 73(10):1291-1297.

(167) Bleeker MC, Hogewoning CJ, van den Brule AJ, Voorhorst FJ, Van Andel RE, Risse EK et al. Penile lesions and human papillomavirus in male sexual partners of women with cervical intraepithelial neoplasia. Journal of the American Academy of Dermatology 2002; 47(3):351-357.

(168) Hogewoning CJ, Bleeker MC, Van den Brule AJ, Voorhorst FJ, Snijders PJ, Berkhof J et al. Condom use promotes regression of cervical intraepithelial neoplasia and clearance of human papillomavirus: a randomized clinical trial. Int.J.Cancer 107, 811-816. 2003.

(169) Manhart LE, Koutsky LA. Do condoms prevent genital HPV infection, external genital warts, or cervical neoplasia? A meta-analysis. Sexually Transmitted Diseases 2002; 29(11):725-735.

(170) Sokal DC, Hermonat PL. Inactivation of papillomavirus by low concentrations of povidone-iodine. Sexually Transmitted Diseases 1995; 22(1):22-24.

(171) Howett MK, Neely EB, Christensen ND, Wigdahl B, Krebs FC, Malamud D et al. A broad-spectrum microbicide with virucidal activity against sexually transmitted viruses. Antimicrobial Agents & Chemotherapy 1999; 43(2):314-321.

(172) Christensen ND, Reed CA, Culp TD, Hermonat PL, Howett MK, Anderson RA et al. Papillomavirus microbicidal activities of high-molecular-weight cellulose sulfate, dextran sulfate, and polystyrene sulfonate. Antimicrobial Agents & Chemotherapy 2001; 45(12):3427-3432.

(173) Coutlee F, Voyer H. Effect of nonionic detergents on amplification of human papillomavirus DNA with consensus primers MY09 and MY11. Journal of Clinical Microbiology 1998; 36(4):1164.

(174) Anwar H, Coetzee N, Blanchard K, Dangor Y, de Kock A, Friedland B et al. A randomized, placebo-controlled double-blind expanded safety trial of carraguard microbicide gel in South Africa: RTI/STI at Baseline and Follow-up. [Abstract] May 12-15, 2002.Antwerp, Belgium.

(175) Celentano DD, Klassen AC, Weisman CS, Rosenshein NB. The role of contraceptive use in cervical cancer: the Maryland Cervical Cancer Case-Control Study. American Journal of Epidemiology 1987; 126(4):592-604.

(176) Fairley CK, Gay NJ, Forbes A, Abramson M, Garland SM. Hand-genital transmission of genital warts? An analysis of prevalence data. Epidemiology & Infection 1995; 115(1):169-176.

(177) Collins S, Mazloomzadeh S, Winter H, Blomfield P, Bailey A, Young LS et al. High incidence of cervical human papillomavirus infection in women during their first sexual relationship. BJOG: an International Journal of Obstetrics & Gynaecology 2002; 109(1):96-98.

(178) Lowy DR, Frazer IH. Chapter 16: Prophylactic human papillomavirus vaccines. Journal of the National Cancer Institute Monographs 2003;(31):111-116.

(179) Kulasingam SL, Myers ER. Potential health and economic impact of adding a human papillomavirus vaccine to screening programs. JAMA 2003; 290(6):781-789.

(180) Sanders GD, Taira AV. Cost-effectiveness of a potential vaccine for human papillomavirus. Emerging Infectious Diseases 2003; 9(1):37-48.

(181) Koutsky LA, Ault KA, Wheeler CM, Brown DR, Barr E, Alvarez FB et al. A controlled trial of a human papillomavirus type 16 vaccine. New England Journal of Medicine 2002; 347(21):1645-1651.

(182) Kahn JA, Rosenthal SL, Hamann T, Bernstein DI. Attitudes about human papillomavirus vaccine in young women. International Journal of STD & AIDS 2003; 14(5):300-306.

(183) Kiviat NB, Critchlow CW, Holmes KK, Kuypers J, Sayer J, Dunphy C et al. Association of anal dysplasia and human papillomavirus with immunosuppression and HIV infection among homosexual men. AIDS 1993; 7(1):43-49.

(184) Swan J, Breen N, Coates RJ, Rimer BK, Lee NC. Progress in cancer screening practices in the United States: results from the 2000 National Health Interview Survey. Cancer 2003; 97(6):1528-1540.

(185) Seeff LC, McKenna MT. Cervical cancer mortality among foreign-born women living in the United States, 1985 to 1996. Cancer Detection & Prevention 2003; 27(3):203-208.

(186) Saslow D, Runowicz CD, Solomon D, Moscicki AB, Smith RA, Eyre HJ et al. American Cancer Society guideline for the early detection of cervical neoplasia and cancer. Ca: a Cancer Journal for Clinicians 2002; 52(6):342-362.

(187) American College of Obstetricians and Gynecologists. Cervical Cytology Screening. Clinical Management Guidelines for Obstetrician-Gynecologists. ACOG Practice Bulletin, No. 45. August, 2003. 2003.

REPORT TO CONGRESS

Human Papillomavirus: Surveillance and Prevention Research

Julie Louise Gerberding, M.D., M.P.H.
Director
Centers for Disease Control and Prevention
August 2003

Executive Summary

Human papillomavirus (HPV) is a virus that infects the skin and mucous membranes. More than 100 types have been identified. Some infect the hands and feet causing common warts, while others are sexually transmitted and infect the genital area. Over 30 HPV types infect the genital region: some cause clinically apparent genital warts and also low-grade Papanicolaou (Pap) smear abnormalities, but are not associated with cervical cancer and are thus termed "low-risk" types. Other types are considered "high-risk" because they can cause cervical and other anogenital cancers. However, the vast majority of infections with both high and low risk types resolve and do not lead to abnormal growths or cancer.

In the United States, approximately 20 million people are infected with genital HPV, and more than 5 million new infections occur annually. It is estimated that 50-75 percent of sexually active people will acquire genital HPV at some point in their lives making this the most common sexually transmitted infection in the United States. Genital HPV infections are not curable; however the vast majority resolve without long term consequences.

On December 20, 2000, Congress passed Public Law 106-554, which includes new provisions concerning HPV. This legislation requires that the Centers for Disease Control and Prevention (CDC):

Conduct sentinel surveillance and special studies to determine the prevalence of HPV in the United States;
Conduct behavioral and other research on the impact of HPV-related diagnosis on individuals; formative research to assist with the development of educational messages; surveys of physician and public knowledge, attitudes, and practices about genital HPV infection;
Upon the completion of formative research, develop and disseminate educational materials for the public and healthcare providers regarding HPV and its impact and prevention.
Provide a progress and final report to Congress.

Since the law's enactment, the CDC has implemented the following activities:

Initiated sentinel surveillance activities in collaboration with six health departments throughout the country to determine the prevalence in various age groups and populations of specific types of HPV infection in the United States.
Initiated collection of additional HPV prevalence and surveillance information in nationally representative population samples, using CDC's National Health and Nutrition Examination Survey (NHANES) that will provide specific information on HPV 16, one of the most common high-risk types of HPV associated with cervical cancer.

Initiated several formative research activities to assess knowledge and attitudes of the public and HPV-infected individuals about HPV healthcare-seeking and sexual behaviors and HPV information needs.
Completed formative research to develop a provider survey that will assess knowledge, attitudes and practices regarding HPV diagnoses and treatment and developed a draft provider survey and a sampling plan. A package describing the study is under development and will be submitted to the Office of Management and Budget (OMB) by September 2003. The provider survey will assess perceptions, practice barriers, and facilitators regarding HPV risk assessment, testing, treatment, counseling, and partner services.

Centers for Disease Control and Prevention
Report to Congress on Human Papillomavirus:
Surveillance and Prevention Research

Human papillomavirus (HPV) is a virus that infects the skin and mucous membranes. More than 100 types have been identified. Some infect the hands and feet causing common warts, while others are sexually transmitted and infect the genital area. Over 30 HPV types infect the genital region: some cause clinically apparent genital warts and also low-grade Papanicolaou (Pap) smear abnormalities, but are not associated with cervical cancer and are thus termed "low-risk" types. Other types are considered "high-risk" because they can cause cervical and other anogenital cancers. However, the vast majority of infections with both high and low risk types resolve without treatment and do not lead to abnormal growths or cancer.

In the United States, approximately 20 million people are infected with genital HPV, and more than 5 million new infections occur annually. It is estimated that 50-75 percent of sexually active people will acquire genital HPV at some point in their lives making this the most common sexually transmitted infection in the United States. Genital HPV infections are not curable; however the vast majority resolve without long term consequences.

On December 20, 2000, Congress passed Public Law 106-554 which included new HPV provisions. This legislation requires that the Centers for Disease Control and Prevention (CDC):

> Conduct sentinel surveillance and special studies to determine the prevalence of HPV in the United States;
> Conduct behavioral and other research on the impact of HPV-related diagnosis on individuals; formative research to assist with the development of educational messages; surveys of physician and public knowledge, attitudes, and practices about genital HPV infection;
> Upon the completion of research and surveys, develop and disseminate educational materials for the public and healthcare providers regarding HPV and its impact and prevention.
> Provide a progress and final report to Congress.

A copy of this legislation is included as Appendix A.

1. Sentinel Surveillance and Special Research Studies

Surveillance Research Section 317 P (a) (1), authorizes the Secretary, through the Director of CDC, to (A) enter into cooperative agreements with states and other entities to conduct sentinel surveillance or other special studies that would determine the prevalence in various age groups and populations of specific types of HPV at different sites in various regions of the United States ..., and (B) develop and analyze data from the HPV sentinel surveillance system described above."

CDC is determining the prevalence of genital HPV infection in the United States in two ways: (1) conducting sentinel surveillance for HPV infection among women in selected clinical facilities from locations throughout the United States; and (2) conducting a special study incorporating testing for genital HPV infection into the National Health and Nutrition Examination Survey (NHANES).

(a) Sentinel Surveillance

CDC awarded funds to six health departments to conduct surveillance and monitor genital HPV prevalence over time, and examine risk factors associated with genital HPV infection. These six health departments, four state and two local, (i.e., Seattle, Washington; Baltimore, Maryland; Massachusetts, Colorado, Louisiana, and Los Angeles) are enrolling women in this study through 35 clinics. These clinics, which must approve the research before it's initiated, include sexually transmitted disease, family planning, HIV-care, and primary care clinics.

The 35 clinics are monitored by 12 local Institutional Review Boards (IRBs). In November 2002, CDC received approval from its IRB for this research, and from January through July 2003, nine of the 12 local IRB's approved the research in 32 of the 35 clinical sites. Grantees have begun to collect data in the 32 clinics that have received IRB approval. It is expected that data analysis will begin in fall 2004, once 12 months of data are collected from all 35 sites. Data analysis will be completed 6 months thereafter. Currently, CDC has received 588 data records from five of the six grantees. Of these 588 data records, 471 records are complete, providing preliminary data indicating an overall prevalence of 29.7 percent for high-risk types of genital HPV (HR-HPV) with a range from 26.1 percent reported in primary care settings to 38.5 percent reported in HIV care settings. Final analysis of these data are expected to begin in fall 2006, once 36 months of data are collected from all 35 sites. This analysis will be completed six months thereafter.

(b) Special Research Studies

CDC is also conducting a research study on genital HPV prevalence by incorporating HPV testing into the procedures of NHANES. This is an ongoing survey designed to be a representative sample of the non-institutionalized U.S. civilian population. Three years of NHANES data are needed to obtain an adequate sample for estimates of genital HPV prevalence.

The purpose of this study is:

> To determine prevalence of genital HPV DNA, in vaginal specimens, among a nationally representative sample of 14-59 year old women. (Prevalence of genital HPV in men is difficult to determine because HPV sampling methods in men are not well defined. This is currently an area of active research as CDC is collaborating with University of Arizona on a research study to determine which genital specimens are optimal for HPV detection in men.)

To determine seroprevalence of antibody to HPV-16 among a nationally representative sample of 14-59 year old men and women.

Both genital HPV DNA testing (using vaginal swabs to determine currently detectable infection) and blood testing (using serum to determine past infection) are necessary to establish optimal prevalence estimates for the U.S. population. A previous CDC study of stored blood collected from 1991 to 1994 showed that 18 percent of women and 8 percent of men had HPV-16 antibodies. In addition, a recent CDC study of stored blood from men and women attending U.S. STD clinics from 1993 – 1995 found that 30 percent of women and 19 percent of men had HPV-16 antibody. Because fewer than 60 percent of women with HPV-16 DNA have a detectable HPV-16 antibody response and because antibody becomes undetectable over time in some persons who have been infected, measuring antibody prevalence without simultaneously measuring DNA prevalence seriously underestimates total prevalence of HPV-16 infection.

This study includes the use of self-collected vaginal swabs by women participants, a new technique. Therefore, a pilot study was performed to assess the feasibility and evaluation of this new technique before the procedure would be included in the national survey. This study was approved in July 2001 and conducted from September to December 2001. The pilot study demonstrated that self-collected vaginal swabs were acceptable to women; therefore, specimen collection as part of the national survey began in January 2002.

Three years of data collection are required to have a sample size large enough to be appropriately analyzed. In December 2004, the data collection will be completed, and in March 2005, the data will be analyzed.

Prevention Research

Section 317 P (b)(1) directs CDC to conduct prevention research on HPV to include: (a) behavioral and other research on the impact of HPV-related diagnosis on individuals; (b) formative research to assist with the development of educational messages and information for the public, for patients, and for their partners, about HPV; (c) surveys of physician and public knowledge, attitudes, and practices about genital HPV infection; and (d) development and dissemination of educational materials for the public and health care providers regarding HPV and its impact and prevention.

To meet these requirements, CDC has organized three key activities: (a) a multisite behavioral study to better characterize the impact of HPV-related diagnosis on individuals and to assist in development of educational messages for patients and their partners; (b) surveys of physician knowledge, attitudes, and practices about genital HPV infection; and (c) surveys of public knowledge, attitudes, and practices about genital HPV infection. The final activity, development and dissemination of educational materials, will be based on the results of the three key activities.

(a) A multisite behavioral study of the impact of HPV-related diagnosis

In September 2001, CDC funded five, 3-year projects to support different, but complementary, formative research projects among women with high-risk HPV (HR-HPV)-related diagnoses, their partners, and the providers who care for them. Three of the projects are being conducted by the University of South Carolina, University of Oklahoma Health Sciences Center, and the University of South Florida. The other two projects are being conducted by the Los Angeles County Health Department and the State of Washington Health Department. The projects are being conducted in two phases. The qualitative phase (Phase I) uses focus groups and in-depth interviews to assess knowledge, attitudes, behaviors, and the impact of a HR-HPV diagnosis on women and their sexual partners. Preliminary data from Phase I are being used to inform the development of a quantitative questionnaire to be used in Phase II. This questionnaire will assess the impact of a HR-HPV diagnosis on women and differences in impact and health care needs among different populations of women.

The qualitative protocols of all five projects were reviewed and approved by the IRB at CDC and the local university and project data collection sites. The qualitative phase has been completed by two projects (University of South Florida and University of South Carolina). Interim data from the University of South Florida and University of South Carolina sites will be available in fall 2003, and an interim report is expected to be completed by November 2003. This interim report will include data collected from in-depth interviews with African American, Caucasian and Hispanic women. Health care providers will focus on knowledge, attitudes, behaviors and the impact of a HR-HPV diagnosis on women, and health care providers' perceptions of the informational needs of HR-HPV positive patients.

One project (the University of Oklahoma) has been unable to complete the qualitative phase of the study due to changes in medical research partnerships. The two other projects began recruiting for the qualitative phase in July 2003. A final report on the qualitative phase from all five sites is expected in March 2004.

Preliminary qualitative data from the University of South Florida, the University of Oklahoma, and the University of South Carolina indicate a pervasive lack of knowledge about HPV prior to diagnosis. Women are largely unaware of the relationship between Pap tests and genital HPV infection, and few women understand the link between genital HPV and cervical cancer. Women expressed a variety of reactions to their HPV diagnosis, including anger, sadness, fear, concerns about treatment options, anxiety about fertility, concerns about impact on future sexual activity, and questions about follow-up care. Common questions from HPV-positive women related to the nature of, and their acquisition of, HPV: "What is HPV? When did I get HPV? Who did I get it from?" Participants in the study expressed concerns about notifying sexual partners about their HPV diagnosis, but most were willing to do so.

The participants received information about genital HPV from several sources, including providers, friends, family members, and the Internet. Providers were indicated as a trusted source of information, but women acknowledged that they had additional questions remaining after their consultations with providers.

An initial review of the formative data, suggests that educational messages about genital HPV infection must contain simple, understandable definitions of the diagnosis, as well as recommendations for treatment and follow-up testing. Messages should address questions of source of infection, duration of infection, likelihood of progression to cancer, and whether HPV has an impact upon fertility. In addition, messages should include suggestions for disclosure to male sexual partners, recommendations for medical follow-up for men, and messages about the likelihood of, and prevention of, genital HPV transmission to new partners. Finally, messages should include statements of the prevalence of genital HPV and suggestions for identifying a social support network related to HPV.

Two of the projects, University of South Florida and University of South Carolina, have begun Phase II. Interim Phase II data from the University of South Florida and the University of South Carolina sites are expected to be available in summer 2004, and an interim report from these two projects is expected to be completed by October 2004. A final report on Phase II from all five projects is expected in March 2005. The final report will contain data from a quantitative instrument administered by all sites. Common core elements for the instrument were developed from the qualitative research and include the following: HPV knowledge; counseling information received from health care providers after a HR-HPV diagnosis; often used, most trusted, and preferred sources for HPV educational information; disclosure of HPV diagnosis; sexual history, practices and behaviors; partners' responses to HPV diagnosis; emotional impact of a HR-HPV test result; and HPV vaccine acceptability. The study population for Phase II will include African American, Caucasian, Hispanic, Asian and American Indian HR-HPV positive and negative women. Data analysis will compare women by ethnicity, time since HR-HPV diagnosis, and HR-HPV status.

Findings from all five projects will be used to assist with the development of educational messages and information about HR-HPV for the public, patients, and their partners.

(b) Surveys of Physician Knowledge, Attitudes, and Practices about Genital HPV Infection

In September 2001, CDC awarded a contract to assess providers' knowledge, attitudes, and practices related to genital HPV infection; to assess providers' perceptions of risks and benefits of HPV testing and counseling; to determine barriers and facilitators to appropriate HPV prevention, testing, and counseling practices; and to assess perceptions about offering HPV testing and counseling in the future. The survey consists of three phases.

Phase 1, has been completed. This phase included a series of key informant interviews with researchers, clinicians, and representatives from organizations and agencies with an interest in genital HPV.

Phase 2, which has also been completed, included a subsequent series of focus groups and in-depth interviews with health care providers. The purpose of the focus groups and in-depth interviews was to inform the development of Phase 3, a national survey of a large number of physicians from a variety of practice settings. The data from the focus group interviews are currently being analyzed and a summary of the findings will be available in fall 2003.

Phase 3 will focus on health care provider knowledge, attitudes, and practices relative to adult and adolescent men and women who are at risk for HPV infection, those who have genital warts, and those with a positive HR-HPV test. The sample will include primary care providers caring for sexually active patients infected with or at risk for acquiring genital HPV infection, and specialty care providers managing patients with genital warts, patients with genital HPV infection, and women with low-grade cervical cytologic abnormalities. A variety of other provider types, including nurse practitioners, nurse-midwives, and physician assistants will be included. Pilot testing was recently completed and the survey will be ready to submit to OMB for clearance by September 2003. We anticipate the OMB review process to be complete by January 2004, and the initiation of the survey to begin in February 2004. Data collection should be completed by June 2004, with data entry and analysis completed by October 2004. A final report should be available in February 2005.

(c) Surveys of the Public's Knowledge, Attitudes, and Practices about Genital HPV Infection

Across the United States, CDC will conduct focus groups with members of the general public stratified on gender, age, and ethnicity to assess the diversity of perceptions and information needs about genital HPV infection. The focus groups will provide information on knowledge, attitudes, perceptions, and behavioral intent related to genital HPV infection. In addition, the groups will provide preferences for receiving information about genital HPV infection (i.e., communication channels, media, format, frequency, and timing).

In August 2003, focus group testing started in six states: California, Texas, Kansas, Pennsylvania, Georgia, and Florida. Thirty-six focus groups will be held overall, in six states (three in rural areas and three in urban areas). The purpose of the focus groups is to gain an understanding of the diversity in HPV-related knowledge, attitudes, perceptions, and behavioral intent among the general population. In addition, the focus groups will provide information about the general public's preferences for receiving HPV information (i.e., communication channels, media, tone, format, frequency, and timing). It is anticipated that a preliminary report of focus group findings with the general public will be available in November 2003 and a final report available in December 2003.

(d) Development and dissemination of educational materials.

Materials for patients, partners, and the general public

As outlined in the above sections, the formative research related to knowledge, attitudes and practices of patients, partners, and the general public will be available by March 2004. During

April through June 2004, CDC will synthesize the research findings and formulate a plan for developing and disseminating educational information to these three target populations. In addition to educational content, the formative research findings will help determine the types of materials to develop, the "tone" of the materials, the format, communication channels, the timing and frequency of distribution, credible sources of information, etc.

Because of the expense and delay in using the results to develop educational materials, conducting a large national survey of the general population does not appear to be warranted. It is unlikely that this information would add substantially to the information gained through the formative research, and the estimated cost for such a survey would likely exceed $1 million. Also, focus group and in-depth interview information typically provides better information for developing effective educational materials than a large survey. For these reasons, CDC does not recommend conducting a survey of the general public's knowledge, attitudes and practices related to genital HPV infection as a prelude to developing educational materials. The development of education materials for patients, partners, and the general public is expected to be completed by December 2004. Shortly thereafter, CDC will begin to disseminate the educational materials and to evaluate their impact in the primary audiences.

Materials for providers

Determining the HPV knowledge, attitudes, and practices of health care providers is more complicated and detailed than developing materials for patients, partners, and the general public. The health care provider assessment must include knowledge of the etiology of genital HPV, screening practices, treatment recommendations, as well as counseling practices with patients and their partners. Formative research with this group has already been conducted and analyzed, and the quantitative research results will be available in January 2005. Subsequently, the development of appropriate, effective educational materials for health care providers should be completed by June 2005.

3. Final Report

Upon completion of the surveillance, research, and surveys described above, CDC will issue a final report describing significant findings. Using these findings, and other available scientific information, the report will address the best strategies for prevention of future genital HPV infection in the United States. CDC expects that the report should be available in summer of 2007.

A copy of the entire timeline is included in the report as Appendix B.

APPENDIX A

4 STA' 2763AB72 PUBLIC LAW 106-554

SEC. 516. (a) HUMAN PAPILLOMAVIRUS. Part B of title III of the Public Health Services Act (42 U.S.C. 243 et seq.) is amended by inserting before section 318 the following section:

HUMAN PAPILLOMAVIRUS SEC. 317P. (a) SURVEILLANCE.
(1) IN GENERAL. The Secretary, acting through the Centers for Disease Control and Prevention, shall:

(A) enter into cooperative agreements with States and other entities to conduct sentinel surveillance or other special studies that would determine the prevalence in various age groups and populations of specific types of human papillomavirus (referred to in this section as HPV) in different sites in various regions of the United States, through collection of special specimens for HPV using a variety of laboratory-based testing and diagnostic tools; and

(B) Develop and analyze data from the HPV sentinel surveillance system described in subparagraph A

(2) REPORT. ---The Secretary shall make a progress report to the Congress with respect to paragraph (1) no later than 1 year after the effective date of this section.

(b) PREVENTION ACTIVITIES; EDUCATION PROGRAM.

(1) IN GENERAL. The Secretary, acting through the Centers for Disease Control and Prevention, shall conduct prevention research on HPV, including
(A) behavioral and other research on the impact of HPV-related diagnosis on individuals;
(B) formative research to assist with the development of educational messages and information for the public, for patients, and for their partners about HPV;
(C) surveys of physician and public knowledge, attitudes, and practices about genital HPV infection; and
(D) upon the completion of and based on the findings under subparagraphs (A) through (C), develop and disseminate educational materials for the public and health care providers regarding HPV and its impact and prevention.
(2) REPORT; FINAL PROPOSAL. The Secretary shall make a progress report to the Congress with respect to paragraph
(1) not later than 1 year after the effective date of this section, and shall develop a final report not later than 3 years after such effective date, including a detailed summary of the significant findings and problems and the best strategies to prevent future infections, based on available science.

(c) HPV EDUCATION AND PREVENTION.

(1) IN GENERAL: The Secretary shall prepare and distribute educational materials for health care providers and the public that include information on HPV. Such materials shall address

(A) modes of transmission;
(B) consequences of infection, including the link between HPV and cervical cancer;
(C) the available scientific evidence on the effective-ness or lack of effectiveness of condoms in preventing infection with HPV; and
(D) the importance of regular Pap smears, and other diagnostics for early intervention and prevention of cervical cancer purposes in preventing cervical cancer.

(2) MEDICALLY ACCURATE INFORMATION. Educational material under paragraph (1), and all other relevant educational and prevention materials prepared and printed from this date forward for the public and health care providers by the Secretary (including materials prepared through the Food and Drug Administration, the Centers for Disease Control and Prevention, and the Health Resources and Services Administration), or by contractors, grantees, or subgrantees thereof, that are specifically designed to address STDs including HPV shall contain medically accurate information regarding the effectiveness or lack of effectiveness of condoms in preventing the STD the materials are designed to address. Such requirement only applies to materials mass produced for the public and health care providers, and not to routine communications.

Sec. 516 (b) LABELING OF CONDOMS. The Secretary of Health and Human Services shall reexamine existing condom labels that are authorized pursuant to the Federal Food, Drug, and Cosmetic Act to determine whether the labels are medically accurate regarding the overall effectiveness or lack of effectiveness of condoms in preventing sexually transmitted diseases, including HPV.

Appendix B

Human Papillomavirus Timeline for Surveillance and Prevention Research
August 2003

1) **Sentinel Surveillance and Special Research Studies**

(a) Sentinel Surveillance

Preliminary data analysis – fall 2004
Final data analysis - fall 2006
Expected content: Analysis of HPV prevalence over time, and risk factors associated with HPV infection.

(b) Special Research Studies

Data collection completed – December 2004
Data analyzed – March 2005
Expected content: Prevalence of genital HPV DNA, in vaginal specimens, among a nationally representative sample of 14-59 year old women, and seroprevalence of antibody to HPV-16 among a nationally representative sample of 14-59 year old men and women.

2) **Prevention Research**

(a) Multisite behavioral study of the impact of HPV-related diagnosis

Phase I
Data first available – Fall 2003
Interim Report– November 2003
Expected content/Limitations – Results from focus groups and in-depth interviews held at the University of South Florida and University of South Carolina sites only. Will include knowledge, attitudes, behaviors and impact of high risk HPV (HR-HPV) diagnosis on women; and health care providers' perceptions of the informational needs of HR-HPV (+) patients. Population includes African Americans, Caucasians and Hispanics.

Final Data
Final Report – March 2005 (for all sites)
Expected Content – Data will contain information on knowledge, attitudes, behaviors and impact of HR-HPV diagnosis on women and their male sexual partners. Data obtained from focus groups and in depth interviews with African American, Caucasian, Hispanic, Asian, and American Indian women, men and adolescents. Data will also include information on health care providers' perceptions of the informational needs of HR-HPV (+) patients from a focus group conducted with health care providers at the South Carolina site.

Phase 2
Data first available – summer 2004
Interim Report – October 2004
Expected content/limitations – Data will include preliminary findings from University of South Florida and University of South Carolina sites only. Data obtained from common quantitative instrument administered by all sites. Population will include HR-HPV (+) and (-) African American, Caucasian, Hispanic and American Indian women.

Final Data
Final Report – March 2005 (for all sites)
Expected Content – Data will contain information from a common quantitative instrument administered by all sites. Core elements for the instrument were developed from the qualitative research and include the following: HPV knowledge; counseling information received from health care providers after a HR-HPV diagnosis; often used, most trusted, and preferred sources for HPV educational information; disclosure of HPV diagnosis; sexual history, practices and behaviors; partners' responses to HPV diagnosis; emotional impact of HR-HPV (+) and (-) women. Data analysis will compare women by ethnicity, women at varying times since diagnosis, and women by HR-HPV status.

(b) Surveys of Physician Knowledge, Attitudes, and Practices about Genital HPV Infection

Initiation of survey – February 2004
Data collection – June 2004
Data analysis completed – June 2004
Preliminary report – December 2004
Final Report – February 2005
Expected Content – Completion of the provider survey to assess providers' knowledge, attitudes, and practices related to HPV; to assess providers' perceptions of risks and benefits of HPV testing and counseling; to determine barriers and facilitators to appropriate HPV prevention, testing, and counseling practices; and to assess perceptions about offering HPV testing and counseling in the future.

(c) Surveys of the Public's Knowledge, Attitudes, and Practices about Genital HPV Infection

Preliminary Report – November 2003
Final Report – December 2003
Expected Content – Summary of focus group results The report will include information on the general public's HPV-related knowledge, attitudes and current practices, as well as information on preferred communication channels, message tone, and credible sources of information.

Develop and Disseminate Educational Materials

Materials for patients, partners, and the general public
Completion of materials – December 2004

Materials for Providers
Completion of materials – May 2005

3) **Final Report** -
Date of report – summer 2007

Prevention of Genital HPV Infection and Sequelae: Report of an External Consultants' Meeting

Division of STD Prevention

December 1999

DEPARTMENT OF HEALTH AND HUMAN SERVICES
Centers for Disease Control and Prevention
National Center for HIV, STD, and TB Prevention
Division of STD Prevention
Atlanta, Georgia 30333

Copyright Information

Suggested Citation

Division of STD Prevention. Prevention of Genital HPV Infection and Sequelae: Report of an External Consultants' Meeting. Department of Health and Human Services, Atlanta: Centers for Disease Control and Prevention (CDC), December 1999.

Copies can be obtained from the Office of Communications, National Center for HIV, STD, and TB Prevention, Centers for Disease Control and Prevention, 1600 Clifton Road, Mailstop E-06, Atlanta, Georgia 30333.

This report is available by Internet via the CDC home page at:
http://www.cdc.gov/nchstp/dstd/Reports_Publications/99HPVReport.htm

Acknowledgments

This report was prepared by the following staff in the Division of STD Prevention, National Center for HIV, STD, and TB Prevention, Centers for Disease Control and Prevention: John M. Douglas (currently affiliated with the Denver Department of Public Health, Denver, Colorado), Katherine M. Stone, and Michael E. St. Louis; Elizabeth R. Unger in the Division of Viral and Rickettsial Diseases, National Center for Infectious Diseases, Centers for Disease Control and Prevention; and Robert Smith of the American Cancer Society.

Table of Contents

Abbreviations Used in This Report vii

External Consultants viii

Executive Summary 1

Introduction 5

Overview 6

Recommendations From The Workgroups 9

1. Role of HPV testing in cervical cancer screening 9
    - Background 9
    - Workgroup Discussion 10
    - Recommendations for public health/prevention activities 11
    - Research/evaluation priorities 11
2. Cervical cancer screening in adolescents 12
    - Background 12
    - Workgroup discussion 12
    - Recommendations for public health/prevention activities 13
    - Research/evaluation priorities 13
3. Non-vaccine modalities for primary prevention of genital HPV infection 13
    - Background 13
    - Workgroup discussion 14
    - Recommendations for public health/prevention activities 15
    - Research/evaluation priorities 16
4. Preparedness for prophylactic HPV vaccines 16
    - Background 16
    - Workgroup discussion 17
    - Research/evaluation priorities 18
5. Provider, patient, and public awareness 19
    - Background 19
    - Workgroup discussion 19
    - Provider awareness 20
        - Recommendations for public health/prevention activities 20
        - Research/evaluation priorities 20
    - Patient awareness 20
        - Recommendations for public health/prevention activities 20
        - Research/evaluation priorities 20
    - Public awareness 20
        - Research/evaluation priorities 20
6. Anal Cancer 21
    - Background 21
    - Workgroup discussion 21
    - Research/evaluation priorities 22

7. Surveillance for genital HPV infection and sequelae 22
Background 22
Workgroup discussion 23
Recommendations for public health/prevention activities 23
Research/evaluation priorities 24
References 25

Abbreviations Used in This Document

ACS	American Cancer Society
AGUS	Atypical glandular cells of undetermined significance
AIDS	Acquired immunodeficiency syndrome
ALTS	ASCUS-LSIL Triage Study
ASCUS	Atypical squamous cells of undetermined significance
ASIL	Anal squamous intraepithelial lesion
CDC	Centers for Disease Control and Prevention
CIN	Cervical intraepithelial neoplasia
CIS	Carcinoma in situ
CPT	Certified Procedural Terminology
CSTE	Council of State and Territorial Epidemiologists
DCPC	Division of Cancer Prevention and Control
DNA	Deoxyribonucleic acid
DSTD	Division of Sexually Transmitted Diseases Prevention
DVRD	Division of Viral and Rickettsial Diseases
FDA	Food and Drug Administration
GW	Genital warts
HC-II	Hybrid Capture II
HIV	Human immunodeficiency virus
HMO	Health maintenance organization
HPV	Human papillomavirus
HSIL	High-grade squamous intraepithelial lesion
ICD	International Classification of Disease
JORP	Juvenile onset respiratory papillomatosis
LEEP	Loop electrical excision procedure
LSIL	Low-grade squamous intraepithelial lesion
mRNA	Messenger ribonucleic acid
MSM	Men who have sex with men
NCCDPHP	National Center for Chronic Disease Prevention and Health Promotion
NCHSTP	National Center for HIV, STD, and TB Prevention
NCID	National Center for Infectious Diseases
NDTI	National Disease and Therapeutic Index
NHANES	National Health and Nutrition Examination Survey
NIH	National Institutes of Health
NPCR	National Program of Cancer Registries
PCR	Polymerase chain reaction
PID	Pelvic inflammatory disease
PV	Papillomavirus
RCT	Randomized clinical trial
RRP	Recurrent respiratory papillomatosis
SDS	Sodium dodecyl sulfate
SEER	Surveillance Epidemiology and End Results
SIL	Squamous intraepithelial lesion
STD	Sexually transmitted disease
VLP	Virus-like particle

External Consultants

Adaora A. Adimora, M.D., M.P.H., University of North Carolina School of Medicine, Chapel Hill, NC; ***Linda L. Alexander, Ph.D., FAAN,*** The American Social Health Association, Research Triangle Park, NC; ***Thomas M. Becker, M.D., Ph.D.,*** Oregon Health Sciences University, Portland, OR; ***Karl Beutner, M.D., Ph.D.,*** University of California, San Francisco, Vallejo, CA; ***Gail Bolan,*** California Department of Health Services, Berkeley, CA; ***Virginia Caine, M.D.,*** Marion County Health Department and Indiana University School of Medicine, Indianapolis, IN; ***Willard Cates, Jr., M.D., M.P.H.;*** Family Health International, Durham, NC; ***Charles W. Ebel,*** Independent Consultant, Durham, NC; ***Maria Eugenia Fernandez-Esquer, Ph.D.,*** UT-Houston School of Public Health, Houston, TX; ***Dennis Fortenberry, M.D., M.S.,*** Indiana University School of Medicine, Indianapolis, IN; ***Sue J. Goldie, M.D., M.P.H.,*** Harvard School of Public Health, Boston, MA; ***H. Hunter Handsfield, M.D.,*** University of Washington and Seattle-King County Department of Health, Seattle, WA; ***Diane M. Harper, M.D., M.S., M.P.H.,*** Dartmouth Medical School, Hanover, NH; ***Penelope J. Hitchcock, D.V.M.;*** National Institute of Allergy and Infectious Diseases, Bethesda, MD; ***King K. Holmes, M.D., Ph.D.,*** University of Washington, Seattle, WA; ***Edward W. Hook, III, M.D.,*** University of Alabama, Birmingham, AL; ***David Jenkins, M.D.,*** Nottingham University, Nottingham, UK; ***Laura A. Koutsky,*** University of Washington, Seattle, WA; ***Robert J. Kurman, M.D.,*** Johns Hopkins University School of Medicine, Baltimore, MD; ***Attila T. Lorincz, Ph.D.,*** Digene Corporation, Silver Spring, MD; ***M. Michele Manos, Ph.D., M.P.H.;*** Kaiser Permanente Division of Research, Oakland, CA; ***Heather G. Miller, Ph.D.,*** Research Triangle Institute, Washington, DC; ***Anna-Barbara Moscicki, M.D.,*** University of California at San Francisco, San Francisco, CA; ***Evan R. Myers, M.D., M.P.H.,*** Duke University Medical Center, Durham, NC; ***Jorma Paavonen, M.D.,*** University of Helsinki, Helsinki, Finland; ***Joel Palefsky, M.D.,*** University of California at San Francisco, San Francisco, CA; ***Gary A. Richwald, M.D., M.P.H.,*** National Coalition of STD Directors and Institute for Healthcare Advancement, Whittier, CA; ***Michael W. Ross, Ph.D., M.P.H.,*** WHO Center for Health Promotion Research and Development and University of Texas, Houston, TX; ***Debbie Saslow, Ph.D.,*** American Cancer Society, Atlanta, GA; ***John Schiller, Ph.D.,*** National Cancer Institute, NIH, Bethesda, MD; ***Jane R. Schwebke, M.D.,*** University of Alabama, Birmingham, AL; ***Keerti V. Shah, M.D., Dr.P.H.,*** Johns Hopkins School of Public Health, Baltimore, MD; ***Robert Smith, Ph.D.,*** American Cancer Society, Atlanta, GA; ***Diane Solomon, M.D.,*** National Cancer Institute, Rockville, MD; ***Mark L. Welton, M.D.,*** University of California at San Francisco, San Francisco, CA; ***Cosette M. Wheeler, Ph.D.,*** University of New Mexico School of Medicine, Albuquerque, NM; ***Jonathan M. Zenilman, M.D.,*** Johns Hopkins University School of Medicine, Baltimore, MD; ***Gregory D. Zimet, Ph.D.,*** Indiana University School of Medicine, Indianapolis, IN.

CDC Participants

Sevgi O. Aral, Ph.D., Division of STD Prevention (NCHSTP); ***Harrell Chesson, Ph.D.,*** Division of STD Prevention (NCHSTP); ***Susan DeLisle, A.R.N.P., M.P.H.,*** Division of STD Prevention (NCHSTP); ***John M. Douglas, M.D.,*** Division of STD Prevention (NCHSTP) and Denver Department of Public Health, Denver, CO; ***Elamin H. Elbasha, Ph.D.,*** Office of the Director (NCID); ***Ted V. Ellerbrock, M.D., FACOG, Division of HIV/AIDS Prevention (NCHSTP); Lauri Flatt,*** Office of Communications (NCHSTP); ***Rima F. Khabbaz, M.D., Division of Viral and Rickettsial Diseases (NCID); Nancy C. Lee, M.D.,*** Division of Cancer Prevention and Control (NCCDPHP); ***William C. Levine, M.D.,*** Division of STD Prevention (NCHSTP); ***Harold S. Margolis, M.D.,*** Division of Viral and Rickettsial Diseases (NCID); ***Lauri Markowitz, M.D.,*** Division of STD Prevention (NCHSTP); ***Matthew T. McKenna, M.D., M.P.H.;*** Division of Cancer Prevention and Control (NCCDPHP); ***William C. Reeves, M.D.,*** Division of Viral and Rickettsial Diseases (NCID); ***Russell H. Roegner, Ph.D.,*** Division of STD Prevention (NCHSTP); ***Janet St. Lawrence, Ph.D.,*** Division of STD Prevention (NCHSTP); ***Michael E. St. Louis, M.D,*** Division of STD Prevention (NCHSTP); ***Katherine M. Stone, M.D.,*** Division of STD Prevention (NCHSTP); ***Guoyu Tao, Ph.D.,*** Division of STD Prevention (NCHSTP); ***Elizabeth R. Unger, Ph.D., M.D.,*** Division of Viral and Rickettsial Diseases (NCID); ***Suzanne D. Vernon, Ph.D.,*** Division of Viral and Rickettsial Diseases (NCID); ***Judith N. Wasserheit, M.D., M.P.H.;*** Division of STD Prevention (NCHSTP).

Executive Summary

Genital human papillomavirus (HPV) infection is the most common sexually transmitted disease (STD) in the United States and is of increasing public health concern, yet no prevention programs have been established. Certain HPV types cause abnormal Pap smears and are etiologically related to cervical, vulvar, anal, and penile cancers; other types cause genital warts, recurrent respiratory papillomatosis, and low-grade Pap smear abnormalities. Recommendations for programmatic activities, prevention research, and evaluation were developed by a group of invited experts who met in Atlanta on April 13-14, 1999. This consultation on "Prevention of Genital HPV Infection and Sequelae" was cosponsored by CDC's Division of STD Prevention (DSTD), National Center for HIV, STD, and TB Prevention (NCHSTP); Division of Cancer Prevention and Control (DCPC), National Center for Chronic Disease Prevention and Health Promotion (NCCDPHP); Division of Viral and Rickettsial Diseases (DVRD), National Center for Infectious Diseases (NCID); and the American Cancer Society (ACS). Discussions were focused around key questions for seven topics pertinent to prevention of genital HPV infection and sequelae: the role of HPV testing in cervical cancer screening, cancer screening in adolescents, non-vaccine approaches to primary prevention of HPV infection, preparedness for prophylactic HPV vaccines, public and provider awareness, prevention of anal cancer, and surveillance for HPV and cancer. Following a summary of the discussion of the issues in each core topic area, recommendations are listed. These include recommendations (summarized below) for programmatic public health/prevention activities ready for implementation in the near future as well as recommendations for prevention research or other evaluation activities. While these recommendations were made primarily as suggestions for CDC and ACS, many are also relevant for other organizations interested in prevention of genital HPV or related sequelae (e.g., the National Institutes of Health). The intent of this report is to stimulate long-term collaborative efforts among a variety of organizations.

Summary of Recommendations for Public Health/Prevention Activities for Genital HPV Infections and Sequelae

1. Role of HPV testing in cervical cancer screening

a. CDC and ACS should acknowledge usefulness of HPV testing as an option in triage of women with ASCUS Pap smears.

b. CDC or ACS should facilitate a meeting to review cervical cancer prevention modeling and assess cost-effectiveness of different strategies.

2. Cervical cancer screening in adolescents

a. Because the large majority of cervical lesions in adolescents are self-limited, in those with low-grade cytologic abnormalities (e.g., ASCUS, LSIL) consideration should be given to conservative follow-up by repeat Pap smear rather than triage by HPV testing or early colposcopy/biopsy.

b. CDC and ACS should recommend that the cytology should be collected first when Pap smear screening is conducted concurrently with STD testing.

3. Non-vaccine modalities for primary prevention of genital HPV infection

a. Given the uncertainties about prevention of transmission of genital HPV to sexual partners, a standard script for providers to use in education /counseling should be developed and used.

4. Preparedness for prophylactic HPV vaccines - none ready for implementation.

5. Provider, patient, and public awareness

a. CDC, ACS, and other professional organizations should draft and disseminate a consensus statement for use in professional educational materials of what has been scientifically established about genital HPV (as well as what is not known).

b. In conjunction with provider materials, patient educational materials should be developed and distributed.

6. Anal Cancer - none ready for implementation.

7. Surveillance for genital HPV infection and sequelae

a. Routine disease reporting of all genital HPV infections or for any specific types is not recommended at this time.

b. CDC should conduct further analysis of the experience with genital warts reporting in various states to guide future directions in genital warts surveillance.

c. Because routine reporting of CIS could be a useful adjunct to cancer surveillance, especially as HPV vaccine programs are implemented, problems encountered by SEER in the past should be examined and alternative approaches considered.

d. Surveillance for HPV-related cancers should be enhanced in ways that contribute to understanding the causative role of HPV infection and prevention strategies (e.g., special studies using population-based cancer registries to ascertain sexual preference for men with anogenital cancers).

Summary of Research/Evaluation Priorities for Prevention of Genital HPV Infections and Sequelae

1. Role of HPV testing in cervical cancer screening

a. demonstration projects to evaluate feasibility/cost-effectiveness of HPV testing for triage (high priority)

b. HPV testing for triage in targeted high-risk populations (high priority)

c. HPV testing in primary screening in developed countries (high priority)

d. HPV testing in primary screening in developing countries (high priority)

e. HPV testing in follow-up of untreated CIN 1 and treated CIN 2/3 (intermediate priority)

2. Cervical cancer screening in adolescents

a. natural history of CIN 2 (prospective) and CIN 3 (comparative laboratory studies) in adolescents (high priority)

b. long-term reproductive complications of ablative therapy in adolescents (high priority)

c. long-term behavioral complications of ablative therapy in adolescents (intermediate priority)

d. feasibility of recommending initiating Pap smear screening based on coitarche (intermediate priority).

e. relative importance of rapidly progressive cancer in younger women (low priority)

3. Non-vaccine modalities for primary prevention of genital HPV infection

a. assessment of HPV endpoints in ongoing condom and microbicide studies of STD/HIV prevention (high priority)

b. efficacy of promotion of behavior change (reduction of partner number, etc.) to prevent HPV (high priority)

c. definition of laboratory markers of genital HPV infectiousness (intermediate priority)

d. benefit of treatment in preventing HPV transmission (intermediate priority)

e. assessment of risk factors for persistent HPV infection and its role in transmission (intermediate priority)

4. Preparedness for prophylactic HPV vaccines

a. assessment of rates and risk factors for HPV incidence, prevalence, and persistence in men (high priority)

b. development of better sampling/ testing methods for incident HPV infection, including self-sampling (high priority)

c. marketing research among the general public and providers about HPV vaccine acceptability (high priority)

d. modeling studies of HPV transmission to target immunization programs (high priority)

e. cost-effectiveness studies of HPV vaccines, including types 6/11(high priority)

f. studies of more convenient routes of delivery and dosing schedules of HPV vaccines (high priority)

g. following efficacy trials, immunogenicity studies in other groups (men, young teens, STD clinics) (high priority)

h. following licensure, studies of behavioral impact of vaccine use (high priority)

5. **Provider, patient, and public awareness**

a. surveys of provider knowledge, attitude, and practices (intermediate priority)

b. assessment of counseling/education needs of patients/partners and alternative methods (high priority)

c. determination of psychosocial impact of diagnoses of HPV and of disclosure to partners (intermediate priority)

d. surveys of knowledge and attitudes of the general public (intermediate priority)

e. pilot public education programs to assess optimal form and content and drawbacks of messages (high priority)

6. **Anal cancer prevention**

a. multicenter study of natural history and effectiveness/complications of therapy of anal LSIL and HSIL (high priority)

b. anal Pap smear reproducibility, interobserver variability, optimal sampling technique, predictive value (high priority)

c. assessment of role of HPV testing in anal cancer screening and triage of abnormal Pap smears (intermediate priority)

d. assessment of risk factors for anal cancer in women and heterosexual men (intermediate priority)

7. **Surveillance for genital HPV infection and sequelae**

a. population-based serosurveys enhanced by collection of mucosal swabs for DNA detection (high priority)

b. sentinel approach for surveillance of HPV-related disease (high priority)

c. enhance surveillance for JORP to better understand risk factors for transmission (high priority)

d. expand/redefine ICD and CPT codes to capture better data on HPV-related procedures (intermediate priority)

e. collaborate with organizations with electronic clinic databases to monitor genital warts trends (intermediate priority)

Introduction

Genital human papillomavirus (HPV) infections are sexually transmitted infections of increasing public health importance. Known for years as the cause of genital warts, there is a growing body of evidence demonstrating the etiological association with a variety of anogenital cancers. Furthermore, genital HPV infections are widespread among adults who have been sexually active and are estimated to have the highest incidence of any sexually transmitted disease (STD) in the U.S.[1]. Although cervical cancer screening programs have been implemented in the U.S. and other developed countries for decades, public health agencies have not established programs for primary prevention of genital HPV infection nor attempted to modify existing cancer prevention programs to take advantage of the associated role of HPV[2].

With the steady progress being made against bacterial STD and the increasing recognition of the widespread prevalence of viral STD such as genital herpes and genital HPV infection, the Centers for Disease Control and Prevention (CDC) has initiated a Viral STD Prevention Initiative to systematically evaluate possible control strategies and a prevention research agenda for these infections. As part of this process, CDC's Divisions of STD Prevention (DSTD), Cancer Prevention and Control (DCPC), and Viral and Rickettsial Diseases (DVRD) and the American Cancer Society (ACS) co-sponsored an expert consultants' meeting on April 13-14, 1999 on "Prevention of Genital HPV Infection and Sequelae". Invited participants included 36 external consultants and 24 participants from CDC or ACS with expertise in the biology and epidemiology of HPV, clinical management, laboratory sciences, behavioral sciences, health education, health services research, and STD and cancer prevention program implementation and development. The meeting was organized around three workgroups during which participants discussed key questions in seven selected core topic areas pertinent to prevention of genital HPV infection and sequelae: the role of HPV testing in cervical cancer screening, cancer screening in adolescents, non-vaccine approaches to primary prevention of HPV infection, preparedness for prophylactic HPV vaccines, public and provider awareness, prevention of anal cancer, and surveillance for HPV and cancer. It should be noted that other important topic areas were not considered for specific workgroup discussion (e.g., increasing coverage of Pap smear screening in the population, treatment of HPV-related disease) because of lack of time and the perception that they would be more effectively addressed in other settings.

This report is organized around the seven core topic areas and represents the collective deliberations and recommendations from the workgroups and a concluding discussion session including all participants. Following a summary of the discussion of the issues in each core topic area, recommendations are listed. These include recommendations for programmatic public health/prevention activities ready for implementation in the near future as well as recommendations for prevention research or other evaluation activities. While these recommendations were made primarily as suggestions for CDC and ACS, many are also relevant for other organizations interested in prevention of genital HPV or related sequelae (e.g., the National Institutes of Health). The future response to these recommendations will optimally be collaborative among a variety of organizations, and it is hoped that this report will serve as a stimulus for such long-term collaborative efforts.

Overview

Papillomaviruses are members of the papovaviridae family of DNA viruses, all of which are considered tumor viruses because of their ability to immortalize normal cells. They are species-specific and occur in a wide variety of vertebrates, where they cause benign and malignant epithelial proliferations. Because papillomaviruses complete their life cycle only in fully differentiated epithelial cells, they are difficult to propagate in cell culture, which has limited the study of their life cycle, immunology, transmission dynamics, diagnosis, and therapy. The initial lack of well-characterized viral antigens also means that, in contrast to most other viruses, papillomavirus taxonomy is based on DNA homology rather than antigenic diversity[3, 4]. For HPV, more than 100 different types have been detected, over 80 of which have been well-characterized by genomic sequencing, with different types defined as having < 90% homology with DNA sequences of L1 (HPV Nomenclature Committee, 16th International Papillomavirus Conference, Quebec, 1998). Approximately 30 types cause infection of genital mucosal sites, and these genital types are generally characterized as "high-risk" types (e.g., HPV 16, 18, 31, 33, 35, 39, 45, 51, 52), which are associated with low- and high-grade squamous intraepithelial lesions (LSIL and HSIL) and invasive cancer, and "low-risk" types (e.g., HPV 6, 11, 42, 43, 44), which are primarily associated with genital warts, LSIL, and recurrent respiratory papillomatosis (RRP)[3-6].

The sequela of genital HPV infection of greatest public health importance is cervical cancer. For over a century, epidemiologic studies have indicated a relationship between cervical cancer and sexual activity, with consistent associations with age of onset of sexual activity, multiple sexual partners, and contact to "high-risk" males, men with multiple partners or prior partners with genital neoplasia[7-10]. During the past 50 years, there have been ongoing attempts to identify a sexually transmitted agent responsible for these observations, and associations can be found with most sexually transmitted bacteria and viruses. Over the last 15 years, however, the central role of HPV in the pathogenesis of cervical cancer has been firmly established. High-risk types of HPV are found in $\geq$ 93% of cervical cancers worldwide, with HPV 16 present in 50% and HPV 18, 31, and 45 in another 30%[11, 12], and case-control studies from several areas have demonstrated odds ratios for HPV detection in cervical cancer of 15-46[6, 13]. Furthermore, high-grade cervical intraepithelial neoplasia precursor lesions (e.g., CIN 2 and 3) have similarly high rates of the same HPV types (5, 6, 13, 14), and prospective studies have demonstrated a plausible temporal relationship, with infection with high-risk HPV types consistently preceding development of CIN 2/3 13, 15, 16). Finally, the epidemiologic data are supported by laboratory studies demonstrating that high-risk HPV types contain genomic sequences with oncogenic activity, E6 and E7, which are consistently retained and expressed in cancers. Integration of HPV into cellular DNA occurs in the majority of cancers. This event generally disrupts the HPV E2 transcription regulatory gene and enhances stability of HPV mRNA by attaching it to cellular sequences. Either of these events may lead to increased expression of the E6 and E7 proteins. They, in turn, affect cell growth by binding with cellular tumor suppression proteins, E6 with p53 and E7 with the retinoblastoma gene product, causing their inactivation and ultimately the disruption of normal cell cycle control[3, 6, 17].

This body of epidemiologic and laboratory data is sufficiently strong that the International Agency for Research on Cancer and the National Institutes of Health have concluded that high-risk genital HPV types act as carcinogens in the development of cervical cancer[6, 18]. While infection with high-risk types appears to be "necessary" for the development of cervical cancer, it is not "sufficient" in that cancer does not develop in the vast majority of infected women[6, 18], raising questions about other possible co-factors, including smoking, hormonal exposure (e.g., multiparity and prolonged oral contraceptive use), nutritional deficiency, HLA haplotypes, other genital tract infections, and immunodeficiency, especially HIV infection[6]. The data supporting the role of HPV in other anogenital cancers are more limited, although a large proportion of anal, as well as a subset of vulvar, vaginal, and penile cancers are also associated with high-risk HPV[6, 19-22].

Because genital HPV infection is not a reportable condition, assessments of its magnitude are derived by extrapolation from epidemiological studies measuring current infection by detection of HPV DNA, with the most sensitive method being the polymerase chain reaction (PCR) technique, and approximating lifetime infection by measuring HPV antibody in serologic assays. While results have varied by population studied and sampling and detection methods used, overall they indicate that among sexually active women, over 50% have been infected with one or more genital HPV types, approximately 15% have evidence of current infection, 50-75% of which is with high-risk types, and 1% have genital warts[14, 23-26]. These findings are supported by a recent study of incident HPV infection in young women, which documented a 36-month incidence rate of 43%[26]. Men have been less well-studied, in part because sites and methods of mucosal sampling are less well-standardized. Levels of current infection in men as measured by PCR appear to be similar to women[14, 27, 28], while levels of lifetime infection as measured by serum antibody appear to be lower in men, possibly related to gender differences in the development of antibody after infection[24, 29]. A recent assessment of the magnitude of various STD in the U.S. estimated an annual incidence of genital HPV infection of 5.5 million and a prevalence of current infection (detectable HPV DNA) of 20 million[1]. The majority of infections with all types appear to be subclinical, detectable neither by physical exam nor cytology, but only by the use of HPV DNA detection tests[14, 23].

The disease burden created by genital HPV infection is high. Worldwide, there are estimated to be 400,000-500,000 cases of cervical cancer per year[10, 22]. Most cases occur in developing countries without cervical cancer prevention activities; however, even in industrialized countries, where rates have fallen by up to 75% since the introduction of Pap smear screening programs, the disease burden is still considerable[10, 30]. In the U.S., for example, incidence rates are currently 8.3/100,000, with approximately 14,000 cases and 5000 deaths annually, despite the performance of an estimated 50 million Pap smears per year. In addition, as a result of these screening activities, an estimated 2.5 million Pap smears with low-grade abnormalities (e.g., atypical squamous cells of undetermined significance–ASCUS, atypical glandular cells of undetermined significance–AGUS, and LSIL) and 200,000-300,000 Pap smears with HSIL are detected annually in the U.S. While these lesions cause no clinical morbidity apart from that resulting from treatment, their magnitude is important because of the health care costs they generate[31, 32]. Despite the absence of prevention programs, the incidence of other HPV-related cancers are 5-10 fold lower than that of cervical cancer[33], with the exception of anal cancer in homosexual men, which was estimated to be 12-35/100,000 prior to the onset of the AIDS epidemic and which may be higher now[34, 35]. Estimates for genital warts are less precise than those for cancer because of the absence of case reporting and because they often recur after treatment; however, limited data suggest that in the U.S. incidence rates may be as high as 100 per 100,000[36] with a prevalence of 1.4 million[14]. Finally, estimates for RRP, a disease of both children and adults in which papillomas of the larynx and upper respiratory tract cause hoarseness and respiratory obstruction, are similarly imprecise, with estimated incidence rates of 0.4 to 1.2 per 100,000 children[37]. Only limited attempts have been made to estimate the annual cost burden of genital HPV infection in the U.S. Existing estimates range from $1.6 billion to $6 billion, making genital HPV the second most costly STD after HIV infection; these estimates do not include costs for management of RRP, indirect costs (i.e., lost time and wages), or intangible costs (e.g., emotional pain, anxiety, disrupted relationships)[31, 38, 39].

Factors associated with genital HPV infection in women have been evaluated in a large number of cross-sectional studies. Although smoking, pregnancy, and use of oral contraceptives have been variably associated with genital HPV infection, the most consistent predictors have been various parameters of sexual activity. The lifetime number of sex partners has been associated with both current and lifetime infection in most studies which have addressed this question[24, 25, 29, 40-44]. However, several reports have emphasized that number of partners in more recent timeframes is even more highly associated with current infection[45-49] and that the number of partners of the sex partner(s) is an additional risk factor[26, 46]. Studies in men are more limited, but they suggest similar associations with sexual activity[24, 29, 50]. While non-sexual routes of transmission of genital HPV infection via fomites, non-sexual contact, or vertical transmission are plausible[51] and supported by some but not all serological studies in children[52-54], cervical HPV infection has been rarely detected in virginal females[55-57], and it is generally accepted that most genital HPV infections are transmitted by sexual activity[7, 14]. Alternatively, the likely mode of transmission for RRP is upper respiratory tract exposure to infected genital mucosa, at the time of delivery in juvenile-onset disease and presumably through oral-genital sexual contact for adults[58].

Of importance, an increasing body of data suggests that the majority of type-specific genital HPV infections are only transiently detectable by DNA detection techniques. Most studies have noted an inverse relationship of age with infection as measured by detection of HPV DNA. Peak rates are found in women $\leq$ 25 years old, which is speculated to result from clearance of infection over time in most women as an effective immunologic response is induced[7, 14, 26, 45-48, 59-61]. Although questions remain as to whether HPV infection which becomes non-detectable by PCR has completely resolved or may intermittently reactivate[62-64], median duration of incident infection is reported to be 8 months, with rates of persistence of only 30% after 1 year and 9% after 2 years[26]. Because women with persistent infection, especially those with high-risk types, are at greater risk for developing CIN[15, 26, 40, 65] and CIN lesions which persist rather than regress[16], defining determinants of persistence is important in assessing which of the many women with HPV infection are at most risk of subsequent sequelae. Studies to date suggest that infection with high-risk and multiple types of HPV and older age are associated with persistent infection[26, 66].

Recommendations From The Workgroups

1. Role of HPV testing in cervical cancer screening

Background

With the recognition of the etiologic role of high-risk types of genital HPV infection in cervical cancer, there has been an intense focus on the use of HPV diagnostic tests in cervical cancer prevention activities. Interest has focused primarily in three areas: triage of women with low-grade Pap smear abnormalities, primary screening, and follow-up of women with confirmed CIN. All three uses are based upon the association of high-risk HPV types with high-grade precursor lesions. Evaluations of these strategies have used both non-amplified and PCR-based testing, although the recent development and FDA approval of a more sensitive signal amplification assay, Hybrid Capture II (HC-II, Digene), should enhance standardized evaluation of these strategies and make reproducible use in clinical settings more feasible.

The most comprehensively evaluated area is HPV testing for triage of low-grade Pap smear abnormalities (e.g., ASCUS, AGUS, and LSIL). Although the majority of women with these cytologic findings have normal histology or lesions which are likely to regress (CIN 1), a minority (5-20%) will have CIN2/3, representing the majority of high-grade lesions in some settings[67-69]. Current management recommendations for women with low-grade abnormalities offer several options, including follow-up Pap smear evaluation with colposcopy only for those with persistent abnormalities or immediate colposcopy for all women[31]. Neither approach is ideal. Routine colposcopy is costly and generates a large number of unnecessary procedures, while the follow-up Pap smear approach may result in women being lost to follow-up and lower cost-effectiveness, and both approaches may produce anxiety pending completion of the evaluation[31, 70-72].

A third option, HPV testing with colposcopy only for those with high-risk types identified, has also been recommended "for physicians who understand its limitations"[31], but has not been widely accepted[72-76] because of variation of earlier generations of commercially available tests in sensitivity for detection of CIN2/3 (56-93%) and cost-effectiveness[71, 77, 78]. The current generation HC-II test has an expanded number of high-risk HPV types and a lower detection threshold for HPV DNA, giving it a level of sensitivity similar to that of PCR[79]. It uses a battery of probes to detect presence of *any* of a group of 13 high-risk types (16, 18, 31, 33, 35, 39, 45, 51, 52, 56, 58, 59, 68) and *any* of a group of low-risk types (6, 11, 42, 43, 44); it does not allow identification of specific HPV types. Published reports of its performance[67, 80], including the largest evaluation to date of HPV testing for triage[67], demonstrate high sensitivity (approximately 90%) and acceptable specificity (40-65%) for detection of CIN2/3 for women with ASCUS; similar results have been found in women with AGUS[68]. Test specificity and positive predictive value for detecting CIN2/3 are lower in settings where the prevalence of HPV infection is higher, such as younger women or those with LSIL[81-83]. The strategy of obtaining a sample at the time of the initial Pap smear to save for possible HPV testing is feasible using either liquid-based cytology media (PreservCyt fluid, Cytyc Corporation) or a vial of sample transport media specific for HPV testing. This allows "reflex HPV testing" (testing only the samples from women whose Pap smears are found to be abnormal) without a return visit[67, 83, 84], although does require appropriate sample collection and storage procedures. The use of HPV testing for triage is being further evaluated in two large ongoing randomized trials in the U.S. and the U.K. which are comparing the three management strategies and which should provide even more information on their relative clinical value [70, 85]. Because HPV testing for triage largely serves to enhance cost-effectiveness of care and reduce patient anxiety[70, 72], these RCTs will include cost-effectiveness analyses to complement those currently underway[67]. Potential anxiety generated by HPV testing (when a patient and her partner are told they have or have been exposed to an incurable STD) will need to be considered in both clinical use and cost-effectiveness analyses[70, 72].

HPV testing for primary cancer screening is a more complex issue, but one with potentially greater benefit. Used as an adjunct to the Pap smear, it has the potential of increasing sensitivity and specificity of primary screening, and, more importantly, enhancing cost-effectiveness by lengthening the screening interval and determining when screening can be stopped altogether, especially among older women[70, 77, 86-88]. Of even greater importance is the possibility that it could be an alternative to the Pap smear for accessing women not currently being reached by Pap smear screening. In developed countries, ease of collection via vaginal swab could facilitate screening in clinic settings where pelvic examinations are not routinely available or acceptable or in non-clinic-based settings by outreach workers[70]. In developing countries without Pap smear screening programs, intermittent or even once in a lifetime HPV testing might be more feasible and cost-effective than cytologic screening[77, 89], although would require implementation of treatment programs for its benefit to be fully realized. By enhancing population coverage, both of these strategies could not only enhance cost-effectiveness, but also lead to a reduction in cervical cancer incidence and mortality[77, 89]. In the context of primary screening, several studies have reported enhanced sensitivity for detection of CIN2/3 when HPV testing is combined with cytology in comparison to cytology alone[90, 91]. There are a number of ongoing studies of primary screening in developed and developing countries comparing cytology, HPV testing, or both for detection of CIN 2/3, with several preliminary reports describing sensitivities of HC-II of $\geq$ 85%[92-95]. These and other studies, especially those from ongoing RCTs[87], should provide the additional data regarding positive and negative predictive value and optimal age for HPV testing needed to determine its value in primary screening[71].

Lastly, regarding the use of HPV testing to manage women with confirmed CIN, interest stems from natural history studies which indicate that persistent high-risk HPV infection predicts subsequent development of CIN 2/3[15, 65, 96-99], and from studies of women with treated CIN which indicate that persistent HPV is associated with recurrent CIN. Because the large majority of CIN 1 lesions regress without treatment, their routine treatment is not recommended, although close follow-up is required when treatment is deferred[74, 100]. Determination of whether high-risk HPV types are present, and if so, whether they persist, may help select a group in whom closer follow-up and/or treatment may be most useful. Likewise, following ablative treatment of CIN, approximately 10-15% of women will experience a recurrence[81, 101]. Presence of high-risk types of HPV DNA is associated with recurrences, and follow-up HPV testing could enhance identification of those most likely to recur, allowing more intensive follow-up[71, 102-104].

Workgroup Discussion

The workgroup felt that while the ongoing large RCTs evaluating HPV testing for triage would provide the most useful data from which to make definitive recommendations about the relative value of the three management options, recent data on the performance of HC-II in the triage of women with ASCUS (and AGUS) supported its value in this setting. The workgroup also thought that there are insufficient data to recommend HPV testing routinely for other clinical purposes at present, although there was agreement that testing might be of great value in primary screening and other clinical settings and that studies evaluating these possibilities were priorities. It was noted that although there are no data to address the possibility that CIN 2/3 lesions presenting with ASCUS or LSIL cytology have a different (less aggressive) natural history than those presenting with HSIL, this possibility may influence the cost-effectiveness of HPV testing for triage of low-grade abnormalities. The ongoing RCTs should provide some insight into this question, which may also be amenable to evaluation by studies of molecular markers in tissues (e.g., specific HPV type, copy number, physical state and transcriptional activity, as well as other markers as they are discovered).

Recommendations for public health/prevention activities

a. The potential usefulness of HPV testing as an option in the triage of women with ASCUS and AGUS Pap smears should be acknowledged by CDC and other organizations. Formal recommendations about the use of HPV testing in this setting should be made after ongoing RCTs have been completed. HPV testing for other purposes is not currently recommended.

b. CDC, ACS, and/or other organizations interested in prevention of genital HPV infection and sequelae should facilitate a meeting to review cervical cancer prevention modeling and assess cost-effectiveness of different strategies. This meeting could contribute to interchange of ideas regarding different approaches and development of a unified model and of common instruments to collect data for model calibration to enhance consistency of modeling efforts. The meeting should also attempt to develop and distribute simple cost-effectiveness modules for use by local programs.

Research/evaluation priorities

a. Demonstration projects should be initiated to evaluate feasibility and cost-effectiveness of HPV testing for triage of ASCUS Pap smears in various "real-world" settings. Such analyses should consider direct costs of providing counseling and education for patients who test HPV-positive and their partners, as well as indirect costs (e.g., lost wages and productivity) and intangible costs (e.g., anxiety, psychosocial burden of being diagnosed with HPV infection). (High priority)

b. If ongoing RCTs confirm that HPV testing improves clinical management of women with ASCUS Pap smears, focused studies should be performed among high-risk women who may not be adequately represented in multicenter trials (e.g., STD and family planning clinics, minority populations, HIV+ women, adolescents, older women). (High priority)

c. Additional studies should be performed in U.S. populations to evaluate HPV testing as an adjunct to the Pap smear in primary screening for cervical cancer as a method of enhancing sensitivity and lengthening screening intervals. These should involve evaluation of self-collected samples for HPV testing as a means of increasing coverage of screening programs in difficult-to-access populations and should be supplemented by modeling studies to assess cost-effectiveness. (High priority)

d. Studies should be performed to evaluate HPV testing as a potentially cheaper and easier to implement alternative to cytology in developing countries that presently lack comprehensive cervical cancer screening programs. (High priority)

e. Studies should be performed to assess clinical utility of HPV testing in follow-up of women with untreated CIN 1 (i.e., more intensive follow-up and/or earlier treatment for those with persistent high-risk HPV infection) and following treatment of HSIL (as a test-of-cure). (Intermediate priority)

2. Cervical cancer screening in adolescents

Background

Since the early 1980s, U.S. guidelines for cervical cancer prevention have recommended initiating Pap smear screening at age 18 or with the onset of sexual activity[74, 105-107]. In contrast, because the latency period of cervical cancer after onset of sexual activity is lengthy and rates of cervical cancer are very low in adolescents[33], guidelines in various European countries recommend starting routine screening between the ages of 20 and 30 years. There are several arguments in favor of beginning screening in adolescence. Despite low cancer rates, there are indications that increasing sexual activity in adolescents has resulted in increased rates of CIN[108, 109]. There is also evidence that the incidence of cervical cancer has increased in younger women (<35 years old) in some countries[108, 110-112], although the trend in the U.S. is less clear[33, 113]. Additionally, questions remain about a possibly increased risk in younger women of "rapidly progressive" lesions which can evolve over a much shorter time than the usual latency period[114, 115]. Finally, there are concerns that HPV transmission to pre-adolescents as a result of sexual activity or abuse could be underestimated and represent an important problem[57, 116, 117].

On the other hand, initiating screening at such a young age raises several problems[116, 118-121]. First, screening in adolescents is likely to be less cost-effective than in older women, both because the development of high-grade lesions within the first several years after the onset of intercourse is infrequent and because the latency period of those which do occur is generally long enough to allow their detection if screening is initiated in the early-mid 20s[30, 107]. Furthermore, modeling studies suggest that CIN has a higher probability of regression in younger than older women[122], which is likely a result of higher rates of recently acquired genital HPV infection in young women, whose manifestations are usually transient, in contrast to the greater likelihood of persistent infection in older women. These considerations suggest a greater potential for detecting transient low-grade abnormalities in younger women, which lead to additional unnecessary management costs[89, 118, 122]. Second, there are concerns that adolescents may have a higher rate of post-treatment complications than older women, both physiologic and behavioral. Although the data regarding long-term effects of the therapeutic modalities for CIN in current widespread use (e.g., cryosurgery, LEEP, and laser) do not suggest an increase in problems related to fertility or pregnancy, the studies have had relatively short follow-up periods and have been too small to evaluate age-specific outcomes[123]. One recent report of complications of cryosurgery in adolescents reported PID in 9%, cervical stenosis in 3%, and cervical narrowing in 30%[124]. It has also been suggested that the anxiety engendered as a result of undergoing a pelvic exam or of being informed of a "pre-cancerous" Pap smear result may be greater in adolescents than in older women[118, 119].

Workgroup discussion

The workgroup agreed that several questions were important to address regarding Pap smear screening of adolescents. It was not felt that current recommendations about age of onset of screening should be changed. However, because of the likelihood of a more benign natural history of CIN 2/3 lesions and limited data on long-term complications in younger women, the workgroup felt that screening in adolescents may have low cost-effectiveness and thus bears reconsideration. There was consensus that it would be useful and ethical to learn more about the natural history of CIN 2 lesions in adolescent women and that, in young women in whom follow-up could be assured, it would be appropriate to follow such lesions without treatment in research settings. In those undergoing both Pap smear and STD testing, it was felt that bleeding induced by cervical swabs was potentially a greater problem for cytology than for cervical gonorrhea or chlamydia tests and that the Pap smear should be collected first.

Recommendations for public health/prevention activities

a. Because the large majority of cervical lesions in adolescents are self-limited, in those with low-grade cytologic abnormalities (e.g., ASCUS, LSIL) consideration should be given to conservative follow-up by repeat Pap smear rather than triage by HPV testing (since predictive value in adolescents is not well-characterized) or by early colposcopy/biopsy.

b. CDC and ACS should recommend that the cytology sample be collected first when Pap smear screening is conducted simultaneously with STD testing. If STD tests are run on single samples collected as part of liquid-based cytology testing, sequence questions will not be an issue.

Research/evaluation priorities

a. Prospective studies of the natural history of untreated CIN 2 in adolescents should be performed in carefully monitored research settings. Although similar natural history studies of untreated CIN 3/CIS would be difficult to perform for ethical reasons, comparative molecular studies (e.g., specific HPV type, copy number, physical state and transcriptional activity, as well as other markers as they are discovered) of these lesions in younger versus older women would be useful in assessing possible differences in natural history. (High priority)

b. Studies should be performed to better characterize the incidence and type of long-term reproductive complications of ablative therapy of CIN in adolescents. (High priority)

c. Studies should be conducted to determine if the experience of undergoing ablative therapy of CIN influences future health-care seeking behavior of adolescents (e.g., makes them less likely to return for follow-up to avoid pain or complications). (Intermediate priority)

d. Studies should be conducted to determine the feasibility of recommending initiation of Pap smear screening a certain number of years after acknowledged first sexual activity rather than at a specific age (e.g., determine rate of abnormality by years of stated activity, willingness to discuss age of onset of sexual activity). (Intermediate priority)

e. Multicenter studies should be performed comparing younger and older women with invasive cervical cancer to determine whether rapid onset disease is more common in younger women and, if so, to assess associated risk factors (e.g., HPV type, histologic type, age of onset of sexual activity, presence of other co-factors). (Low priority)

3. Non-vaccine modalities for primary prevention of genital HPV infection

Background

The reproductive rate of a sexually transmitted infection in a susceptible population is a function of three parameters: the efficiency of transmission per sexual partnership, the duration of infectivity, and the number of new partners an infected person has per unit of time[125, 126]. In the absence of measures to reduce susceptibility (e.g., effective vaccines), strategies to reduce each of these parameters can reduce transmission of infection: the efficiency of transmission by strategies to reduce infectivity (e.g., condoms, microbicides), the duration of infectivity by treatment, and new partnerships by behavior change approaches. There is limited understanding about the value of each of these approaches for prevention of genital HPV infection.

Theoretically, barrier contraceptives such as condoms are less likely to be effective in preventing infections such as genital HPV, which can involve the external genital skin, than they are for infections which are limited to specific mucosal areas and spread by semen (e.g., chlamydia or gonorrhea), although estimation of potential benefit of condoms for HPV is hindered by absence of measures of infectivity. Studies which have attempted to assess male condom benefit for women have generally found no evidence of protection against infection[26, 28, 43, 45, 46]. However, existing reports have not adequately assessed consistency and correctness of condom use, and, in cross-sectional studies, HPV infection may have preceded condom use. There are data suggesting a benefit of condom use for men, although the studies are limited[29, 50] and no data available for female condoms for either women or men. Some reports have suggested a benefit in prevention of HPV-related disease (e.g., genital warts, SIL, cervical cancer)[50, 127-130], possibly by reducing viral inoculum, repeated viral exposure, or exposure to other co-factors which might be involved in development of disease. However, a protective effect has not been seen consistently[131, 132], and the cross-sectional and case control studies published to date are limited by recall bias and the difficulty in controlling for a variety of important variables[132, 133].

There are also reports of a potential protective effect of spermicides in the prevention of cervical cancer[127, 128, 131, 132], which is of interest because of the microbicidal properties of such agents[134]. Evaluation of the activity of microbicides has been hampered by the difficulties with in vitro cultivation of HPV, which is needed to screen potential products. However, recent work with various papillomaviruses in animal systems indicates that while nonoxynol-9, which functions largely as a detergent that disrupts lipid envelopes, has no activity against non-enveloped viruses like papillomaviruses, other agents such as povidone-iodine and the detergent sodium dodecyl sulfate (SDS), which also denatures proteins, inactivate papillomaviruses including HPV[135-137]. Since SDS is a common ingredient in toothpaste and shampoo, it may be a promising agent for clinical trial evaluation in the future should human toxicity studies indicate lack of mucosal irritation with prolonged use.

In contrast to bacterial STD, for which transmission can be prevented through curative treatment, there is no evidence that treatment of HPV-associated lesions is useful in prevention of transmission. There are no effective systemic therapies for genital HPV, as there are for bacterial and other viral STD, and current treatment options include a variety of locally destructive approaches for both genital warts and SIL, as well as topical use of cytotoxic and immunomodulating agents for genital warts[138]. It has been speculated that treatment of genital warts might be useful in reducing infectiousness[138]. This premise is difficult to test because of the lack of assays for infectivity, but is supported by observations that treatment of genital warts with the imunomodulating agent imiquimod reduces viral DNA and mRNA in post-treatment biopsies[139] and that therapy of CIN results in clearance of HPV in follow-up cervical swabs in 70-80% of women[102, 104]. However, clinically normal skin and mucosa in the vicinity of HPV-associated lesions often contain HPV[140, 141]. This reservoir is thought to explain the typical recurrence rates of 10-20% after treatment for CIN[81, 103] and 20-50% after treatment of genital warts[142] and the fact that treatment of partners does not influence recurrence rates of genital warts[143]. Thus, based on limited existing data, currently available therapies for HPV-related lesions may reduce but probably do not eliminate infectiousness, and whether the reduction in viral load which occurs with treatment impacts future transmission remains unclear.

Workgroup discussion

The workgroup agreed that existing data were not supportive of a benefit of male condoms, especially for women, but that because existing studies had serious methodologic limitations, an RCT would be the only study design by which the issue could be clarified. However, such a trial would be difficult and expensive to conduct, and because of the low probability of documenting benefit, a trial specifically designed to evaluate the value of condoms for HPV prevention would not be a high priority. A more efficient approach would be to include HPV outcomes in prevention trials being undertaken for prevention of HIV or other STD, in which use of condoms or microbicides could be carefully documented. There was also agreement that comparison of the efficacy of existing treatments for genital warts, development of new therapies for genital warts and CIN, and a better understanding of the impact of existing and new therapies on transmission were important issues.

Finally, there was extensive discussion about the merits of trying to reduce genital HPV transmission by focusing on behavior change approaches. As noted, the most consistent risk factor for HPV prevalence in cross-sectional studies and HPV incidence in observational studies is number of partners and, secondarily, partners' number of partners[25, 28, 29, 40-49]. It was pointed out that although HPV-related mortality is at least twice that of HIV for women in the U.S., the predominant STD/HIV prevention messages promoted are those pertaining to HIV risk reduction, and that, in contrast to HIV[144], no attempts have been made to look at benefit of counseling strategies for HPV prevention. Since most women and men do not understand the prevalence of genital HPV infection or its role in cervical cancer, such knowledge might give them reasons to modify behavior. Increased awareness that HPV infection is widespread, that it might not be fully prevented by condom use, and that it can have rare but serious sequelae might help stimulate and sustain efforts to reduce exposure to HPV and other STD. Such strategies could include delay in initiation of sexual intercourse, a reduction in the number of partners, and selection of partners perceived to have had fewer partners.

Options for prevention trials to evaluate the benefit of a behavior change approach could include individualized counseling or health education messages delivered at the community level, with a focus on the magnitude of genital HPV infection, its association with cancer, and the benefit of reducing partners and selecting less sexually experienced partners. However, concern was expressed that, although an intuitively promising approach, such a strategy would have a number of potential problems, including stigmatization and exaggerated fear about what would likely continue to be a very common STD, difficulty in using this approach for the large number of women in the population with very few sex partners[145], a likely increased emphasis on and requests for HPV tests, whose meaning would be difficult to interpret, and a potential to undermine condom use, possibly enhancing acquisition of other STD (e.g., HIV, gonorrhea) which are more effectively prevented by condom use.

Recommendations for public health/prevention activities

a. Given the uncertainties about prevention of transmission of genital HPV to sexual partners, promulgation of a "standard script" for providers to use in education/counseling of patients with HPV infection (e.g., genital warts or CIN) would be helpful. Key messages should include the following:

   - Persons with genital warts or CIN should be informed about the high prevalence of HPV infection among adults who have been sexually active and the likely persistence of infection after treatment for an indefinite period of time.
   - Those with monogamous partners should be counseled that partners may already have been infected.
   - No scientific data support condom use specifically for genital HPV prevention; however, condoms should be recommended for prevention of other STDs.
   - Because duration of infectiousness is unknown and because genital HPV is so common among persons who have been sexually active, the value of disclosing a past diagnosis of HPV infection to future sex partners is unclear, although candid discussions about past STD should be attempted whenever possible.

- Given the complexity of counseling messages, clinicians should be encouraged to refer patients to educational materials, hotlines, and other appropriate resources.

Research/evaluation priorities

a. Randomized clinical trials designed specifically to assess prevention of genital HPV infection by male and female condoms in both women and men would be desirable; however, these will be difficult and expensive to perform. Thus, attempts should be made to include HPV outcomes (e.g., incident infection defined by HPV DNA detection in mucosal samples or by seroconversion; development of cervical SIL lesions) in ongoing/planned RCTs of various primary prevention modalities (e.g., condoms, microbicides, behavior change) for prevention of HIV and /or other STD. (High priority)

b. Because of the limited confidence in condoms for prevention of genital HPV infection, studies of behavior change (e.g., reduction in number of partners, selection of less sexually experienced partners, and delayed onset of intercourse, and which focus in part on the high prevalence and relative difficulty of preventing HPV infection) to prevent HPV outcomes should be considered. Although it was recognized that such studies would be difficult to perform and could have the unintended consequence of increasing the stigma and anxiety associated with HPV infection, they could also have other STD prevention benefits. These studies would also need to address the potential of such behavior change approaches to undermine condom use, possibly enhancing acquisition of STD (e.g., HIV, gonorrhea) more effectively prevented by condom use. (High priority)

c. Additional studies of the role of treatment in preventing transmission should be performed including assessment of persistence of detectable HPV DNA after treatment of GW and SIL. (Intermediate priority)

d. In order to inform patient counseling (especially as HPV testing becomes more common), transmission modelling, and intervention assessment/planning, studies to better define laboratory markers of genital HPV infectivity (e.g., viral load, mRNA detection, viral capsid protein detection, etc.) in different anatomic sites and lesion types should be performed. (Intermediate priority)

e. Additional studies of risk factors of persistent HPV infection should be performed because of the potential role of persistent infection in transmission dynamics in women and men, as well as in predicting subsequent neoplasia. (Intermediate priority).

4. Preparedness for prophylactic HPV vaccines

Background

The difficulty with non-vaccine modalities of primary prevention and the large global burden of HPV-related disease make the development of effective prophylactic vaccines an important public health priority[32]. Initial barriers to development of promising candidate HPV vaccines included the difficulties in propagating the virus in vitro, the potential hazard of a vaccine containing an oncogenic viral genome, and the lack of an animal model of HPV infection suitable for challenge experiments[32, 146-148]. The development of L1 virus-like particle (VLP) subunit vaccines through molecular biologic techniques has remedied the first two problems. L1, the major capsid protein and the site of the primary neutralizing epitopes of HPV, self-assembles into particles resembling authentic virions after expression in eukaryotic cells, thus retaining the native conformation required for induction of neutralizing antibody. The lack of an animal model for studying HPV remains an issue, although challenge studies with species-specific papillomaviruses and parenteral injection of VLPs have demonstrated a consistently high level of protection (90-100%) against infection in three animal systems, one cutaneous (cottontail rabbit PV) and two oral mucosal (bovine PV type 4 and canine oral PV)[146]. These results have stimulated great enthusiasm about the potential of VLP vaccines to prevent infection in humans. Several Phase I trials sponsored by industry and by the NIH with monovalent HPV 6, 11, and 16 VLP vaccines are underway, with subsequent larger clinical trials likely if the initially promising immunogenicity and safety results are confirmed[32, 147].

Although there is cause for optimism about the potential value of VLPs as prophylactic HPV vaccines, several important issues remain to be addressed. First, the animal challenge studies, although encouraging, have not used natural routes of mucosal infection, and vaccination strategies which produce greater levels of mucosal immunity may ultimately be required to prevent human infection. Second, while trials of monovalent vaccines are appropriate for initial proof of concept studies, polyvalent vaccines will ultimately be preferable because of the large number of HPV types found in cervical cancer and genital warts and the apparent lack of cross-type immunity produced by L1 vaccines, adding to the time required for full evaluation. Third, cervical cancer will not be a feasible endpoint to study because of its long latency, and clinical trials will need to focus on shorter-term (and more indirect for cancer prevention) measures such as HPV infection and CIN. Fourth, initial studies will need to be conducted in females in order to assess CIN outcomes and while studying those without prior genital HPV exposure is desirable, trials may need to focus on young adults rather than adolescents for ethical reasons. This presents an issue of translating clinical trials into practice, since the ideal target for an STD with a high incidence soon after onset of sexual activity would be pre-sexually active adolescents or children, including males as well as females. Ultimately, a vaccine which has therapeutic value in early infection as well as prophylactic value would be optimal, providing benefit to those who are already infected as well as those uninfected; this may allow a greater flexibility of populations who could be targeted, and thus possibly earlier public health benefit in terms of cancer prevention[32, 147, 148].

Workgroup discussion

Effective HPV vaccines would represent a major public health advance and their development was strongly endorsed by experts across multiple disciplines as a high priority research initiative. The workgroup participants thought that industry and the NIH should continue to play the primary role in developing new candidate vaccines and assessing their efficacy in clinical trials. In addition, there are a number of important issues which will need to be addressed both prior to as well as following licensure of effective vaccines which might appropriately involve CDC or other organizations interested in prevention of genital HPV infection. Several issues were felt to be important for upcoming clinical trials. Of immediate concern was a better understanding of the incidence and natural history of HPV infection in men, since they will likely be included in clinical trials at some point. Also, because serologic measures of incident infection are insensitive and, after VLP immunization, nonspecific for natural infection versus vaccine response, another priority of relevance for clinical trials is development of cheaper and less intrusive methods to establish incident HPV infection through samples collected from mucosal surfaces in order to permit less costly and more frequent assessment of outcomes. Additional issues would become important if initial trials indicated the likelihood of vaccine efficacy. For example, because cost analyses have been important in driving other vaccine implementation efforts and also in influencing pricing decisions, cost-effectiveness studies of vaccines for both high-risk and low-risk types of HPV would be useful and could lead to collection of specific cost data during final trials in order to refine analyses. Also, transmission modeling studies could help assess the level of vaccine efficacy required for a population-based benefit[149] and could also be of value in assessing different age and gender mixes in vaccine implementation strategies. Of particular concern are issues of gaining acceptance among the general public and healthcare providers for an HPV vaccine. The experience with hepatitis B immunization, the only STD for which an effective vaccine exists, showed that implementation was limited in the general population until a universal immunization approach was recommended, and even with hepatitis B, because of other routes of transmission, the "STD connection" has not been emphasized. The workgroup felt that effective ways of presenting an HPV vaccine to the public, including parents who would need to consent if the vaccine were administered to minors not yet sexually active, and also to providers need to be explored, preferably in collaboration with industry. These assessments should include whether the vaccine is best described as one to prevent a common STD, which would be applicable to both females and males, versus a vaccine to prevent cancer, which would be largely relevant for females.

Research/evaluation priorities

a. More extensive population-based studies should be performed of rates and risk factors for genital and anal HPV incidence, prevalence, and persistence in men. These studies should include adolescent and young adult heterosexuals as well as men who have sex with men (MSM) and should be conducted in both developed and developing countries. (High priority)

b. Improved sampling and testing methods are needed to detect incident genital HPV infection as a study outcome, including assays sensitive enough to detect HPV infections in men, sensitive and specific methods to detect type-specific (and quantitative) HPV infection, and methods amenable to self-sampling (to allow more frequent and less expensive measurements of outcomes). (High priority)

c. Given that there is no experience with implementing immunization programs for infections transmitted predominantly by sexual activity, marketing research about HPV vaccine acceptability in adolescents, their parents, and their health care providers should be encouraged by and/or carried out by CDC. (High priority)

d. Mathematical modeling studies of genital HPV transmission should be performed in order to assess optimal targets for immunization programs (e.g., age and gender mix). (High priority)

e. Cost-effectiveness studies of HPV vaccines should be carried out from a societal perspective, including assessment of indirect and intangible costs. These should include studies of HPV 6/11 to further encourage industry efforts to develop and test vaccines for these types, both as a means of preventing their sequelae (e.g., genital warts, CIN 1, and recurrent respiratory papillomatosis) in women as well as to offer benefit to men. (High priority)

f. Studies of alternative, potentially more convenient routes of delivery and dosing schedules of HPV vaccines should be conducted. (High priority)

g. Following successful efficacy trials of HPV vaccines in young adult women, immunogenicity studies should be performed in other populations (e.g., heterosexual men and MSM, young adolescent men and women, higher risk patients such as those attending STD clinics). (High priority)

h. Following licensure of an effective vaccine, studies should be performed to assess behavioral implications of its use (e.g., increases in risky sexual behavior due to misperceptions about vaccine protection against other STD, reduced compliance with cancer screening recommendations, etc.). (Intermediate priority)

5. Provider, patient, and public awareness

Background

Improvement in awareness by health care providers and the general public has been an important strategy in response to widespread public health problems such as HIV infection. Greater provider understanding can improve management of patients and provision of information to them and their families (or partners in the case of STD), and awareness in the general public can enhance responsiveness to prevention activities, such as screening or immunization. Data on provider understanding about genital HPV infection are limited. They suggest that providers are broadly aware of the sexually transmitted nature of the infection and its relationship to cervical cancer, but are less clear about the relationship of genital warts to cancer, the indication for use of various management strategies, transmission-related issues, and the indications for partner evaluation[150-152]. This lack of clarity, coupled with discomfort over discussion of issues related to STD and sexuality and limited time for counseling/education, is often perceived by patients as inadequate information and advice[152-154]. Limited data from selected populations show substantial levels of emotional distress among patients with a diagnosis of genital HPV infection (genital warts or abnormal Pap smears), which can far exceed the level of physical distress. These include feelings of shock, shame, anger at partners and providers, depression, and fear about sequelae and ongoing contagiousness[152, 153, 155-157]. Fear of or actual experience of rejection in future sexual relationships was reported by 67% and 19% of patients, respectively[153].

Workgroup discussion

The workgroup felt that the awareness of cervical cancer and of Pap smear screening as a prevention strategy are widely recognized and supported by the general public in the U.S. However, the linkage of genital HPV infection to cervical cancer is much less widely recognized, and understanding of genital HPV as an STD is limited, with STD awareness only slightly greater among women with multiple partners than other women[154]. Promoting public awareness in these areas is appealing, but represents a complex situation. On the one hand, a policy of consistently informing the public about strongly documented scientific findings is likely to be the most ethical and effective policy in the long run, and may help to lessen stigma and increase sympathy for persons suffering from sequelae of STDs. Such messages could also be useful in enhancing future acceptance of HPV immunization programs[32]. Furthermore, STD prevention messages that have been underutilized to date because of concerns over their likely benefit (e.g., reducing the number of sex partners and choosing safer sex partners) might become more acceptable strategies for many individuals if there were greater awareness of the magnitude of genital HPV infection.

On the other hand, promotion of greater awareness that cervical cancer is linked to an STD could conceivably undermine general support for Pap smear screening programs or could lead women or providers to decide that a woman considered to be at low risk for an STD does not need a Pap smear. Directing prevention messages to the general public is further complicated by the lack of clarity of what the most appropriate health care and prevention strategies are for HPV infection, given that most infected persons are asymptomatic, the overwhelming majority will not suffer any adverse consequences, no data document that condoms are effective for HPV prevention, diagnostic services are relatively expensive, and diagnosis of HPV infection has not yet been demonstrated to lead to improvement in health outcomes. Therefore, it may be counterproductive to promote messages that increase anxiety in the absence of effective strategies to reduce risk for infection. The workgroup emphasized that messages must be carefully crafted to deal with these complexities and that assessment of such prevention messages should be a critical element of research. Audiences must at least be segmented into providers, persons with known HPV infection, and the general population. When messages are directed to patients or to the general public, it is important that parallel efforts be made to inform providers at same time.

Provider awareness

Recommendations for public health/prevention activities

CDC, ACS, and other organizations interested in prevention of genital HPV infection and sequelae should draft a consensus statement for use in professional educational materials of what has been scientifically established about HPV (as well as what is not known). This statement should address currently available diagnostic, treatment, prevention, and counseling/education strategies and should be widely disseminated (e.g., published, put on websites, etc) and updated on a regular basis.

Research/evaluation priorities

Although methodologically challenging, surveys of provider knowledge, attitudes, and practices should be conducted to guide future targeting of educational efforts. (Intermediate priority)

Patient awareness

Recommendations for public health/prevention activities

In conjunction with development of professional educational materials, patient educational materials should be developed and distributed widely, and their use and/or adaptation by groups involved in patient education strongly encouraged.

Research/evaluation priorities

a. Efforts should be made to assess counseling/educational needs for patients (and partners) with HPV-related diagnoses and to develop alternatives to physicians as primary providers of education/counseling. These might include other types of patient educators (e.g., nurse clinicians who provide diabetes education, which is now a billable non-physician service), brochures, web-based material, hotlines, etc. (High priority)

b. Studies should be performed on the behavioral/psychosocial impact of HPV-related diagnoses on persons with genital warts and CIN and their partners and the impact of disclosure about these conditions on current and future sexual partnerships. (Intermediate priority)

Public awareness

Research/evaluation priorities

a. Knowledge and attitude surveys should be performed to assess information needs of various populations within the general public and to help guide existing and possible future public awareness activities. (Intermediate priority)

b. Pilot public education programs should be carried out in selected areas to assess optimal form and content of public awareness messages as well as potential drawbacks (e.g., stigmatization of Pap smear screening programs, competition with other public health prevention messages), both to respond to the increased public concern likely to occur with wider use of HPV testing and also to enhance prevention activities related to HPV and sequelae (i.e., Pap smear screening, vaccine preparedness, general understanding of relationship of HPV to cervical cancer) . (High priority)

6. Anal Cancer

Background

Anal cancer is a relatively uncommon malignancy, with a current U.S. incidence rate of only 0.9/ 100,000[33]. However, incidence rates are reported to have increased over the past 20-30 years in several countries[19, 33, 34, 158], including the U.S., where rates increased by 96% for men and 39% for women from 1973-97[33]. This increase has been partly ascribed to changes in sexual activity. There is a growing body of data linking anal cancer to sexual behavior, especially anal intercourse, and HPV infection[19, 159, 160]. The highest incidence is reported in MSM, with rates 12 to 50 times higher than in heterosexual men[159-162] and an overall annual incidence rate of up to 35/100,000[159], similar to rates of cervical cancer among women in the absence of Pap smear screening[163]. Women with previous cervical cancer are also at higher risk for anal cancer, an association likely attributable to the presence of HPV infection at both sites[164].

An additional factor in this increase may be the HIV epidemic. Prevalence rates of anal SIL (ASIL) of 20-45% have been reported in HIV+ MSM, substantially higher than in HIV- MSM, with ASIL most strongly correlated with HPV infection[163, 165-168]. Two prospective studies have documented a higher incidence of anal HSIL lesions in HIV+ vs. HIV- men, with incident HSIL associated with persistent HPV infection in both HIV+ and HIV- men[166, 168]. Finally, rates of anal cancer are estimated to be 30-80 fold higher in patients with AIDS than in the general population, although the proportion of this increase attributable to the higher overall rates seen in MSM versus the effect of HIV-related immunodeficiency has not been determined[162, 167, 169]. These data have lead to consideration of the potential benefit of anal cancer prevention programs[163, 170, 171] through cytologic screening, since evaluations to date suggest that anal Pap smears may be similar in sensitivity to cervical smears[172, 173]. This approach is supported by modeling studies of anal cancer screening in MSM, which indicate that the cost-effectiveness of screening could be similar to that for other prevention interventions. However, the models are most sensitive to assumptions about the natural history of anal LSIL, about which there are limited data, and the natural history of HSIL and the effectiveness of ablative therapy, about which there are virtually no data[35, 174]. Furthermore, little is known about the complications of ablative treatment, either in terms of medical costs or effect on quality of life. An additional consideration is the uncertain impact of the use of highly active antiretroviral therapy in HIV+ MSM, in that it could possibly lead to either an increased risk of anal cancer owing to greater longevity or a reduced risk owing to better control of HPV infection and regression of SIL lesions as a result of improved immune function[175].

Workgroup discussion

Despite the relative infrequency of anal cancer at the population level, the workgroup thought that pursuing prevention strategies for high-risk groups (primarily HIV+ MSM, but also HIV+ women and HIV- MSM) was important, and that studies to obtain better information about natural history and effectiveness of treatment of anal SIL lesions were high priorities. There were differences of opinion on how best to conduct these studies. On the one hand, because so many key questions about a potentially important prevention strategy remain unanswered and because lack of widespread implementation of anal cancer screening programs to date mean that "standards of care" have not been established, most of the workgroup felt that it would be ethical and appropriate for these studies to be implemented as RCTs. Such studies could provide much-needed unbiased data on rates of progression and regression of HSIL, and if follow-up were performed at close intervals, could minimize the risk of those anal cancers which did occur developing beyond an early stage.

Likewise, they could provide the best information on the effectiveness and complications associated with ablative therapy. On the other hand, there was also an opinion that, because of the biologically plausible analogy with the cervix and the risk of untreated HSIL progressing to cancer, it would be ethically problematic not to offer therapy to those with such lesions. An alternative evaluation methodology could thus involve a demonstration project of anal cancer screening, with follow-up of those electing no treatment for HSIL to assess natural history and of those choosing treatment to assess efficacy and complications of therapy. This approach would also provide the opportunity to assess operational feasibility and training needs of an anal cancer screening program and help to further refine cost-effectiveness analyses.

Research/evaluation priorities

a. Multicenter projects (RCTs or demonstration projects) should be initiated to assess parameters of importance in anal cancer screening programs in MSM, especially a better understanding of the natural history of LSIL and HSIL in HIV+ and HIV- MSM and the efficacy and complications of ablative therapy of anal HSIL in HIV+ and HIV- MSM. (High priority)

b. Studies should be performed to determine reproducibility, interobserver variability, optimal sampling technique, and predictive value of anal Pap smears. (High priority)

c. Analogous to studies of cervical cancer prevention, studies should be performed to evaluate performance of HPV testing in triage of abnormal anal Pap smears and in primary screening. (Intermediate priority)

d. Studies should be performed to determine risk factors for women and heterosexual men with anal cancer as a possible guide to future screening programs. (Intermediate priority)

7. Surveillance for genital HPV infection and sequelae

Background

The term "surveillance" in public health encompasses a range of activities. Surveillance for STDs in the U.S. includes three categories of activities: case notification (e.g., reporting of individual cases of notifiable conditions by providers or laboratories), prevalence monitoring (e.g., monitoring the prevalence of infection in settings where screening occurs systematically), and other special studies (e.g., sentinel surveillance activities, supplemental testing which may provide information about the incidence or prevalence of an STD). To avoid unnecessary workloads for providers and laboratories, case notification is recommended for STD with case management implications (e.g., curative treatment, partner notification), with planned or ongoing prevention programs (e.g., screening, immunizations), or in the setting of an outbreak. Case notification of STDs for these purposes is currently recommended nationally by the Council of State and Territorial Epidemiologists (CSTE) only for syphilis, gonorrhea, chlamydia, hepatitis B, and chancroid. All three categories of surveillance activity are reflected in current U.S. surveillance data for STDs[176].

HPV infections and their sequelae pose many challenges for routine public health surveillance efforts. The estimated number of new infections with genital HPV is substantially higher than those of the reportable STD[1], and they are largely undiagnosed given the limitations of routine diagnostics. Although there have been no national recommendations encouraging case notification of HPV infection, a number of states have made genital warts a reportable condition. Preliminary analysis of these reports indicate that they did not provide representative data since the vast number came from public clinics and were of warts in men, despite the widespread occurrence of genital warts in women (DSTD, unpublished observations). Special surveillance studies for genital HPV infection include assessment through the National Disease and Therapeutic Index (NDTI) of the number and proportion of ambulatory care visits in the U.S. accounted for by genital warts[176], a sentinel surveillance system for RRP[37], and a population-based national household survey, the National Health and Nutrition Examination Survey (NHANES), which has provided valuable information about trends in infection with genital herpes[177] and from which pilot seroprevalence surveys for HPV 16 and 6/11 are planned.

At the other end of the natural history spectrum, surveillance for cervical and other anogenital cancers is through cancer registries. National cancer surveillance in the U.S. has been carried out through the NIH National Cancer Institute's Surveillance Epidemiology and End Results (SEER) Program since 1973, comprising 11 geographic areas covering about 14% of the U.S. population. Extrapolations from these data are used to determine rates and trends in various types of cancers and are also the basis for annual estimates of cancer incidence compiled by the American Cancer Society. To supplement data collected through SEER on a broader geographic basis, CDC initiated the National Program of Cancer Registries (NPCR) in 1992, which will cover over 95% of the population when fully operational.

Workgroup discussion

The workgroup concluded that at the current time public health surveillance for genital HPV infection is best done through prevalence monitoring and special studies rather than through case reporting, because of the absence of the rationale for such as discussed above. There was discussion about a range of potential new surveillance activities for HPV infection and related sequelae in the U.S., focusing particularly on events in the natural history of HPV infection that are intermediate between first acquisition of infection at one extreme, and diagnosis of cancer at the other extreme. For high-risk HPV types, such events might include: development of persistent genital HPV infection, given its association with development of CIN; detection of serologic evidence of type-specific infection, given its association with persistent mucosal infection[25]; and detection of cervical carcinoma in situ (CIS). There was consensus that CIS, as the most advanced pre-cancerous precursor lesion, would be extremely useful to follow at a population-based level as an early indicator of the impact of an HPV immunization program. It was noted that since this diagnosis is increasingly made in outpatient settings, it had become difficult to capture through traditional cancer registry programs which focus on hospital-based care, and that because of this problem, the SEER Program had recently chosen to discontinue collection of this diagnosis. Suggestions about alternative systems, albeit not population-based, from which to collect data on rates of CIS include sentinel surveillance within managed care organizations or the Indian Health Service. For low-risk HPV types, key events for surveillance include not only genital warts, which may be possible to track through clinic-based and administrative datasets more effectively than is currently the case through NDTI, but also juvenile-onset RRP, which is as common as neonatal herpes infection but much less widely recognized.

Recommendations for public health/prevention activities

a. Routine disease reporting (e.g., case notification) of all genital HPV infections or of any specific HPV disease or type (e.g., genital warts, HPV 16 infection) is not practical and thus not recommended at this time.

b. CDC should conduct further analysis of the experience with genital warts reporting in various states to guide future directions in genital warts surveillance. Although data from the NDTI have limitations, their continued analysis by CDC is recommended until superior data, preferably population-based, become available.

c. Routine reporting of CIS could represent a valuable adjunct to cancer surveillance, especially as HPV immunization programs are implemented. However, because of past problems encountered by SEER, future efforts to report and interpret data on CIS should examine this experience and consider alternative approaches to monitor this diagnosis.

d. Surveillance for HPV-related cancers should be enhanced in ways that contribute to understanding the causative role of HPV infections and to prevention strategies. Such enhancements could include recording the sexual preference of men with anogenital cancers (recognizing that this will depend upon the consistency with which this variable is recorded in the medical record).

Research/evaluation priorities

a. Pilot NHANES seroprevalence studies by CDC should be continued and other subpopulations for similar studies should be identified, since monitoring serologic evidence of infection with HPV 16 and/or other high risk types may be an efficient method of prevalence monitoring. These studies should also be expanded to include self-collected samples such as vaginal swabs and urine samples for HPV DNA studies, with a focus on specific types likely to be included in vaccines, since these may enhance data provided by serologic studies in monitoring levels of type-specific infection over time. (High priority)

b. A sentinel approach, possibly in areas where other sentinel surveillance activities (e.g., SEER or one of the NPCR sites) have been established, should be considered in order to evaluate the spectrum and trends of HPV-related disease and as a foundation for subsequent population-level prevention activities such as immunization programs. Such activities might include monitoring specific types and type-variants of HPV infection and population-based Pap smear registries. (High priority)

c. The current CDC sentinel surveillance for juvenile-onset RRP should be strengthened and expanded (e.g., additional sites; more data related to acquisition of infection, including maternal HPV status and other risk factors for mother-child transmission; consideration of case control and/or observational studies to better define risk factors for transmission and potential benefit of interventions such as C-section). (High priority)

d. Because ICD and CPT codes do not accurately capture HPV-related diagnoses, treatments, or procedures, CDC should explore efforts to redefine these codes. Such changes would enhance prevalence monitoring of HPV-related outcomes and ongoing assessments of HPV-related healthcare costs in large administrative databases (e.g., Medicaid, Medstat, etc.). (Intermediate priority)

e. CDC should make efforts to collaborate with organizations that have electronic databases of patient encounters which include variables such as reason for visit and primary diagnosis (e.g., STD clinics, group model HMOs, etc.) in order to monitor trends in and assess burden of health care related to the prevalence of genital warts. (Intermediate priority)

REFERENCES

1. Cates W, American Social Health Association Panel. Estimates of the incidence and prevalence of sexually transmitted diseases in the United States. *Sex Transm Dis*. 1999;26(suppl):52-57.
2. Lytwyn A, Sellors J. Sexually transmitted human papillomaviruses: current concepts and control issues. *Can J Hum Sex*. 1997;6:113-126.
3. Galloway DA. Biology of Human Papillomaviruses. In: Holmes K, Mardh P, Sparling P, et al., eds. *Sexually Transmitted Diseases*. 3rd ed. New York: McGraw-Hill; 1999:335-346.
4. Richart R, Masood S, Syrjanen K, et al. Human papillomavirus IAC Task Force Summary. *Acta Cytol*. 1998;42:50-58.
5. Lorincz A, Reid R, Jenson A, Greenberg M, Lancaster W, Kurman R. Human papillomavirus infection of the cervix: relative risk associations of 15 common anogenital types. *Obstet Gynecol*. 1992;79:328-337.
6. World Health Organization. *IARC Monograph on the Evaluation of Carcinogenic Risks to Humans: Human Papillomaviruses*. Vol. 64; Lyons: IARC; 1995.
7. Schiffman M. Recent progress in defining the epidemiology of human papillomavirus infection and cervical neoplasia. *J Natl Cancer Inst*. 1992;84:394-398.
8. Beral V. Cancer of the cervix: a sexually transmitted infection? *Lancet*. 1974(i):1037-1040.
9. Kessler I. Venereal factors in human cervical cancer: evidence from marital clusters. *Cancer*. 1977;39:1912-1919.
10. Kiviat N, Koutsky L, Paavonen J. Cervical Neoplasia and Other STD-Related Genital Tract Neoplasias. In: Holmes K, Mardh P, Sparling P, et al., eds. *Sexually Transmitted Diseases*. 3rd ed. New York: McGraw-Hill; 1999:811-832.
11. Bosch FX, Manos MM, Munoz N, et al. Prevalence of human papillomavirus in cervical cancer: a worldwide perspective. *J Natl Cancer Inst*. 1995;87:796-802.
12. Walboomers J, Jacobs M, Manos M, et al. Human papillomavirus is a necessary cause of invasive cervical cancer worldwide. *J Pathol*. 1999;189:12-19.
13. Munoz N, Bosch F. The causal link between HPV and cervical cancer and its implications for prevention of cervical cancer. *Bull PAHO*. 1996;30(4):362-377.
14. Koutsky L. Epidemiology of genital human papillomavirus infection. *Am J Med*. 1997;102 (5A):3-8.
15. Koutsky L, Holmes K, Critchlow M, et al. A cohort study of the risk of cervical intraepithelial neoplasia grade 2 or 3 in relation to papillomavirus infection. *N Engl J Med*. 1992;327:1272-1278.
16. Ho G, Burk R, Klein S, et al. Persistent genital human papillomavirus infection as a risk factor for persistent cervical dysplasia. *J Natl Cancer Inst*. 1995;87:1365-1371.
17. Southern S, Herrington C. Molecular events in uterine cervical cancer. *Sex Transm Dis*. 1998;74:101-109.
18. National Institutes of Health. Cervical Cancer. *NIH Consensus Statement*. 1996;14(1):1-38.
19. Frisch M, Glimelius B, van den Brule J, Wohlfahrt J, Meijer C, Walboomers J. Sexually transmitted infection as a cause of anal cancer. *N Engl J Med*. 1997;337:1350-1358.
20. Bjorge T, Dillner J, Anttila T, et al. A prospective seroepidemiological study of the role of human papillomavirus in non-cervical anogenital cancers. *Br Med J*. 1997;15:646-649.
21. Maden C, Sherman K, Beckmann A, Hislop T, Teh C, Daling J. History of circumcision, medical conditions, and sexual activity and risk of penile cancer. *J Natl Cancer Inst*. 1993;85:19-24.
22. Pisani P, Parkin D, Munoz N, Ferlay J. Cancer and infection: estimates of the attributable fraction in 1990. *Cancer Epidemiol Biomarkers and Prev*. 1997;6:387-400.

23. Koutsky L, Kiviat NB. Genital Human Papillomaviruses. In: Holmes K, Mardh P, Sparling P, et al., eds. *Sexually Transmitted Diseases*. 3rd ed. New York: McGraw-Hill; 1999:347-360.

24. Svare EK, SK, Nonnemacher B, Worm A, et al. Seroactivity to human papillomavirus type 16 virus-like particles is lower in high-risk men than in high-risk women. *J Infect Dis*. 1997;176:876-883.

25. Wideroff L, Schiffman M, Hoover R, et al. Epidemiologic determinants of seroactivity to human papillomavirus (HPV) type 16 virus-like particles in cervical HPV-16 DNA-positive and -negative women. *J Infect Dis*. 1996;174:937-943.

26. Ho G, Bierman R, Beardsley L, Chang C, Burk R. Natural history of cervicovaginal papillomavirus infection in young women. *N Engl J Med*. 1998;338:423-428.

27. Baken L, Koutsky L, Kuypers J, et al. Genital human papillomavirus infection among male and female sex partners: prevalence and type-specific concordance. *J Infect Dis*. 1995;171:429-432.

28. Svare E, Kjaer S, A W, et al. Risk factors for HPV infection in women from sexually transmitted disease clinics: comparison between two areas with different cervical cancer incidence. *Cancer*. 1998;75:1-8.

29. Strickler H, Kirk G, Figueroa J, et al. HPV 16 antibody prevalence in Jamaica and the United States reflects differences in cervical cancer rates. *Int J Cancer*. 1999;80:339-344.

30. Eddy D. Screening for cervical cancer. *Ann Intern Med*. 1990;113:214-226.

31. Kurman R, Henson D, Herbst A, Noller K, Schiffman M. Interim guidelines for management of abnormal cervical cytology. *JAMA*. 1994;271:1866-1869.

32. World Health Organization. The current status of development of prophylactic vaccines against human papillomavirus infection. 1999. Report No.: WHO/V&B/99.04.

33. Ries L, Kosery C, Hankey B, Miller B, Clegg L, Edwards B. SEER Cancer Statistics Review 1973-1996. Vol. NIH Pub. No. 99-2789. Bethesda, MD: National Cancer Institute; 1999.

34. Melbye M, Rabkin C, Frisch M, Biggar R. Changing patterns of anal cancer incidence in the United States, 1940-1989. *Am J Epidemiol*. 1994;139:772-780.

35. Goldie S, Kuntz K, Weinstein M, Freedberg K, Welton M, Palefsky J. The clinical effectiveness and cost-effectiveness of screening for anal squamous intraepithelial lesions in homosexual and bisexual HIV-positive men. *JAMA*. 1999;281:1822-1829.

36. Chuang TY. Condyloma acuminatum in Rochester, Minnesota, 1950—1978. I. Epidemiology and clinical features. *Arch Dermatol*. 1984;120:469-475.

37. Armstrong L, Preston E, Reichert M. Incidence and prevalence of recurrent respiratory papillomatosis (RRP) among juveniles in the Atlanta and Seattle areas. . 15th International Papillomavirus Conference. Siena, Italy; 1997.

38. American Social Health Association. Sexually Transmitted Diseases in America: How Many Cases and at What Cost? 1998.

39. Siegal J. The economic burden of sexually transmitted diseases in the United States. In: Holmes K, Mardh P, Sparling P, et al., eds. *Sexually Transmitted Diseases*. 3rd ed. New York: McGraw-Hill; 1999:1367-1380.

40. Kotloff K, Wasserman S, Russ K, et al. Detection of genital human papillomavirus and associated cytological abnormalities among college women. *Sex Transm Dis*. 1998;25:243-250.

41. Munoz N, Kato I, Bosch F, et al. Risk factors for HPV DNA detection in middle-aged women. *Sex Transm Dis*. 1996;23:504-510.

42. Wheeler C, Parmenter C, Hunt W, et al. Determinants of genital human papillomavirus infection among cytologically normal women attending the University of New Mexico student health center. *Sex Transm Dis*. 1993;20:286-289.

43. Karlsson R, Jonsson M, Edlund K, et al. Lifetime number of partners as the only independent risk factor for human papillomavirus infection: a population-based study. *Sex Transm Dis*. 1995;22:119-126.

44. Kjellberg L, Wang Z, Wiklund F, et al. Sexual behavior and papillomavirus exposure in cervical intraepithelial neoplasia: a population-based case-control study. *J Gen Virol.* 1999;80:391-398.

45. Burk RD, Kelly P, Feldman J, et al. Declining prevalence of cervicovaginal human papillomavirus infection with age is independent of other risk factors. *Sex Transm Dis.* 1996;23:333-341.

46. Burk RD, Ho GYF, Beardsley L, Lempa M, Peters M, Bierman R. Sexual behavior and partner characteristics are the predominant risk factors for genital human papillomavirus infection in young women. *J Infect Dis.* 1996;174:679-689.

47. Figueroa J, Ward E, Luthi T, Vermund S, Brathwaite A, Burk R. Prevalence of human papillomavirus among STD clinic attenders in Jamaica: association of younger age and increased sexual activity. *Sex Transm Dis.* 1995;22:114-118.

48. Hildesheim A, Gravitt P, Schiffman M, et al. Determinants of genital human papillomavirus infection in low-income women in Washington, D.C. *Sex Transm Dis.* 1993;20:279-285.

49. Fairley C, Chen S, Ugoni A, Tabrizi S, Forbes A, Garland S. Human papillomavirus infection and its relationship to recent and distant sexual partners. *Obstet Gynecol.* 1994;84:755-759.

50. Hippelainen M, Syrjanen S, Hippelainen M, et al. Prevalence and risk factors of genital human papillomavirus (HPV) infections in healthy males: a study on Finnish conscripts. *Sex Transm Dis.* 1993;20(321):328.

51. Roden R, Lowy D, Schiller J. Papillomavirus is resistant to desiccation. *J Infect Dis.* 1997;176:1076-9.

52. Rice P, Cason J, Best J, Banatvala J. High risk genital papillomavirus infections are spread vertically. *Rev Med Virol.* 1999;9:15-21.

53. Cubie H, Plumstead M, Zhang W, de Jesus O, Duncan L, Stanley M. Presence of antibodies to human papillomavirus virus-like particles (VLPs) in 11-13 year-old schoolgirls. *J Med Virol.* 1998;56:210-216.

54. af Geijersstam V, Eklund C, Wang Z, et al. A survey of seroprevalence of HPV types 16, 18, and 33 among children. *Int J Cancer.* 1999;80:489-493.

55. Ley C, Bauer H, Reingold A, et al. Determinants of genital human papillomavirus infection in young women. *J Natl Cancer Inst.* 1991;83:997-1003.

56. Fairley C, Chen S, Tabrizi S, al e. The absence of genital human papillomavirus infection in virginal women. *International Journal of STD and AIDS.* 1992;3:414-417.

57. Gutman L, St Claire K, Herman-Giddens M, Johnston W, Phelps W. Evaluation of sexually abused and nonabused young girls for intravaginal human papillomavirus infection. *Am J Dis Child.* 1992;146(6):694-699.

58. Kashima H, Shah F, Lyles A, et al. A comparison of risk factors in juvenile-onset and adult-onset recurrent respiratory papillomatosis. *Laryngoscope.* 1992;102:9-13.

59. Bauer HM, Ting Y, Greer CE, et al. Genital human papillomavirus infection in female university students as determined by a PCR-based method. *JAMA.* 1991;265:472-477.

60. Bauer HM, Hildesheim A, Schiffman MH, et al. Determinants of genital human papillomavirus infection in low-risk women in Portland, Oregon. *Sex Transm Dis.* 1993;20:274-278.

61. Melkert PJ, Hopman E, van den Brule J, Risse E, Van Diest P, Bleker O. Prevalence of HPV in cytomorphlogically normal cervical smears, as determined by the polymerase chain reaction, is age-dependent. *Int J Cancer.* 1993;53:919-923.

62. Schneider A, Kirchhoff T, Meinhardt G, Gissmann L. Repeated evaluation of human papillomavirus 16 status in cervical swabs of young women with a history of normal papanicolaou smears. *Obstet Gynecol.* 1992;79:683-688.

63. Moscicki A, Palefsky J, Smith G, Siboshski S, Schoolnik G. Variability of human papillomavirus DNA testing in a longitudinal cohort of young women. *Obstet Gynecol.* 1993;82:578-585.

64. Wheeler C, Greer C, Becker T, Hunt W, Anderson S, Manos M. Short-term fluctuations in the detection of cervical human papillomavirus DNA. *Obstet Gynecol.* 1996;88:261-268.

65. Nobbenhuis M, Walboomers J, Helmerhorst T, et al. Relation of human papillomavirus status to cervical lesions and consequences for cervical-cancer screening: a prospective study. *Lancet.* 1999;354:20-25.

66. Hildesheim A, Schiffman M, Gravitt P, et al. Persistence of type-specific human papillomavirus infection among cytologically normal women. *J Infect Dis.* 1994;169:235-240.

67. Manos M, Kinney W, Hurley L, et al. Identifying women with cervical neoplasia: using human papillomavirus DNA testing for equivocal papanicolaou results. *JAMA.* 1999;281:1605.

68. Ronnett B, Manos M, Ransley J, et al. Atypical glandular cells of undetermined significance (AGUS): cytopathologic features, histopathologic results, and HPV DNA detection. *Hum Pathol.* 1999;30:816-25.

69. Kinney W, Manos M, Hurley L, Ransley J. Where's the high-grade cervical neoplasia? the importance of minimally abnormal Papanicolaou diagnoses. *Obstet Gynecol.* 1998;85:202-210.

70. Jenkins D, Sherlaw-Johnson C, Gallivan S. Assessing the role of HPV testing in cervical cancer screening. *Papillomavirus Rep.* 1998;9:89-101.

71. Cox J. Clinical role of HPV testing. *Obstet Gynecol Clinics NA.* 1996;23:811-851.

72. Cox J. Evaluating the role of HPV testing for women with equivocal papanicolaou test findings. *JAMA.* 1999;281:1645-1647.

73. Centers for Disease Control and Prevention. 1998 Guidelines for Treatment of Sexually Transmitted Diseases. *MMWR.* 1998;47(RR-1):1-116.

74. American College of Obstetrics and Gynecology. Cervical Cytology: Evaluation and management of abnormalities. *ACOG Technical Bulletin.* 1993(183):1-8.

75. Johnson K, The Canadian Task Force on the Periodic Health Examination. Periodic health examination, 1995 update: 1. Screening for human papillomavirus infection in asymptomatic women. *Can Med Assoc J.* 1995;152(4):483-493.

76. Kaufman R, Adam E. Does typing of human papillomavirus assist in the triage of women with repeated low-grade, cervical cytologic abnormalities? *Gynecol Oncol.* 1998;70:317-318.

77. Jenkins D, Sherlaw-Johnson C, Gallivan S. Can papilloma virus testing be used to improve cervical cancer screening? *Int J Cancer.* 1996;65:768-773.

78. Kaufman R, Adam E, Icenogle J, et al. Relevance of human papillomavirus screening in management of cervical intraepithelial neoplasia. *Am J Obstet Gynecol.* 1997;176:87-92.

79. Peyton C, Schiffman M, Lorincz A, et al. Comparison of PCR- and hybrid capture-based human papillomavirus detection systems using multiple cervical specimen collection strategies. *J Clin Microbiol.* 1998;36:3248-3254.

80. Ferris D, Wright Jr. T, Litaker M, et al. Comparison of two tests for detecting carcinogenic HPV in women with papanicolaou smear reports of ASCUS and LSIL. *J Fam Pract.* 1998;46:136-141.

81. Cox J. Management of cervical intraepithelial neoplasia. *Lancet.* 1999;353:857-859.

82. Chesebro M, Everett W, Lorincz A. High-risk human papillomavirus testing of women with cytological low-grade squamous intraepithelial lesions. *J Lower Genital Tract Dis.* 1997;1:234-239.

83. Wright Jr T, Lorincz A, Ferris D, et al. Reflex human papillomavirus deoxyribonucleic acid testing in women with abnormal papanicolaou smears. *Am J Obstet Gynecol.* 1998;178:962-966.

84. Sherman M, Schiffman M, Lorincz A, et al. Cervical specimens collected in liquid buffer are suitable for both cytologic screening and ancillary human papillomavirus testing. *Cancer.* 1997;81:89-97.

85. Schiffman M, Adrianza E, Group. TAS. The ASCUS-LSIL Triage Study (ALTS): design, methods, and characteristics of trial participants. [manuscript in preparation]. .

86. Meijer C, van den Brule A, Snijders P, Helmerhorst T, Kenemans P, Walboomers J. Detection of human papillomavirus in cervical scrapes by the polymerase chain reaction in relation to cytology: possible implications for cervical cancer screening. In: Munoz N, Bosch F, Shah K, Meheus A, eds. *The*

Epidemiology of Cervical Cancer and Human Papillomavirus. Lyons: International Agency for Research on Cancer; 1992:271-281.

87. Dillner J. Can cervical cancer screening programs be improved by incorporating screening for human papillomavirus infection? *The Cancer Journal*. 1998;11:272-275.

88. van Ballegooijen M, van den Akker-van Marie M, Warmerdam P, Meijer C, Walboomers J, Habbema J. Present evidence on the value of HPV testing for cervical cancer screening: a model-based exploration of the (cost-)effectiveness. *Br J Cancer*. 1997;76(5):651-657.

89. Ponten J, Adami H, Bergstrom R, et al. Strategies for global control of cervical cancer. *Int J Cancer*. 1995;60:1-26.

90. Cuzick J, Beverley E, Ho L, et al. The value of HPV testing in primary screening of older women. *Br J Cancer*. 1999;81:554-558.

91. Schneider A, Zahm D, Kirchmayr R, Schneider V. Screening for cervical intraepithelial neoplasia grade 2/3: validity of cytologic study, cervicography, and human papillomavirus detection. *Am J Obstet Gynecol*. 1999;174:1534-1541.

92. Ratnam S, Ghatage P, Franco E, Ferenczy A. Utility of HPV testing in combination with papanicolaou smear in primary cervical cancer screening. *17th International Papillomavirus Conference, Charleston, SC*. 1999.

93. Hill R, Kuhn L, Denny L, Wright T, Sun X, Lorincz A. Use of HPV DNA testing for cervical cancer screening: results from the Khayelitsha study, South Africa. *17th International Papillomavirus Conference, Charleston, SC*. 1999.

94. Clavel C, Masure M, Bory JP, et al. Hybrid Capture II-based human papillomavirus detection, a sensitive test to detect in routine high grade cervical lesions: a preliminary study on 1518 women. *Br J Cancer*. 1999;80:1306-11.

95. Schiffman M, Herrero R, Hildesheim A, et al. HPV DNA testing for cervical cancer screening: results from 9,000 women in the NCI Guanacaste project. *JAMA*. 2000 (in press).

96. Campion M, Cuzick J, McCance D, Singer A. Progressive potential of mild cervical atypia: prospective cytological, colposcopic, and virological study. *Lancet*. 1986;ii:237-240.

97. Hording U, Junge J, Rygaard C, Lundvall F. Management of low-grade CIN: follow-up of treatment? *Eur J Obstet Gynecol Reprod Biol*. 1995;62:49-52.

98. Liu T, Seng-jaw S, Alvarez R, Butterworth Jr. C. A longitudinal analysis of human papillomavirus 16 infection, nutritional status, and cervical dysplasia progression. *Cancer Epidemiology, Biomarkers, and Prevention*. 1995;4:373-380.

99. Remmink A, Walboomers J, TJM H, et al. The presence of persistent high-risk HPV genotypes in dysplastic cervical lesions is associated with progressive disease: natural history up to 36 months. *Int J Cancer*. 1995;61:306-311.

100. Nasiell K, Roger V, Nasiell M. Behavior of mild cervical dysplasia during long-term follow-up. *Obstet Gynecol*. 1986;67:665-669.

101. Mitchell H, Medley G. Age and time trends in the prevalence of cervical intraepithelial neoplasia on Papanicolaou smear tests, 1970-1988. *Med J Aust*. 1990;152:252-255.

102. Elfgren K, Bistoletti P, Dillner L, Walboomers J, Meijer C, Dillner J. Conization for cervical intraepithelial neoplasia is followed by disappearance of human papillomavirus deoxyribonucleic acid and a decline in serum and cervical mucus antibodies against human papillomavirus antigens. *Am J Obstet Gynecol*. 1996;174:937-942.

103. Mitchell M, Tortolero-Luna G, Cook E, Whittaker L, Rhodes-Morris H, Silva E. A randomized clinical trial of cryotherapy, laser vaporization, and loop electrosurgical excision for treatment of squamous intraepithelial lesions of the cervix. *Obstet Gynecol*. 1998;92(5):737-744.

104. Bollen L, Tjong-a-Hung S, van der Velden J, et al. Prediction of recurrent and residual dysplasia by human papillomavirus detection among patients with abnormal cytology. *Gynecol Oncol.* 1999;72:199-201.

105. American Cancer Society . *Guidelines for the cancer-related checkup: an update* Atlanta: American Cancer Society; 1993.

106. Hawkes A, Kronenberger C, MacKenzie T, et al. Cervical cancer screening: American College of Preventive Medicine practice policy statement. *Am J Prev Med.* 1996;12:342-344.

107. Woolf S. Screening for cervical cancer. In: DiGuiseppi C, Atkins D, Woolf S, eds. *Guide to Clinical Preventive Services: Report of the U.S. Preventive Services Task Force.* 2nd ed. Alexandria, Virginia: International Medical Publishing; 1996.

108. Crowther M. Is the nature of cervical carcinoma changing in young women? *Obstet Gynecol Surv.* 1994;50:71-82.

109. Mangan S, Legano L, Rosen C, et al. Increased prevalence of abnormal Papanicolau smears in urban adolescents. *Arch Pediatr Adolesc Med.* 1997;151:481-484.

110. Cook GA, Draper GJ. Trends in cervical cancer and carcinoma in situ in Great Britain. *Br J Cancer.* 1984;3:367-375.

111. Bourne RG, Grove W. Invasive carcinoma of the cervix in Queensland. Change in incidence and mortality, 1959-1980. *Med J Aust.* 1983;138:156-158.

112. Walton R, Allen H, Anderson G, et al. Cervical cancer screening programs: Summary of the 1982 Canadian Task Force Report. *Can Med Assoc J.* 1983;127:581-589.

113. Devesa S, Young J, Brinton L, JF F. Recent trends in cervix uteri cancer. *Cancer.* 1989;64:2184-2190.

114. Silcocks B, Moss S. Rapidly progressive cervical cancer: is it a real problem? *Br J Obstet Gynaecol.* 1988;95:1111-1116.

115. Hildesheim A, Hadjimichael O, Schwartz P, et al. Risk factors for rapid-onset cervical cancer. *Am J Obstet Gynecol.* 1999;180:571-577.

116. Perlman S, Kahn J, Emans S. Should pelvic examinations and papanicolaou cervical screening be part of preventive health care for sexually active adolescent girls? *J Adol Health.* 1998;23:62-67.

117. Siegfried E, Rasnick-Conley J, Cook S, Leonardi C, Monteleone J. Human papillomavirus screening in pediatric victims of sexual abuse. *Pediatrics.* 1998;101:43-47.

118. Shafer M. Annual pelvic examination in the sexually active adolescent female: what are we doing and why are we doing it? *J Adol Health.* 1998;23:68-73.

119. Hillard P, Brown R. Adolescent pap smear screening: yes or no. *J Ped Adol Gynecol.* 1996;9:93-97.

120. Olamijulo J. Is cervical cytology screening of teenagers worthwhile? *Br J Obstet Gynaecol.* 1995;102:515-516.

121. O'Mahony C. There is no longer a place for underage cytology in genitourinary medicine clinics. *Genitourin Med.* 1996;70:433-434.

122. Van Oortmarssen G, Habbema J. Epidemiological evidence for age-dependent regression of pre-invasive cervical cancer. *Br J Cancer.* 1991;64:559-565.

123. Montz F. Impact of therapy for cervical intraepithelial neoplasia on fertility. *Am J Obstet Gynecol.* 1996;175:1129-1136.

124. Hillard P, Biro F, Wildey L. Complications of cervical cryotherapy in adolescents. *J Reprod Med.* 1991;36:711-716.

125. Brunham RC, Plummer FA. A general model of STD epidemiology and its implications for control. *Med Clin North Am.* 1990;74:1339-1352.

126. Garnett G, Anderson R. Sexually transmitted diseases and sexual behavior: insights from mathematical models. *J Infect Dis.* 1996;174(Suppl2):S150-S161.

127. Peters R, Thomas D, Hagan D, Mack T, Henderson B. Risk factors for invasive cervical cancer among Latinas and Non-Latinas in Los Angeles County. *J Natl Cancer Inst.* 1986;77:1063-1077.

128. Slattery M, Overall Jr J, Abbott T, French T, Robison L, Gardner J. Sexual activity, contraception, genital infections, and cervical cancer: support for a sexually transmitted disease hypothesis. *Am J Epidemiol.* 1989;130:248-258.

129. Grimes D, Economy K. Primary prevention of gynecologic cancers. *Am J Obstet Gynecol.* 1995;172:227-235.

130. Shlay J, McGill W, Masloboeva H, Douglas Jr J. Pap smear screening in an urban STD clinic: yield of screening and predictors of abnormalities. *Sex Transm Dis.* 1998;25:468-475.

131. Celentano DD, Klassen AC, Weisman CS, Rosenshein NB. The role of contraceptive use in cervical cancer: the Maryland cervical cancer case-control study. *Am J Epidemiol.* 1987;126:592-604.

132. Hildesheim A, Brinton L, Mallin K, et al. Barrier and spermicidal contraceptive methods and risk of invasive cervical cancer. Epidemiol. 1990;1:266-272.

133. Daling J, Weiss N. Are barrier methods protective against cervical cancer? *Epidemiol.* 1990;1:261-262.

134. Rosenthal S, Cohen S, Stanberry L. Topical microbicides: current status and research considerations for adolescent girls. *Sex Transm Dis.* 1998;25:368-377.

135. Hermonat P, Daniel R, Shah K. The spermicide nonoxynol-9 does not inactivate papillomavirus. *Sex Transm Dis.* 1992;19:203-205.

136. Sokal D, Hermonat P. Inactivation of papillomavirus by low concentrations of povidone-iodine. *Sex Transm Dis.* 1995;22:22-24.

137. Howett M, Neely E, Christensen N, et al. A broad-spectrum microbicide with virucidal activity against sexually transmitted viruses. *Antimicrob Agents Chemother.* 1999:314-321.

138. Beutner KR, Richwald GA, Wiley DJ, Reitano MV, AMA Expert Panel on External Genital Warts. External genital warts: report of the American Medical Association Consensus Conference. *Clin Infect Dis.* 1998;27:796-806.

139. Tyring S, Arany I, Stanley M, et al. A randomized, controlled, molecular study of condylomata acuminata clearance during treatment with imiquimod. *J Infect Dis.* 1998;178:551-555.

140. Ferenczy A, Mitao M, Nagai N, Silverstein S, Crum C. Latent papillomavirus and recurring genital warts. *N Engl J Med.* 1985;313:784-788.

141. Colgan TJ, Percy ME, Suri M, Shier RM, Andrews DF, Lickrish GM. Human papillomavirus infection of morphologically normal cervical epithelium adjacent to squamous dysplasia and invasive carcinoma. *Hum Pathol.* 1989;20:316-319.

142. Beutner KR, Ferenczy A. Therapeutic approaches to genital warts. *Am J Med.* 1997;102 (5A):28-37.

143. Krebs H, Helmkamp F. Treatment failure of genital condylomata acuminata in women: role of the male sexual partner. *Am J Obstet Gynecol.* 1991;165:337-340.

144. Kamb M, Fishbein M, Douglas J. Efficacy of risk-reduction counseling to prevent human immunodeficiency virus and sexually transmitted diseases. *JAMA.* 1998;280:1161-1167.

145. Laumann E, Gagnon J, Michael R, Michaels S. The number of partners. *The Social Organization of Sexuality.* Chicago: The University of Chicago Press; 1994:172-224.

146. Schiller J, Okun M. Papillomavirus vaccines: current status and future prospects. *Adv Derm.* 1996;11:355-381.

147. Galloway D. Is vaccination against human papillomavirus a possibility? *Lancet.* 1998;351(suppl III):22-24.

148. Hines J, Ghim S, Jenson A. Prospects for human papillomavirus vaccine development: emerging HPV vaccines. *Curr Opin Infect Dis.* 1998;11:57-61.

149. Anderson RM, Garnett GP. Low-efficacy HIV vaccines: potential for community-based intervention programmes. *Lancet.* 1996;348:1010-1013.

150. Linnehan M, Andrews S, Groce N. College health providers' knowledge, attitudes, and management practices of genital HPV infection. *Nurse Pract.* 1996;21:122 -129.

151. McClean H, Hillman R. Anogenital warts and condom use—a survey of information giving. *Genitourin Med.* 1997;73:203-206.

152. Reitano M. Counseling patients with genital warts. *Am J Med.* 1997;102(5A):38-43.

153. Clarke P, Ebel C, Catotti DN, Stewart S. The psychosocial impact of human papillomavirus infection: implications for health care providers. *Internat J STD AIDS.* 1996;7:197-200.

154. Institute of Medicine. *The Hidden Epidemic: Confronting Sexually Transmitted Diseases.* Washington, D.C.: National Academy Press; 1997. Eng T, Butler W, eds.

155. Campion MJ, Brown JR, McCance DJ, et al. Psychosexual trauma of an abnormal cervical smear. *Br J Obstet Gynaecol.* 1988;95:175-181.

156. Persson G, Dahlof L, Krantz I. Physical and psychological effects of anogenital warts on female patients. *Sex Transm Dis.* 1993;20:10-13.

157. Bell S, Porter M, Kitchener H, Fraser C, Fisher P, Mann E. Psychological response to cervical screening. *Prev Med.* 1995;24:610-616.

158. Goldman S, Glimelius B, Nilsson B, Pahlman L. Incidence of anal epidermoid carcinoma in Sweden, 1970-1984. *Acta Chir Scand.* 1989;155:191-197.

159. Daling J, Weiss N, Klopfenstein L, Cochran L, Chow W, Daifuku R. Correlates of homosexual behavior and the incidence of anal cancer. *JAMA.* 1982;247:1988-1990.

160. Daling J, Weiss N, Hislop T, et al. Sexual practices, sexually transmitted diseases, and the incidence of anal cancer. *N Engl J Med.* 1987;317:973-977.

161. Holly E, Whittemore A, Aston D, Ahn D, Nickoloff B, Kristiansen J. Anal cancer incidence: genital warts, anal fissure or fistula, hemorrhoids, and smoking. *J Natl Cancer Inst.* 1989;81:1726-1731.

162. Koblin B, Hessol N, Zauber A, et al. Increased incidence of cancer among homosexual men, New York City and San Francisco, 1978-1990. *Am J Epidemiol.* 1996;144:916-923.

163. Palefsky J. Anal human papillomavirus infection and anal cancer in HIV-positive individuals: an emerging problem. *AIDS.* 1994;8:283-295.

164. Rabkin C, Biggar R, Melbye M, Curtis R. Second primary cancers following anal and cervical carcinoma: evidence of shared etiologic factors. *Am J Epidemiol.* 1992;136:54-8.

165. Palefsky J, Holly E, Gonzales J, Lamborn K, Hollander H. Natural history of anal cytologic abnormalities and papillomavirus infection among homosexual men with group IV HIV disease. *J Acquir Immune Defic Syndr Hum Retroviro.* 1992;5:1258-1265.

166. Critchlow C, Surawicz C, Holmes K, et al. Prospective study of high grade anal squamous intraepithelial neoplasia in a cohort of homosexual men: influence of HIV infection, immunosuppression and human papillomavirus infection. *AIDS.* 1995;9:1255-1262.

167. Goedert J, Cote T, Virgo P, et al. Spectrum of AIDS-associated malignant disorders. *Lancet.* 1998;351:1833-1839.

168. Palefsky J, Holly E, Ralston M, Jay N, Berry M, Darragh T. High incidence of anal high-grade squamous intra-epithelial lesions among HIV-positive and HIV-negative homosexual and bisexual men. *AIDS.* 1998;12:495-503.

169. Melbye M, Cote T, Kessler L, Gail M, Biggar R, AIDS/Cancer Working Group. High incidence of anal cancer among AIDS patients. *Lancet.* 1994;343:636-639.

170. Vernon S, Holmes K, Reeves W. Human papillomavirus infection and associated disease in persons infected with human immunodeficiency virus. *Clin Infect Dis.* 1995;21 (suppl 1):S121-S124.

171. Centers for Disease Control. 1999 USPHS/IDSA guidelines for the prevention of opportunistic infections in persons infected with human immunodeficiency virus. *MMWR*. 1999;48(RR-10):1-87.

172. de Ruiter A, Carter P, Katz D, et al. A comparison between cytology and histology to detect anal intraepithelial neoplasia. *Genitourin Med*. 1994;70:22-25.

173. Palefsky J, Holly E, Hogeboom C, Berry J, Jay N, al e. Anal cytology as a screening tool for anal squamous intraepithelial lesions. *Lancet*. 1997;351:1833-1839.

174. Goldie S, Kuntz K, Weinstein M, Freedberg K, Palefsky J. Cost-effectiveness of screening for anal squamous cell cancer in homosexual and bisexual men. *Am J Med*. 2000 (in press).

175. Heard I, Schmitz V, Costagliola D, Orth G, Kazatchkine M. Early regression of cervical lesions in HIV-seropositive women receiving highly active antiretroviral therapy. *AIDS*. 1998;12:1459-1464.

176. Centers for Disease Control, Division of STD Prevention. Sexually Transmitted Diseases Surveillance 1997. 1998.

177. Fleming D, McQuillan G, Johnson R, et al. Herpes simplex virus type 2 in the United States, 1976 to 1994. *N Engl J Med*. 1997;337(16):1105-1111.

7. American Cancer Society Detailed Guide on Cervical Cancer

American Cancer Society®

Cancer Reference Information

print
close

Detailed Guide: Cervical Cancer

What Are the Risk Factors for Cervical Cancer?

A risk factor is anything that increases your chance of getting a disease such as cancer. Different cancers have different risk factors. For example, exposing skin to strong sunlight is a risk factor for skin cancer. Smoking is a risk factor for cancers of the lung, mouth, larynx, bladder, kidney, and several other organs. But having a risk factor, or even several, does not mean that a person will get the disease.

Several risk factors increase your chance of developing cervical cancer. Women without any of these risk factors rarely develop cervical cancer. Although these risk factors increase the odds of developing cervical cancer, many women with these risks do not develop this disease. When a woman develops cervical cancer or precancerous changes, it is not possible to say with certainty that a particular risk factor was the cause.

In considering these risk factors, it helps to focus on those that you can change or avoid (such as smoking and sexual behaviors that can lead to human papillomavirus infection), rather than those that you cannot (such as differences in age and family history). However, understanding risk factors that cannot be changed is still important because it can convince women with these factors to get a Pap test for early detection of cervical cancer. Cervical cancer risk factors include:

Human papillomavirus infection: The most important risk factor for cervical cancer is infection by the human papillomavirus (HPV). Doctors feel that a woman must be infected with this virus before they develop cervical cancer. HPVs are a group of more than 100 types of viruses called papillomaviruses because they can cause warts, or papillomas. Certain types, however, cause cancer of the cervix. These are called "high-risk" HPV types and include HPV 16, HPV 18, HPV 31, HPV 33, and HPV 45, as well as some others. About half of all cervical cancers are caused by HPV 16 and 18.

Other HPV types cause different types of warts in different parts of your body. Some types cause common warts on the hands and feet. Other types tend to cause warts on the lips or tongue. Certain HPV types can infect the female and male genital organs and the anal area. These HPV types are passed from one person to another during sexual contact.

When HPV infects the skin of the external (outer) genital organs and anal area, it often causes raised bumpy warts. These may be barely visible or they may be several inches across. The medical term for genital warts is condyloma accuminatum. Most genital warts are caused by two HPV types: HPV 6 and HPV 11. These seldom are associated with cervical cancer and are called "low-risk" viruses. However, other sexually transmitted HPVs have been linked with genital or anal cancers in both men and women.

HPVs can also cause flat warts on the cervix or vagina that are not visible and cause no symptoms. Flat warts caused by low-risk HPV types have little or no effect on cancer risk. Flat warts caused by high-risk HPV types can develop into cervical or vaginal cancers. Most health care professionals do not determine the HPV type because these warts are usually treated.

There is currently no cure for papillomavirus infection. However, the warts and abnormal cell growth caused by these viruses can be treated effectively. These treatments can destroy flat warts on the cervix and vagina and prevent them from developing into cancers.

Most women with HPV infection do not develop cervical cancer. Usually the infection disappears without any treatment, because the woman's immune system has been successful in fighting the virus.

Precancerous changes are diagnosed when abnormal cells are found in specimens (samples) taken from a Pap test or biopsy (these are discussed further in "Can Cervical Cancer Be Prevented?"). HPV infection can cause changes in cells of the cervix that can be detected by the Pap test. New tests can directly identify HPVs by finding their DNA in the cells. Many doctors are now testing for HPV if the Pap smear result is mildly abnormal (doctors refer to these findings as atypical squamous cells, or ASC). If a high-risk type of HPV is present, they will perform a colposcopy and consider further treatment.

Certain types of sexual behavior increase a woman's risk of getting HPV infection:

- intercourse at an early age
- having many sexual partners
- having sex with uncircumcised males

HPV can be present for years with no symptoms, and HPV infection does not always produce warts or other symptoms; so you can be infected with HPV and pass it on without knowing it. Recent studies show that condoms ("rubbers") do not protect well against HPV infection. This is because HPV can be passed from person to person by skin-to-skin contact with any HPV-infected area of the body, such as skin of the genital or anal area not covered by the condom. The absence of visible warts cannot be used to decide whether caution is needed, because HPV can be passed to another person even when there are no visible warts or other symptoms.

Although condoms do not protect against HPV, it is still important, though, to use condoms to protect against AIDS and other sexually transmitted diseases that are passed on through some body fluids.

Although it is necessary to be infected with HPV for cervical cancer to develop, most women with this infection do not develop cancer. Doctors feel that other factors must come into play for cancer to develop. Some of the known factors are listed below.

Smoking: Women who smoke are about twice as likely as nonsmokers to get cervical cancer. Smoking exposes the body to many cancer-causing chemicals that affect more than the lungs. These harmful substances are absorbed by the lungs and carried in the bloodstream throughout the body. Tobacco by-products have been found in the cervical mucus of women who smoke. Researchers believe that these substances damage the DNA of cells in the cervix and may contribute to the development of cervical cancer.

Human immunodeficiency virus (HIV) infection: HIV is the virus that causes the acquired immunodeficiency syndrome(AIDS). Because this virus damages the body's immune system, it makes women more susceptible to HPV infections, which may increase the risk of cervical cancer. Scientists believe that the immune system is important in destroying cancer cells and slowing their growth and spread. In women infected with HIV, a cervical precancer might develop into an invasive cancer faster than it normally would.

Chlamydia infection: Chlamydia is a relatively common kind of bacteria that can infect the female reproductive system. It is spread by sexual contact. Although infection may cause symptoms, many women do not know they are infected unless samples taken at the time of their Pap test are analyzed for this type of bacteria.

Some recent studies suggest that women whose blood test results indicate past or current chlamydia infection are at greater risk for cervical cancer than are women with a negative blood test. Although further studies are needed to confirm this finding, there is already good reason to avoid this infection and to have it treated with antibiotics promptly after diagnosis. Long-term chlamydia infection is well known as a cause of pelvic inflammation that can lead to infertility.

Diet: Women with diets low in fruits and vegetables may be at increased risk for cervical cancer. Also overweight women are more likely to develop this cancer.

Oral contraceptives: There is evidence that long-term oral contraceptive (OC) use increases the risk of cancer of the cervix. Some research suggests a relationship between using OCs for 5 or more years and an increase in the risk of cervical cancer. In one study the risk was increased four fold in women who used OCs longer than 10 years.

In the meantime, the American Cancer Society believes that a woman and her doctor should discuss whether the benefits of using OCs outweigh this very slight potential risk. A woman with multiple sexual partners should use condoms to lower her risk of sexually transmitted diseases no matter what form of contraception she uses.

Multiple pregnancies: Women who have had many full term pregnancies have an increased risk of developing cervical cancer.

Low socioeconomic status: Low socioeconomic status is also a risk factor for cervical cancer. Many women with low incomes do not have ready access to adequate health care services, including Pap tests and treatment of precancerous cervical disease. Such women may also be undernourished, which may play a role in increasing their risk.

Diethylstilbestrol (DES): DES is a hormonal drug that was prescribed between 1940 and 1971 for some women thought to be at increased risk for miscarriages. Of every 1,000 women whose mother took DES when pregnant with them, about 1 develops clear-cell adenocarcinoma of the vagina or cervix. Stated another way, about 99.9% of "DES daughters" do not develop these cancers.

Clear cell adenocarcinomas are more common in the vagina than the cervix. The risk appears to be greatest in those whose mothers took the drug during their first 16 weeks of pregnancy. The average age at diagnosis of DES-related clear-cell adenocarcinoma is 19 years. Most DES daughters are now between 30 and 60, so the number of new cases of DES-related cervical and vaginal clear-cell adenocarcinoma has been decreasing during the past 2 decades. However, this type of cancer has recently been found in a woman in her early 40s, and doctors still do not know exactly how long women remain at risk for DES-related cancers.

Although DES daughters have an increased risk of developing clear cell carcinomas, about 40% of women with this cancer have not been exposed to DES or related medications. Some of these patients' mothers might have taken DES but did not recall the name of the drug. It is certain, however, that women don't have to be exposed to DES for clear cell carcinoma to develop since some cases of the disease were diagnosed before DES was invented. Some studies suggest that DES daughters are also at somewhat increased risk of developing squamous cell cancer of the cervix and precancerous changes of cervical squamous cells.

Family history of cervical cancer: Recent studies suggest that women whose mother or sisters have had cervical cancer are more likely to develop the disease themselves. Some researchers suspect this familial tendency is caused by an inherited condition that makes some women less able to fight off HPV infection than others.

Revised 10-21-03

8. NIH Consensus Statement on Cervical Cancer

NIH Consensus Statement

Volume 14, Number 1
April 1–3, 1996

Cervical Cancer

This statement reflects the panel's assessment of medical knowledge available at the time the statement was written. Thus, it provides a "snapshot in time" of the state of knowledge on the conference topic. When reading the statement, keep in mind that new knowledge is inevitably accumulating through medical research.

National Institutes Of Health
Continuing Medical Education

NATIONAL INSTITUTES OF HEALTH
Office of the Director

Abstract

Objective

To provide physicians and the general public with a responsible assessment of current screening, prevention, and treatment approaches to cervical cancer.

Participants

A non-Federal, nonadvocate, 13-member panel representing the fields of obstetrics and gynecology, gynecologic oncology, radiation oncology, and epidemiology. In addition, 28 experts in obstetrics and gynecology, gynecologic oncology, radiation oncology, gynecologic surgery, and psychology presented data to the panel and a conference audience of 500.

Evidence

The literature was searched through Medline and an extensive bibliography of references was provided to the panel and the conference audience. Experts prepared abstracts with relevant citations from the literature. Scientific evidence was given precedence over clinical anecdotal experience.

Consensus Process

The panel, answering predefined questions, developed its conclusions based on the scientific evidence presented in open forum and the scientific literature. The panel composed a draft statement that was read in its entirety and circulated to the experts and the audience for comment. Thereafter, the panel resolved conflicting recommendations and released a revised statement at the end of the conference. The panel finalized the revisions within a few weeks after the conference.

Conclusions

Carcinoma of the cervix is causally related to infection with the human papillomavirus (HPV). Reducing the rate of HPV infection by changes in sexual behaviors in young people and/or through the development of an effective HPV vaccine would reduce the incidence of this disease. Pap smear screening remains the best available method of reducing the incidence and mortality of invasive cervical cancer. Persons with stage IA1 disease have a high cure rate with either simple hysterectomy or, where fertility preservation is an issue, by cone biopsy with clear margins. For patients with other stage I and stage IIA disease, radical surgery and radiation are equally effective treatments. These patients should be carefully selected to receive one treatment or the other but not both, as their combined use substantially increases the cost and morbidity of treatment. Women with more advanced, nonmetastatic disease should be treated with radiation. Recurrent cervical cancer confined to the pelvis should be treated with the modality not previously received. Radiation is recommended to palliate symptoms in patients with metastatic disease.

Introduction

Carcinoma of the cervix is one of the most common malignancies in women, accounting for 15,700 new cases (6 percent of all cancers) and 4,900 deaths in the United States each year. Worldwide, cervical cancer is second only to breast cancer as the most common malignancy in both incidence and mortality. More than 471,000 new cases are diagnosed each year, predominantly among the economically disadvantaged, in both developing and industrialized nations. During the last 50 years in the United States, the utilization of screening programs based on the Papanicolaou (Pap) smear and pelvic examination has led to a steep decline in incidence and deaths from cervical cancer.

Both invasive cervical cancers and precursor lesions have been firmly associated with the presence of human papillomavirus (HPV) DNA. It has also been well established that the majority of squamous cell cancers of the cervix progress through a series of well-defined preinvasive lesions and that during this usually lengthy process, the disease can be easily detected by Pap smear screening. During this preinvasive stage, cervical squamous intraepithelial lesions (SIL) can be controlled with nearly uniform success and with the retention of fertility.

Many treatment and quality-of-life issues remain unresolved for women with cervical cancer. For women with early-stage disease, key issues include determining guidelines for the extent of treatment, the pathologic and clinical indicators for the intensity of therapy, and the selection of a treatment modality among several competing options. For women with advanced-stage disease, critical issues include optimal radiotherapy techniques, whether chemotherapy or combined modality regimens improve outcome, the morbidity and benefit of salvage therapy for recurrent disease, and palliative treatment. Additional topics include advances in screening technology, the implementation of The Bethesda System for Pap smears, the role of HPV testing and subtyping, treatment selection for patients with preinvasive disease, advances in laparoscopic surgical staging and therapy techniques, and the application of newer imaging techniques such as magnetic resonance. Prospects for both prophylactic and therapeutic vaccines against HPV offer hope for fundamental alterations in the prevention and management of this disease.

To address these and related issues, the National Cancer Institute and the NIH Office of Medical Applications of Research convened a Consensus Development Conference on Cervical Cancer. The conference was cosponsored by the National Institute of Nursing Research, the National Institute of Allergy and Infectious Diseases, the Office of Research on Minority Health and the Office of Research on Women's Health of the NIH, and the Centers for Disease Control and Prevention.

After 1 1/2 days of presentations and audience discussion, an independent, non-Federal consensus panel weighed the scientific evidence and developed a draft statement that addressed the following key questions:

- How can we strengthen efforts to prevent cervical cancer?
- What is the appropriate management of low-stage cervical cancer (FIGO stages I–IIA)?
- What is the appropriate management of advanced-stage and recurrent cervical cancer?
- What are new directions for research in cervical cancer?

How Can We Strengthen Efforts to Prevent Cervical Cancer?

A strong causal relationship between HPV and cervical cancer and its precursors has been established. The evidence for this statement is as follows:

- HPV DNA is present in virtually all cases (93 percent) of cervical cancer and its precursor lesions.
- Multiple epidemiological studies indicate that HPV infection is the major risk factor for squamous intraepithelial lesions (SIL) and invasive cervical carcinoma.
- Studies have demonstrated that the HPV genes E6 and E7 are integrated into the host genome and that the transforming proteins encoded by these genes are tumorigenic.

More than 70 types of HPV have been identified. However, only 23 of these infect the uterine cervix; of these, only one-half are associated with SIL or invasive cervical cancer. These are further classified into low-risk types, HPV 6 and 11, and high-risk types, most commonly 16, 18, 31, and 45, which account for more than 80 percent of all invasive cervical cancers. An unknown percentage of women infected with HPV will develop either low-grade SIL (LSIL) or high-grade SIL (HSIL). One-third of all grades of SIL will regress, whereas 41 percent persist and 25 percent progress. Of lesions that progress, 10 percent progress to carcinoma in situ and 1 percent to invasive cancer. Three-quarters of all grades of SIL will not progress.

This virus is transmitted through sexual intercourse, with a peak prevalence of infection in women in the 22–25-year age group. The prevalence of infection decreases with increasing age suggesting that most infections in women and men resolve over time through host immune responses.

Epidemiologic studies are now focusing on cofactors and host factors that may explain the natural history of HPV infections and their associated lesions. Factors under investigation include smoking; use of hormonal contraceptives; number of live births; young age at first sexual intercourse;

use of vitamins such as carotenoids, vitamin C, and folic acid; co-infection with other sexually transmitted diseases (e.g., herpes simplex, HIV, chlamydia); growth factors; cytokines; and humoral and cellular immunity.

Screening

Squamous cell cervical cancer is an ideal disease for screening because of the typically long preclinical phase, which permits early detection. Use of the Pap smear is effective in reducing morbidity and mortality from cervical cancer. Despite the recognized benefits of Pap smear screening, substantial subgroups of American women have not been screened or are not screened at regular intervals. One-half of the women with newly diagnosed invasive cervical carcinoma have never had a Pap smear, and another 10 percent have not had a smear in the past 5 years.

The unscreened populations include older women, the uninsured, ethnic minorities, especially Hispanics and elderly blacks, and poor women, particularly those in rural areas. One-fourth of the cases of cervical cancer and 41 percent of the deaths occur in women age 65 and older. Data from the 1992 National Health Interview Survey indicate that one-half of all women age 60 and older have not had a Pap smear in the past 3 years. Although older women are screened less frequently, they have the same number of recent physician visits as younger women, which indicates the need to educate older women and their health care providers about the importance of Pap smear screening. For patients who are not involved in routine screening programs, any health care encounter should be an opportunity to obtain a Pap smear and offer other screening modalities. On the other hand, recent evidence demonstrates that the gap in the incidence of cervical cancer between black and white women under age 50 is disappearing, suggesting that the rate of screening has increased among young black women.

To improve outreach to unscreened populations, reasons for nonparticipation in screening must be determined and addressed with appropriate interventions. Community-based approaches to reaching diverse ethnic populations are recommended and should include using community leaders and members to assess attitudes and concerns prior to instituting screening programs, and as part of the process of education and awareness. Culturally sensitive and linguistically compatible staffing for outreach and screening is a key component.

Logistical problems associated with screening in both metropolitan and rural settings should be addressed during outreach planning (e.g., transportation, child care, duration of appointments, multiple site referrals, accessible screening sites). Options such as mobile screening services and incentives should be considered.

A concerted effort to standardize Pap smear terminology resulted in The Bethesda System (TBS) (Table 1). TBS evaluates the specimen for adequacy, uses diagnostic terminology, and makes recommendations pertaining to the smear when necessary. Determining the adequacy of the specimen is a major contribution, because retrospective reviews of smears from women with cervical cancer have shown that many were unsatisfactory. Smears may be unsatisfactory for a variety of reasons, the most common of which are obscuring blood or inflammation. Evaluation of others may be less than optimal because of factors such as absence of sampling from the transformation zone.

Among the diagnostic terminologies are LSIL and HSIL. Another category of abnormal squamous cells is atypical squamous cells of undetermined significance (ASCUS). Management modalities for HSIL are established and include colposcopy-directed biopsy and endocervical curettage followed by conization with scalpel, cautery, laser, or loop electrocautery excision procedure. Management modalities for ASCUS and LSIL are not as uniform. A large clinical trial is currently under way to determine whether HPV testing can effectively triage these patients, to develop clinical management guidelines and provide prognostic information, and to identify areas for cost reduction in screening and treatment. The glandular cell abnormalities are divided into two categories, atypical glandular cells of undetermined significance (AGUS) and adenocarcinoma.

Table 1

The 1991 Bethesda System

Adequacy of the Specimen

Satisfactory for evaluation
Satisfactory for evaluation but limited by (specify reason)
Unsatisfactory for evaluation (specify reason)

General Categorization (Optional)

Within normal limits
Benign cellular changes; see descriptive diagnosis
Epithelial cell abnormality; see descriptive diagnosis

Descriptive Diagnoses

- Benign cellular changes
  - Infection
    - *Trichomonas vaginalis*
    - Fungal organisms morphologically consistent with Candida sp
    - Predominance of coccobacilli consistent with shift in vaginal flora
    - Bacteria morphologically consistent with Actinomyces sp
    - Cellular changes associated with herpes simplex virus
    - Other
  - Reactive changes
  - Reactive cellular changes associated with:
    - Inflammation (includes typical repair)
    - Atrophy with inflammation ("atrophic vaginitis")
    - Radiation
    - Intrauterine contraceptive device (IUD)
    - Other
- Epithelial cell abnormalities
  - Squamous cell
    - Atypical squamous cells of undetermined significance (ASCUS): qualify*
  - Low-grade squamous intraepithelial lesion (LSIL) encompassing HPV** mild dysplasia/CIN 1
  - High-grade squamous intraepithelial lesion (HSIL) encompassing moderate and severe dysplasia, CIS/CIN 2, and CIN 3
    - Squamous cell carcinoma
  - Glandular cell
    - Endometrial cells, cytologically benign, in a postmenopausal woman
    - Atypical glandular cells of undetermined significance: qualify*
    - Endocervical adenocarcinoma
    - Endometrial adenocarcinoma
    - Extrauterine adenocarcinoma
    - Adenocarcinoma, not otherwise specified
- Other malignant neoplasms: specify
- Hormonal evaluation (applies to vaginal smears only)
  - Hormonal pattern compatible with age and history
  - Hormonal pattern incompatible with age and history; specify
  - Hormonal evaluation not possible due to...(specify)

*Atypical squamous or glandular cells of undetermined significance should be further qualified as to whether a reactive or a premalignant/malignant process is favored.

**Cellular changes of HPV (previously termed "koilocytotic atypia" or "condylomatous atypia") are included in the category of low-grade squamous intraepithelial lesion.

Methods of specimen acquisition, preparation, and evaluation of the Pap smear have changed little since its introduction in the 1940's. Although it is highly effective in screening for preinvasive lesions of the cervix, a single test has a false-negative rate estimated to be 20 percent. One-half of the false negatives are due to inadequate specimen sampling, and the other half are attributed to a failure to identify the abnormal cells or to interpret them accurately. Pap smears should be obtained in conjunction with a pelvic examination. If a gross lesion is visualized, it should be biopsied, as a Pap smear alone is inadequate in this situation.

To improve the adequacy of the cervical smear specimen, a variety of sampling devices is available (e.g., spatula, endocervical brush, broom, and cotton swab). Liquid-based specimen collection methods are currently being evaluated to improve sampling and cell preservation and presentation.

In fall 1995, the Food and Drug Administration (FDA) approved two automated instruments for rescreening smears evaluated as negative on the initial screen. Data from clinical trials suggest that these could reduce the rate of false–negative smears. Neither the efficacy in routine practice nor the cost-benefit of these devices has been determined. In addition, these and other devices are being evaluated for use as primary screening instruments.

In 1988 a group of experts recommended that annual Pap smears and pelvic examinations begin at onset of sexual activity or age 18. After three consecutive normal examinations, the interval between screenings may increase at the discretion of the physician and patient. In 1995, the American College of Obstetricians and Gynecologists (ACOG) recommended that patients with one or more risk factors for cervical cancer (e.g., HIV or HPV infection, a history of LSIL, high-risk behavior) be screened annually. Women over the age of 65 should continue to be screened.

Prevention

Primary prevention of HPV infection will require (1) directing education efforts toward adolescents and health care providers regarding the strong causal link between acquisition of

HPV as a sexually transmitted disease and development of cervical cancer and its precursors, (2) encouraging delayed onset of sexual intercourse, (3) developing an effective prophylactic vaccine, and (4) developing effective vaginal microbicides. The data on the use of barrier methods of contraception to prevent the spread of HPV are controversial but do not support this as an effective method of prevention.

Secondary prevention efforts must focus on (1) developing effective antiviral agents to treat HPV and/or prevent transformation by E6/E7, (2) developing therapeutic vaccines to prevent HPV progression, (3) improving the sensitivity and specificity of screening for the precursors of cervical cancer, and (4) expanding education and screening programs to target underreached populations.

9. NIH Workshop Executive Summary on Condom Effectiveness

Workshop Summary:

Scientific Evidence on Condom Effectiveness

for Sexually Transmitted Disease (STD) Prevention

June 12-13, 2000

Hyatt Dulles Airport

Herndon, Virginia

This summary report was prepared by the National Institute of Allergy and Infectious Diseases, National Institutes of Health, Department of Health and Human Services.

July 20, 2001

EXECUTIVE SUMMARY

Background

Sexually transmitted diseases (STDs), including HIV, are common, important, and preventable causes of morbidity, mortality, disability, lost-productivity, and health care costs. In the United States, more than 65 million individuals are living with an STD, the majority of which are incurable viral infections. Approximately 15 million new sexually transmitted infections occur annually in the U.S. In the United States, approximately 493,000 individuals have died from AIDS, and 800,000-900,000 people are living with HIV disease. Many sexually transmitted infections can cause adverse pregnancy outcomes including miscarriages, stillbirths, intrauterine growth restriction and perinatal (mother-to-infant) infections. Some STDs can cause infertility or lead to ectopic pregnancy among women and one, the human papillomavirus, can cause cervical and anogenital cancer. Furthermore, other STDs facilitate HIV transmission.

The Problem and the Process

Primary prevention of STD infection is an important health priority. Unfortunately there are no STD vaccines, except for hepatitis B vaccine, and topical microbicides to prevent STDs are not available. Beyond mutual lifelong monogamy among uninfected couples, condom-use is the only method for reducing the risk of HIV infection and STDs available to sexually active individuals.

Recently, a number of Federal agencies sponsored a workshop to answer the following question: "What is the scientific evidence on the effectiveness of latex male condom-use to prevent STD transmission during vaginal intercourse?" This workshop was attended by 180 persons, and the data from numerous peer-reviewed published studies were discussed. Following the workshop, a panel of 28 experts worked to develop this report.

The sessions included review of published information on the properties and user patterns of the male latex condoms for vaginal intercourse and included data from studies on pregnancy prevention. Focused research studies have documented the high effectiveness of condoms for prevention of pregnancy. The data associated with condom use in eight specific STDs were considered in detail, including HIV infection, gonorrhea, chlamydial infection (including gonococcal and chlamydial pelvic inflammatory disease), syphilis, chancroid, trichomoniasis, genital herpes, and genital HPV infection and associated diseases (i.e. cervical dysplasia, cervical cancer and genital warts).

The meeting was not intended to make public health policy recommendations regarding the role of condoms in HIV/STD prevention policy and programs.

Assessment of the Data

In general, the Panel found the published epidemiology literature to be inadequate to definitively answer the question posed to the workshop participants. Most studies reviewed did not employ a prospective design, which is the optimal method to assess the effectiveness of condoms in preventing infection.

Conclusions on STDs Transmitted by Genital Secretions

The published data documenting effectiveness of the male condom were strongest for HIV. The Panel concluded that, based on a meta-analysis of published studies "always" users of the male condom significantly reduced the risk of HIV infection in men and women. These data provided strong evidence for the effectiveness of condoms in preventing HIV transmission in both men and women who engage in vaginal intercourse.

The Panel also concluded that the consistency of findings across four epidemiological studies of gonorrhea indicated that the latex male condom could reduce the risk of gonorrhea for men.

The strongest evidence for potential effectiveness of condoms on other STDs transmitted by genital secretions (i.e. gonorrhea in women, chlamydial infection and trichomoniasis) was the laboratory-based studies on the properties of the male latex condom and the strength of the evidence for condom use reducing the risk of HIV transmission in men and women and gonorrhea in men. The Panel concluded, however, that because of limitations in study designs there was insufficient evidence from the epidemiological studies on these diseases to draw definite conclusions about the effectiveness of the latex male condom in reducing the transmission of these diseases.

Conclusions on Genital Ulcer Diseases

The Panel agreed that the published epidemiologic data were insufficient to draw meaningful conclusions about the effectiveness of the latex male condom to reduce the risk of transmission of genital ulcer diseases (genital herpes, syphilis and chancroid).

Conclusions on HPV

For HPV, the Panel concluded that there was no epidemiologic evidence that condom use reduced the risk of HPV infection, but study results did suggest that condom use might afford some protection in reducing the risk of HPV-associated diseases, including warts in men and cervical neoplasia in women.

Summary

The Panel stressed that the absence of definitive conclusions reflected inadequacies of the evidence available and should not be interpreted as proof of the adequacy or inadequacy of the condom to reduce the risk of STDs other than HIV transmission in men and women and gonorrhea in men. To definitely answer the remaining questions about condom effectiveness for preventing STD infections will require well-designed and ethically sound clinical studies.

10. NCI Letter to House Subcommittee on Health and Environment

DEPARTMENT OF HEALTH & HUMAN SERVICES

Public Health Service

National Institutes of Health
National Cancer Institute
Bethesda, Maryland 20892

APR 8 1999

The Honorable Michael Bilirakis
Chairman
House Committee on Commerce
Subcommittee on Health and Environment
Washington, D.C. 20515

Dear Mr. Chairman:

I am responding to your letter of March 19, 1999, in which you pose twelve questions as a follow-up to my testimony before the Subcommittee on Health and Environment on March 16, 1999.

As requested, the questions have been restated below. The answer follows each numbered question.

1. **The National Cancer Institute (NCI) is in the process of conducting a randomized trial to establish the best way to manage abnormalities that are discovered during Pap smear tests. This study is often referred to as ASCUS/LSIL Triage Study or ALTS. Please explain the purpose and significance of this trial?**

NCI is conducting a large randomized trial to find the best way to manage the mild abnormalities that often show up on Pap tests and may, in rare instances, progress to cancer if left untreated. The ALTS trial is comparing three approaches: 1) immediate colposcopy (a procedure in which a physician examines the cervix through a magnifying instrument and biopsies any abnormal area; 2) repeating the Pap test every six months (because most abnormalities return to normal without treatment); and 3) testing for cancer-associated types of HPV as a means to differentiate between abnormalities that need immediate colposcopy and those that can be best followed with repeat Pap tests. Researchers will compare the three different groups to assess the effectiveness of each management option in detecting the serious abnormalities that can progress to cancer, the acceptability of each option to patients, and the cost effectiveness of each option.

2. **When do you estimate the NCI will develop a vaccine for human papillomavirus (HPV)? Can you describe all of the different HPV vaccines that are being tested?**

There are both preventative and therapeutic HPV vaccines which have been developed by the NCI that are currently being tested in clinical trials. They seek to prevent infection or to induce regression of established infection via immune recognition of specific HPV-encoded proteins or peptides. Such vaccines can be delivered either directly as a protein or by viral vectors derived from organisms of a different but related species.

3. What effect, if any, does HPV have on men?

Scientists have found an association between several types of HPV and the development of anal cancer and cancer of the penis (a rare cancer). HPV also frequently causes benign warts.

4. In addition to cervical cancer, what other effects can HPV have on the body?

Genital warts (condylomata acuminata or venereal warts) are caused by only a few of the many types of HPV. Other common types of HPV infections, such as those that cause warts on the hands and soles of the feet, only rarely cause genital warts. In women, the warts occur on the outside and inside of the vagina, on the cervix, or around the anus. In men, genital warts are less common. If present, they are seen on the tip of the penis or the urethra; however, they also may be found on the shaft of the penis, on the scrotum, or around the anus. Rarely, genital warts also can develop in the mouth or throat of a person who has had oral sexual contact with an infected person.

5. Please provide the number of HPV cases in the U.S. Is this number increasing or decreasing? To what can this trend be attributed?

It is important to remember that estimating the prevalence of HPV is difficult. Prevalence depends on many factors which include: the population screened, the sexual habits of those screened, what is classified as HPV infection at the time of screening, etc. Estimates for the number of HPV cases varies. In November of 1996 the CDC estimated that 24 million Americans were infected with HPV. The incidence of HPV infection has increased with changing sexual mores starting in the 1960's. It is difficult to know whether variations in incidence and prevalence reported during the 1990's represent an actual change in the number of cases of HPV.

6. What, if any symptoms are associated with HPV? If it is asymptomatic, how would one know one is infected?

HPV may cause warts with many different characteristics. They may appear small or large, flat or raised, single or multiple; sometimes the warts may not even be visible to the naked eye. The most common places to notice genital warts are outside the vagina, on the penis, and around the anus. In women, HPV can lead to the development of warts inside the vagina and on the cervix as well. For many people who have HPV infection, there are no obvious signs of infection. However, if warts are present, a doctor can diagnose HPV infection by their characteristic appearance and the history of how they developed. In women, to look for warts on the cervix or in the vagina, a doctor may use a colposcope, which is like a telescope. In addition, Pap smear results may be suggestive of HPV infection. There is currently no blood test that has proven reliable in the diagnosis of HPV infection and it is not possible to routinely culture HPV. However, there are sensitive DNA based assays which can be used to diagnose symptomatic and asymptomatic HPV infection.

7. How widespread or common is HPV? Of the women who have HPV, what is the percentage of those women who will develop cervical cancer?

More than 80 types of HPV have been identified. However, approximately 25 types infect the uterine cervix; of these, only some are associated with invasive cervical cancer. They are therefore classified into low-risk types, HPV 6 and 11, and high-risk types, most commonly 16, 18, 31, and 45, which account for more than 80 percent of all invasive cervical cancers. Less than 15 percent of women infected with HPV will develop either low-grade squamous intraepithelial lesions (LSIL) or high-grade squamous intraepithelial lesions (HSIL). At least one-third of all grades of SIL will fade, whereas less than half persist and approximately one-quarter progress. Of lesions that progress, approximately 10 percent progress to carcinoma in situ and 1 percent to invasive cancer.

Since the virus is transmitted primarily through sexual intercourse, there seems to be a peak prevalence of infection in sexually active women who are younger than 25 years of age. The prevalence of infection decreases with increasing age, suggesting that most infections in women and men resolve over time through host immune responses.

8. The NCI has identified risk factors, such as the human papillomavirus, in the development of cervical cancer. What work has NCI done to coordinate a Federal response to the prevention of cervical cancer? Specifically, what has NCI done to coordinate with the Department of Health and Human Services (HHS) Office of Population Affairs and the HHS Health Resources and Services Administration (HRSA) to alert women concerning the risk factors associated with cervical cancer?

Federal agencies are designated to serve the United States in specific ways. The National Institutes of Health (NIH), of which NCI is a part, is a research agency. In its mission to protect and improve human health, the NIH (and NCI) conducts and supports basic, applied, and clinical and health services research to understand the processes underlying human health and to acquire new knowledge to help prevent, diagnose, and treat human disease and disabilities. This may include developing an information campaign such as the **Pap Tests: A healthy habit for life** campaign and evaluating its effectiveness at achieving its goal. NCI also has a mandate to disseminate research findings so that when the development and evaluation are completed, other Federal and state agencies, and private sector organizations, may take this information and apply it accordingly. NCI, therefore, plays an integral role in these activities.

The NCI disseminates research findings widely through scientific publication, press conferences, press statements, clinical alerts, patient education materials, meetings of professional societies, television and radio, the World Wide Web, our toll-free Cancer Information Service, our PDQ databases, and the Information Associates Program. Our staff has many contacts within agencies for a variety of programs and issues. Through these personal contacts, and those mechanisms mentioned above, Federal agencies and offices have direct access to information pertinent to their programs. In addition, we maintain and foster close working relationships with other Institutes that have formal collaborative relationships with the Office os Population Affairs-our projects and programs are thus included in that broad knowledge base. NCI has several partnerships with other federal agencies and non-federal groups to enhance our information dissemination activities. Following are examples of two specific information campaigns on cervical cancer:

Pap Tests: A healthy habit for life: In May 1998 the Office of Cancer Communications began a campaign to alert the public of the results of a survey that showed that older women were unaware of their continued risk for cervical cancer. National activities have included focusing on minority media outreach and the distribution of a media packet that focused on cervical cancer and older women. Additionally, NCI collaborated with the Healthcare Financing Administration (HCFA) to reprint an NCI cervical cancer publication with Medicare information for older women to be distributed through HCFA and NCI networks. Other activities have included conducting research with physicians to identify their attitudes and perceptions of Pap test screening among women 65 and older. Based on this research, a print public service announcement and newsletter article are being developed that encourage physicians to talk to their older patients about Pap test screening. These materials will be promoted through physician publications and newsletters.

The Pap Test and Cervical Cancer Video: An intertribal video on the early detection of cervical cancer for American Indian Women was produced by the NCI in conjunction with the Nebraska Department of Health. The video comes with educational material to help inform American Indian women of the importance of regular Pap tests.

9. **Please name the NCI liaisons with CDC, HRSA, and the Office of Population Affairs. Has NCI coordinated activity with the Title V Abstinence Education Grant Program or the Title XX programs within those agencies?**

As previously stated, NCI staff has many contacts within agencies for a variety of programs and issues. Liaisons with CDC, HRSA and the Office of Population Affairs vary on the program and issue involved.

NCI has not formally collaborated specifically on Title V Abstinence Education Grant program or the Title XX programs. As a research agency, NCI's role is to conduct and support research, then disseminate widely, new knowledge gained. This is done through information campaigns like the **Pap Tests: A healthy habit for life** campaign.

Page 5 - The Honorable Michael Bilirakis

10. What is the amount of research dollars spent by NCI on HPV as compared to the virus that causes AIDS? How many women die annually in the United States from cervical cancer? How many women die annually in the United States from AIDS?

There are over 80 types of HPV, about 15 of which are associated with cancer of the cervix. NCI estimates that it will spend about $38 million on cervical cancer-related HPV research, and about $235 million on AIDS related cancers, in FY 1999. There are about 5,000 deaths in the U.S. from cervical cancer each year, and more than 200,000 deaths world wide. Over 90 percent of these cancers are HPV-related. There were about 4,600 female deaths in the U.S., and 900,000 worldwide, from HIV-related illness in FY 1997.

11. On January 12, 1999, Chairman Bliley sent a letter to the NCI on women's health issues, including cervical cancer. In response to that letter, NCI estimated the number of Americans with HPV to be 24 million. In testimony before this committee by Dr. Ronald Valdiserri, of the Centers for Disease Control and Prevention (CDC), on March 16, 1999, he indicated that number is 45 million. Can you explain the discrepancy in numbers?

The NCI estimated number of Americans with HPV came from the CDC website. The entry title is "The Challenge of STD Prevention in the U.S." and it was written in November 1996. CDC was not contacted by NCI for verification of this number and the CDC testified using an estimated number that may be more current than the one posted. Once again, it is important to remember that estimating the prevalence of HPV is difficult. Prevalence depends on many factors which include: the population screened, the sexual habits of those screened, what is classified as HPV infection at the time of screening, etc.

12. In the above referenced letter from NCI to Chairman Bliley, NCI stated that, "*Condoms are ineffective against HPV because the virus is prevalent not only in mucosal tissue (genitalia) but also on dry skin of the surrounding abdomen and groin and it can migrate from those areas into the vagina and cervix.*" That letter went on to say that "*additional research efforts by NCI on the effectiveness of condoms in preventing HPV transmission are not warranted.*" To the contrary, Dr. Ronald Valdiserri of CDC testified on March 16, 1999 that "Several studies have shown condoms to provide some protection against cervical cancer. . ." Can you explain the difference in conclusions made by CDC and NCI?

The NCI conclusion that condoms are ineffective against HPV infection is based on the results of several long term studies which have failed to show that barrier contraceptives prevent cervical HPV infection, dysplasia, or cancer (Attachment 1, 2, 3). Dr. Valdiserri's testimony might be based on studies that show that while condoms are ineffective in preventing transmission of HPV, they are quite effective at preventing transmission of HIV and other sexually transmitted diseases. CDC would be able to provide insight into the basis of Dr. Valdiserri's statement.

Please do not hesitate to contact me if you have further questions.

Sincerely,

Dr. Douglas Lowy
Deputy Director
Division of Basic Sciences, NCI

Enclosures

ATTACHMENT 1

Original Articles

Barrier and Spermicidal Contraceptive Methods and Risk of Invasive Cervical Cancer

Allan Hildesheim,[1] Louise A. Brinton,[1] Katherine Mallin,[2] Herman F. Lehman,[3] Paul Stolley,[4] David A. Savitz,[5] and Robert Levine[6]

The effects of barrier and spermicidal methods of contraception on cervical cancer risk were examined by studying 479 cases of histologically confirmed invasive cervical cancer cases and 788 random digit dialing controls. In addition to a detailed history of contraceptive practices, information was available on numerous potential confounders, including demographic characteristics, sexual behavior, reproductive factors, Pap smear screening history, and smoking. After adjustment for relevant confounders, diaphragm and condom use were found not to be significantly associated with risk of cervical cancer. Although there was a small reduction in risk (OR = 0.8) associated with long-term use (5+ years) of the diaphragm, the effect appeared to relate to concomitant spermicide use, since there was evidence of further decreases in risk for women using spermicides alone for extended periods (OR = 0.7 for 5+ years). Effects were only seen among subjects of higher income and education levels, suggesting that patterns of usage may be important. The potential ability of spermicides to reduce cervical cancer risk by neutralizing viral agents warrants further attention. (Epidemiology 1990;1:266–272)

Keywords: Cervical cancer, contraception.

The strong and consistent association between sexual behavior and invasive cervical cancer (1) has led to the suggestion that a sexually transmitted agent is involved in the etiology of this disease. Two agents in particular have been extensively studied: herpes simplex virus type 2 and human papillomaviruses (2,3).

Given the possible infectious nature of cervical cancer, it is of interest to examine the possible protective effect of contraceptive methods. Specifically, barrier methods of contraception (mainly the diaphragm and/or condom) provide a physical barrier that could reduce the likelihood of infection by sexually transmitted agents and consequently reduce the risk of developing cervical cancer. Also likely is that use of spermicides (foam, jelly, and/or cream) reduce the risk of cervical cancer by protecting users from acquiring sexually transmitted diseases. Spermicides contain surfactants, mainly nonoxynol-9 (4), which have been shown to neutralize HSV-2 (5,6), as well as other venereal agents (7,8). In addition to the role of each contraceptive method in isolation, use of spermicidal agents in conjunction with barrier methods might further protect against cancer of the cervix.

Previous studies of barrier contraceptives and spermicides in relation to invasive and preinvasive cervical cancer have yielded conflicting results. Many studies (9–16), but not all (17–19), have reported an inverse relation between diaphragm and/or condom use and cervical cancer risk. In addition, four studies (9,12,14,17) have detected a negative relation between vaginal spermicide use and cervical cancer, although one study that also examined this issue did not detect an association (19).

Of the studies mentioned above, only two were capable of controlling for potential confounding by both sexual and screening behavior (12,17). Both of these were studies of invasive cervical cancer. Celentano et al (17) reported a 70% reduced risk of invasive cervical cancer among women who reported ever use of a vaginal spermicide compared with never users of spermicides. Unfortunately, this study was unable to assess the effect of duration of spermicide use on risk of cervical cancer. Peters et al (12) reported a 7% reduction in risk of invasive cervical cancer per year of use of a barrier method of contraception (defined as condom, diaphragm, and/or spermicide). Although results are not

[1]Environmental Epidemiology Branch, National Cancer Institute, Executive Plaza North, Room 443, Bethesda, MD 20892 (address reprint requests to Allan Hildesheim). [2]Illinois Cancer Council, Comprehensive Cancer Center for the State of Illinois, Chicago, IL. [3]Department of Epidemiology, School of Public Health, University of Alabama at Birmingham, Birmingham, AL. [4]Department of Medicine, University of Pennsylvania, Philadelphia, PA. [5]School of Medicine, University of Colorado Health Sciences Center, Denver, CO. (Currently at the Department of Epidemiology, School of Public Health, University of North Carolina, Chapel Hill, NC.) [6]Papanicolaou Comprehensive Cancer Center, Miami, FL 33136. (Currently at the Department of Internal Medicine, Our Lady of Mercy Medical Center, Bronx, NY.)

presented in detail, Peters et al also noted that women who used vaginal spermicides without a diaphragm appeared to be at a lower risk of invasive cervical cancer than those who used the diaphragm without vaginal spermicides.

In an attempt to assess the effect of barrier and spermicide methods of contraception on risk of cervical cancer, we obtained information regarding lifetime birth control practices from invasive cervical cancer cases and community controls in five regions of the United States. The availability of information on numerous potential confounders, including demographic characteristics, sexual and reproductive factors, Pap smear screening history, smoking, and use of other contraceptive methods, allowed us to examine the effects of barrier and spermicide use independent of other known cervical cancer risk factors.

Methods

Between April 1982 and January 1984, women 20–74 years of age with newly diagnosed invasive cervical cancer were recruited from 24 participating hospitals in 5 areas reporting to the Comprehensive Cancer Patient Data System (Birmingham, Chicago, Denver, Miami, and Philadelphia).

Community controls were obtained through random digit dialing techniques (20). Controls were individually matched to cases on age (within 5 years), race, and telephone exchange. Two controls were selected per case. More details of the selection process are provided elsewhere (21).

A total of 658 eligible cases and 1114 controls were ascertained. Home interviews were conducted by trained interviewers who obtained information on contraceptive practices, sociodemographic characteristics, pregnancy history, menstrual history, hygiene practices, sexual behavior, medical events, smoking, diet, marital history, and family history of cancer. Information on birth control use was obtained by using lifetime calendars to record usage of specific methods on a monthly basis in the context of other relevant life events such as age at menarche, age at first intercourse, pregnancies, and age at menopause.

Interviews were successfully obtained from 481 cases (73.1%) and 801 controls (71.9%). Nonresponse was accounted for by refusal (9.7% of cases, 21.9% of controls), subjects having moved or being unlocatable (3.8%, 3.4%), death (5.0%, 0.5%), illness (2.1%, 1.1%), and other problems (1.7%, 1.1%). In addition, physician consent was not obtained for 4.6% of cases. The final groups used in the analysis consisted of 479 cases and 788 controls for whom complete contraceptive history was available.

The odds ratio (OR), as an estimator of the relative risk, was the measure of association used to determine the relation between contraceptive usage and cervical cancer. Unconditional logistic regression analysis provided adjusted ORs and 95% confidence intervals (CI) (22). Conditional logistic regression (23) that retained the matching of cases and controls yielded similar estimates. We present results from unconditional logistic regression in this report, since use of conditional regression analyses involved the exclusion of 22% of study subjects owing to missing matches.

Results

Table 1 describes the contraceptive practices among the 610 (77%) community controls enrolled in the study who reported use of contraceptive methods and illustrates the frequent use of combinations of birth control methods. Seven methods of contraception were examined: vaginal spermicides, the diaphragm, condoms, oral contraceptives, intrauterine devices (IUDs), female sterilization, and vasectomy. The majority of these controls (75%) reported use of two or more methods. A total of 22% of users reported the use of four or more different methods in their lifetime.

Among 293 women reporting ever use of vaginal spermicides, only 10 (3%) used it as the sole method of birth control, while 227 (77%) also reported use of barrier methods of contraception. Less than 1% of 164 women reporting diaphragm use and 15% of 287 women reporting condom use used these methods exclusively.

Tables 2 and 3 present the risk of cervical cancer associated with use of specific birth control methods. Initially, barrier methods of contraception appeared to be associated with reduced risks of cervical cancer. However, after controlling for age, race, education, income, interval since last Pap smear, and lifetime number of sexual partners, the effect nearly disappeared. Thus, the risk associated with ever use after adjustment was 1.2 (95% CI = 0.9,1.6). In addition, after adjustment, no significant trend was observed with increased duration of use of barrier methods (p for trend = 0.68), short-term users (<5 years) having an OR of 1.4 and long-term users an OR of 0.9. Further adjustment for duration of oral contraceptive use or smoking did not alter these or any other observed estimates.

When barrier methods of contraception were separated into diaphragm and condom use (Table 2), there was no effect on risk for condom use, but some evidence of decreased risk associated with diaphragm use. Risk

TABLE 1. Contraceptive Practices among 610 Community Controls Reporting Birth Control Use

			Pairwise Birth Control Use with						
	Total	Only	Vaginal Spermicide	Diaphragm	Condom	Oral Contraceptive	IUD	Female Sterilization	Vasectomy
Vaginal spermicides	293	10	—	154	157	199	82	64	37
Diaphragm	164	1	154	—	87	99	44	28	25
Condom	287	44	157	87	—	183	64	51	41
Oral contraceptives	403	56	199	99	183	—	113	90	64
IUD	151	10	82	44	64	113	—	43	18
Female sterilization	151	29	64	28	51	90	43	—	1
Vasectomy	85	5	37	25	41	64	18	1	—

	Number of Birth Control Methods Used in Lifetime						
	1	2	3	4	5	6	TOTAL
Number of women	155	174	148	86	39	8	610
Percentage	25.4	28.5	24.3	14.1	6.4	1.3	100

TABLE 2. Risk of Invasive Cervical Cancer Associated with Barrier Contraceptive Use

	Cases*	Controls*	OR†	OR‡	CI
Barrier methods§					
Never	281	418	1.0	1.0	
Ever	182	356	0.8	1.2	[0.9,1.6]
Never	281	418	1.0	1.0	
<5 years	124	223	0.9	1.4	[1.0,1.8]
5+ years	58	133	0.6	0.9	[0.6,1.4]
Trend			$p = 0.004$	$p = 0.68$	
Diaphragm§					
Never	401	613	1.0	1.0	
<5 years	46	123	0.6	0.9	[0.6,1.3]
5+ years	16	38	0.6	0.8	[0.4,1.6]
Trend			$p = 0.002$	$p = 0.36$	
Condom§					
Never	317	494	1.0	1.0	
<5 years	104	189	1.0	1.2	[0.9,1.7]
5+ years	42	91	0.6	1.0	[0.6,1.5]
Trend			$p = 0.05$	$p = 0.62$	

* Women with missing values are excluded from analysis.
† Adjusted for age.
‡ Adjusted for age, race, education, income, interval since last Pap smear, and lifetime number of sexual partners.
§ Many users of barrier methods also used spermicides, either synchronously or asynchronously.

decreased slightly with increasing duration of use, but the trend was not statistically significant (p for trend = 0.36).

Table 3 presents the risk of cervical cancer associated with use of vaginal spermicides. After adjusting for confounding factors, spermicide users were at a similar risk of disease as nonusers (OR = 1.0; 95% CI = 0.7,1.3). When duration of use was examined, no significant trend of risk with increasing duration of use was observed (p for trend = 0.71), long-term users having an OR of 0.9 (95% CI = 0.5,1.4). However, when spermicide use was restricted to those women who reported

TABLE 3. Risk of Invasive Cervical Cancer Associated with Vaginal Spermicide Use

	Cases*	Controls*	OR†	OR‡	CI
Vaginal spermicides§					
Never	331	486	1.0	1.0	
Ever	132	288	0.7	1.0	[0.7,1.3]
Never	331	486	1.0	1.0	
<5 years	102	216	0.8	1.0	[0.7,1.4]
5+ years	30	72	0.6	0.9	[0.5,1.4]
Trend			$p = 0.009$	$p = 0.71$	
Spermicide without barrier					
Never	383	605	1.0	1.0	
<5 years	69	140	0.9	1.0	[0.7,1.4]
5+ years	11	29	0.7	0.7	[0.3,1.5]
Trend			$p = 0.19$	$p = 0.51$	

* Women with missing values are excluded from analysis.
† Adjusted for age.
‡ Adjusted for age, race, education, income, interval since last Pap smear, and lifetime number of sexual partners.
§ Includes women who used vaginal spermicides alone, as well as women who used vaginal spermicides with the diaphragm or condom.

using vaginal spermicides without the simultaneous use of a barrier method (vaginal spermicide only use), long-term users had a slightly reduced cervical cancer risk (OR = 0.7; 95% CI = 0.3,1.5), although the test for trend was not significant ($p = 0.51$).

Given the possibility that timing, in addition to duration, of birth control use might be of importance, the period of contraceptive usage was examined in relation to the date of diagnosis of the case (and comparable data for controls). Five-year periods of time were constructed starting from the date of diagnosis of the case and moving backwards in time. Within each 5-year period, women reporting 6 or more months of use of a given method were compared with those reporting no use of the same method during the same period. No time periods could be identified where the varying methods of birth control had distinct effects.

Women who report never having used any birth control may be an inappropriate reference for comparison with women who report using methods of contraception, owing to wide differences in patterns of health care, sexual behavior, and socioeconomic status (SES). This concern led us to investigate the issue more closely. A total of 31% of the cases reported never using any method of birth control compared with 23% of the controls, yielding an OR of 1.5. When controls who reported no contraceptive usage were investigated, they were found to be more likely than controls who reported having used contraceptives to be poor, uneducated, black, and never to have been screened for cervical cancer. We detected significant differences with regard to number of lifetime sexual partners. Despite these differences, excluding women who never used contraceptives from the analyses did not markedly alter the adjusted estimates of risk, and conclusions drawn from the data remained unchanged.

The effect of excluding women who had ever used oral contraceptives was examined in analyses comparing users of nonhormonal contraceptives with each other. Although no significant trends were observed, long-term vaginal spermicide only users were found to be at a 70% decreased risk of disease (OR = 0.3; 95% CI = 0.06,1.1).

Because of concerns regarding the accuracy and consistency of use of contraceptive methods, we examined contraceptive users and nonusers within different categories of income and education (Table 4). Women with 0–11 years of education and ≤$20,000 yearly income were classified as low SES. Those with 12+ years of education and income >$20,000 were classified as high SES, and the remainder were classified as medium SES. When analysis was performed stratified by SES, barrier and spermicidal contraceptive use among low and medium SES women did not appear to be associated with reduced risks. Among low SES women, long-term vaginal spermicide users were at a 1.7-fold excess risk, but this effect was not statistically significant. Among high SES women, a significant dose response of decreasing risk with increasing duration of use was observed among spermicide users (OR = 0.5 for long-term users; p for trend = 0.03). Furthermore, the reduction in risk was strongest among women who reported use of vaginal spermicides without simultaneous use of barrier methods (OR = 0.3 for long-term users; P for trend = 0.05).

TABLE 4. Risk of Invasive Cervical Cancer Associated with Birth Control Use, by Socioeconomic Status

	Low SES*		Medium SES		High SES	
	OR†	Cases‡	OR	Cases	OR	Cases
Vaginal spermicides						
Never used	1.0	(148)	1.0	(92)	1.0	(73)
<5 years	1.1	(31)	1.1	(39)	0.7	(30)
5+ years	1.7	(10)	1.0	(8)	0.5	(11)
p for trend	$p = 0.40$		$p = 0.72$		$p = 0.03$	
Vaginal spermicide alone						
Never used	1.0	(157)	1.0	(110)	1.0	(97)
<5 years	1.3	(28)	1.1	(25)	0.7	(14)
5+ years	1.1	(4)	0.9	(4)	0.3	(3)
p for trend	$p = 0.52$		$p = 0.88$		$p = 0.05$	
Diaphragm						
Never used	1.0	(174)	1.0	(121)	1.0	(86)
<5 years	2.4	(11)	0.6	(14)	0.7	(21)
5+ years	1.1	(4)	1.1	(4)	0.6	(7)
p for trend	$p = 0.27$		$p = 0.40$		$p = 0.12$	
Condom						
Never used	1.0	(150)	1.0	(88)	1.0	(64)
<5 years	1.3	(29)	1.2	(35)	1.2	(36)
5+ years	0.7	(10)	1.1	(16)	1.0	(14)
p for trend	$p = 0.89$		$p = 0.62$		$p = 0.68$	

* Low SES = 0–11 years education and ≤20K yearly income. Medium SES = (0–11 years education and >20K income) or (12+ years education and ≤20K income). High SES = 12+ years education and >20K income.
† Adjusted for age, race, interval since last Pap smear, and lifetime number of sexual partners.
‡ Women with missing values are excluded from analysis.

Among high SES women, there was also evidence of decreased risk associated with long-term diaphragm use. The trend, however, was not statistically significant ($p = 0.12$). Among condom users, no protective effect was detected.

Analysis was also conducted stratifying by number of lifetime sexual partners, under the assumption that women who report multiple partners would have greater benefits from use of barrier and spermicidal contraceptive methods. No differences were observed when ORs obtained from the main analysis and those obtained from the stratified analysis were compared (data not shown).

Discussion

Previous studies have reported reduced risks of cervical cancer associated with barrier (9–16) as well as spermicide (9,12,14,17) methods of contraception. Few studies, however, have been able to adjust appropriately for confounding variables (12,17). Adjustment for Pap smear screening history, SES, and sexual behavior is essential when assessing the effect of birth control methods on risk of cervical cancer, as has been shown in our previous report of the effect of oral contraceptive use on risk of invasive cervical cancer (21).

Indeed, education and interval since last Pap smear were strong confounders of the association of birth control use and cervical cancer, while lesser confounders were income and number of sexual partners. Adjustment for these factors brought the estimates of risk associated with barrier and spermicidal methods of contraception close to unity. Additional adjustment for duration of oral contraceptive use and smoking had little effect on the risk estimates. Thus, although both condom and diaphragm use appeared initially to be associated with a reduced risk of cervical cancer, these effects were essentially eliminated by adjustment for confounding factors.

Initial examination of spermicide use showed an apparent protective effect on the risk of invasive cervical cancer, although adjustment for confounding factors eliminated this association. Further assessment of usage within categories of SES, however, revealed that women of high SES who used vaginal spermicides were at a significantly reduced risk of invasive cervical cancer. Although a similar, but nonsignificant effect was observed for diaphragm users, the observation that high

SES women who used vaginal spermicides without concomitant use of a barrier methods were at a lower risk than those who used spermicides with a barrier method suggests that the spermicide and not the diaphragm protects against disease. Furthermore, 92% of diaphragm users reported also using vaginal spermicides, indicating that the nonsignificant decrease in risk observed among women of high SES who reported diaphragm use could result from the effect of the spermicide on risk. In addition, our finding that long-term vaginal spermicide only users were at a 70% decrease in risk when compared with other nonhormonal contraceptive users further strengthens the hypothesis that the reduction in risk is from spermicide rather than diaphragm use.

A possible explanation for this subgroup effect is that women of higher SES and those who use spermicides alone are more likely to use the spermicide consistently or more likely to use larger quantities of spermicide. Also, data obtained from higher SES women might be more accurate and ORs obtained from this subset of women might be better estimators of the association of birth control use and cervical cancer. Caution, however, must be exercised in interpreting these results, given the small numbers of women involved and also the possibility of confounding by sexual behavior of the male partners of women, a variable not assessed in this study.

The lack of a significant protection provided by the diaphragm might also be explained by the fact that the diaphragm traps some of the spermicide close to the cervix, reducing the effectiveness of the spermicide to protect against viral infection of the vaginal vault. Various agents, including those believed to be linked causally to cervical cancer (HSV-2 and HPV), are capable of infecting the vagina and vulva (24–28). The vaginal vault may thus become infected during intercourse, and the infection may spread to the cervix after removal of the diaphragm.

Condom use has traditionally been regarded as a physical barrier that protects the vaginal vault from infection during sexual intercourse. Our observation that condom use does not reduce the risk of cervical cancer might be interpreted as indicating that the condom is not always used appropriately. Sexual contact prior to the placement of the condom would eliminate its protective effect. In this study we were unable to assess directly the reliability of use of condoms. Stratification by SES variables did not suggest any differential use patterns among high and low SES women. Another possible explanation for the lack of protection provided by the condom is that areas of the base of the penile shaft may not be shielded by the condom, and any infections in this area may be transmitted to the female partner. A previous report (29) has demonstrated that high proportions of male HPV infections occur in the penile shaft.

In summary, after adjustment for confounding in this study, neither diaphragm nor condom use appeared to reduce substantially the risk of invasive cervical cancer. A protective effect of vaginal spermicide use among high SES women was suggested by the data; the effect was strongest among women who used spermicides without the diaphragm. Although a reduction in cervical cancer risk among women reporting spermicide use is biologically plausible based on its proven antiviral effects, further investigations are needed to confirm the relationship.

References

1. Brinton LA, Fraumeni JF Jr. Epidemiology of uterine cervical cancer. J Chron Dis 1986;39(12):1051–65.
2. Kaufman RH, Adam E. Herpes simplex virus and human papilloma virus in the development of cervical cancer. Clin Obstet Gynecol 1986;29(3):678–92.
3. Reeves WC, Rawls WE, Brinton LA. Epidemiology of genital papillomaviruses and cervical cancer. Rev Infect Dis 1989;11(3):426–39.
4. New developments in vaginal contraception. Population Reports 1984;XII(1):H-157–H-190.
5. Postic B, Singh B, Squeglia NL, Guevarra LO. Inactivation of clinical isolates of herpesvirus hominis, types 1 and 2, by chemical contraceptives. Sex Transm Dis 1978;5(1):22–4.
6. Singh B, Postic B, Cutler JC. Virucidal effect of certain chemical contraceptives on type 2 herpesvirus. Am J Obstet Gynecol 1976;126(4):422–4.
7. Singh B, Cutler JC. Vaginal contraceptives for prophylaxis against sexually transmissible diseases. In: Zatuchni GI et al, ed. Vaginal contraception: new developments. Hagerstown, Maryland: Harper & Row, 1979.
8. Porter J. Contraception and sexually transmissible diseases. Healthright 1984;3(4):12–5.
9. Slattery ML, Overall JC, Abbott TM, French TK, Robison LM, Gardner J. Sexual activity, contraception, genital infections, and cervical cancer: Support for a sexually transmitted disease hypothesis. Am J Epidemiol 1989;130:248–58.
10. Harris RW, Brinton LA, Cowdell RH, et al. Characteristics of women with dysplasia or carcinoma in situ of the cervix uteri. Br J Cancer 1980;42:359–69.
11. Wright NH, Vessey MP, Kenward B, McPherson K, Doll R. Neoplasia and dysplasia of the cervix uteri and contraception: a possible protective effect of the diaphragm. Br J Cancer 1978;38:273–9.
12. Peters RK, Thomas D, Hagan DG, Mack TM, Henderson BE. Risk factors for invasive cervical cancer among latinas and nonlatinas in Los Angeles County. J Natl Cancer Inst 1986;77:1063–77.
13. Fasal E, Simmons ME, Kampert JB. Factors associated with high and low risk of cervical neoplasia. J Natl Cancer Inst 1981;66:631–6.
14. Swan SH, Brown WL. Oral contraceptive use, sexual activity, and cervical carcinoma. Am J Obstet Gynecol 1981;139:52–7.
15. Richardson AC, Lyon JB. The effect of condom use on squamous cell cervical intraepithelial neoplasia. Am J Obstet Gynecol 1981;140:909–13.

16. Molina R, Thomas DB, Dabancens A, et al. Oral contraceptives and cervical carcinoma in situ in Chile. Cancer Res 1988;48:1011–5.
17. Celentano DD, Klassen AC, Weisman CS, Rosenheim NB. The role of contraceptive use in cervical cancer: The Maryland cervical cancer case-control study. Am J Epidemiol 1987;126(4):592–604.
18. Melamed MR, Flehinger BJ. Early incidence rates of precancerous cervical lesions in women using contraceptives. Gynecol Oncol 1973;1:290–8.
19. Thomas DB. Relationship of oral contraceptives to cervical carcinogenesis. Obstet Gynecol 1972;40:508–18.
20. Hartge P, Brinton LA, Rosenthal JF, Cahill JI, Hoover RN, Waksberg J. Random digit dialing in selecting a population-based control group. Am J Epidemiol 1984;120:825–33.
21. Brinton LA, Huggins GR, Lehman HF, et al. Long-term use of oral contraceptives and risk of invasive cervical cancer. Int J Cancer 1986;38:339–44.
22. Breslow NE, Day NE. Statistical methods in cancer research, vol. 1. The analysis of case-control studies. Lyon, France: IARC, 1980.
23. Lubin JH. A computer program for the analysis of matched case-control studies. Comput Biomed Res 1981;14:138–43.
24. Koutsky LA, Galloway DA, Holmes KK. Epidemiology of genital human papillomavirus infection. Epidemiol Rev 1988;10:122–63.
25. Spitzer M, Krumholz BA, Seltzer VL. The multicentric nature of disease related to human papillomavirus infection of the female lower genital tract. Obstetrics and Gynecology 1989;73:303–7.
26. Beckmann AM, Kiviat NB, Daling JR, Sherman KJ, McDougall JK. Human papillomavirus type 16 in multifocal neoplasia of the female genital tract. International Journal of Gynecological Pathology 1988;7:39–47.
27. Reid R, Greenberg M, Jenson AB, et al. Sexually transmitted papillomaviral infections I. The anatomic distribution and pathologic grade of neoplastic lesions associated with different viral types. Am J Obstet Gynecol 1987;156:212–22.
28. McCance DJ, Clarkson PK, Dyson JL, Walker PG, Singer A. Human papillomavirus types 6 and 16 in multifocal intraepithelial neoplasias of the female lower genital tract. Br J Obstet Gynaecol 1985;92:1093–100.
29. O'Brien WM, Jenson AB, Lancaster WD, Maxted WC. Human papillomavirus typing of penile condyloma. J Urol 1989;141:863–5.

ATTACHMENT 3 Jdnn

ARTICLES

Epidemiologic Correlates of Cervical Neoplasia and Risk of Human Papillomavirus Infection in Asymptomatic Women in Brazil

Luisa Lina Villa, Eduardo Luis Fabiano Franco, Ludwig Institute for Cancer Research Human Papillomavirus Study Group*

To investigate whether the epidemiologic correlates of cervical cancer are predictors of infection with genital human papillomavirus (HPV), we performed a prevalence survey in two metropolitan areas of Brazil, Recife and São Paulo. The data records of four randomly selected HPV-negative women were matched on the basis of age, clinic, and admission period with those of each of 136 patients with positive HPV DNA hybridizations. Anal intercourse [prevalence rate ratio (PRR) = 1.7] and current pregnancy (PRR = 2.3) were the only variables associated with HPV 6/11 infection ($P < .10$). Only the frequency of gynecologic consultations was associated (negatively) with risk of HPV 16/18 infection ($P = .0175$). Our data failed to provide evidence for the existence of shared risk factors for genital HPV infection and cervical cancer. The frequency of mixed HPV infections was 13 times higher than expected, a finding suggestive of the existence of additional determinants of HPV infection not akin to the general behavioral characteristics of women that are probed in the study. [J Natl Cancer Inst 81:332-340, 1989]

Epidemiologic studies have consistently shown that the main determinants of risk for cervical neoplasia are correlates of sexual activity. The characteristics generally identified in such investigations are (*a*) early onset of sexual activity, (*b*) multiple sex partners, and (*c*) promiscuity of the partner (*1-3*). In addition, other studies have suggested that wives of patients with penile cancer are at an increased risk of developing cervical cancer later in life (*4,5*). Such findings are further supported by results from population correlation studies, in which strong associations have been found between the development of cervical cancer and penile cancer with the use of mortality and morbidity data (*6,7*). These epidemiologic associations suggest a role for a sexually transmitted infectious agent in the etiology of cervical cancer.

Human papillomaviruses (HPVs) have been implicated as the most likely causal agents of cervical neoplasia, since much experimental and histopathologic evidence has been obtained in regard to the oncogenic potential of this group of viruses (*8,9*). HPV nucleic acid sequences have been found in a substantial proportion of specimens from cervical carcinomas occurring in different populations (*10*). Other investigations including surrogate control groups representative of asymptomatic women have demonstrated that, although HPV DNA sequences are also found in normal cervical epithelia, they are detected at rates that are much lower than those found in cervical cancer cases (*11-13*).

The above model of a single-agent causation for cervical cancer has two drawbacks. First, the mere statistical association between the HPV detection rate and the occurrence of disease is also consistent with another possible role for this group of viruses. On the basis of the hypothesis that abnormally proliferating epithelia would be more prone to infection by HPV, one would also observe a higher detection rate among women with cervical abnormalities than among normal controls. Secondly, cervical cancer appears to be a disease with a multifactorial pattern of occurrence, since other determinants (e.g., oral contraceptive use, parity, and tobacco smoking) have also consistently emerged as independent risk

---

Received October 5, 1988; revised November 21, 1988; accepted November 29, 1988.

Ludwig Institute for Cancer Research, São Paulo Branch, São Paulo, Brazil.

The following institutions, constituting the Human Papillomavirus Study Group, participated in the study: Ludwig Institute for Cancer Research, São Paulo, Brazil (*Luisa Lina Villa, Eduardo L. F. Franco, Humberto Torloni, Maria Cecilia Costa, Affonso Novello-Netto, Maria Estela Silva, Raimunda Pereira, Lindelcy Andrade*); Hospital Vila Nova Cachoeirinha, São Paulo (*Alcides Vara*); Instituto Materno-Infantil de Pernambuco, Recife, Brazil (*Evaldo Costa, Mercez Cunha*); and Hospital do Cancer de Pernambuco, Recife (*Jayro Poggi*).

**Correspondence to:* Dr. Eduardo L. F. Franco, Department of Epidemiology, Ludwig Institute for Cancer Research, São Paulo Branch, R. Prof. Antonio Prudente, 109, 01509 São Paulo, Brazil.

factors in epidemiologic investigations (*14*). Only prospective studies can disentangle the similarity of effects between the two models because, unlike cross-sectional or retrospective surveys, follow-up studies provide the correct time perspective needed for establishing causation. However, most prospective studies of HPV-infected women are in the initial stages; thus, their results are only preliminary and lack statistical power to provide conclusive evidence for the role of HPV as a causal agent for cervical cancer.

In the present investigation we propose an alternative study design for assessing the role of HPV in cervical neoplasia. Our investigation is based on the hypothesis that the sexual activity correlates of the disease are in reality determinants of genital infection with HPV. As such, these correlates should be directly measured in an epidemiologic study of behavioral predictors of the HPV prevalence rates in asymptomatic women.

Methods

Study Populations

Two Brazilian metropolitan areas were selected for the study: Recife and São Paulo. The capital of Pernambuco State, Recife is in Brazil's northeastern region and is considered to be a high-risk area for cervical cancer. The average annual incidence rate for this neoplasm (invasive disease) in Recife during the most recent survey period of 1976-1979 was 96.5 new cases per 100,000 women, age-adjusted by the world population (*15*). São Paulo, the capital of São Paulo State, is in southeastern Brazil and is considered to be an intermediate-risk area for cervical cancer, with an age-standardized incidence rate for 1978 of 35.1 (*16*).

Study subjects were selected by stratified random sampling of the adult female populations attending three family-planning and maternal and child health clinics, two in Recife [Instituto Materno-Infantil de Pernambuco (IMIP) and Hospital do Cancer de Pernambuco (HCP)] and the third in São Paulo [Hospital de Vila Nova Cachoeirinha (HVNC)]. The reasons given for attending the clinics included (*a*) routine medical examinations for women using contraceptive methods, (*b*) child immunization, and (*c*) general pediatric and gynecologic care. The nationwide health and social security system maintained by the Brazilian Government is billed directly for all health delivery services. Additional funding is provided under contracts by the municipal and state governments. These clinics maintain for their communities active screening programs for cervical cancer. During the study period (April 1986 through April 1988), the combined biennial accrual for these clinics was 29,000 women. On the basis of this dynamic population, we selected 2,050 as the target sample size, to allow sufficient statistical power to detect at least a 50% difference in HPV infection rate above the expected prevalence level of 2% that was obtained during a pretest phase conducted in São Paulo in 1986.

Informed consent was obtained from all patients. None of the selected patients refused to participate. A routine Papanicolaou cytology examination was done on all subjects. The cotton-tipped swabs used for harvesting cervical cell specimens were immersed in phosphate-buffered saline (PBS) and refrigerated at 2-8 °C for, at most, 3 days before they were shipped in wet ice to the laboratory in São Paulo, where HPV DNA analyses were performed. After specimens were collected from the patients, the patients were subjected to a standardized, structured interview that lasted 30-40 minutes. The trained female interviewers elicited information on socioeconomic and demographic variables, smoking and alcohol drinking habits, personal hygiene practices, access to health care, reproductive history, and sexual practices. The interviewers were not aware of the study hypotheses or of any current or past cytologic results for the patients. Since the questionnaire dealt with sensitive information, the interviewers were asked to grade the responses of the patients on the basis of their willingness to cooperate in answering all questions.

HPV DNA Hybridization Analysis

Detection of HPV DNA sequences of subtypes 6, 11, 16, and 18 (provided by Professor Harald zur Hausen, German Cancer Research Center, Heidelberg, Federal Republic of Germany) was performed by the filter in situ hybridization method (*17*) with the following modifications. The cervical cell suspensions were centrifuged for 2 minutes at 1,500 *g*, resuspended in 1 mL of PBS, and counted in a hemocytometer to establish the number of cells delivered onto nitrocellulose filters (Millipore, 0.45-μm porosity, 25 mm in diameter). Cell-containing filters were overlaid on Whatman 3MM paper that had been soaked in denaturing solution (0.5 *N* NaOH, 1.5 *M* NaCl) for 5 minutes and then overlaid on Whatman paper that had been soaked in 1.5 *M* Tris-HCl and 0.5 *M* NaCl for 5 minutes. The filters were then air dried and baked at 80 °C for 2 hours. Only highly stringent conditions (18 °C below the melting temperature) were used for both hybridization and washing of the filters. The two halves of each filter were separately prehybridized in a solution containing 50% formamide, 5× Denhardt's solution (0.1% Ficoll, 0.1% polyvinylpyrrolidone, 0.1% bovine serum albumin), 5× SSPE [0.9 *M* sodium chloride, 50 m*M* sodium phosphate buffer (pH 7.4), 5 m*M* EDTA], 0.1% sodium dodecyl sulfate, and 100 μg of denatured salmon sperm DNA/mL at 42 °C for 12-18 hours and hybridized with radiolabeled HPV DNA sequences of subtypes 6, 11, 16, and 18. Probes were nick translated in the presence of ^{32}P-labeled deoxynucleotides to specific activities of 1-5 $\times 10^8$ cpm/μg and added (combinations 6/11 and 16/18) to the hybridization mixture (5 $\times 10^6$ cpm of ^{32}P-labeled DNA probe/mL). After 36-48 hours at 42 °C, filters were washed twice in 2× SSC (300 m*M* sodium chloride, 30 m*M* sodium citrate) and 0.1% sodium dodecyl sulfate at 68 °C for 30 minutes and exposed for 5 days at −70 °C to x-ray film (Kodak, X Omat, XK 1). Autoradiographs were read by a single observer (L. L. Villa), who was totally unaware of both the cytology results and the risk factor profiles of the patients. HPV DNA hybridization results were classified on the basis of the signal intensity of the autoradiographs into three categories: negative, borderline, and frankly positive. HPV-positive cell scrapings from cervical condylomata were used as positive controls in every hybridization batch.

Statistical Analysis

The total study sample accrued during the investigation was 2,618 patients. Excluded from the study were 253 patients whose cervical cell specimens could not be evaluated and an additional 35 patients whose questionnaires were judged to be of poor quality by the interviewers. For the remaining 2,330 women, HPV infection rates were calculated according to each study variable. The search for variables predictive of the likelihood of a positive HPV DNA result followed a two-step analysis. Initially, we estimated group-specific HPV prevalence rate ratios (PRRs) by computing crude and clinic-adjusted Mantel-Haenszel odds ratios and their 95% confidence intervals (CIs). Adjusted trend effects in the relationship between factor dose and magnitude of risk were evaluated by Mantel's extension to the Mantel-Haenszel method (*18*).

Because of the risk factor heterogeneity of the populations sampled in the study, a nested case-control analysis was subsequently performed to allow better control of confounding. The data records of four randomly selected patients with HPV-negative or borderline results were matched on the basis of clinic, 5-year age group, and trimester of admission with those of each of the 141 women with a frankly positive HPV result (either subtype). The process of computerized, random record linkage to generate the nested case-control matched sets eliminated five patients because fewer than four controls were available in their matching strata. The resulting case-control data set, consisting of 136 cases and 544 controls, was analyzed according to the subset determined by the HPV group: 89 HPV 6/11 cases with their corresponding 356 controls and 96 HPV 16/18 cases with their corresponding 384 controls. For each matched case-control subset, crude PRRs for all variables were computed by conditional logistic regression (*19,20*). The likelihood ratio chi-square statistics from each univariate matched analysis were used to build multivariate models containing all factors that were associated with risk of HPV infection at the 10% significance level. The most predictive models for each subset were then obtained by stepwise elimination of all variables not reaching the above significance level.

Results

None of the statistical correlates of a frankly positive HPV specimen were associated with the risk of having a borderline result (data not shown). If borderline results from autoradiographs represented for the most part true intermediate results, because of lower numbers of viral copies or lower frequencies of infected cells per specimen, their statistical correlates would be similar to those of frankly positive specimens. The number of epithelial cells per filter used in the hybridization was the most important determinant for our finding a borderline result. Frequencies of such results were two to four times higher among specimens containing >330,000 cells per filter than among specimens with lower cell counts. However, frankly positive specimens were only 1.2 times more frequently observed among lysates with higher numbers of cells. In addition, frequencies of HPV infection, as judged by frankly positive results, were much higher in the Recife clinics than in the São Paulo clinic, whereas the frequency of borderline results was higher in the clinic in São Paulo. Therefore, we considered borderline specimens as due mostly to background reactivity, and all subsequent analyses included these results among the clearly negative ones.

HPV infection rates according to HPV group and clinic are shown in table 1. Since the São Paulo population has many migrant groups from other Brazilian regions and, in particular, from the northeastern region, PRRs are presented both as crude estimates and after adjustment for the geographic origin of patients. Infection rates for both HPV groups were considerably higher in the Recife clinics than in the São Paulo clinic. There were no statistically significant differences in infection rates between the two Recife clinics, regardless of HPV group. The magnitude of the HPV 6/11 PRRs for study clinics was confounded by the geographic origin of the subjects. Geographically adjusted PRRs for HPV 6/11 were substantially higher than the crude estimates. The same was not observed for HPV 16/18, because adjusted estimates were not materially different from univariate PRRs (table 1).

Table 2 shows the frequencies of group-specific HPV infection according to selected socioeconomic and demographic factors. Because of the strong association seen with

Table 1. PRRs* and 95% CIs for HPV infection according to HPV group and study clinic

HPV group	Study clinic	Infection rate (%)	Crude analysis		Adjusted for geographic origin of patient	
			PRR	95% CI†	PRR	95% CI†
6/11	HVNC (São Paulo)	2.4	1.0	(ref)	1.0	(ref)
	IMIP (Recife)	5.5	2.4	1.4–4.0	4.4	1.5–10.4
	HCP (Recife)	4.7	2.0	1.0–3.8	3.9	1.2–11.1
	Both clinics (Recife)	5.2	2.3	1.4–3.8	4.1	1.4–8.7
16/18	HVNC (São Paulo)	2.0	1.0	(ref)	1.0	(ref)
	IMIP (Recife)	5.4	2.8	1.6–5.0	3.0	2.0–7.0
	HCP (Recife)	7.0	3.8	2.0–7.0	4.1	1.6–10.1
	Both clinics (Recife)	5.9	3.1	1.8–5.4	3.3	1.4–7.1

*Mantel-Haenszel odds ratio estimates.
†(ref) = reference category.

Table 2. Group-specific HPV infection rates (%) and PRRs* with 95% CIs according to selected socioeconomic, demographic, and related factors

Variable	No.†	HPV 6/11			HPV 16/18		
		%	PRR	95% CI‡	%	PRR	95% CI‡
Age (yr)							
≤25	561	3.9	1.0	(ref)	5.0	1.0	(ref)
26–32	631	4.1	1.2	0.6–2.2	4.4	0.9	0.5–1.7
33–41	571	4.4	1.3	0.7–2.4	4.0	0.8	0.5–1.5
≥42	567	3.7	1.1	0.5–2.0	3.5	0.7	0.4–1.4
Chi-square for trend (*P*):			0.001 (.9771)			1.735 (.1878)	
Race							
White	962	2.8	1.0	(ref)	2.6	1.0	(ref)
Mulatto	1,254	5.1	1.3	0.7–2.2	5.8	1.5	0.8–2.6
Black	103	2.9	1.0	0.2–3.6	1.0	0.3	0.0–2.2
Schooling (yr)							
≤4	1,191	4.1	1.0	(ref)	3.9	1.0	(ref)
5–8	941	3.4	1.0	0.6–1.6	4.1	1.4	0.9–2.2
≥9	198	6.6	1.6	0.8–3.1	7.1	1.8	0.9–3.5
Chi-square for trend (*P*):			0.961 (.3271)			4.287 (.0384)	
Monthly income (U.S. dollars)							
≤140	1,018	3.8	1.0	(ref)	5.1	1.0	(ref)
>140	1,036	3.9	1.5	0.9–2.5	3.6	1.1	0.7–1.8
Unknown	276	5.4	1.3	0.7–2.5	3.6	0.6	0.3–1.3
Marital status							
Never married	185	3.2	1.0	(ref)	7.0	1.0	(ref)
Ever married	2,145	4.1	1.4	0.6–3.5	4.0	0.6	0.3–1.2
Geographic origin							
Northern/northeastern region	1,685	4.5	1.0	(ref)	5.1	1.0	(ref)
Southern/southeastern region	625	3.0	2.1	0.7–5.1	2.1	1.0	0.4–2.7
Distance from clinic (km)							
1–10	1,256	3.2	1.0	(ref)	3.1	1.0	(ref)
≥11	979	4.8	0.9	0.5–1.7	5.3	1.0	0.6–1.7

*Mantel-Haenszel odds ratio estimates adjusted by study clinic.
†Missing values excluded from some analyses.
‡(ref) = reference category.

study clinic, PRRs are presented after we controlled for this variable. Group-specific infection rates and adjusted PRRs exhibited opposite directions of association with age, as measured in approximate quartiles of the distribution for this variable. However, neither the trends observed nor the level-specific PRRs reached statistical significance. Likewise, although mulattoes seemed to experience a 30%–50% increase in risk of HPV infection, the magnitude of the differences could be attributed to chance. Of the remaining variables, only years of schooling seemed to exert a risk effect for HPV 16/18. A trend test for this variable in regard to the association with HPV 16/18 was significant ($P = .0384$).

Similarly, table 3 displays equivalent information in regard to associations with selected variables for reproductive history. Most of these factors failed to be associated with risk of a positive HPV result, regardless of the HPV group. Patients who reported that they were pregnant during the interview seemed to experience a twofold higher risk of infection with HPV 6/11, a marginally significant association. Parity, a variable frequently associated with risk of cervical cancer, failed to correlate with the likelihood of HPV infection in either group.

The interviewer elicited information with respect to a number of health-related and personal hygiene practices (table 4). Of those, only the lifetime frequency of visits to a gynecologist was associated with risk of HPV infection, most notably for infection by HPV 16/18. Risk of infection was negatively associated with frequency of visits ($P = .0172$). None of the women with an altered Papanicolaou smear cytology (class III or higher) had a positive specimen for HPV 6/11. On the other hand, patients with abnormal smears had twice the risk of infection with HPV 16/18 than did women with cytology classes I and II. In neither case, however, did the association between cytology class and HPV infection risk reach statistical significance because of the small number of women with abnormal smears in the survey. Cigarette smoking or other forms of tobacco smoking were not predictors of the risk of HPV infection. Likewise, when cumulative exposure was calculated as number of pack-years of cigarette smoking, no dose–response relationship was found with risk of HPV infection (table 4).

Table 5 shows the association between risk of HPV infection and four surrogate measures of sexual activity and promiscuity. Most of these variables failed to exhibit important correlations with the likelihood of finding a positive HPV specimen of either viral group. Although women reporting more than five sex partners had a 30%–70% increase in risk of HPV infection when compared with the risk found in monogamous patients, the differences were not significant. Likewise, patients reporting having had their first intercourse

Table 3. Group-specific HPV infection rates (%) and PRRs* with 95% CIs according to selected reproductive history factors

Variable	No.†	HPV 6/11 %	HPV 6/11 PRR	HPV 6/11 95% CI‡	HPV 16/18 %	HPV 16/18 PRR	HPV 16/18 95% CI‡
Age at menarche (yr)							
≤12	840	4.0	1.0	(ref)	3.0	1.0	(ref)
>12	1,479	4.0	0.9	0.6–1.5	4.6	1.3	0.8–2.0
Parity							
0	242	5.8	1.0	(ref)	5.4	1.0	(ref)
1–2	819	3.5	0.7	0.3–1.4	4.8	1.0	0.5–1.9
≥3	1,268	4.0	0.7	0.4–1.4	3.7	0.7	0.4–1.4
Chi-square for trend (*P*):			0.287 (.5921)			1.921 (.1658)	
No. of abortions							
0	1,347	4.2	1.0	(ref)	4.4	1.0	(ref)
1	553	4.2	1.0	0.6–1.6	4.5	1.0	0.6–1.7
≥2	429	3.5	0.8	0.4–1.5	3.5	0.8	0.4–1.4
Chi-square for trend (*P*):			0.497 (.4810)			0.768 (.3807)	
Current pregnancy							
No	2,227	3.8	1.0	(ref)	4.2	1.0	(ref)
Yes	85	9.4	2.1	0.9–4.8	5.9	1.2	0.4–3.3
Use of oral contraceptives							
Never used	909	4.1	1.0	(ref)	4.4	1.0	(ref)
Ever used	1,421	4.0	1.1	0.7–1.7	4.2	1.1	0.7–1.7
Use of condoms							
Never used	1,983	4.0	1.0	(ref)	4.3	1.0	(ref)
Ever used	347	4.0	1.5	0.8–2.9	3.7	1.5	0.7–2.9
Use of intrauterine contraceptive device							
Never used	2,160	4.2	1.0	(ref)	4.3	1.0	(ref)
Ever used	170	2.4	0.7	0.2–2.1	3.5	1.2	0.5–3.1

*Mantel-Haenszel odds ratio estimates adjusted by study clinic.
†Missing values excluded from some analyses.
‡(ref) = reference category.

below the age of 16 were at 1.3 to 1.4 times higher risk of infection, but the confidence bounds for these estimates included the null value (unity). Conversely, lower risks were observed in patients with more active lifetime sexual activities after we controlled for the study clinic. However, as with the preceding analyses, no statistically important associations were seen. There were five virgins among the women surveyed. One of them was infected with both HPV 6/11 and HPV 16/18. The remaining four had no HPV infections.

The practice of anal intercourse was reported more frequently among women who had a positive HPV specimen. The clinic-adjusted PRR for this variable in regard to HPV 6/11 (1.9) was statistically significant at the 5% level.

The search for the most explanatory set of variables was based on the nested case–control subset, in which the matching criteria were maintained during the analysis by multiple logistic regression with the use of conditional maximum likelihood estimation. Table 6 shows the final models with predictive properties with respect to risk of HPV infection by groups 6/11 and 16/18. Both models were determined on the basis of conservative statistical criteria (10% significance level). The independent factors associated with risk of infection by HPV 6/11 included practice of anal intercourse and current pregnancy. For HPV 16/18, only one variable (i.e., frequency of visits to a gynecologist) exhibited a strong independent association with risk. When used as a single-term, ordinal variable, this variable caused the best improvement in fit. Additional independent explanatory effects were seen for number of cells per filter and age at first intercourse, both of which were used as dichotomous variables.

The dissimilarity between the above profiles of predictor variables prompted us to verify whether the distribution of group-specific infections was independent or exhibited a pattern that could reflect a joint mechanism favoring the occurrence of mixed (both HPV 6/11 and HPV 16/18) infections. Table 7 shows such an analysis as stratified by study clinic, the strongest determinant of the likelihood of finding a positive HPV specimen in this survey. The frequency of mixed infections was 13 times higher than that expected by chance alone, if one assumes independent distributions for group-specific infections. Higher observed frequencies were apparent for all three study clinics. The Recife clinics exhibited a similar pattern of joint distribution for HPV groups. The observed number of mixed infections in the São Paulo clinic was at an even higher level than that in the Recife clinics (ratio of observed to expected = 18).

Discussion

This study failed to provide strong evidence for the association between epidemiologic correlates of cervical cancer and risk of HPV infection of either subtype. With the exception of the study clinic and, by extension, the metropolitan area, determinants of risk for HPV infection with virus group 6/11 were not the same as those found for infection with group 16/18. Different subsets of predictor variables

Table 4. Group-specific HPV infection rates (%) and PRRs* with 95% CIs according to selected hygienic and health-related factors

Variable	No.†	HPV 6/11			HPV 16/18		
		%	PRR	95% CI‡	%	PRR	95% CI‡
Use of tampons							
Never used	2,307	4.0	1.0	(ref)	4.2	1.0	(ref)
Ever used	23	4.3	1.6	0.1–11.5	4.3	1.7	0.1–12.4
Vaginal douching							
Never	1,035	4.8	1.0	(ref)	4.8	1.0	(ref)
Ever	1,295	3.4	0.7	0.4–1.0	3.8	0.7	0.5–1.1
No. of visits to gynecologist							
0	192	7.8	1.0	(ref)	8.3	1.0	(ref)
1–2	491	3.9	0.6	0.3–1.4	5.5	0.8	0.4–1.7
≥3	1,637	3.7	0.6	0.3–1.1	3.4	0.6	0.3–1.1
Chi-square for trend (*P*):			2.068 (.1504)			5.673 (.0172)	
History of genital sores							
Never	2,072	3.9	1.0	(ref)	4.1	1.0	(ref)
Ever	240	5.4	1.2	0.6–2.2	5.4	1.1	0.6–2.0
Frequency of Papanicolaou smears							
1	723	4.8	1.0	(ref)	5.0	1.0	(ref)
2–4	1,008	3.8	0.8	0.5–1.4	4.5	1.1	0.7–1.7
≥5	599	3.5	0.9	0.5–1.6	3.0	0.8	0.4–1.5
Chi-square for trend (*P*):			0.226 (.6349)			0.339 (.5603)	
Smear class							
I–II	2,301	4.1	1.0	(ref)	4.2	1.0	(ref)
≥III	28	0.0	0.0	0.0–3.9	10.7	2.0	0.5–7.4
Smoking history							
Never smoked	1,173	3.8	1.0	(ref)	4.3	1.0	(ref)
Current smoker	806	4.8	1.4	0.9–2.2	4.2	1.0	0.6–1.6
Ex-smoker	350	3.1	0.8	0.4–1.6	4.0	0.9	0.4–1.6
Cumulative tobacco exposure (pack-years)							
<1	1,442	4.1	1.0	(ref)	4.6	1.0	(ref)
1–10	630	4.1	1.0	0.6–1.7	3.7	0.8	0.5–1.4
>10	239	3.3	0.9	0.4–2.0	2.5	0.6	0.2–1.4
Chi-square for trend (*P*):			0.042 (.8382)			0.451 (.5020)	

*Mantel-Haenszel odds ratio estimates adjusted by study clinic.
†Missing values excluded from some analyses.
‡(ref) = reference category.

were obtained with the use of conditional logistic regression on each group and its matched controls. Despite conflicting results for clinic-adjusted PRRs according to measures of sexual activity, age at first intercourse emerged as an explanatory variable for HPV 16/18 in the more controlled nested case–control analysis. However, both the magnitude of the PRR estimate for the latter variable and its statistical precision lacked strength of association. Other known correlates of cervical cancer risk (e.g., number of sex partners, parity, oral contraceptive use, and tobacco smoking) failed to exhibit any independent associations with infection by either HPV group. The strongest risk factor (protective effect) for HPV 16/18 was represented by the reported frequency of visits to a gynecologist. It is unlikely that this finding represents an indirect association due to differences in study populations, since controlling for age and clinic had been performed in the design and had been maintained during the analysis.

Besides study clinic and geographic origin, the only two predictors of risk of infection with HPV 6/11 were of marginal statistical significance. Practice of anal intercourse was positively associated with risk. We used this variable in the study to obtain an additional proxy variable for promiscuity. Although only a few women reported being pregnant during specimen collection and interview (85 patients, 3.7%), a relatively impressive proportion harbored HPV 6/11 DNA sequences in their cervices (9.4%). We had originally anticipated that such a finding would be a result of confounding by differences in fertility rates and age distributions between women in Recife and São Paulo, which could have influenced the proportion of pregnant women among the survey subjects. However, further adjustment by study clinic and the analysis of the finely matched strata of the case–control subset revealed an independent explanatory risk effect for current pregnancy. A similar finding has been shown in a previous study (*21*).

The number of epithelial cells used in the assay exerted a nonnegligible effect on the likelihood of finding a positive HPV 16/18 specimen. A preliminary exploratory analysis of factors associated with the likelihood of obtaining borderline and frankly positive specimens revealed a strong role for the cell counts only with respect to borderline hybridizations. Therefore, in the interest of conservative interpretation and because borderline results did not differ in frequency among

Table 5. Group-specific HPV infection rates (%) and PRRs* with 95% CIs according to selected sexual activity variables

Variable	No.†	HPV 6/11			HPV 16/18		
		%	PRR	95% CI‡	%	PRR	95% CI‡
Age at first sexual intercourse (yr)							
≥20	750	4.0	1.0	(ref)	3.6	1.0	(ref)
16–19	1,079	3.3	0.8	0.5–1.4	4.0	1.1	0.7–1.9
≤15	491	5.3	1.3	0.7–2.3	5.3	1.4	0.8–2.5
Chi-square for trend (*P*):			0.572 (.4494)			0.920 (.3375)	
No. of sex partners							
1	1,441	4.0	1.0	(ref)	4.0	1.0	(ref)
2–5	781	3.8	1.0	0.6–1.5	4.6	1.2	0.7–1.8
≥6	94	6.4	1.7	0.6–4.1	5.3	1.3	0.5–3.6
Chi-square for trend (*P*):			0.261 (.6094)			0.490 (.4837)	
Lifetime occasions of sexual intercourse							
≤410	428	4.7	1.0	(ref)	5.6	1.0	(ref)
411–900	490	3.5	0.7	0.4–1.5	4.7	0.8	0.4–1.5
901–1,560	489	3.3	0.7	0.3–1.4	3.3	0.5	0.3–1.1
1,561–2,600	438	4.3	0.9	0.5–1.8	3.2	0.5	0.3–1.1
≥2,601	450	4.0	0.8	0.4–1.6	3.8	0.6	0.3–1.2
Chi-square for trend (*P*):			0.021 (.8849)			1.989 (.1584)	
Practice of anal intercourse							
Never practiced	1,954	3.5	1.0	(ref)	3.9	1.0	(ref)
Ever practiced	366	6.3	1.9	1.1–3.1	5.2	1.4	0.8–2.3

*Mantel-Haenszel odds ratio estimates adjusted by study clinic.
†Virgins and unknowns excluded.
‡(ref) = reference category.

Table 6. Variables most associated with the risk of HPV infection in 680 cytologic specimens (136 cases and 544 controls)*

Variable	Relative risk	95% CI	*P* value†
HPV 6/11 (89 cases and 356 controls)			
Anal intercourse (ever vs. never)	1.69	0.95–3.01	.0795
Current pregnancy (yes vs. no)	2.31	0.88–6.08	.0877
HPV 16/18 (96 cases and 384 controls)			
Frequency of visits to gynecologist (0, 1–2, ≥3)	0.65	0.45–0.93	.0175
No. of cells per filter (×1,000) (>200 vs. ≤200)	1.58	0.96–2.61	.0675
Age at first intercourse (≤15 yr vs. >15 yr)	1.67	0.99–2.83	.0817

*Matched on clinic, 5-yr age group, and trimester of admission. Results obtained by conditional logistic regression with the use of stepwise elimination of terms based on a significance level of 10%.

†Likelihood ratio chi-square between current model and a reduced one excluding the variable.

the study clinics, we decided to use only frankly positive specimens as equating with HPV infection (22).

A striking finding from the present study was represented by the marked joint distribution of group-specific infections. Since the sets of predictor variables found for the two HPV groups were distinct, we expected that study clinic or city alone could explain the high number of mixed infections seen in this investigation. Prevalence rates had been much higher in the Recife clinics; thus, one could speculate that the observed number of combined infections was caused by a "concentration" effect that was due to the higher risk experienced by women from Recife. This situation was not the case, however, since the ratio of observed to expected cases was abnormally high for all clinics. This finding suggests the existence of a strong common determinant for group-specific HPV infections.

The choice of methods for viral DNA detection is far from resolved (23). The filter in situ hybridization method is con-

Table 7. Frequencies of HPV-infected women according to HPV group and study clinic

Study clinic	No. of women not infected with HPV*	No. of women infected with			Infection with both HPV 6/11 and HPV 16/18	
		HPV 6/11 only	HPV 16/18 only	Both HPV 6/11 and HPV 16/18	Expected	Ratio† of observed to expected
HVNC (São Paulo)	935	14	10	9	0.5	18.0
IMIP (Recife)	860	23	22	28	2.7	10.4
HCP (Recife)	394	5	15	15	1.4	10.7
All clinics	2,189	42	47	52	4.0	13.0

*Based on the subtypes used in the study.
†Ratio of actual frequency of combined infections (HPV 6/11 and HPV 16/18) to that expected by chance alone.

sidered to be less sensitive than the Southern blot analysis according to some studies (22). Nevertheless, under stringent conditions, the filter in situ hybridization technique has a specificity comparable to that of the latter method and is more conveniently adapted to population surveys. A recent study has attributed comparable sensitivity and specificity to the two methods (24). However, it is still premature for one to judge the diagnostic performance of the two major methods from isolated studies while many different technical variants are being practiced, as reported in the literature. Case ascertainment in the present survey relied exclusively on the filter in situ hybridization test, which could have represented a possible source of error. Important random misclassification of cases and controls would have resulted if the number of false-positive and -negative hybridizations had reached a substantial proportion among all study subjects. In this situation, the PRR estimates would have been biased toward the null value. Because most of our study's findings were based on the absence or weakness of associations between epidemiologic correlates of cervical cancer and risk of HPV infection, one cannot immediately rule out the hypothesis of random misclassification. However, the sensitivity of the filter in situ hybridization assay by the present set of results may be judged as comparable to that of other prevalence studies (22,25). Likewise, if a substantial number of random misclassifications had occurred, the proportions of mixed infections as analyzed above would have fluctuated markedly and a smaller frequency of co-positive hybridizations would have been observed. In addition, a high degree of specificity is contributed by the high stringency conditions with which cell-containing filters were hybridized with the viral probes.

Lack of associations with most study variables would also have emerged if there had been random misclassification of exposure levels for factors correlated with cervical cancer. If this problem had occurred, one would fail to observe associations between key study variables and risk of an abnormal cervical cytology. However, despite the low frequency of the latter results (28 patients), we found significant ($P < .05$) associations (data not shown) for schooling and frequency of Papanicolaou smears (negative) as well as for number of lifetime occasions of sexual intercourse (positive). In addition, marginal associations were seen for parity (positive) and family income (negative).

The evidence suggesting an etiologic role for certain subtypes of HPV in regard to cervical malignancy is more concrete than that for most other microbial agents, such as *Trichmonas*, *Chlamydia*, cytomegalovirus, and herpes simplex virus. Strong support for the oncogenic role of HPV in the genital tract has stemmed mostly from four types of observations: (*a*) most genital cancers harbor HPV DNA sequences; (*b*) the physical state of the viral DNA differs (i.e., viral DNA is mostly integrated in invasive tumors and extrachromosomal in benign and premalignant lesions) (26,27); (*c*) transcriptionally active viral genomes are frequently found in cervical tumors and their cell lines maintained in culture (28,29); and (*d*) malignant transformation is obtained when viral DNA is transfected into mammalian cells in culture (30,31). However, recent reports have challenged the consistency of some of these lines of evidence. In different populations, HPV DNA has been found in surprisingly high frequency among women with normal cervices (32). In addition, some studies have shown that the within-specimen distribution of the viral DNA and its transcriptional activity in cervical tumors exhibit a "patchy" pattern of occurrence (33,34).

With the exception of the above fourth line of evidence, all other observations are also consistent with an additional activity that could explain the association between HPV and cervical cancer. HPVs are a group of viruses with strong epitheliotropic properties; thus, by merely claiming such properties, one could accommodate the findings of their statistical association with abnormal cervical proliferation. The physical state and expression differences found between advanced and precursor lesions could also be a consequence of long-lasting infection by the virus. Another tenable model would accommodate both hypotheses by the assumption that viral infection may not represent a necessary and sufficient single etiologic component. Neoplastic changes in the cervix could begin and progress without the presence of either the HPV DNA or its transcriptional activity, but it would be plausible for one to assume that the virus has an important role as promoter (27). The proper distinction among these etiologic models must be obtained through sensible epidemiologic study designs. Unfortunately, most of the clinico-epidemiologic investigations of HPV and genital cancer have been plagued by a number of problems affecting their validity (23).

In the present investigation, we provided results from an alternative epidemiologic study design. Although the difficulty resides in researchers obtaining an identifiable time perspective in regard to appearance of viral infection and onset of malignancy, it is simple to obtain histories of behavioral and other characteristics of women that would be conducive to risk of infection. As such, our study was based on the assumption that HPV infection is in the causal pathway represented by female sexual activity correlates and cervical cancer.

The prevalence survey design was selected for our study because of its inherent advantage in allowing an a posteriori definition for the control group. This advantage eliminated possible biases with self-selection and lack of comparability of control patients. Another advantage of the nested case-control approach of analysis is that the controls can be matched to cases on the basis of factors that could potentially confound the interpretation of results. Matching criteria controlled for characteristics that could fluctuate over time (e.g., diagnostic ascertainment quality and specimen collection technique) and factors that are associated with the balance of putative risk factors for the disease (e.g., age and clinic).

We found higher HPV infection rates in Recife than in São Paulo, a finding in agreement with the observed differences in cervical cancer incidence rates between the two cities. However, this observation is purely ecologic and should not be construed as evidence for an association between HPV infection and cervical neoplasia. In fact, the bulk of the results generated by the present study suggests that HPV infection and cervical cancer are elicited by different risk factor profiles. Our findings regarding a higher than expected frequency of infections with both HPV groups (6/11 and 16/18) are also suggestive of the existence of additional common determinants for the risk of HPV infection. These determinants are not akin to the general behavioral characteristics of women that are typically probed in epidemiologic studies of cervical cancer.

References

(1) Brinton LA, Hamman RF, Huggins GR, et al: Sexual and reproductive risk factors for invasive squamous cell cervical cancer. JNCI 79:23-29, 1987

(2) La Vecchia C, Franceschi S, Decarli A, et al: Sexual factors, venereal diseases, and the risk of intraepithelial and invasive cervical neoplasia. Cancer 58:935-941, 1986

(3) Zunzunegui MV, King MC, Coria CF, et al: Male influences on cervical cancer risk. Am J Epidemiol 123:302-307, 1986

(4) Graham S, Prioré R, Graham M, et al: Genital cancer in wives of penile cancer patients. Cancer 44:1870-1874, 1979

(5) Smith PG, Kinlen LJ, White GC, et al: Mortality of wives of men dying with cancer of the penis. Br J Cancer 41:422-428, 1980

(6) Franco EL, Campos Filho N, Villa LL, et al: Correlation patterns of cancer relative frequencies with some socioeconomic and demographic indicators in Brazil: An ecologic study. Int J Cancer 41:24-29, 1988

(7) Yao-Li J, Li FP, Blot WJ, et al: Correlation between cancers of the uterine cervix and penis in China. JNCI 69:1063-1065, 1982

(8) Broker TR, Botchan M: Papillomaviruses: Retrospectives and prospectives. *In*: Cancer Cells 4/DNA Tumor Viruses (Botchan M, Grodzicker T, Sharp PA, eds). Cold Spring Harbor, NY: Cold Spring Harbor Laboratory, 1986, pp 17-36

(9) Pfister H: Relationship of papillomaviruses to anogenital cancer. Obstet Gynecol Clin North Am 14:349-361, 1987

(10) Pfister H: Human papillomaviruses and genital cancer. Adv Cancer Res 48:113-147, 1987

(11) Lorincz A, Temple GF, Kurman RJ, et al: Oncogenic association of specific human papillomavirus types with cervical neoplasia. JNCI 79:671-677, 1987

(12) Wickenden C, Malcolm ADB, Byrne M, et al: Prevalence of HPV DNA and viral copy numbers in cervical scrapes from women with normal and abnormal cervices. J Pathol 153:127-135, 1987

(13) Reeves WC, Caussy D, Brinton LA, et al: Case-control study of human papillomaviruses and cervical cancer in Latin America. Int J Cancer 40:450-454, 1987

(14) Brinton LA, Fraumeni JF Jr: Epidemiology of uterine cervical cancer. J Chronic Dis 39:1051-1065, 1986

(15) Carvalho MRC, Franco EL, eds: Cancer Incidence in Recife County, Brazil (1967-1979). Ludwig Institute for Cancer Research Monogr Ser in Cancer Epidemiol, vol 2. São Paulo: LICR, 1986

(16) Mirra AP, Franco EL, eds: Cancer Incidence in São Paulo County, Brazil (1969, 1973, 1978). Ludwig Institute for Cancer Research Monogr Ser in Cancer Epidemiol, vol 1. São Paulo: LICR, 1985

(17) Wagner D, Ikenberg H, Bohm N, et al: Identification of human papillomavirus in cervical smears by deoxyribonucleic acid in situ hybridization. Obstet Gynecol 64:767-772, 1984

(18) Mantel N: Chi-square tests with one degree of freedom: Extensions of the Mantel-Haenszel procedure. J Am Stat Assoc 58:690-700, 1963

(19) Gail MH, Lubin JH, Rubinstein LV: Likelihood calculations for matched case-control studies and survival studies with tied death times. Biometrika 68:703-707, 1981

(20) Campos-Filho N, Franco EL: A microcomputer program for multiple logistic regression by unconditional and conditional maximum likelihood methods. Am J Epidemiol, 1989. In press

(21) Schneider A, Hotz M, Gissmann L: Increased prevalence of human papillomaviruses in the lower genital tract of pregnant women. Int J Cancer 40:198-201, 1987

(22) de Villiers EM, Wagner D, Schneider A, et al: Human papillomavirus infections in women with and without abnormal cervical cytology. Lancet 2:703-705, 1987

(23) Muñoz N, Bosch X, Kaldor JM: Does human papillomavirus cause cervical cancer? The state of the epidemiological evidence. Br J Cancer 57:1-5, 1988

(24) Caussy D, Orr W, Daya AD, et al: Evaluation of methods for detecting human papillomavirus deoxyribonucleotide sequences in clinical specimens. J Clin Microbiol 26:236-243, 1988

(25) Schneider A, Sterzik K, Buck G, et al: Colposcopy is superior to cytology for the detection of early genital human papillomavirus infection. Obstet Gynecol 71:236-241, 1988

(26) Lehn H, Krieg P, Sauer G: Papillomavirus genomes in human cervical tumors: Analysis of their transcriptional activity. Proc Natl Acad Sci USA 82:5540-5544, 1985

(27) Lehn H, Villa LL, Marziona F, et al: Physical state and biological activity of human papillomavirus genomes in precancerous lesions of the female genital tract. J Gen Virol 69:187-196, 1988

(28) Schwarz E, Freese UK, Gissmann L, et al: Structure and transcription of human papillomavirus sequences in cervical carcinoma cells. Nature 314:111-114, 1985

(29) Shirasawa H, Tomita Y, Sekiya S, et al: Integration and transcription of human papillomavirus type 16 and 18 sequences in cell lines derived from cervical carcinomas. J Gen Virol 68:583-591, 1987

(30) Pirisi L, Yasumoto S, Feller M, et al: Transformation of human fibroblasts and keratinocytes with human papillomavirus type 16 DNA. J Virol 61:1061-1066, 1987

(31) Matlashewski G, Schneider J, Banks L, et al: Human papillomavirus type 16 DNA cooperates with activated ras in transforming primary cells. EMBO J 6:1741-1746, 1987

(32) Anonymous: Human papillomaviruses and cervical cancer: A fresh look at the evidence. Lancet 1:725-726, 1987

(33) Stoler MH, Broker TR: In situ hybridization detection of human papillomavirus DNAs and messenger RNAs in genital condylomas and a cervical carcinoma. Hum Pathol 17:1250-1258, 1986

(34) Nagai N, Nuovo G, Friedman D, et al: Detection of papillomavirus nucleic acids in genital precancers with the in situ hybridization technique. Int J Gynecol Pathol 6:366-379, 1987

11. Medical Institute for Sexual Health HPV Prevention Report

THE MEDICAL INSTITUTE January 22, 2004

1101 S. Capital of Texas Hwy.
Bldg. B, Suite 100
Austin, TX 78746
Phone: (512) 328-6268
Fax: (512) 328-6269

Human Papilloma Virus: A Major Unrecognized Epidemic

W. David Hager, M.D., F.A.C.O.G.
Freda McKissic Bush, M.D., F.A.C.O.G.
Joe S. Mcilhaney, Jr., M.D., F.A.C.O.G.

Patricia Thickstun, Ph.D., Editor
Kate Hendricks, M.D., M.P.H. & T.M., Editor

Table of Contents

Page

Table of Contents i

I. Background Information 1

II. Morbidity and Mortality 1

III. Course of Infection, Susceptibility, and Prevalence 2-3

A. Multiple strains
B. Oncogenic strains

IV. Pathophysiology of Disease 3-4

A. The mechanism by which HPV causes cervical dysplasia/cancer

V. PAP Smear Screening in the United States 4-5

A. The possibility of HPV becoming a reportable disease

VI. Prevention 5-6

VII. Conclusion 7

References 8

Human Papillomavirus: A Major Unrecognized Epidemic

I. Background Information

Infection with human papillomavirus (HPV) has become a significant health problem in the United States as well as in the rest of the world. This DNA virus causes acute infection as well as infection-related disease among sexually active men and women. Although disease caused by this virus has been known for centuries, it is only relatively recently that HPV has been recognized as a cause of cervical cancer. During the past 20 years, HPV infection and the genital warts and cervical cancer it causes have escalated to alarming levels.

II. Morbidity and Mortality

HPV infection is the most prevalent of all viral sexually transmitted infections, even more common than herpes and HIV combined. It is estimated that 5.5 million people are infected by HPV every year in the United States.[1] Every year, 3.5 million American women have abnormal PAP smears; 13,400 are diagnosed with cervical cancer, and 4,100 die of cervical cancer. Worldwide, more than 500,000 cases of cervical cancer and 200,000 deaths are caused by HPV each year. [2]

III. Course of Infection, Susceptibility, and Prevalence

Of the more than 100 HPV strains identified so far, around 35 can infect the human genital tract. HPV infection with "benign" strains that do not cause cancer may lead to genital warts, which may be associated with itching, burning, or pain. In contrast, most infections with "oncogenic" or cancer-causing strains of HPV may cause no symptoms at all and are asymptomatic. Persons infected with cancer-causing strains are generally unaware that they are infected and that they are putting their unsuspecting sex partners at risk of infection with these potentially lethal viruses. Overall, more than 90% of HPV infections are asymptomatic. Unlike non-sexually transmitted viral infections such as the common cold, influenza, or measles that last only a week or two, HPV infections can last for months and occasionally for years.

The prevalence[a] of HPV infection has increased at an astonishing rate. Over the past two decades millions of people have been diagnosed with this viral infection. Recent estimates indicate that 50–75% of sexually active adults are HPV positive. In a study during the late 1990s, 43% of college coeds who were HPV negative at the beginning of the study developed HPV infection over the 3 years of the study.[3] In general, factors that put sexually active people at risk for HPV infection include early age

[a] Prevalence is defined as the total number of cases of a specific disease in existence at a certain time in a particular population

Risk Factors for HPV Infection and Cervical Cancer

HPV infection and cervical cancer risk is increased by:

- Beginning sexual intercourse at an early age—especially age 16 or younger
- Having multiple sexual partners
- Sex with partners who engage in high-risk sexual behavior (because of partner's risk of having a sexually transmitted infection)

["Human Papillomaviruses and Cancer," National Cancer Institute, October 15, 2002]

Available at: http://cis.nci.nih.gov/fact/3_20.htm

[Joffe GP, Foxman B, Schmidt AJ, et.al. Multiple partners and partner choice as risk factors for sexually transmitted disease among female college students. *Sex Trans Dis 1992;19:272-78]*

at sexual debut, multiple sexual partners, and sex with partners who engage in high-risk sexual behavior. Adolescent and young adult females are biologically more susceptible to HPV disease because the cervix has not reached its mature, adult state.[b] The cells of the cervix that are susceptible to infection with bacteria and viruses are more vulnerable in young females than in mature women. This leaves them far more susceptible to infection with sexually transmitted pathogens such as chlamydia, gonorrhea, and HPV. In addition to being more susceptible to infection, the cells on the surface of the immature cervix can be transformed into precancerous cells (cervical dysplasia),[c] and these precancerous cells may further develop into potentially lethal cervical cancer.[4]

IV. Pathophysiology of Disease

Infection with HPV is markedly different from infection with the other persistent viral sexually transmitted infections. Herpes simplex virus, or HSV, invades the skin and

[b] In *all women* the vagina is lined with epithelial (skin-like) cells, and the cervix is covered with two cell types---epithelial cells and columnar (like the cells lining the intestine) cells. In mature females, the outer part of the cervix (ie, the part from which cells are obtained for a PAP smear) is covered with hardy epithelial cells, and the upper (ie, inner) part is lined with fragile columnar cells. The location of the junction of the two cell types (squamocolumnar [SC] junction) varies considerably between adolescents/young women and mature women. Adolescents/young women have a condition referred to as ectopy. With ectopy, the junction between the two cell types is somewhere on the outer cervix rather than somewhere on the upper (inner) cervix. The more ectopy there is, the larger the diameter of fragile columnar cells on the outer exposed surface of the cervix. In addition to being highly susceptible to STIs, the exposed columnar and SC junction cells are easily transformed into precancerous cells or into cancer.

[c] Dysplasia is an alteration in the size, shape, and organization of adult cells

migrates to nerves where it lies dormant between outbreaks. The human immunodeficiency virus (HIV) persists in the bloodstream after entering a host through breaks in the skin or mucus membranes. In contrast, although HPV infects superficial skin cells called keratinocytes, it never migrates beyond these superficial skin cells.

The mechanism through which HPV causes cancer is unique and is related to special parts of the virus's genetic structure called oncogenes. HPV has two important oncogenes—E7 and E6—that take over normal cell mechanisms to cause cancer. The E7 oncogene attaches to the host cell's retinoblastoma (Rb) gene and interferes with its usual function of controlling cell growth. The E6 oncogene binds to the P53 gene, interfering with the cell's ability to repair cell damage. Thus, infection with cancer-causing HPV strains can lead to uncontrolled cell growth and can also prevent the repair of damaged cells. This can result in a precancerous change, called dysplasia, or an even more serious change, squamous cell cancer of the cervix. This same process can damage and transform cells of the external genitalia (vulva) and the anus in females and cells of the penis and the anus in males.

External genital warts are cauliflower-like lesions of the external genitalia. Although genital warts are visible to the naked eye, only about 10% of patients infected with HPV have such lesions. The incubation period between HPV infection and the development of genital warts ranges from 30 days to 9 months. The changes resulting from cancer-causing or oncogenic strains of HPV are usually not visible to the naked eye. Once a person is infected, the virus persists for an average of 8 months (range of 3–15 months).[3] While most women have strong enough immune systems to clear even "high-risk" or cancer-causing infections, approximately 10–12% of women will have persistent infections. Persistence has been identified as a significant risk factor for the development of cervical dysplasia and cancer.[5] Unfortunately, HPV infection with a cancer-causing strain rarely causes symptoms, so unless a woman undergoes regular PAP smear screening she will not know that she is infected with a cancer-causing strain and is at risk of dying from undiagnosed cervical cancer if it is present.

Of the 35 HPV types that cause genital infections, 18 are known to be oncogenic or cancer-causing "high-risk" types.[d] Just two types, 16 and 18, are responsible for more than 70% of all cervical dysplasia and cancer.[6] With current PAP smear screening technology it is possible to not only detect the cellular abnormalities of the cervix but also to sort abnormal specimens into low- and high-risk categories. Because low-risk types do not lead to cervical cancer, patients with these types do not require medical treatment, but do need continued screening. Patients with high-risk types require microscopic evaluation of the cervix (colposcopy) to identify the abnormal areas so that cervical biopsies can be obtained for pathologic evaluation.

V. PAP Smear Screening in the United States

In the United States more than 50 million PAP smears are evaluated annually. Of these, 45 million are normal, 1.5 million show benign inflammatory changes, and 2 million

[d] The high-risk types include 16, 18, 31, 33, 35, 39, 45, 51, 53, 56, 58, 59 and 68. Low-risk types include 6, 11, 42, 43, and 44.

show atypical cells of the cervix. A total of 1.5 million show precancerous changes known as squamous intraepithelial lesions, 1.2 million have low-grade squamous intraepithelial lesions (LGSIL), and 300,000 have high-grade squamous intraepithelial lesions (HGSIL). Sadly, 13,400 cases of cancer are diagnosed every year.[7] Low-grade squamous intraepithelial lesions (SIL) include atypia[e] and mild dysplasia, while high-grade lesions (HGSIL) include moderate and severe dysplasia and carcinoma-in-situ[f] of the cervix. Current estimates of HPV infection come from PAP smear data and limited prospective data. Currently HPV is not a reportable sexually transmitted infection and there are no mechanisms yet in place to track infected persons or their sexual partners.

Approximately two-thirds (68%) of males whose female sexual partners are diagnosed with cervical dysplasia have microscopic HPV lesions of the penis. These males are almost always asymptomatic and thus are unaware that they can transmit this disease. Infection of the penis or anus with high-risk HPV types predisposes these men to cancer of those organs.

VI. Prevention

Because HPV is a viral infection, no curative treatment is available. For the past several decades most national efforts to reduce sexually transmitted infections have focused on the promotion of condom use among sexually active individuals. However, it was not until 2000 that a national panel was convened by NIH to investigate condom effectiveness. This panel found that condoms do not provide any protection from HPV infection in females, although their use may reduce the risk of HPV-associated diseases, such as genital warts in men and cervical dysplasia in women. The panel also found that consistent and correct use of condoms reduces the risk of HIV infection by approximately 85% in males and females, but the risk of gonorrhea infection is reduced by only 25–75 % in males.[8] Later data also showed some reduction in transmission of herpes simplex virus in women.[9] Although condom usage rates have recently increased among high school age males,[10] sexually transmitted infection rates, particularly for HIV and chlamydia, have continued to increase in this age group. Because genital warts and asymptomatic HPV infection may be outside the area covered by a condom, consistent and correct condom use still leaves a significant chance for transmitting these and other sexual diseases.

Research on HPV vaccines is underway. Testing of a monovalent vaccine against just one HPV strain (type 16) has been promising.[12] Evaluation of a polyvalent vaccine that contains types 16,18, 6 and 11 is in progress. Unknowns include the duration of protection, whether reimmunization will be necessary, how well received the vaccine will be, and how effective the polyvalent vaccine will be.

Obviously the best way to prevent transmission of any sexually transmitted infection (STI) is to abstain from sexual intercourse outside a long-term, mutually monogamous relationship such as marriage. Add Health, the nationwide adolescent

[e] atypia is defined as deviation from the normal or typical state
[f] carcinoma-in-situ is a superficial cancer that has not yet invaded underlying tissues

Condoms Do Not Provide Effective Protection Against HPV

"HPV can be present for years with no symptoms, and HPV infection does not always produce warts or other symptoms; so you can be infected with HPV and pass it on without knowing it. Recent studies show that condoms ("rubbers") do not protect well against HPV infection. This is because HPV can be passed from person to person by skin-to-skin contact with any HPV-infected area of the body, such as skin of the genital or anal area not covered by the condom."

["Detailed Guide: Cervical Cancer, What Are the Risk Factors for Cervical Cancer?" American Cancer Society website, October 20, 2003]

Available at:
http://www.cancer.org/docroot/CRI/content/CRI_2_4_2X_What_are_the_risk_factors_for_cervical_cancer_8.asp?rnav=cri

"Condoms are ineffective against HPV because the virus is prevalent not only in the mucosal tissue (genitalia) but also on dry skin of the surrounding abdomen and groin, and it can migrate from those areas into the vagina and the cervix. Additional research efforts by NCI on the effectiveness of condoms in preventing HPV transmission are not warranted."

[Dr. Richard Klausner, Director of the National Cancer Institute, correspondence to U.S. House Commerce Committee, February 19, 1999]

"....the Panel concluded that there was no epidemiological evidence that condom use reduced the risk of HPV infection, but study results did suggest that condom use might afford some protection in reducing the risk of HPV-associated diseases, including warts in men and cervical neoplasia in women."

[Workshop Summary: Scientific Evidence on Condom Effectiveness for Sexually Transmitted Disease (STD) Prevention, June 12-13, 2000]

Available at: http://www.niaid.nih.gov/dmid/stds/condomreport.pdf

health study, found that the best deterrents to sexual activity among adolescents involve parental influence, moral and religious training, community influences, and appropriate peer influences.[11]

VII. Conclusion:

HPV is a preventable disease that continues to cause adverse health effects and death in our country and around the world. We must initiate methods to track the incidence and prevalence of disease. We must take steps to stop the alarming increase in this disease among teens and young adults. We must stop promoting methods that are known to have high failure rates in preventing HPV transmission, notably the condom, and be honest in informing young people about this fact. We must continue to emphasize highly effective methods of prevention, namely abstinence, whenever possible.

Best Strategies for HPV Prevention:

- Delaying the onset of sexual activity
- Abstinence
- Mutual monogamy with an uninfected lifetime partner
- Reduction in the number of sexual partners

REFERENCES:

1. NIAID Fact Sheet, *NIH, December 1998.*

2. Porten J, Adam HO, Bergstrom R, et.al. Strategies for global control of cervical cancer. *Am J Cancer 1995;60:1-26.*

3. Ho, GYF, Gierman R, Beardsley L., et.al. Natural history of cervicovaginal papillomavirus infection in young women. *N Engl J Med 1998;338:423-8.*

4. Joffe GP, Foxman B, Schmidt AJ, et.al. Multiple partners and partner choice as risk factors for sexually transmitted disease among female college students. *Sex Trans Dis 1992;19:272-78.*

5. Schlecht NF, Kulaga S, Robitaille J, Ferreira S, Santos M, et.al. Persistent human papilloma virus infection as a predictor of cervical intraepithelial neoplasia.*JAMA 2001;286:3106-14*

6. Clifford GM, Smith JS, Plummer M, et.al. Human papilloma virus types in invasive cervical cancer worldwide: a meta analysis. *Br J Cancer 2003;88:63-73.*

7. American Cancer Society data on cervical cancer/PAP smears

8. Workshop Summary: Scientific Evidence on Condom Effectiveness for Sexually Transmitted Disease (STD) Prevention. July 20, 2001. National Institute of Allergy and Infectious Diseases, National Institute of Health, Department of Health and Human Services. Cassette tapes of the June 12-13, 2000 conference can be obtained from Audio Transcripts, Ltd., 3660-B Wheeler Avenue, Alexandria, VA 22304, Conference #1561. (703) 370-8273, (800) 338-2111. The "Open Discussion" tape is tape #13 or 13-1561.

9. Wald A, Langengerg AG, Kexel E, Izu AE, Ashley R, Corey L. Condoms protect men and women against Herpes Simplex Virus Type 2 (HSV-2 Acquisition). Abstract BO93, 2002 National STD Prevention Conference, San Diego, CA , March 4-7, 2002. Available at http://www.stdconference.org.

10. Centers for Disease Control and Prevention. Youth Risk Behavior Surveillance – United States – 2001. *MMWR. 2002;51:1-64.*

11. Add Health and Add Health 2000: A National Longitudinal Study of Adolescent Health. J. Richard Udry. http://www.cpc.unc.edu/addhealth.

12. Koutsky L, Ault KA, Wheeler CM, et.al. A controlled trial of a human papilloma virus Type-16 vaccine. *N Engl J Med. 2002;347:1645-51.*

12. Studies on HPV

ARTICLES

Sexually Transmitted Diseases Among American Youth: Incidence and Prevalence Estimates, 2000

By Hillard Weinstock, Stuart Berman and Willard Cates, Jr.

Hillard Weinstock is medical epidemiologist, and Stuart Berman is chief of the Epidemiology and Surveillance Branch, both at the Division of STD Prevention, Centers for Disease Control and Prevention, Atlanta. Willard Cates, Jr., is president, Institute for Family Health, Family Health International, Research Triangle Park, North Carolina.

CONTEXT: *In the United States, young people aged 15–24 represent 25% of the sexually experienced population. However, the incidence and prevalence of sexually transmitted diseases (STDs) among this age-group are unknown.*

METHODS: *Data from a variety of sources were used to estimate the incidence and prevalence of STDs among 15–24-year-olds in the United States in 2000. The quality and reliability of the estimates were categorized as good, fair or poor, depending on the quality of the data source.*

RESULTS: *Approximately 18.9 million new cases of STD occurred in 2000, of which 9.1 million (48%) were among persons aged 15–24. Three STDs (human papillomavirus, trichomoniasis and chlamydia) accounted for 88% of all new cases of STD among 15–24-year-olds.*

CONCLUSIONS: *These estimates emphasize the toll that STDs have on American youth. More representative data are needed to help monitor efforts at lowering the burden of these infections.*

Perspectives on Sexual and Reproductive Health, 2004, 36(1):6–10

Sexually transmitted diseases (STDs) are among the most common infections in the United States. According to national estimates for 1996, more than 15 million new STD cases occur each year.[1] However, the annual STD incidence among young Americans is not known, even though 15–24-year-olds represent 25% of the sexually experienced population aged 15–44.[2]

Accurately monitoring the incidence and prevalence of STDs among the population, and particularly among young people, is important in measuring the effects of disease control and prevention efforts. However, a major obstacle to the diagnosis, treatment and surveillance of STDs is that many of these infections—including chlamydia, genital herpes, trichomoniasis and human papillomavirus (HPV) infection—have few, if any, recognizable symptoms. If STDs are not detected because infected persons have no symptoms and therefore do not get tested, these infections cannot be reported and counted. Even when STDs are diagnosed, health care providers may not always report nationally notifiable ones, such as syphilis, gonorrhea and chlamydia. Furthermore, some STDs, such as genital herpes, trichomoniasis and HPV infection, are not nationally reportable; our knowledge about these infections is based on prevalence surveys conducted among various populations that may not be representative of the general population.

As a result of expanded screening programs and improved detection tests, the ability to monitor the occurrence of STDs, especially asymptomatic infections, has increased since 1996. In this article, we examine available evidence and provide estimates for the incidence and prevalence of STDs among 15–24-year-olds in the United States in 2000.

METHODS

We studied relevant data and estimates of STD incidence and prevalence in the available literature, focusing on the eight main STDs. For each STD, we adjusted the available information to estimate the incidence and prevalence among 15–24-year-olds in the United States for the year 2000. Sources were case reports of nationally notifiable diseases, national surveys, literature reviews and the World Health Organization (WHO).

Building on prior efforts,[1] we categorized the quality and reliability of our estimates as good (level I), fair (level II) or poor (level III). Table 1 summarizes the criteria for these ratings. Our estimates were made using the available information with the highest-quality evidence.

RESULTS

Chlamydia

Chlamydia trachomatis infection is the most commonly reported notifiable disease in the United States. In 2000—the year in which all 50 states and the District of Columbia required that cases of chlamydia be reported—the Centers for Disease Control and Prevention (CDC) received 702,093 reports of chlamydial infection.[4] Of reported cases that included the age of the infected individual, 74%—that is, 439,041 infections—occurred in persons aged 15–24. Nevertheless, because of the asymptomatic nature of this disease, incomplete screening coverage[5] and underreporting, this figure most likely reflects a substantial underestimate of the true incidence of chlamydia among young people.

Using data from the Regional Infertility Chlamydia Prevalence Monitoring Project, Groseclose and colleagues estimated that three million new cases of genital chlamydia occurred among 15–44-year-olds in 1996.[6] In 2000, the same project included women of reproductive age attending almost 2,400 family planning clinics in all 50 states, the District of Columbia, the Virgin Islands and Puerto Rico.[7] To estimate the incidence and prevalence of chlamydia, we adjusted the 2000 data for state, age, and race and ethnicity, and used a similar calculation method to that of Groseclose and colleagues (which assumes that the incidence of chlamydial infection is its prevalence divided by the duration of infection, that infection lasts 0.96 years among women and 0.40 years among men, and that the incidence among men equals that among women). From this procedure, we estimate that 2.8 million new cases of chlamydia occurred in 2000 and that the prevalence was 1.9 million. Furthermore, on the basis of data for women aged 15–24, the estimated annual incidence of chlamydia among all men and women in this age-group was 1.5 million infections (54% of the total), and the prevalence was 1.0 million infections. These estimates assume that approximately 50% of people aged 15–19 have never had sexual intercourse and that 15–24-year-olds make up 25% of the population aged 15–44 who have ever had intercourse.[8] Because of the assumptions applied and because the Regional Infertility Chlamydia Prevalence Monitoring Project is not a population-based survey, we classified the quality of evidence and our estimates for chlamydia as level II.

Gonorrhea

Following a 74% decrease from 1975 through 1997, the rate of *Neisseria gonorrhoeae* infection increased in 1998 and remained essentially unchanged through 2000. In 2000, a total of 358,995 new cases of gonorrhea were reported to the CDC, of which 60% were among persons aged 15–24.[9] Previous estimates of gonorrhea incidence have assumed a 50% underdiagnosis and underreporting rate.[10] Applying this assumption to the available level II national surveillance data, we estimate that 718,000 new cases of gonorrhea occurred in 2000 and that 431,000 cases occurred among persons aged 15–24. Data were unavailable to allow the calculation of prevalence rates.

Syphilis

Syphilis rates decreased dramatically during the 1990s among both women and men. The greatest declines were among black Americans and persons living in the South, where rates historically have been the highest. In 2000, some 5,979 cases of primary and secondary syphilis (i.e., early stages of symptomatic *Treponema pallidum* infection) were reported to the CDC—the lowest yearly number ever recorded.[11] However, in the same year, the CDC also received 9,470 reports of early latent syphilis, in which infection was probably acquired in the preceding year. A further 15,597 reports were of late latent disease, in which infection probably occurred more than one year before diagnosis, making a total of 31,046 new cases of syphilis. Between 1997 and 2000, some 45–50% of all syphilis cases reported were late latent, indicating that a substantial proportion of syphilis cases were not diagnosed within one year of infection.

TABLE 1. *Criteria used to rate estimates of incidence and prevalence of STDs*

Rating level	Criteria
I (good)	Representative national surveys Complete national reporting
II (fair)	Consistent and widespread prevalence data from convenience samples
	Consistent and widespread, although incomplete, national reporting
	Extrapolations and assumptions based on representative national surveys
III (poor)	Inconsistent, nonrepresentative prevalence data Estimates based on rough extrapolations

Source: reference 1.

Of the 15,449 cases that were reported in 2000 and acquired in the previous year (primary, secondary or early latent syphilis), 3,399 cases were among 15–24-year-olds.[12] If 50% of all reported syphilis cases are diagnosed and reported more than one year after infection and 20% of infections are never diagnosed or reported,[13] then approximately 8,200 new syphilis infections occurred among persons aged 15–24 in 2000. Because of the incomplete national reporting of syphilis, this figure represents a level II estimate. Data were unavailable to allow the calculation of syphilis prevalence rates.

Genital Herpes

The incidence and prevalence of genital herpes—both symptomatic and asymptomatic—have increased dramatically during the past three decades.[14] The number of clinically diagnosed cases of symptomatic genital herpes in the 1980s was 11 times that in the 1970s, and it has remained relatively constant ever since.[15] Reports from a variety of clinical settings in the United States show that genital herpes accounts for a large majority of patient requests for treatment of symptomatic genital ulcers.[16] Genital herpes accounts for the majority of symptomatic ulcers outside the United States as well.[17]

Symptomatic herpes infections are merely the tip of the iceberg. Surveys have shown that only a minority of infections with herpes simplex virus type 2 (HSV-2), the main virus that causes genital herpes, are recognized as symptomatic by those who are infected. In the early 1990s, an estimated 45 million Americans were infected with HSV-2, but only 9% of them reported a history of genital herpes.[18] Using age-specific incidence curves and assuming that the rate of genital herpes in 2000 remained the same as the rate in 1985,[19] we estimate that 1.6 million new HSV-2 infections occurred in the United States in 2000. Adjusting this figure for the age distribution of persons newly infected with HSV-2 to account for those aged 15–24—40% in models based on the National Health and Nutrition Examination Survey[20]—we estimate that youth acquire 640,000 new HSV-2 infections each year.

TABLE 2. Estimated incidence and prevalence of selected STDs among 15–24-year-olds, and strength of evidence, United States, 2000

STD	Incidence	Prevalence	Strength of evidence*
Total	**9.1 million**	u	
Chlamydia	1.5 million	1.0 million	II
Gonorrhea	431,000	u	II
Syphilis	8,200	u	II
Genital herpes	640,000	4.2 million	II
HPV	4.6 million	9.2 million	III
Hepatitis B	7,500	u†	II
Trichomoniasis	1.9 million	u	III
HIV	15,000	u	II

*Rated according to criteria shown in Table 1. †Estimated prevalence of chronic hepatitis B virus infection is not available. *Note:* u=unavailable.

Assuming that the prevalence of HSV-2 infection remained stable between the early 1990s and 2000, at 45 million, we estimate that 4.2 million persons aged 15–24 (11% of the population aged 15–24) have been infected. It is important to note that although our estimates of incidence and prevalence of genital herpes among youth are derived from level I data on HSV-2, we classify them as level II because of the assumptions we made. In addition, our calculations ignore the sizable proportion of genital herpes infections caused by HSV-1; thus, our figures should be considered minimum estimates.

HPV

Comprehensive surveillance data are not available for genital HPV infection. If we suppose that age-specific incidence estimates for cervical HPV infection among women[21] reflect the HPV incidence rates among men, then approximately 6.2 million new HPV infections occurred in 2000 among Americans aged 15–44; of these infections, 74% (4.6 million) occurred among 15–24-year-olds.

Using an estimated female HPV prevalence of 33% (derived from a survey of sexually active women attending a university health service[22]), assuming an equal prevalence among sexually active men and applying these figures to the number of sexually active 15–24-year-olds in the population, we estimate that in 2000, some 9.2 million persons in this age-group were infected with HPV and hence were capable of spreading the virus. We classify the estimated incidence and prevalence of HPV as level III because of the limited evidence and crude extrapolations used.

Hepatitis B

Hepatitis B remains a prominent STD despite the availability of a preventive vaccine for more than two decades. By adjusting the reported number of cases to account for underreporting and asymptomatic infection,[23] the CDC has estimated that 81,000 new infections with the hepatitis B virus occurred in the United States in 2000, of which 15,000 occurred in persons aged 15–24.[24] Approximately half of these cases were among individuals who reported high-risk sexual activity.[25] Hence, the estimated incidence of sexually acquired hepatitis B among 15–24-year-olds is 7,500. Because of the assumptions and adjustments underlying this estimate, we classified it as level II.

Young people bear an even larger proportion of the burden from chronic infection: Of the estimated 5,000 new chronic infections in the United States in 2000, some 1,200—nearly one-quarter—occurred among 15–24-year-olds. Individuals with chronic infection not only remain infectious for most or all of their lives, but also have an approximately 25% lifetime risk of developing cirrhosis or liver cancer.[26]

Trichomoniasis

Vaginal infections caused by *Trichomonas vaginalis* are among the most common conditions transmitted sexually. Worldwide, more than 180 million cases of trichomoniasis are estimated to occur each year, accounting for nearly 20% of all cases of symptomatic vaginitis.[27] In the United States, depending on the type of clinical facility and the level of STD risk, between 5% and 60% of women and men screened for trichomonas will be infected with the parasite.[28] According to WHO, approximately 8.2 million new *T. vaginalis* infections occurred in the United States and Canada in 1999.[29] Assuming that 90% of these were in the United States and that the incidence remained the same in 2000, we estimate that 7.4 million new cases of trichomoniasis occurred in this country in 2000. If these infections were evenly distributed among sexually active persons of all age-groups,[30] 25% of them—1.9 million—occurred among persons aged 15–24. Because this figure is based on a rough extrapolation, we classify it as level III. Moreover, *T. vaginalis* infection may be underdiagnosed in the United States because of reliance on the relatively insensitive wet-mount procedure for diagnosis.[31]

HIV

The annual number of new HIV infections in the United States appears to have stabilized during the 1990s, although the introduction of highly active antiretroviral therapy has increased the prevalence of HIV by extending the life of HIV-infected people. The CDC has estimated that 800,000–900,000 persons in the United States are infected with HIV and approximately 40,000 new infections occur each year.[32] In particular, the incidence of HIV and other STDs among men who have sex with men has remained high.[33]

Assuming that 50% of HIV infections are contracted by persons younger than 25,[34] we expect that about 20,000 new HIV infections occur each year among youth. In 2000, according to the distribution of AIDS cases in the United States by the recorded route of infection, an estimated 75% of HIV infections were acquired through sexual intercourse. Thus, approximately 30,000 new infections were contracted through sexual intercourse in 2000, and 15,000 of these were contracted by persons aged 15–24. Being based on assumptions about HIV incidence in the United States, this estimate is level II.

Total STD Incidence

Despite decreases in the rates of some reportable STDs during the 1990s, we estimate that 18.9 million new cases of STD occurred in 2000, of which 9.1 million (48%) were among young people aged 15–24 (Table 2). These estimates emphasize this age-group's particular vulnerability to STDs. Of the STDs examined, HPV was the most commonly acquired, followed by trichomoniasis and chlamydia. Together, these three STDs accounted for 88% of all new cases of STD among 15–24-year-olds in 2000; HPV and trichomoniasis accounted for 72% of new infections.

DISCUSSION

Estimates of the national incidence and prevalence of STDs are based on various sources of data, each with its own limitations. Information about infections that are reportable to state and local health departments are affected by the completeness of diagnosis and reporting. We assumed that only 50% and 80% of all gonorrhea and syphilis infections, respectively, are diagnosed and reported; however, few studies have been done to substantiate these assumptions, and those that have been conducted have small samples.[35] Because so many STDs, including HIV, are asymptomatic, infected individuals may not seek medical care. In particular, young, apparently healthy persons may not have routine contact with health care practitioners.

Estimates based on prevalence surveys, such as those for chlamydia and HPV, are subject to limitations of representativeness. For example, although women attending family planning clinics were surveyed for chlamydia in all 50 states and the District of Columbia, they may not have an STD prevalence that is generalizable to the entire population of sexually active women.[36] Additionally, our chlamydia estimates depended on assumptions about duration of infection among both men and women.[37] As the coverage of chlamydia screening increases over time, this duration may decrease; as a result, our estimated incidence of chlamydia would be an underestimation of the true incidence of this disease.

HPV infection and trichomoniasis accounted for 72% of all new cases of STD among the 15–24-year age-group in 2000; however, the quality of the evidence—level III—was poor. For all other STDs, we graded the evidence as level II. Thus, while information about STDs—particularly for chlamydia and HPV—has improved somewhat since incidence and prevalence estimates were last made, in 1996, the overall reliability of the supporting data remains weak.

Our estimate of 18.9 million new STDs in 2000 among the general population is somewhat higher than the 1996 estimate of 15 million infections. This increase may be attributable to our improved ability to screen and detect STDs; however, it may also reflect the imprecision of the estimates themselves. More representative data are needed, especially for those infections of highest incidence and greatest morbidity.

Nevertheless, given the available information about the burden of STDs among sexually active young people, our estimate of 9.1 million new infections in 2000 among 15–24-year-olds demonstrates the tremendous toll these infections continue to have on youth in America: Representing one-quarter of the ever–sexually active population aged 15–44,[38] young people acquire nearly one-half of all new STDs. This burden is reflected not only in morbidity among the individuals affected but also in economic and psychological costs. The estimates provided here are the best numbers to date on which to base policy decisions, outreach and educational efforts. We encourage other researchers to refine these estimates and thereby help monitor national efforts at lowering the burden of STDs, especially among young Americans.

REFERENCES

1. Cates W. Jr., and American Social Health Association Panel, Estimates of the incidence and prevalence of sexually transmitted diseases in the United States, *Sexually Transmitted Diseases*, 1999, 26(Suppl. 4):S2–7.

2. Sonenstein FL et al., Changes in sexual behavior and condom use among teenaged males: 1988 to 1995, *American Journal of Public Health*, 1998, 88(6):956–959; Abma J et al., Fertility, family planning, and women's health: new data from the 1995 National Survey of Family Growth, *Vital and Health Statistics*, 1997, Vol. 23, No. 19; and Laumann EO et al., *National Health and Social Life Survey, 1992*, Chicago and Ann Arbor, MI: National Opinion Research Center and Inter-University Consortium for Political and Social Research, 1995.

3. Cates W, Jr., and American Social Health Association Panel, 1999, op. cit. (see reference 1).

4. Centers for Disease Control and Prevention (CDC), *Sexually Transmitted Disease Surveillance, 2000*, Atlanta: CDC, 2001.

5. Levine WC et al., Indirect estimation of chlamydia screening coverage using public health surveillance data, *American Journal of Public Health*, 2004 (forthcoming).

6. Groseclose SL et al., Estimated incidence and prevalence of genital *Chlamydia trachomatis* infection in the United States, 1996, *Sexually Transmitted Diseases*, 1999, 26(6):339–344.

7. CDC, *Chlamydia Prevalence Monitoring Project Annual Report 2000. Sexually Transmitted Disease Surveillance 2000 Supplement*, Atlanta: CDC, 2001.

8. Sonenstein FL et al., 1998, op. cit. (see reference 2); Abma J et al., 1997, op. cit. (see reference 2), and Laumann EO et al., 1995, op. cit. (see reference 2).

9. CDC, 2001, op. cit. (see reference 4).

10. Cates W, Jr., and American Social Health Association Panel, 1999, op. cit. (see reference 1).

11. CDC, 2001, op. cit. (see reference 4).

12. Ibid.

13. Cates W, Jr., and American Social Health Association Panel, 1999, op. cit. (see reference 1).

14. Johnson R et al., A seroepidemiologic survey of the prevalence of herpes simplex virus type 2 infection in the United States, *New England Journal of Medicine*, 1989, 321(1):7–12; Fleming DT et al., Herpes simplex virus type 2 in the United States, 1976–1994, *New England Journal of Medicine*, 1997, 337(16):1105–1111; Armstrong G et al., Incidence of herpes simplex virus type 2 infection in the United States, *American Journal of Epidemiology*, 2001, 153(9):912–920; and Fisman DN et al., Projection of the future dimensions and costs of the genital herpes simplex type 2 epidemic in the United States, *Sexually Transmitted Diseases*, 2002, 29(10):608–622.

15. CDC, 2001, op. cit. (see reference 4).

16. Tao G, Kassler W and Rein D, Medical care expenditures for genital herpes in the United States, *Sexually Transmitted Diseases*, 2000, 27(1):32–38; and Corey L and Wald A, Genital herpes, in: Holmes KK et al., eds., *Sexually Transmitted Diseases*, New York: McGraw-Hill, 1999, pp. 285–312.

17. Corey L and Handsfield H, Genital herpes and public health: addressing a global problem, *Journal of the American Medical Association*, 2000, 283(6):791–794.

18. Fleming DT et al., 1997, op. cit. (see reference 14).

19. Armstrong G et al., 2001, op. cit. (see reference 14).

20. Ibid.

21. Myers ER, Mathematical model for the natural history of human papillomavirus infection and cervical carcinogenesis, *American Journal Epidemiology*, 2000, 151(12):1158–1171.

22. Bauer HM et al., Genital human papillomavirus infection in female university students as determined by a PCR-based method, *Journal of the American Medical Association*, 1991, 265(4):472–477.

23. Coleman PJ et al., Incidence of hepatitis B virus infection in the United States, 1976–1994: estimates from the National Health and Nutrition Examination Surveys, *Journal of Infectious Diseases*, 1998, 178(4):954–959.

24. Armstrong G, CDC, Atlanta, personal communication, Sept. 9, 2003.

25. Goldstein ST et al., Incidence and risk factors for acute hepatitis B in the United States, 1982–1998: implications for vaccination programs, *Journal of Infectious Diseases*, 2002, 185(6):713–719.

26. Margolis HS et al., Prevention of hepatitis B virus transmission by immunization: an economic analysis of current recommendations, *Journal of the American Medical Association*, 1995, 274(15):1201–1208.

27. World Health Organization (WHO), *Global Prevalence and Incidence of Selected Curable Sexually Transmitted Infections: Overview and Estimates*, Geneva: WHO, 2001.

28. Krieger JN and Alderete JF, *Trichomonas vaginalis* and trichomoniasis, in: Holmes KK et al., 1999, op. cit. (see reference 16), pp. 587–604.

29. WHO, 2001, op. cit. (see reference 27).

30. Lossick JG, Epidemiology of urogenital trichomoniasis, in: Honigberg BM, ed., *Trichomonads Parasitic in Humans*, New York: Springer-Verlag, 1989, pp. 311–323; and Cotch MF et al., Demographic and behavioral predictors of *Trichomonas vaginalis* infection among pregnant women, *Obstetrics & Gynecology*, 1991, 78(6):1087–1092.

31. Krieger JN and Alderete JF, 1999, op. cit. (see reference 28).

32. Karon JM et al., HIV in the United States at the turn of the century: an epidemic in transition, *American Journal of Public Health*, 2001, 91(7):1060–1068; and Karon JM et al., Prevalence of HIV infection in the United States, 1984 to 1992, *Journal of the American Medical Association*, 1996, 276(2):126–131.

33. CDC, HIV among young men who have sex with men, *Morbidity and Mortality Weekly Report*, 2001, 50(21):440–444; and CDC, Primary and secondary syphilis—United States, 2002, *Morbidity and Mortality Weekly Report*, 2003, 52(46):1117–1120.

34. Rosenberg PS and Biggar RJ, Trends in HIV incidence among young adults in the United States, *Journal of the American Medical Association*, 1998, 279(23):1894–1899.

35. Doyle TJ, Glynn MK and Groseclose SL, Completeness of notifiable infectious disease reporting in the United States: an analytical review, *American Journal of Epidemiology*, 2002, 155(9):866–874.

36. Frost JJ, Public or private providers? U.S. women's use of reproductive health services, *Family Planning Perspectives*, 2001, 33(1):4–12.

37. Groseclose SL et al., 1999, op. cit. (see reference 6).

38. Sonenstein FL et al., 1998, op. cit. (see reference 2); Abma J et al., 1997, op. cit. (see reference 2); and Laumann EO et al., 1995, op. cit. (see reference 2).

Acknowledgments

The authors thank Debra Mosure, Linda Webster Dicker, Greg Armstrong, Fujie Xu, Kathleen Irwin, Rachel Jones, Katherine Stone and Akbar Zaidi for their contributions to the manuscript and helpful suggestions. The University of North Carolina School of Journalism and Mass Communication Panel on Youth, Sexually Transmitted Diseases and the Media also contributed to the manuscript and included the following members: Tracey A. Adams, Jane D. Brown, Virginia Caine, Jacqueline E. Darroch, Ralph DiClemente, Lloyd J. Kolbe, Jonathan Stacks, Susan L. Rosenthal, Felicia Stewart, James Trussell, Richard A. Crosby, Laura F. Salazar, Joan R. Cates, Felicia E. Mebane, Nancy Herndon and Susan Schulz. The panel's work was supported by the William T. Grant Foundation.

Author contact: hsw2@cdc.gov

NIAID NEWS Office of Communications and Public Liaison

National Institute of Allergy and Infectious Diseases • National Institutes of Health

FOR RELEASE
Wednesday, Feb. 11, 1998

Cheryl Parrott
(301) 402-1663
cparrott@nih.gov

Sexually Active Younger Women are at Higher Risk for Infection with Human Papillomavirus

Sexually active college-age women have a high incidence of human papillomavirus (HPV) infection according to a study supported by the National Institute of Allergy and Infectious Diseases (NIAID) and reported in the Feb. 12, 1998 issue of *The New England Journal of Medicine*.

"Genital infection with HPV is one of the most common sexually transmitted diseases, with its prevalence in young women ranging from 20 percent to 46 percent in different countries," says Study Director Robert D. Burk, M.D., of the Department of Pediatrics, Microbiology and Immunology, and the Department of Epidemiology and Social Medicine at the Albert Einstein College of Medicine. "The public health impact of this infection is compounded by the recognized causal relationship between genital infections with certain types of HPV and cell abnormalities of the cervix and cervical cancer."

"The incidence of HPV infection in sexually active young college women is alarming. Furthermore, we currently have no effective way to prevent infection. The need for topical microbicides and effective vaccines is urgent," says Penny Hitchcock, D.V.M., chief of the sexually transmitted diseases branch in NIAID's Division of Microbiology and Infectious Diseases. "It is certainly reassuring that only a small number of women will develop cervical cell changes or cancer. However, until we have more precise diagnostic tests, it is important for young women to have regular Pap smears."

Through campus-wide advertisements at a state university in New Brunswick, N.J., the study team enrolled 608 young women. Their average age was 20 years, and the ethnic distribution was 57 percent white, 13 percent Hispanic, 12 percent black and 18 percent other. Twenty-six percent were diagnosed with HPV infection at the beginning of the study. Each of the women had pelvic examinations and Pap smears at the study outset and annually. For a maximum of three years, the women responded at six-month intervals to questionnaires on lifestyle and sexual behavior. At the same visits, samples of cells from the cervix and vagina were taken to ascertain whether or not HPV was present and to determine the type, or strain, of HPV. If the same type of HPV was present during two consecutive visits, the infection was defined as persistent. The average duration of HPV infection was eight months.

The cumulative incidence of HPV infection in the women who were HPV-negative at baseline was 43 percent. The investigators noted, however, that this incidence decreased with time: it was 20 percent in the first 12 months; 14 percent in the second 12 months; and only 9 percent in the final 12 months.

"The encouraging news," says Dr. Hitchcock, "is that this study suggests that the body's response to infection plays an important role in limiting persistence of the virus and disease progression. If this is mediated by the immune response, it could indicate that development of prophylactic and therapeutic vaccines would play an important role in prevention and control."

Higher risk and incidence of HPV infection are associated with younger age, ethnic minority subgroups, increased frequency of alcohol consumption, anal sex or a high frequency of vaginal sex. A woman was less likely to have an HPV infection last for six months if it had been her first infection. The longer an infection endured from previous visits, the more likely it was to persist.

One of the consequences of HPV infection is the presence of various types of abnormal cells. One such type, squamous intraepithelial lesion, a potentially pre-cancerous condition, is caused by HPV infection of cervical cells, and is usually first detected as an abnormal Pap smear.

The authors caution that because of the six-month interval between medical visits, the study results may underestimate the incidence and overestimate the duration of HPV infection. They also warn that it is uncertain whether these data apply to older women.

In addition to Dr. Burk, collaborators included Gloria Y. F. Yo, Ph.D., and Chee J. Chang, Ph.D., both of the Albert Einstein College of Medicine, Bronx, N.Y.; and Robert Bierman, M.D., and Leah Beardsley, N.P., both of Rutgers University Student Health Service, New Brunswick, N.J.

NIAID is a component of the National Institutes of Health (NIH). NIAID conducts and supports research to prevent, diagnose and treat illnesses such as HIV disease and other sexually transmitted diseases, tuberculosis, malaria, asthma and allergies. NIH is an agency of the U.S. Department of Health and Human Services.

Press releases, fact sheets and other NIAID-related materials are available on the Internet via the NIAID home page at http://www.niaid.nih.gov.

Search | Home | News Releases

NIAID
AIDS agenda

June 1996 - Page 8

Increased Risk of Cervical Abnormalities Among HIV-Infected African Women

In a study in Malawi, HIV-infected women were three times more likely than uninfected women to have persistent human papillomavirus infections (HPV), and twice as likely to have cervical abnormalities, according to NIAID-supported investigators and their colleagues. HPV infection is causally associated with cervical cancer, the most common malignancy among women in the developing world. Scientists estimate that worldwide 500,000 new cases of cervical cancer and 300,000 related deaths occur annually.

As reported in the March 1996 *Journal of Infectious Diseases*, the researchers found squamous epithelial lesions in 15 percent of 116 HIV-positive women, and 7 percent of 152 HIV-negative women. This heightened occurrence of cervical lesions probably resulted from a greater overall frequency of HPV infections (48 percent vs. 23 percent) in the HIV-positive group, write Paolo G. Miotti, M.D., of NIAID's Division of AIDS, Keerti V. Shah, M.D., of The Johns Hopkins University School of Hygiene and Public Health, and their colleagues.

Two high-risk types of HPV associated with cervical cancer--HPV-16 and HPV-18--accounted for half of the HPV types identified in the study.

HIV-positive women were three times more likely than HIV-negative women to have an HPV infection that persisted from a first clinic visit to a second visit a year later. The most immunosuppressed women--those with fewer than 300 CD4+ T cells/mm^3--were most likely to have persistent HPV infections.

"The strong correlation between HPV detection and immunosuppression levels suggests that HIV-induced immunosuppression may increase the susceptibility to HPV infection, its reactivation or duration," the authors write.

Previous studies have shown that HIV-infected women in the United States and Europe have elevated rates of HPV infection, cervical abnormalities and cervical cancer. In sub-Saharan Africa, however, data about the association between HIV, HPV and cervical abnormalities are largely lacking.

"This study adds to growing evidence that early detection of HPV and regular monitoring of HPV-related cervical lesions are especially important in HIV-infected women, in developing as well as developed countries," says Penny Hitchcock, D.V.M., chief of the sexually transmitted diseases branch of NIAID's Division of Microbiology and Infectious Diseases.

--Greg Folkers

Do Condoms Prevent Genital HPV Infection, External Genital Warts, or Cervical Neoplasia?

A Meta-Analysis

LISA E. MANHART, MPH,*† AND LAURA A. KOUTSKY,† PhD

From the Departments of *Medicine and †Epidemiology, University of Washington, Seattle, Washington

Background: **Although condoms most likely prevent HIV infection, evidence of their effectiveness against other sexually transmitted diseases is mixed.**

Goal: **The goal of the study was to determine whether condom use prevents genital human papillomavirus (HPV) infection and HPV-related conditions.**

Study Design: **We conducted a literature review and meta-analysis of the effect of condom use on the prevention of genital warts, subclinical HPV infection, cervical intraepithelial neoplasia (CIN), and invasive cervical cancer (ICC).**

Results: **Among 27 estimates from 20 studies, there was no consistent evidence that condom use reduces the risk of becoming HPV DNA–positive. However, risk for genital warts, CIN of grade II or III (CIN II or III), and ICC was somewhat reduced.**

Conclusions: **Available data are too inconsistent to provide precise estimates. However, they suggest that while condoms may not prevent HPV infection, they may protect against genital warts, CIN II or III, and ICC.**

HUMAN PAPILLOMAVIRUS (HPV) is a common sexually transmitted infection, and it is estimated that over 50% of sexually active men and women aged 15 to 49 years have been infected with one or more genital HPV types at some point in their lives.[1] Of the over 38 different types of this small DNA virus known to infect the genital tract,[2] only two types (HPV 6 and 11) are clearly linked with genital warts, whereas virtually all types have been linked with squamous intraepithelial lesions (SILs) of the uterine cervix. Furthermore, genital HPV types play an etiologic role in the development of virtually all cases of invasive cervical cancer (ICC).[3] Invasive cancers of the vagina, vulva, penis, and anus have also been linked with genital HPV infection, but compared with cervical cancer, these cancers are rare.[4] Papanicolaou (Pap) smear screening has allowed for early detection and treatment of HPV-associated cervical lesions, dramatically decreasing cervical cancer incidence and mortality among women.

As with other infections that cause significant morbidity and mortality, preventing the spread of the infectious agent throughout a susceptible population is generally more cost-effective than approaches involving early detection and treatment. In the absence of a vaccine, abstinence, mutual monogamy, and condoms are options for preventing genital HPV infection. In response to the recent congressional mandate to provide the public with more accurate information on the efficacy of condoms in preventing HPV infection,[5] a comprehensive review of the literature was undertaken and a meta-analysis performed.

The strongest evidence of the role of male condoms in preventing disease transmission is for HIV. A meta-analysis of 25 studies of HIV-serodiscordant heterosexual couples provided a summary efficacy estimate of 87% (95% CI, 60–95%).[6] The evidence is less clear, however, for other STDs. In vitro testing has shown that condoms provide 100% protection as a physical barrier to chlamydia, herpes simplex virus-2 (HSV-2), and HIV,[7] and some reports indicate protection against gonorrhea, chlamydia, and HSV-2.[8–10] However, a study of Baltimore STD clinic attendees revealed that condom use was not associated with any reduction in the incidence of gonorrhea, chlamydia, trichomoniasis, or syphilis.[11] Although no studies have been conducted explicitly to assess the effectiveness of condoms in preventing HPV infections, numerous publications present

The authors thank Connie Nelson for her assistance in preparing Figure 1.

Supported by grants from the National Institutes of Allergy and Infectious Diseases (AI38383) and Cancer (CA34493) and a training grant to Ms. Manhart from the National Institute of Allergy and Infectious Diseases (NIAID 5T32AI07140).

Reprint requests: Laura A. Koutsky, PhD, HPV Research Group, 1914 North 34th Street, Suite 300, Seattle, WA 98103. E-mail: kouts@u.washington.edu

Received for publication October 29, 2001, revised February 6, 2002, and accepted February 21, 2002.

data on the relationship between condom use and HPV-related conditions. The present analysis examines the existing evidence on the effectiveness of condoms against HPV infections and HPV-related conditions (e.g., genital warts, subclinical HPV infection, cervical intraepithelial neoplasia [CIN], and ICC).

Methods

We examined the peer-reviewed literature on condoms and HPV-related conditions published in the English language since 1980 to identify studies for inclusion in this analysis. The search was limited to the past 20 years of published literature because before the mid-1980s HPV DNA testing was not available, and before the late 1970s classification schemes of HPV-related cervical pathology were not standardized. After initial discussions with experts in the field to identify appropriate studies, we engaged in a MEDLINE search and reviewed reference lists from published articles to identify other publications not already selected. The following search terms were used: human papillomavirus (HPV) and condoms, cervical cancer and condoms, SIL or cervical intraepithelial neoplasia (CIN) and condoms, and warts and condoms, as well as each of these search terms independently. Only studies that examined use of the male condom were included. To date, there have been no studies of the female condom and HPV.

Inclusion Criteria

Studies were included in this analysis if they met the following criteria: (1) a clear definition of the endpoint (HPV infection; HPV type; warts, SIL, CIN; cancer), (2) an exclusive definition of condom use, and (3) an appropriate comparison group. Nine studies that examined the effect of barrier contraceptive methods lumped together (condom, diaphragm, cervical cap) were excluded, as it was not possible to disentangle the effect of condoms from the other methods. Two studies conducted in populations with high rates of HIV infection were also excluded because the presented data did not allow for assessment of condom use and prevention of HPV-related conditions in the absence of immunosuppression. Compared with individuals who are not infected with HIV, those who are infected tend to have more evidence of HPV-related disease.[4] In case–control studies, we required controls to be selected from the same populations that gave rise to the cases[12]; two studies did not meet this criterion. Four other studies were excluded because of inadequate assessment of either condom use or outcome.

Because of the instability of estimates derived from studies of small sample size, we also excluded all studies that had fewer than 20 cases and/or controls or less than 20 condom users (2 studies). When more than one publication reported on the same study population, we included only the one with the clearest presentation of data on the relationship between condom use and the outcome of interest. When several definitions of condom use were evaluated or more than one comparison was reported, we elected to present only one comparison, giving higher priority to the definition of "always use versus never use" and less priority to definitions suggesting occasional use. For many studies, however, condom use was measured as only "yes versus no" or "ever versus never."

For biologic homogeneity, separate evaluations were performed for the five outcomes of interest: (1) external genital warts, (2) HPV DNA detection in genital samples, (3) cervical warts and SIL, or CIN (grade I or unspecified), (4) CIN II or III, and (5) ICC (squamous cell carcinoma and adenocarcinoma not differentiated). Cervical SIL (Bethesda classification system) and CIN (Richart's classification scheme) define the same set of lesions, although the SIL category includes cellular features of HPV infection (e.g., koilocytosis) alone, as well as classic cellular features of CIN with or without koilocytosis.[4]

Whenever the odds ratio (OR) or relative risk (RR) presented in the publication was calculated from a clear baseline category, we utilized that estimate and corresponding 95% confidence intervals in our analysis. Because most of these studies were not designed to assess the relationship between HPV-related conditions and condom use, in some cases the OR presented in the publication did not reflect always-versus-never use of condoms. For those studies, we recalculated the OR and CI, from data presented in the publication[13] or data obtained from the investigators themselves.[14,15] We also calculated ORs and 95% CIs for studies that presented percentages.[16,17] In all instances, Epi-Info (version 6.04b; Centers for Disease Control and Prevention, Atlanta, GA) was used in the calculation of the 95% CIs.[18] When provided, adjusted ORs (OR_{adj}) or adjusted RRs (RR_{adj}) were presented.

We conducted a chi-square test of homogeneity[19] for each outcome and concluded that substantial heterogeneity was present in each group. Therefore, we elected not to calculate pooled odds ratios and have presented only the individual estimates.

Results

A total of 20 studies met all the inclusion criteria (Tables 1 and 2). Five of these studies assessed more than one outcome, providing a total of 27 different estimates on the relationship between HPV-related conditions and condom use. Two studies included data on the relationship between condom use and external genital warts[13,17]; in 6 studies the primary outcome was detection of HPV DNA in cervical samples[14,18–24]; 4 studies examined cervical SIL, cervical warts, or CIN (grade I or unspecified)[16,25–27]; 6 studies used CIN grade II or III as the outcome[25,27–31]; and 5 studies

TABLE 1. Studies Included in Analysis, Stratified by Outcome and Ordered by Date

Date*	Study†	N	Location	Gender	Design
External genital warts					
1992	Hippelainen (17)	432	Finland	Males	Cross-sectional
1996	Wen (13)	1298	Australia	Males	Case–control
1996	Wen (13)	656	Australia	Females	Case–control
Cervical HPV DNA					
1988–1990	Davidson (20)	1126	U.S.	Females	Cross-sectional
1989–1990	Jamison (21)	634	U.S.	Females	Cross-sectional
1992–1993	Kjaer (22)	182	Denmark	Females	Cross-sectional
1992–1995	Young (24)	1477	Canada	Females	Cross-sectional
1994–1997	Ho (14)	608	U.S.	Females	Cohort
1997‡	Kjaer (23)	956	Denmark	Females	Cross-sectional
Cervical warts and SIL or CIN (grade I or unspecified)					
1968–1974	Zondervan§ (25)	1749	England/Scotland	Females	Nested case-control
1981–1985	Kataja (26)	1397	Finland	Females	Case–control
1984‡	Syrjanen (16)	292	Finland	Females	Case–control
2000‡	Adam‖ (27)	430	U.S.	Females	Cross-sectional
CIN II or III					
1968–1974	Zondervan§ (25)	1331	England/Scotland	Females	Nested case–control
1985–1987	Munoz (28)	207	Spain	Females/husbands	Case–control
1985–1988	Munoz (28)	187	Colombia	Females/husbands	Case–control
1989–1991	Becker (29)	538	U.S.	Females	Case–control
1991–1994	Wang (31)	723	Taiwan	Females/husbands	Case–control
1992–1994	Ho (30)	258	U.S.	Females	Cross-sectional
2000‡	Adam‖ (27)	530	U.S.	Females	Cross-sectional
Invasive cervical cancer					
1968–1974	Zondervan§ (25)	354	England/Scotland	Females	Nested case–control
1979–1988	Thomas (15)	522¶	Thailand	Females/husbands	Case–control
1982–1984	Hildesheim (34)	1267	U.S.	Females	Case–control
1984–1987	Slattery (32)	638	U.S.	Females	Case–control
1987–1988	Kjaer (33)	131	Denmark	Females/husbands	Case–control

*Date study was conducted.
†First author (reference number).
‡Publication date (study date not indicated).
§Single study with three different outcomes: invasive cervical cancer (n = 33), carcinoma in situ (n = 121), and dysplasia (n = 159), by ICD-8 definitions. Ten controls per case from cohort of 17,032 (women with no cervical abnormalities), with the exception of 1 case of invasive cervical cancer for which only 1 control was available.
‖Single study with two different outcomes; compared women with no lesions and no HPV DNA (n = 269) with women with CIN I (n = 161) and women with CIN II/III (n = 261). All diagnoses biopsy-confirmed.
¶N represents a subset of the larger study reported in the article (n = 1016); N of 522 includes only those subjects (1) who reported monogamy and (2) whose husbands were interviewed and reported visiting a prostitute at least once.

focused on ICC.[15,25,32–34] The majority of studies measuring HPV DNA as the primary outcome were cross-sectional, with the exception of one cohort study. In contrast, all publications on cervical cancer were reports of case–control studies. Studies assessing (1) external genital warts, (2) cervical SIL, cervical warts, or CIN (grade I or unspecified), and (3) CIN II or III represented a mixture of case–control and cross-sectional designs.

The overwhelming majority of these studies were conducted among women, with one study of men only and another of both men and women. Three of the studies on women, however, gathered condom use data directly from their husbands.[15,28,33] Although the age range of all subjects was large, in general, studies of genital warts, HPV DNA detection, or SIL were conducted among men and women in their twenties and early thirties, while studies of ICC were conducted among slightly older women.

Several different condom measures were used in these studies, but all relied on self-report, which can sometimes result in misclassification. Time intervals were rarely stated, and only four studies specified a defined measurement period for condom use. Two studies compared users for 5 or fewer years with those who had used condoms for greater than 5 years, 1 assessed condom use in the past 4 months, and 1 compared users for 6 or more months with those who had used them for fewer than 6 months. The type of condom (latex versus nonlatex) was not specified in any of the studies.

External Genital Warts

Only two studies assessed the relationship between condom use and external genital warts, and both found protective effects (Figure 1). One analysis examined young male military recruits, while the other evaluated men and women attending an STD clinic. Among military recruits, those who reported always using condoms were 70% less likely to have genital warts or subclinical HPV infection of the penis than male recruits who occasionally or never used them

TABLE 2. Summary Estimates, Condom Measures, and Potential Confounders Examined for Studies Included in the Analysis, Ordered By Magnitude of the Odds Ratio (OR)

Study[*]	Population Source	Risk Estimate (95% CI)	Condom Measure	Potential Confounders Examined in Analyses
External genital warts				
Hippelainen[†] (17)	Military recruits (men)	0.3 (0.2–0.5)[‡]	Always vs. never/occasionally	History of STDs, casual sex contacts (tested, but not significant)
Wen (13)	STD clinic			Crude ORs and 95% CIs presented. Data in article allowed for calculation of adjusted ORs but not 95% CIs.
	Men	0.3 (0.2–0.4)[‡]	Always vs. never	Men: OR = 0.4 after adjustment for age group, no. of lifetime partners, smoking
	Women	0.6 (0.4–0.9)[‡]	Always vs. never	Women: OR = 0.4 after adjustment for age group, marital status, occupation
Cervical HPV DNA				
Kjaer (22)	Female sex workers in Copenhagen, Denmark	0.2 (0.1–0.6)	Current always vs. never (w/private partners, past 4 mo)	Age (continuous), no. of private partners in past 4 mo, ever gonorrhea
Ho (14)	University health center	0.8 (0.4–1.4)[§]	Always vs. never	Age, race, alcohol consumption, no. of sex partners in prior 6 mo, no. of sex partners in prior 7–12 mo, anal sex, frequency of vaginal sex, male partner's no. of lifetime partners, main partner currently in school (in model) Income; lifestyle; use of cigarettes, recreational drugs, oral contraceptives; no. of casual sex partners, regular partners, new regular partners; frequency of oral sex; sex with alcohol or drugs; postcoital bleeding; sex during menstruation; douching (tested & not significant)
Davidson (20)	Alaska Native medical center + random sample from Alaska Native population	0.9 (0.5–1.5)[§]	Always vs. never (within past 2 y)	Age, lifetime no. of sex partners, oral contraceptive use (tested & not significant)
Jamison (21)	Adolescent clinics	1.2 (0.7–2.1)	>75% of time vs. <25% (prior 6 mo)	Ethnicity, age, pregnancy, smoking, oral contraceptives, gonorrhea/chlamydial infection, no. of sex partners in past 6 mo (tested & not significant)
Young (24)	Community health center (43% Aboriginal)	1.5 (1.1–2.0)	Most/always vs. never (during past 1 y)	Aboriginal, smoking, marital status, age, oral contraceptives, age at first sex, lifetime no. of partners, no. of partners in past 1 y, no. of past pregnancies, Pap test results
Kjaer (23)				
Oncogenic	General female population in Copenhagen	1.6 (0.8–3.3)	Current vs. never	Age (significant); lifetime no. of partners, no. of regular partners (≥3 mo), age at first intercourse, years since first intercourse, history of chlamydia, history of any STD, years of diaphragm use, years of oral contraceptive use, no. of live births, smoking (tested)
Nononcogenic	General female population in Copenhagen	3.8 (1.2–11.6)	Current vs. never	Age, lifetime no. of partners, no. of live births, history of chlamydia (significant), no. of partners (≥3 mo), age at first intercourse, years since first intercourse, history of any STD, years of diaphragm use, years of oral contraceptive use, smoking (tested)
Cervical warts and SIL or CIN (grade I or unspecified)				
Zondervan[‖] (25)	Family planning clinics	1.0 (0.7–1.4)	Ever vs. never[¶]	Husband's social class, smoking, age at first birth, ever use of oral contraceptives, ever use of diaphragm
Adam[**] (27)	Colposcopy clinic	1.1 (0.7–1.8)	Ever vs. never	Referral for Pap test result, age, race, high-risk HPV, pregnancies, smoking
Syrjanen (16)	Outpatient OB/GYN university hospital	1.4 (0.7–2.9)[‡]	Yes vs. no[¶]	—
Kataja[††] (26)	Communal health centers	1.8 (1.4–2.4)	Yes vs. no[¶]	Pap smear result, no. of sex partners in past 2 years, age, intrauterine device, regular use of any contraception, hygiene, smoking, warts in partners, frequency of sex per week
CIN II or III				
Ho (30)	Colposcopy clinics	0.3 (0.1–0.8)	Most/always vs. never	Age, education, ethnicity, no. of Pap smears in last 3 years, oncogenic HPV type (significant)
CIN III vs. I[‡‡]				Lifetime no. of partners, no. of partners in past 6 mo, age at first coitus, frequency of vaginal sex, douching after sex, current & past oral contraceptive use, no. of pregnancies (tested & not significant)
Wang[‡‡] (31)	Cervical cancer screening sites	0.3 (0.1–0.9)	Any use vs. none	No. of sex partners, age at first sex, husband's frequency of visiting prostitutes, HPV infection, oral contraceptive use, ≥4 vaginal deliveries, ≥2 induced abortions
Adam[**] (27)	Colposcopy clinic	0.6 (0.4–0.9)	Ever vs. never	Referral for Pap test result, age, race, high-risk HPV, pregnancies, smoking
Ho (30)	Colposcopy clinic	0.7 (0.3–1.8)	Most/always vs. never	Age, education, ethnicity, no. of Pap smears in past 3 y, oncogenic HPV type (significant)
CIN II vs. I[‡‡]				Lifetime no. of partners, no. of partners in past 6 mo; age at first coitus; frequency of vaginal sex; douching after sex; current & past oral contraceptive use; no. of pregnancies (tested & not significant)

TABLE 2. *Continued*

Study*	Population Source	Risk Estimate (95% CI)	Condom Measure	Potential Confounders Examined in Analyses
Becker[§§] (29)	University maternal/infant care clinics	0.8 (0.5–1.3)	Ever vs. never	Age, age at first sex, lifetime no. of partners, ethnicity, HPV
Munoz[‡‡] (28)	Hospitals, pathology labs, screening clinics (cases: Spain, Colombia)			
	Family planning clinics (Spain) [controls]	0.8 (0.6–1.7)	Ever vs. never[¶] (husband's response)	Age, diagnostic center, no. of sex partners, age at first sex, HPV, chlamydia, no. of husband's sex partners (Spain)
	Screening clinics (Colombia) [controls]	0.8 (0.5–2.7)	Ever vs. never[¶] (husband's response)	Age, diagnostic center, no. of sex partners, age at first sex, HPV, chlamydia, smoking (Colombia)
Zondervan[‖] (25)	Family planning clinics	1.2 (0.8–1.8)	Ever vs. never[¶]	Husband's social class, smoking, age at first birth, ever use of oral contraceptives, ever use of diaphragm
Invasive cervical cancer				
Kjaer (33)	Monogamous women (1 or 2 lifetime partners) Cancer registry (cases) General population (controls)	0.2 (0.1–0.6)	Ever vs. never (husband's response)	Age, ever genital warts (significant - husband's characteristics) Male partner's no. of partners, visits to prostitutes, age at first sex, circumcision status, number of genital washes per month (not significant)
Thomas (15)	Monogamous women whose husbands ever visited prostitutes Hospitals (cases & controls)	0.5 (0.2–1.0)	Always/frequently vs. rarely/never (husband w/ prostitutes)	Woman's age, center, husband's no. of partners, husband's no. of STD episodes
Slattery (32)	Cancer registry (cases) RDD (controls)	0.7 (0.5–1.2)	≥6 mo vs. <6 mo[¶]	Age, years of education, church attendance, cigarette smoking, no. of sex partners of woman
Zondervan[‖] (25)	Family planning clinics	0.8 (0.3–2.0)	Ever vs. never[¶]	Husband's social class, smoking, age at first birth, ever use of oral contraceptives, ever use of diaphragm
Hildesheim (34)	Hospitals (cases) RDD (controls)	1.0 (0.6–1.5)	≥5 y vs. never[¶]	Age, education, income, interval since last Pap, lifetime no. of partners, socioeconomic status

*First author (reference number).
†Outcome is defined as "HPV-suggestive infection" (n = 113), including (1) typical peniscopical pattern of exophytic warts and/or typical flat lesions (44%), (2) aceto-white lesions without genital warts (48.6%), or (3) HPV positivity by PCR only (7.4%).
‡OR calculated from data presented in article.
§Relative risk. All other risk estimates presented are ORs.
‖Single study with three different outcomes: invasive cervical cancer (n = 33), carcinoma in situ (n = 121), and dysplasia (n = 159), by ICD-8 definitions. Ten controls per case from cohort of 17,032 (women with no cervical abnormalities), with the exception of 1 case of invasive cervical cancer for which only 1 control was available.
¶Condom use specified as a contraceptive method.
**Single study with two different outcomes. Compared women with no lesions and no HPV DNA (n = 269) with women with CIN I (n = 161) and women with CIN II/III (n = 261). All diagnoses biopsy-confirmed.
††Biopsy-confirmed SIL. All women included as cases "had a clinically manifest HPV lesion, i.e., flat, inverted, or papillomatous condyloma, with or without concomitant cervical intraepithelial neoplasia."
‡‡Biopsy-confirmed CIN.
§§"High-grade dysplasia" defined as "moderate dysplasia/severe dysplasia/carcinoma in situ of the cervix," diagnosed on colposcopic examination (biopsy-confirmed). No detail given on number of subjects with moderate dysplasia, severe dysplasia, or carcinoma in situ.

(OR, 0.3; 95% CI, 0.2–0.5).[17] Investigators tested potential confounding factors, but none influenced the association. Among both men and women attending an STD clinic, reported condom use (always versus never) reduced the likelihood of genital warts by approximately 60% (OR_{adj}, 0.4). Although 95% CIs were not presented for these estimates, the crude ORs with 95% CIs were similar to the adjusted estimates (men: crude OR of 0.3 and 95% CI of 0.2–0.4; women: crude OR of 0.6 and 95% CI of 0.4–0.9).[13]

Cervical HPV DNA

All six studies measuring HPV DNA detection as the outcome were conducted among women, and only one showed a statistically significant protective effect for condom use. Among Danish sex workers who reported always using condoms with their commercial partners, those who also always used them with their private partners during the past 4 months were 80% less likely to have HPV DNA detected than those who never did (OR_{adj}, 0.2; 95% CI, 0.1–0.6).[23]

The odds ratios for the four other cross-sectional studies assessing condom use and HPV DNA detection ranged from 0.8 to 1.6, with the exception of the study reported by Kjaer et al. Among a random sample of women from the general population of Denmark, those who reported current use of condoms were almost four times more likely to have a nononcogenic HPV type detected than women who reported never using condoms (OR_{adj}, 3.8; 95% CI, 1.2–11.6).[22] A similar effect, but of lower magnitude, was reported for oncogenic HPV types (OR_{adj}, 1.6; 95% CI, 0.8–3.3). Of the four remaining studies, only one showed a statistically sig-

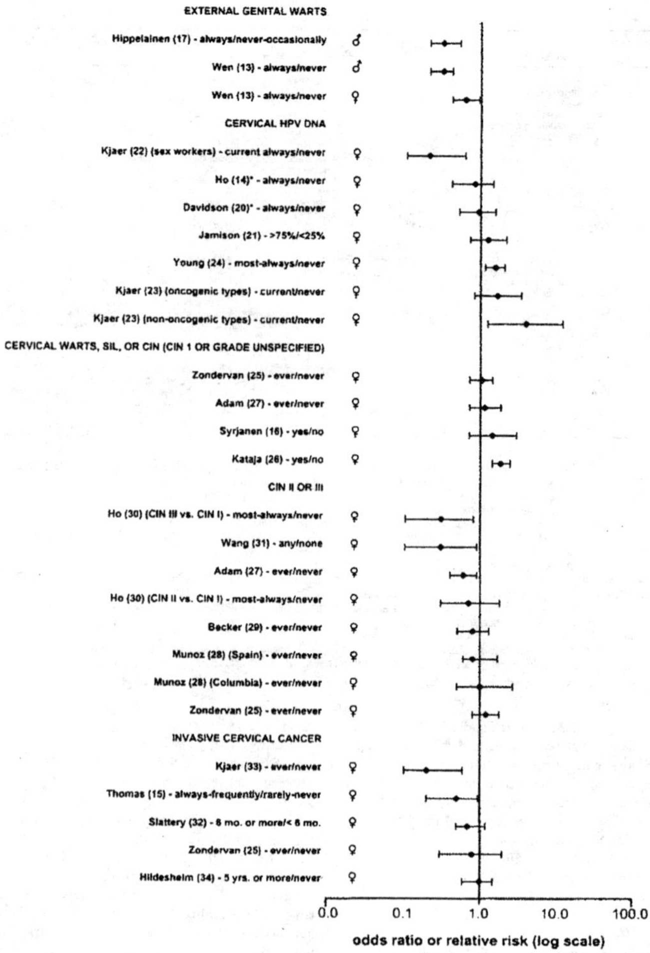

Fig. 1. Effect of condom use on prevention of external genital warts; detection of HPV DNA in cervical samples; cervical SIL, cervical warts, or CIN (grade I or unspecified); and CIN II/III and invasive cervical cancer. Asterisk indicates studies reporting relative risk estimates.

nificant elevated risk for HPV DNA detection among women who reported condom use. Young et al[24] found that women who reported using condoms "most of the time" or "always" were 50% more likely to have HPV DNA detected than those who reported never using condoms (OR_{adj}, 1.5; 95% CI, 1.1–2.0). Among female adolescents, Jamison et al[21] found a slight, nonsignificant increase in risk of HPV DNA detection for women who used condoms >75% of the time in comparison with those who used them <25% of the time (OR, 1.2; 95% CI, 0.7–2.1). However, Davidson et al[20] reported virtually no effect among native Alaskan women (RR_{adj}, 0.9; 95% CI 0.5–1.5).

In the sole cohort study, Ho et al[14] found that, compared with women who reported never using condoms, those who reported always using them were slightly less likely to become HPV DNA–positive, but the effect was not statistically significant (RR_{adj}, 0.8; 95% CI, 0.4–1.4).

Cervical Warts and SIL or CIN (Grade I or Unspecified)

Four studies examined the effect of condom use among women in whom cervical SIL, cervical warts, CIN I, or CIN of an unspecified grade had been detected. In two of these studies there was no effect of condom use on CIN I (grade I or unspecified) after adjustment for confounding factors.[25,27] Zondervan et al[25] enrolled women attending family planning clinics and found no relationship between ever having used condoms (as a contraceptive method) and dysplasia (OR_{adj}, 1.0; 95% CI, 0.7–1.4). Similarly, Adam et al[27] studied women referred to colposcopy clinics with abnormal Pap smears and found no association between ever using condoms and CIN I (OR_{adj}, 1.1; 95% CI, 0.7–1.8).

In contrast, two Finnish studies reported increased risk of cervical SIL with condom use as a contraceptive method. Syrjanen et al[16] found a slight, nonsignificant increase in risk for women attending an outpatient OB/GYN unit who reported using condoms compared with those who did not (OR, 1.4; 95% CI, 0.7–2.9). Kataja et al[26] showed an 80% increased risk of SIL among women who reported using condoms (OR, 1.8; 95% CI, 1.4–2.4), but the final estimate was not adjusted for potential confounding factors, and cases were significantly younger than controls.

CIN II or III

Six studies assessed the relationship between condom use and CIN II or III. All of these studies adjusted for confounding factors, but no two studies adjusted for the same factors. Zondervan et al,[25] Munoz et al,[28] Becker et al,[29] Wang et al,[31] and Adam et al[27] compared women with either CIN II or III with women who had normal cervical cytology. Two of these investigative teams found a significant protective effect, yet three others reported no significant effect of condom use. Wang et al[31] interviewed women and their husbands and determined that women attending cervical cancer screening sites who reported any use of condoms were 70% less likely to have CIN II or III than women who reported no use of condoms (OR_{adj}, 0.3; 95% CI, 0.1–0.8). Adam et al[27] estimated that among women referred to colposcopy clinics for abnormal Pap smears, those who reported ever having used condoms were 40% less likely to have CIN II or III than those who had never used condoms (OR_{adj}, 0.6; 95% CI, 0.4–0.9).

Becker et al[29] surveyed women attending university-based women's and maternal/infant care clinics and found that, compared with women who had never used condoms, those who reported ever using condoms were slightly less likely to have high-grade lesions (OR_{adj}, 0.8; 95% CI, 0.5–1.3). Munoz et al[28] conducted parallel studies in Spain and Colombia and interviewed women with and without CIN II or III and their husbands. In Spain a slight protective effect for condom use (ever versus never) was observed, although this was not statistically significant (OR_{adj}, 0.8; 95% CI, 0.6–1.7). In Colombia, no relationship between condom use and CIN II or III was found (OR_{adj}, 1.0; 95% CI, 0.5–2.7). A slightly elevated, nonsignificant risk of CIN II or III among women who had ever used condoms compared with those who had never used them (OR_{adj}, 1.2; 95% CI, 0.8–1.8) was reported by Zondervan et al.[25]

In contrast to the above studies, which compared women with CIN II or III with women with no cervical pathology, Ho et al[30] enrolled only women with histologically confirmed CIN and compared those with CIN II or III with those with CIN I. Compared with women who reported never using condoms, those who reported using condoms most or all of the time were approximately 30% less likely to have CIN II (OR_{adj}, 0.7; 95% CI, 0.3–1.8) and nearly 70% less likely to have CIN III (OR_{adj}, 0.3; 95% CI, 0.1–0.8). However, the comparison for women with CIN II was not statistically significant.

Invasive Cervical Cancer

A further five studies evaluated condom use as a risk factor for ICC. Four of the five studies showed a range of protective effects for condom use, while the fifth showed no effect. None of the studies showed any increased risk.

Two studies revealed a significant protective effect for condom use. Kjaer et al[33] selected women with cervical cancer from the Danish Cancer Registry and compared them with women from the general population. The analysis was restricted to "monogamous women" (women with one or two lifetime sex partners), and data on condom use were collected from the husband. Women whose husbands had ever used condoms were 80% less likely to have cervical cancer than those whose husbands had never used condoms (OR_{adj}, 0.2; 95% CI, 0.1–0.6). Thomas et al[15] also gathered data on the husband's use of condoms and found a significantly reduced risk for cervical cancer. Monogamous Thai women whose husbands always or frequently used condoms in their visits to prostitutes were 50% less likely to have cervical cancer than women whose husbands rarely or never used condoms with prostitutes (OR_{adj}, 0.5; 95% CI, 0.2–1.0).

Slattery et al[32] studied women from the Utah Cancer registry and compared them with women selected by random-digit dialing who had not been diagnosed with cancer. Women who reported using condoms for 6 or more months were 30% less likely to have cervical cancer than women who had used them for less than 6 months (OR_{adj}, 0.7; 95% CI, 0.5–1.2). Among women attending family planning clinics, Zondervan et al[25] found that ever using condoms was associated with a slight decreased risk (20%) of cervical cancer (OR_{adj}, 0.8; 95% CI, 0.3–2.0). Hildesheim et al,[34] however, found no effect on risk of cervical cancer when comparing women who had used condoms as a contraceptive method for at least 5 years with those who had never used them (OR_{adj}, 1.0; 95% CI, 0.6–1.5).

Discussion

Condoms are known to be effective in preventing HIV among both men and women,[6,35–37] but data on their protective effect against other STDs are less consistent.[11] The studies included here represent the best available data describing the relationship between condoms and HPV-related conditions. Although the absence of nonpublished studies raises the question of publication bias, exclusive reference to the peer-reviewed literature ensures the highest quality of data. Nevertheless, it was difficult to compare results from these studies because of the variety of different measures of condom use and the numerous different outcomes. All of the studies we evaluated had at least one of two problems: (1) they were not designed to evaluate condom use and therefore did not include precise measures of consistent or correct usage and/or (2) the temporal sequence was not established.

Generally, condom use was asked about in the context of contraception and only of female subjects (rather than of their male partners, who are the actual users). Previous studies have shown that important modifiers of condom efficacy include measures of user experience such as frequency and consistency of use and correct coverage. Individuals who often use condoms report fewer problems with breakage or slippage than infrequent users,[38,39] yet even experienced users report episodes where problems (putting it on inside out, application after penetrative intercourse has begun, breakage, and slippage) resulted in potential transmission risk.[40,41]

Other investigators have determined that the level of reported condom use varies, depending on the type of survey questions used. "Always use" versus "never use" is a popular epidemiologic measure, because the exclusive categories clearly define opportunity for exposure to HPV. However, a comparative study determined that "always use" rarely covered use for more than a year,[42] which is inadequate for infections such as HPV that can be present for longer intervals before progressing to CIN II or III or ICC. The type of sex partner also determines the frequency of condom use, with condoms being more often used with new and casual partners than with regular partners.[43] However, questions regarding partner type were rarely posed in these studies: only one study included questions about condom use with prostitutes, and another asked commercial sex workers about use with clients and regular partners.

Temporal sequence is an important criterion in making causal inference, yet only one study[14] was designed to look at new acquisition of HPV. For all other studies, it was impossible to determine whether condoms were used before or after acquisition of HPV. Without determining that individuals began using condoms while they were still infection-free, it is impossible to accurately assess the role that condoms play in preventing new infections. However, it is possible (but unknown) that condom use with the same partner after acquisition of a new HPV infection might reduce the total amount of virus transmitted and the number of genital sites infected.

Despite design problems inherent in the studies available for review, some observations may be made. Although only two studies were conducted among men, both suggested good protection against development of external genital warts. The sole study of external genital warts among women also showed protection; however, the level of protection was somewhat lower among these women than among men included in the same study. The limited data on heterosexual men suggest that, compared with young men who do not always use condoms with vaginal intercourse, those who do may be less likely to develop external genital warts. The evidence among women for protection from external genital warts and other HPV-related conditions is less clear because it is based on only one study.

There was no consistent evidence of a protective effect of condom use on HPV DNA detection, and in some studies, condom use was associated with a slightly increased risk for these lesions. Only among Danish commercial sex workers was there a strong, statistically significant reduction in risk with report of condom use with private partners. The fact that these sex workers also reported always using condoms with their clients suggests that they were experienced users, and as has been reported following other studies of sex workers,[44] they may have been able to ensure their partners used condoms correctly and consistently.

The studies grouped together under the heading "cervical warts and SIL or CIN (grade I or unspecified)" represent a mixture of conditions that are often indicative of transient infections. Therefore, this group may be composed of women who have a more recently acquired HPV infection. In the study by Kjaer et al, condom use was associated with a substantially increased risk of detecting nononcogenic HPV types. Common nononcogenic types are HPV 6 and 11, which are the same types associated with external genital warts. Kjaer et al also measured condom use as current versus never use. It may be that women opted to use condoms after noticing genital warts on their male partner. Because the virus was probably present before the warts appeared, condom use then may have begun after transmission had already occurred, thus giving the impression that condom use increased risk for the nononcogenic HPV types associated with genital warts. Alternatively, condoms may do little to protect against initial infection with HPV and subsequent transient conditions, a supposition that may be supported by the slightly increased risk seen for HPV DNA detection.

The individual odds ratios, and thus evidence of a protective role for condoms, varied for studies of CIN II or III. Two studies demonstrated a protective effect of 70% for condom use, four showed only slight protection (20–40%), and two showed either no effect or a slightly increased risk. Ho et al[30] showed a strong protective effect of condoms for CIN III (compared with CIN I). The effect was attenuated for CIN II, perhaps indicating the indistinct nature of CIN II as an intermediate category of cervical intraepithelial neoplasia. Whereas CIN III is a cervical cancer precursor lesion with a high probability of progression to invasion, CIN I appears to be the acute manifestation of cervical HPV infection and has a high likelihood of spontaneous resolution.[45]

Among the available data on condom use and prevention of cervical cancer is a hint that a subset of women was at least partially protected. Notably, the two studies that demonstrated a statistically significant protective effect of condoms against ICC were conducted among monogamous women and collected condom use data from the male sex partners of these women. This rigorous study design accounts for the sexual behavior of both partners and comes closer to approximating a true measure of condom use. Although the three other studies of ICC did not demonstrate statistically significant protective effects of condom use, they used less rigorous condom use definitions, and all but one demonstrated a small reduction in risk associated with condom use.

Some level of protection from HPV-related conditions was observed among 17 of the 27 populations studied; however, in most studies, protection was not substantial. It is unlikely that condoms offer the same level of protection against genital HPV infection as they do for HIV. These data suggest that condoms may prevent progression to lesions (warts, high-grade intraepithelial neoplasia), but perhaps not actual infection by HPV. We hypothesize this may be due to a reduction in the amount of virus transmitted with condom use, which could decrease the probability of developing a clinical lesion.

The data also indicate that condoms may provide more protection for a susceptible man than for a susceptible woman. All studies that were conducted among men or incorporated data collected from men on condom use showed significant and substantial protective effects. Thus, it may be that susceptible men who use condoms are more likely to be protected from infectious women than the reverse. We hypothesize that, in the process of putting on a condom, an infected man may touch the shaft of the penis, transferring virus onto his fingertips and subsequently depositing it onto the exterior of the condom as he rolls it down the penis. He would then infect his susceptible female partner during intercourse through the same vehicle designed to protect her. Sonnex et al[46] showed that HPV DNA could be detected in fingertip samples from 64% of men with external genital warts. A susceptible man using condoms correctly and consistently might be better protected from an infectious woman because she would be less likely to contaminate the condom.

Complete protection from genital HPV infection may be impossible because infections may occur at epithelial sites not covered by the condom. Also, when condoms are used primarily for contraceptive purposes, the condom may not be put on until after external genital contact has occurred. The least protective estimates for cervical SIL, warts, CIN I, and ICC were from studies that evaluated condom use as a contraceptive method only.[16,25,26,31,33]

Due to the inclusion of inadequate measures of condom use and the lack of information on temporal sequence, it is not possible to use available data to draw definitive conclusions on the efficacy of condoms in the prevention of HPV-related conditions. With the potential for HPV vaccines on the horizon,[47–49] one may ask whether there is a need to collect more conclusive data. Based on what we currently know, the answer is yes. Even if an HPV vaccine becomes available within the next 10 years, the benefits of such a vaccine would not accrue for at least another 10 to 20 years. In addition, as HPV DNA testing becomes more widely used in the management of women with Pap smears showing borderline abnormalities, an increasing percentage of women will be told they have an HPV infection. Both men and women need accurate information on how they can protect themselves and their partners from transmitting or acquiring genital HPV infection.

As suggested in a report from the American College of Obstetricians and Gynecologists,[5] there is a need for studies expressly designed and powered to determine the degree to which condoms prevent acquisition of HPV infection or development of HPV-related sequelae. These studies must incorporate accurate measures of condom use (including correct and consistent use), and they must be designed to show a temporal sequence. Unfortunately, the ethical concern associated with randomizing individuals to not using condoms precludes the use of the most rigorous study design: a randomized controlled trial. Given the nature of sexually transmitted diseases, more partner studies similar to those conducted by Kjaer et al[33] and Thomas et al[15] are necessary to accurately measure condom use and sexual behavior among both members of the sexual partnership.

References

1. Koutsky LA, Kiviat NB. Genital human papillomavirus. In: Holmes KK, Sparling PF, Mardh P-A, et al, eds. Sexually Transmitted Diseases. New York: McGraw-Hill, 1999:347–359.
2. Galloway DA. Biology of genital human papillomaviruses. In: Holmes KK, Sparling PF, Mardh P-A, et al, eds. Sexually Transmitted Diseases. New York: McGraw-Hill, 1999:335–346.
3. Bosch FX, Manos MM, Munoz N, et al. Prevalence of human papillomavirus in cervical cancer: a worldwide perspective. International Biological Study On Cervical Cancer (IBSCC) Study Group. J Natl Cancer Inst 1995; 87:796–802.
4. Kiviat NB, Koutsky LA, Paavonen J. Cervical neoplasia and other STD-related genital tract neoplasias. In: Holmes KK, Sparling PF, Mardh P-A, et al, eds. Sexually Transmitted Diseases. New York: McGraw-Hill, 1999:811–832.
5. American College of Obstetricians and Gynecologists. Human Papillomavirus (HPV): Make Decisions About Human Papillomavirus Based on Sound Medicine, Rather than Politics. 3/30/01. Available at: http://www.acog.org/from_home/departments/dept_notice.cfm?recno=11&bulletin=1083, 2001.
6. Davis KR, Weller SC. The effectiveness of condoms in reducing heterosexual transmission of HIV. Fam Plann Perspect 1999; 31:272–279.
7. Judson FN, Ehret JM, Bodin GF, Levin MJ, Rietmeijer CA. In vitro evaluations of condoms with and without nonoxynol 9 as physical and chemical barriers against *Chlamydia trachomatis*, herpes simplex virus type 2, and human immunodeficiency virus. Sex Transm Dis 1989; 16:51–56.
8. Fennema JS, van Ameijden EJ, Coutinho RA, Van den Hoek A. Clinical sexually transmitted diseases among human immunodeficiency virus–infected and noninfected drug-using prostitutes: associated factors and interpretation of trends, 1986 to 1994. Sex Transm Dis 1997; 24:363–371.
9. Cates WC Jr, Holmes KK. Condom efficacy against gonorrhea and nongonococcal urethritis. Am J Epidemiol 1996; 143:843–844.
10. Wald A, Langenberg AG, Link K, et al. Effect of condoms on reducing the transmission of herpes simplex virus type 2 from men to women. JAMA 2001; 285:3100–3106.
11. Zenilman JM, Weisman CS, Rompalo AM, et al. Condom use to prevent incident STDs: the validity of self-reported condom use. Sex Transm Dis 1995; 22:15–21.
12. Rothman KJ, Greenland S. Case-control studies. In: Rothman KJ, Greenland S, eds. Modern Epidemiology. Philadelphia: Lippincott-Raven, 1998:93–114.
13. Wen LM, Estcourt CS, Simpson JM, Mindel A. Risk factors for the acquisition of genital warts: are condoms protective? Sex Transm Infect 1999; 75:312–316.
14. Ho GY, Bierman R, Beardsley L, Chang CJ, Burk RD. Natural history of cervicovaginal papillomavirus infection in young women. N Engl J Med 1998; 338:423–428.
15. Thomas DB, Ray RM, Pardthaisong T, et al. Prostitution, condom use, and invasive squamous cell cervical cancer in Thailand. Am J Epidemiol 1996; 143:779–786.
16. Syrjanen K, Vayrynen M, Castren O, et al. Sexual behavior of women with human papillomavirus (HPV) lesions of the uterine cervix. Br J Vener Dis 1984; 60:243–248.
17. Hippelainen M, Syrjanen S, Koskela H, Pulkkinen J, Saarikoski S, Syrjanen K. Prevalence and risk factors of genital human papillomavirus (HPV) infections in healthy males: a study on Finnish conscripts. Sex Transm Dis 1993; 20:321–328.
18. Centers for Disease Control and Prevention, World Health Organization. Epi-Info Version 6.04b. Atlanta: Centers for Disease Control and Prevention, 1997.
19. Greenland S. Meta-analysis. In. Rothman KJ, Greenland S, eds. Modern Epidemiology. Philadelphia: Lippincott-Raven, 1998:643–674.
20. Davidson M, Schnitzer PG, Bulkow LR, et al. The prevalence of cervical infection with human papillomaviruses and cervical dysplasia in Alaska native women. J Infect Dis 1994; 169:792–800.
21. Jamison JH, Kaplan DW, Hamman R, Eagar R, Beach R, Douglas JM Jr. Spectrum of genital human papillomavirus infection in a female adolescent population. Sex Transm Dis 1995; 22:236–243.
22. Kjaer SK, van den Brule AJ, Bock JE, et al. Determinants for genital human papillomavirus (HPV) infection in 1000 randomly chosen young Danish women with normal Pap smear: are there different risk profiles for oncogenic and nononcogenic HPV types? Cancer Epidemiol Biomarkers Prev 1997; 6:799–805.
23. Kjaer SK, Svare EI, Worm AM, Walboomers JM, Meijer CJ, van den Brule AJ. Human papillomavirus infection in Danish female sex workers: decreasing prevalence with age despite continuously high sexual activity. Sex Transm Dis 2000; 27:438–445.
24. Young TK, McNicol P, Beauvais J. Factors associated with human papillomavirus infection detected by polymerase chain reaction among urban Canadian aboriginal and non-aboriginal women. Sex Transm Dis 1997; 24:293–298.
25. Zondervan KT, Carpenter LM, Painter R, Vessey MP. Oral contraceptives and cervical cancer–further findings from the Oxford Family Planning Association contraceptive study. Br J Cancer 1996; 73:1291–1297.
26. Kataja V, Syrjanen S, Yliskoski M, et al. Risk factors associated with cervical human papillomavirus infections: a case-control study. Am J Epidemiol 1993; 138:735–745.
27. Adam E, Berkova Z, Daxnerova Z, Icenogle J, Reeves WC, Kaufman RH. Papillomavirus detection: demographic and behavioral characteristics influencing the identification of cervical disease. Am J Obstet Gynecol 2000; 182:257–264.
28. Munoz N, Bosch FX, de Sanjose S, et al. Risk factors for cervical intraepithelial neoplasia grade III/carcinoma in situ in Spain and Colombia. Cancer Epidemiol Biomarkers Prev 1993; 2:423–431.
29. Becker TM, Wheeler CM, McGough NS, et al. Contraceptive and reproductive risks for cervical dysplasia in southwestern Hispanic and non-Hispanic white women. Int J Epidemiol 1994; 23:913–922.
30. Ho GY, Kadish AS, Burk RD, et al. HPV 16 and cigarette smoking as risk factors for high-grade cervical intra-epithelial neoplasia. Int J Cancer 1998; 78:281–285.
31. Wang PD, Lin RS. Risk factors for cervical intraepithelial neoplasia in Taiwan. Gynecol Oncol 1996; 62:10–18.
32. Slattery ML, Overall JC Jr, Abbott TM, French TK, Robison LM, Gardner J. Sexual activity, contraception, genital infections, and cervical cancer: support for a sexually transmitted disease hypothesis. Am J Epidemiol 1989; 130:248–258.
33. Kjaer SK, de Villiers EM, Dahl C, et al. Case-control study of risk factors for cervical neoplasia in Denmark. I: role of the "male factor" in women with one lifetime sexual partner. Int J Cancer 1991; 48:39–44.
34. Hildesheim A, Brinton LA, Mallin K, et al. Barrier and spermicidal contraceptive methods and risk of invasive cervical cancer. Epidemiology 1990; 1:266–272.
35. Deschamps MM, Pape JW, Hafner A, Johnson WD Jr. Heterosexual transmission of HIV in Haiti. Ann Intern Med 1996; 125:324–330.
36. de Vincenzi I. A longitudinal study of human immunodeficiency virus transmission by heterosexual partners. European Study Group on Heterosexual Transmission of HIV. N Engl J Med 1994; 331:341–346.
37. Saracco A, Musicco M, Nicolosi A, et al. Man-to-woman sexual transmission of HIV: longitudinal study of 343 steady partners of infected men. J Acquir Immun Defic Syndr 1993; 6:497–502.

38. Macaluso M, Kelaghan J, Artz L, et al. Mechanical failure of the latex condom in a cohort of women at high STD risk. Sex Transm Dis 1999; 26:450–458.
39. Messiah A, Dart T, Spencer BE, Warszawski J. Condom breakage and slippage during heterosexual intercourse: a French national survey. French National Survey on Sexual Behavior Group (ACSF). Am J Public Health 1997; 87:421–424.
40. de Visser RO, Smith AM. When always isn't enough: implications of the late application of condoms for the validity and reliability of self-reported condom use. AIDS Care 2000; 12:221–224.
41. Warner L, Clay-Warner J, Boles J, Williamson J. Assessing condom use practices: implications for evaluating method and user effectiveness. Sex Transm Dis 1998; 25:273–277.
42. Weir SS, Roddy RE, Zekeng L, Ryan KA, Wong EL. Measuring condom use: asking "do you or don't you" isn't enough. AIDS Educ Prev 1998; 10:293–302.
43. Macaluso M, Demand MJ, Artz LM, Hook EW 3rd. Partner type and condom use. AIDS 2000; 14:537–546.
44. Albert AE, Warner DL, Hatcher RA, Trussell J, Bennett C. Condom use among female commercial sex workers in Nevada's legal brothels. Am J Public Health 1995; 85:1514–1520.
45. Holowaty P, Miller AB, Rohan T, To T. Natural history of dysplasia of the uterine cervix. J Natl Cancer Inst 1999; 91:252–258.
46. Sonnex C, Strauss S, Gray JJ. Detection of human papillomavirus DNA on the fingers of patients with genital warts. Sex Transm Infect 1999; 75:317–319.
47. Galloway DA. Is vaccination against human papillomavirus a possibility? Lancet 1998; 351:22–24.
48. Hilleman MR. Overview of vaccinology with special reference to papillomavirus vaccines. J Clin Virol 2000; 19:79–90.
49. Schiller J, Lowy D. Papillomavirus-like particle vaccines. J Natl Cancer Inst Monogr 2001; 28:50–54.

Seroprevalence and Correlates of Herpes Simplex Virus Type 2 Infection in Five Sexually Transmitted–Disease Clinics

Sami L. Gottlieb,[1,2] John M. Douglas, Jr.,[1,2] D. Scott Schmid,[3] Gail Bolan,[4] Michael Iatesta,[3] C. Kevin Malotte,[5] Jonathan Zenilman,[6] Mark Foster,[2] Anna E. Barón,[1] John F. Steiner,[1] Thomas A. Peterman,[3] and Mary L. Kamb,[3] for the Project RESPECT Study Group[a]

[1]*University of Colorado Health Sciences Center and* [2]*Denver Public Health Department, Denver, Colorado;* [3]*Centers for Disease Control and Prevention, Atlanta, Georgia;* [4]*San Francisco Department of Public Health, San Francisco, and* [5]*California State University, Long Beach, California;* [6]*Baltimore City Health Department, Baltimore, Maryland*

The seroprevalence of herpes simplex virus type 2 (HSV-2) infection was studied among 4128 patients from sexually transmitted disease (STD) clinics who were enrolled in a randomized controlled trial of human immunodeficiency virus and STD counseling efficacy. HSV-2 seroprevalence was 40.8% and was higher in women than in men (52.0% vs. 32.4%; $P<.0001$) and higher in blacks than in nonblacks (48.1% vs. 29.6%; $P<.0001$). Among 14–19-year-old patients, 36.8% of black women and 25.8% of nonblack women were infected with HSV-2. Independent predictors of HSV-2 seropositivity included female sex, black race, older age, less education, more lifetime sex partners, prior diagnosis of syphilis or gonorrhea, and lack of HSV-1 antibody. The majority of HSV-2–seropositive persons (84.7%) had never received a diagnosis of genital herpes. HSV-2 infection is common in STD clinic attendees in the United States, even among young age groups, especially among women. Efforts to prevent genital herpes should begin at an early age. The high rate of undiagnosed HSV-2 infection likely contributes to ongoing transmission.

Herpes simplex virus type 2 (HSV-2) is the main cause of genital herpes and a leading cause of genital ulcer disease throughout the world [1, 2]. Although HSV-2 may cause painful genital blisters and ulcerations, most HSV-2 infections are unrecognized or asymptomatic [3–5] yet can still be transmitted to a sex partner [4]. Furthermore, there is mounting evidence that HSV-2 facilitates the transmission of human immunodeficiency virus (HIV) infection [6, 7]. In the United States, large national surveys such as the National Health and Nutrition Examination Surveys (NHANES) II and III have shown that the prevalence of HSV-2 antibody in the general US population has increased since 1978, with 22% of US adults being infected by the early 1990s [8]. However, in high-risk settings such as sexually transmitted disease (STD) clinics, where patients are more likely than the general population to be at risk of both HSV-2 and HIV infection, HSV-2 prevalence data are less complete. Most large HSV-2 seroprevalence studies in STD clinics have been performed outside the United States [9–11] or primarily among US women [5, 12]. Project RESPECT was a large randomized controlled trial in 5 urban STD clinics, which demonstrated that HIV and STD risk-reduction counseling can result in behavioral change and the prevention of new bacterial STDs [13]. The purpose of the present study was to use enrollment data from Project RESPECT to determine the seroprevalence and correlates of HSV-2 infection in a geographically dispersed population of US STD clinic patients.

Methods

Study design and procedures. We performed a cross-sectional seroprevalence analysis, using questionnaire data and serum samples obtained during the Project RESPECT enrollment visit. The complete methodology for Project RESPECT has been described in detail elsewhere [13]. In brief, the trial was conducted from July 1993 through September 1996, at public, inner-city STD clinics in Baltimore, Denver, Long Beach, Newark, and San Francisco. All English-speaking patients aged ≥14 years who came for STD examinations during the study period and had had vaginal intercourse in the preceding 3 months were asked to participate in the study. Men who identified themselves as homosexual or who had had a male sex partner during the preceding 12 months were excluded from the study, as were those patients found to be HIV positive at

Received 3 August 2001; revised 13 May 2002; electronically published 23 October 2002.

Presented in part: National STD Prevention Conference, Milwaukee, 4–7 December 2000 (abstract A6).

Informed consent was obtained from all patients participating in the study. Human experimentation guidelines of the US Department of Health and Human Services and those of participating institutions were followed in the conduct of this research. The Project RESPECT protocol was reviewed and approved by the institutional review board at each participating site.

Financial support: National Research Service Award grant 5 T32 PE10006 08; cooperative agreements with state and local health departments and the Centers for Disease Control and Prevention, National Center for HIV, STD, and TB Prevention.

Reprints or correspondence: Dr. John M. Douglas, Jr., Denver Public Health, 605 Bannock St., Mail Code 2600, Denver, CO 80204 (john.douglas @dhha.org).

The Journal of Infectious Diseases 2002;186:1381–9

0022-1899/2002/18610-0001$15.00

enrollment. Participants were then randomized to 4 arms with varying intensities of safer-sex counseling. Participants in arms 1–3 were scheduled for quarterly follow-up visits over the next 12 months; arm 4 participants had no routine follow-up scheduled. Unlike participants in the first 3 arms, arm 4 participants did not consistently undergo serum testing for HSV-2 at baseline enrollment and thus were excluded from this seroprevalence analysis.

At the enrollment visit, participants were interviewed to obtain information on sociodemographic characteristics, sexual history and behavior, and STD history, including the question "Have you ever been told by a doctor or nurse that you had genital herpes?" No data were available on previous symptoms suggestive of genital HSV (e.g., undiagnosed genital blisters or ulcerations) or contact with a sex partner known to have genital herpes. Genital examinations and laboratory testing for STDs were performed for all patients and included serologic testing for HSV-1 and HSV-2.

Laboratory methods. Stored serum samples were tested for antibodies to HSV-1 and HSV-2 by a type-specific strip immunoblot assay (Chiron) based on recombinant antigen bands for glycoproteins gB1, gD2, gG1, and gG2 [14]. The sensitivity of the strip immunoblot assay has been found to be >98% for HSV-2 and 95% for HSV-1, with a specificity of >99% for both, compared with Western blot analysis [15]. All tests were performed in the same laboratory, with the manufacturer's automated processor. For patients with symptoms or signs of genital herpes, a diagnosis of primary or recurrent infection was made in each STD clinic, on the basis of the examiner's clinical impression of the patient's history and physical condition, without the standardized use of confirmatory HSV culture or other virologic testing. Infection with *Neisseria gonorrhoeae* was defined as a positive culture or, for men, as gram-negative intracellular diplococci on a Gram stain of a urethral swab. Infection with *Chlamydia trachomatis* was defined as a positive result of polymerase chain-reaction assay on endocervical swabs (women) and urine samples (men). Syphilis was diagnosed by positive treponemal and nontreponemal antibody tests. Infection with *Trichomonas vaginalis* in women was defined by a positive culture result or by trichomonads seen on a wet mount from a vaginal swab.

Statistical analysis. Point prevalences, 95% confidence intervals (CIs), and odds ratios (ORs) were calculated by SAS software, version 6.12 (SAS Institute). Univariate and bivariate analyses were performed to examine the association between HSV-2 seropositivity and demographic, sexual behavior, and current and past STD variables by the χ^2 test ($P < .05$). Multiple logistic regression was used to determine independent predictors of HSV-2 seropositivity, by a manual backward-elimination process. All demographic, sexual-behavior, and STD variables with crude associations at $P < .20$ were first entered into a model. A manual stepwise process then removed nonsignificant variables that were not significant confounders, according to the likelihood ratio test using the χ^2 distribution for significance (>95%). Independent predictors in the final model were retained variables with a significance level of $P < .05$. Separate models for men and women were used to assess variables obtained for only 1 sex. An additional multiple logistic regression model was created in the same fashion among only HSV-2–seropositive persons to determine independent predictors of remaining undiagnosed with genital herpes despite having HSV-2 antibodies.

Results

From July 1993 through June 1995, 13,471 eligible patients were asked to participate in Project RESPECT, and 5833 (43%) agreed to enroll. Study participants and those who refused were similar in age, racial or ethnic background, and education level, although, compared with those who refused, participants were more likely to be women (OR, 1.49; 95% CI, 1.44–1.55), to have had an STD at enrollment (OR, 1.19; 95% CI, 1.14–1.24), and to have been previously tested for HIV (OR, 1.13; 95% CI, 1.08–1.18). After exclusion of patients with a positive baseline HIV test result ($n = 75$) and of arm 4 participants who did not routinely receive HSV testing ($n = 1430$), 4328 baseline enrollees remained for this seroprevalence analysis. HSV-2 test results were available for 4128 (95.4%) of these participants. Results were unavailable for 200 participants because of insufficient quantities of serum for HSV testing and the loss of serum samples during transportation, storage, or processing.

Of 4128 total participants, 2348 (56.9%) were male and 1780 (43.1%) were female. The study population was 60.7% black, 20.6% white, 11.3% Hispanic, and 7.4% other racial or ethnic group. The median age was 25 years (range, 14–76 years). Study participants were predominantly low income, and fewer than one-third of respondents had an education beyond high school. All of the study participants had had at least 1 sex partner; the median number of lifetime sex partners was 10 for women and 20 for men. The median age at first sexual intercourse was 15 years. Almost two-thirds (62.7%) of subjects reported prior treatment for at least 1 STD, with gonorrhea being the most commonly reported past STD.

Overall, 1686 (40.8%) of the 4128 participants were positive for HSV-2 antibody (table 1). HSV-2 seroprevalence was higher among women (52.0%) than among men (32.4%; $P < .0001$). HSV-2 seroprevalence among blacks was 48.1%, significantly higher than that among whites (30.1%; $P < .0001$). HSV-2 seroprevalence in Hispanics and other racial or ethnic groups did not differ significantly from that in whites. Black females had the highest overall seroprevalence, 62.8% (95% CI, 59.7–65.9), whereas black males had a seroprevalence of 39.0% (95% CI, 36.5–41.4), with very little variation by study site, for either black women (59%–68%) or black men (37%–42%). Similar to the frequency seen in black males, 40.8% (95% CI, 36.0–41.0) of white females were HSV-2 seropositive, whereas white males had the lowest overall seroprevalence, at 19.7% (95% CI, 15.9–23.6). HSV-2 seroprevalence increased with older age and with less education. Seroprevalence was lowest in San Francisco (33.2%) and highest in Baltimore (50.1%), with differences largely attributable to the proportion of black participants at each study site.

Figure 1 shows HSV-2 seroprevalence, by age, for black and nonblack males and females. Whites, Hispanics, and other races or ethnicities were grouped as nonblacks, because they were not significantly different from each other. HSV-2 seroprevalence increased with age, for all sex and racial groups (χ^2 for

Table 1. Herpes simplex virus type 2 (HSV-2) seroprevalence, by selected participant characteristics.

Variable	No.[a]	HSV-2 prevalence, % (95% CI)	Unadjusted OR (95% CI)
Total	4128	40.8 (39.3–42.3)	
Sex			
Male	2348	32.4 (30.5–34.4)	1.0
Female	1780	52.0 (49.7–54.4)	2.3 (2.0–2.6)
Racial or ethnic group			
White	850	30.1 (27.0–33.3)	1.0
Black	2506	48.1 (46.1–50.1)	2.1 (1.8–2.5)
Hispanic	467	26.8 (22.6–30.9)	0.8 (0.7–1.1)
Other	305	32.5 (27.0–37.9)	1.1 (0.8–1.5)
Age (years)			
14–19	724	23.6 (20.5–26.8)	1.0
20–24	1198	34.3 (31.6–37.0)	1.7 (1.4–2.1)
25–29	802	42.5 (39.0–46.0)	2.4 (1.9–3.0)
30–39	977	49.9 (46.7–53.0)	3.2 (2.6–4.0)
≥40	427	64.6 (60.0–69.3)	5.9 (4.5–7.7)
Education			
Some college	1212	35.4 (32.7–38.1)	1.0
High school graduate	1503	45.6 (43.1–48.2)	1.5 (1.3–1.8)
Less than high school	804	49.8 (46.2–53.3)	1.8 (1.5–2.2)
Still in school	609	28.1 (24.4–31.7)	0.7 (0.6–0.9)
Site			
San Francisco	735	33.2 (29.7–36.7)	1.0
Baltimore	774	50.1 (46.5–53.7)	2.0 (1.6–2.5)
Denver	1015	38.4 (35.4–41.5)	1.3 (1.0–1.5)
Long Beach	754	38.5 (34.9–42.0)	1.3 (1.0–1.6)
Newark	850	44.0 (40.6–47.4)	1.6 (1.3–1.9)
Income during preceding year ($)			
<5000	1733	40.6 (38.3–43.0)	1.0
5000–14,999	1384	41.0 (38.3–43.6)	1.0 (0.9–1.2)
≥15,000	881	39.8 (36.6–43.1)	1.0 (0.8–1.1)
Age at first sex (years)			
≤12	756	45.1 (41.5–48.7)	1.5 (1.2–1.8)
13–14	1138	42.2 (39.3–45.1)	1.3 (1.1–1.6)
15–16	1238	41.2 (38.4–44.0)	1.3 (1.1–1.5)
≥17	996	35.6 (32.6–38.7)	1.0
Sex partners (lifetime number)			
≤5	784	30.1 (26.8–33.4)	1.0
6–10	884	39.8 (36.5–43.1)	1.5 (1.2–1.9)
11–20	921	39.1 (35.9–42.3)	1.5 (1.2–1.8)
21–50	894	42.1 (38.8–45.4)	1.7 (1.4–2.1)
>50	645	56.1 (52.2–60.0)	3.0 (2.4–3.7)
Prior diagnosis of herpes			
No	3884	38.2 (36.7–39.7)	1.0
Yes	234	84.2 (79.3–89.1)	8.6 (6.0–12.7)
Prior diagnosis of chlamydial infection			
No	3239	38.5 (36.8–40.2)	1.0
Yes	868	49.3 (45.9–52.7)	1.6 (1.3–1.8)
Prior diagnosis of gonorrhea			
No	2653	32.5 (30.7–34.3)	1.0
Yes	1460	55.9 (53.3–58.5)	2.6 (2.3–3.0)
Prior diagnosis of syphilis			
No	3876	38.9 (37.4–40.5)	1.0
Yes	238	71.0 (65.0–77.0)	3.8 (2.9–5.2)
Prior diagnosis of trichomoniasis (women)			
No	1314	44.0 (41.3–46.7)	1.0
Yes	450	74.4 (70.3–78.6)	3.7 (2.9–4.8)
HSV-1 antibody			
Absent	1210	37.9 (35.2–40.7)	1.0
Present	2918	42.0 (40.2–43.9)	1.2 (1.0–1.4)
Circumcised (on examination) (men)			
Yes	1645	30.8 (28.5–33.0)	1.0
No	698	36.4 (32.7–40.0)	1.3 (1.1–1.6)

NOTE. CI, confidence interval; OR, odds ratio.

[a] In some cases, data were not available for all participants.

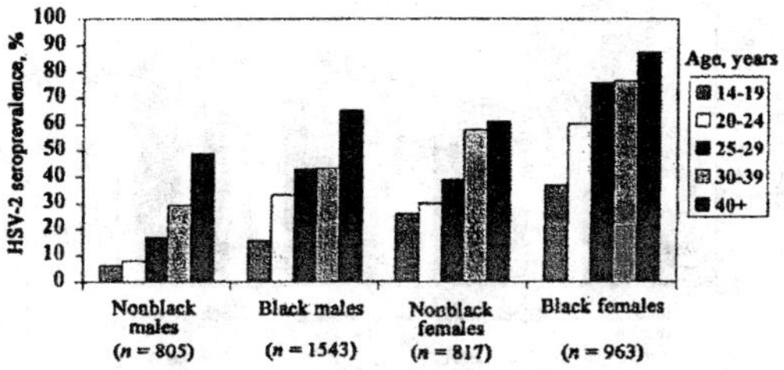

Figure 1. Herpes simplex virus type 2 (HSV-2) seroprevalence according to age, race, and sex. HSV-2 seroprevalence increased with age (χ^2 for trend, $P<.0001$ for all race and sex groups). For each age group, women had higher seroprevalences than did men, and blacks had higher rates than nonblacks ($P<.05$ for all comparisons).

trend, $P<.0001$ for all groups). For each age group, women had higher seroprevalence rates than did men, and blacks had higher rates than did nonblacks ($P<.05$ for each comparison). Within each racial group, women often had higher rates of HSV-2 infection than did substantially older men. For example, nonblack women aged 14–19 years had a higher HSV-2 seroprevalence than did nonblack men aged 25–29 years, and black women aged 20–24 years had a higher rate than did black men aged 30–39 years. Even in the youngest age group (14–19 years old), 25.8% of nonblack women and 36.8% of black women were already infected with HSV-2. It was difficult to determine the age at which HSV-2 seroprevalence first started to increase, because the small number of study participants <17 years old made estimates of seroprevalence during these early adolescent years unreliable. However, among 91 females who were 17 years old, the HSV-2 seroprevalence was already 33.0% (95% CI, 22.8–43.2). In the oldest age group (⩾40 years old), ~50% of nonblack males, 65% of black males, 60% of nonblack females, and almost 90% of black females had HSV-2 infection.

Sexual-behavior history and past STD history also were associated with HSV-2 seroprevalence (table 1). On univariate analysis, an earlier age at first sexual intercourse was associated with higher seroprevalence rates. The presence of HSV-2 antibody also increased with increasing numbers of lifetime sex partners (χ^2 for trend, $P<.0001$). There were 234 persons who had been given a clinical diagnosis of herpes in the past, of whom 197 (84.2%) had HSV-2 antibodies. Of the 37 persons with a prior herpes diagnosis who lacked HSV-2 antibodies, 29 had HSV-1 antibodies and 8 did not. A prior diagnosis of gonorrhea, chlamydial infection, syphilis, and trichomoniasis (for women) were all associated with HSV-2 infection. Among these past STDs, HSV-2 seroprevalence was highest in participants with a prior diagnosis of syphilis (71.0%) and in women with prior trichomoniasis (74.4%). HSV-2 seroprevalence was slightly higher in those who were positive for HSV-1 antibody (42.0%) than in those who were not (37.9%). Likewise, men who were uncircumcised were slightly more likely to be HSV-2 infected than were those who were circumcised (36.4% vs. 30.8%).

Figure 2 demonstrates HSV-2 seroprevalence according to number of lifetime sex partners, race, and sex. HSV-2 seroprevalence increased with increasing numbers of lifetime sex partners, for all sex and racial groupings (χ^2 for trend, $P<.0001$ for all groups). For each category of lifetime sex partners, women had higher prevalences than did men ($P<.0001$) and blacks had higher rates than did nonblacks ($P<.05$). Black women had the lowest median number of lifetime sex partners (8) but had the highest overall seroprevalence. Even among black women with only 1–5 lifetime sex partners, HSV-2 seroprevalence was 45.7% (95% CI, 40.1–51.1). Among nonblack women with only 1–5 lifetime sex partners, HSV-2 seroprevalence was 24.7% (95% CI, 18.8–30.5). In fact, even with only 1 or 2 lifetime partners, HSV-2 seroprevalence was 33.9% (95% CI, 21.3–46.5) among black women and 17.7% (95% CI, 7.4–28.1) among nonblack women.

Independent predictors of HSV-2 seropositivity, by multiple-logistic-regression analysis, are shown in table 2. After adjustment for other risk factors, women had >4 times the odds of HSV-2 infection that men had (OR, 4.6; 95% CI, 3.8–5.5). Black race was also independently associated with HSV-2, with an overall adjusted OR of 2.5 (95% CI, 2.0–3.2), compared with whites. The odds of HSV-2 also increased with increasing age and numbers of lifetime sex partners. Other independent predictors of HSV-2 seropositivity included less education, a history of gonorrhea, a history of syphilis, and fewer new sex partners in the past 3 months. It is noteworthy that, after we controlled for other risk factors, the relationship between HSV-1 antibody and HSV-2 changed, resulting in an inverse asso-

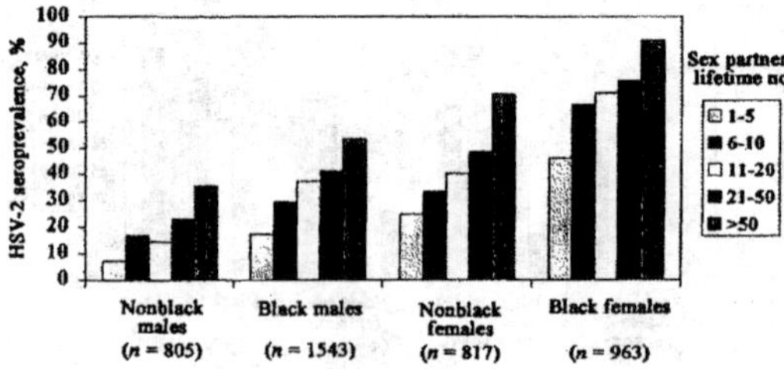

Figure 2. Herpes simplex virus type 2 (HSV-2) seroprevalence by lifetime sex partners, race, and sex. HSV-2 seroprevalence increased with increasing numbers of lifetime partners (χ^2 for trend, $P < .0001$ for all race and sex groups). For each category of lifetime partners, women had higher seroprevalences than did men, and blacks had higher rates than nonblacks ($P < .05$ for each comparison).

ciation (OR, 0.8; 95% CI, 0.7–0.9). Furthermore, in multivariate analysis, both age at first sex and study site were no longer independently associated with HSV-2 infection.

Several variables were available only for women or only for men. When these were considered in separate models for women and men, 4 additional factors predicted HSV-2 infection in women: a prior diagnosis of trichomoniasis (OR, 1.6; 95% CI, 1.2–2.2), a current diagnosis of trichomoniasis (OR, 1.5; 95% CI, 1.1–2.2), a history of prostitution (OR, 1.9; 95% CI, 1.2–2.9), and having had a sex partner who had been in jail (OR, 1.3; 95% CI, 1.0–1.7). The only additional factor predicting HSV-2 infection in men was a history of being in jail (OR, 1.3; 95% CI, 1.0–1.6). It is noteworthy that circumcision was not independently associated with HSV-2 infection, after adjustment for other factors.

Of the 1686 participants with HSV-2 antibodies, only 197 (11.7%) had been previously given the diagnosis of genital herpes, and an additional 60 (3.6%) were diagnosed clinically as having genital herpes during the enrollment visit. Thus, 84.7% of all HSV-2–infected persons remained undiagnosed at the end of the enrollment visit. By univariate analysis, race or ethnicity and HSV-1 status were most strongly associated with having undiagnosed HSV-2 infection. Among those with HSV-2 infection, blacks were significantly more likely than whites to remain undiagnosed (88.8% vs. 74.3%; $P < .001$). Likewise, among HSV-2–infected persons, those who were HSV-1 seropositive were more likely to remain undiagnosed than were those who were HSV-1 seronegative (86.6% vs. 79.7%; $P = .0005$). Table 3 displays the results of a multivariate analysis of factors associated with remaining undiagnosed with genital herpes among HSV-2–infected persons. Factors independently associated with being undiagnosed included black race, female sex, older age, still being in school, attending the Newark clinic, a diagnosis of gonorrhea at enrollment, and being positive for HSV-1 antibody. Thus, black race, female sex, and older age were independently associated not only with HSV-2 seroprevalence but also with the likelihood of remaining undiagnosed with genital herpes once infected.

If both overall HSV-2 seroprevalence and the proportion of infections that remain undiagnosed are taken into account, the percentage of the entire study population with undiagnosed HSV-2 infection can be calculated. This percentage represents the potential yield of serologic screening to detect clinically undiagnosed HSV-2 infection that would not otherwise be found and is shown in table 4, for various race, sex, and age groups. For example, the yield of screening would be >20% in nonblack men ⩾30 years old, black men and nonblack women ⩾20 years old, and black women of any age. Among black men and nonblack women ⩾40 years old, and among black women ⩾20 years old, the yield of screening would be >50%.

Discussion

These data represent the largest evaluation, to date, of HSV-2 seroprevalence in men and women attending STD clinics. The overall seroprevalence of HSV-2 was 41% in this population, predictably higher than the 22% HSV-2 seroprevalence seen in the general US population in the most recent NHANES study [8]. Approximately half of the women and half of the blacks in this study were HSV-2–seropositive. HSV-2 seroprevalence among nonblacks was 20% in men and 39% in women, whereas that among blacks was 39% in men and 63% in women. These findings are consistent with prior studies of women attending US STD clinics [5, 12]; however, similar studies have not previously been performed in heterosexual males. Overall HSV-2 seroprevalence was higher than that previously seen among STD clinic attendees in Europe [9–11].

The disparity in HSV-2 infection by sex was striking; even

Table 2. Independent predictors of herpes simplex virus type 2 (HSV-2) seropositivity, by multivariate analysis.

Variable	Adjusted OR (95% CI)[a]
Sex	
Male	1.0
Female	4.58 (3.84–5.46)
Racial or ethnic group	
White	1.0
Black	2.51 (2.00–3.16)
Hispanic	1.18 (0.88–1.58)
Other	1.22 (0.88–1.68)
Age (years)	
14-19	1.0
20–24	1.77 (1.38–2.26)
25–29	2.77 (2.10–3.64)
30–39	3.22 (2.46–4.23)
≥40	6.46 (4.64–8.99)
Education	
Some college	1.0
High school graduate	1.40 (1.17–1.69)
Less than high school	1.76 (1.40–2.20)
Still in school	1.10 (0.84–1.44)
Sex partners (lifetime number)	
≤5	1.0
6–10	1.86 (1.47–2.36)
11–20	2.06 (1.61–2.63)
21–50	2.43 (1.87–3.16)
>50	3.66 (2.73–4.90)
New sex partners during preceding 3 months	
0	1.0
1	0.86 (0.73–1.02)
≥2	0.74 (0.60–0.91)
Prior diagnosis of gonorrhea	
No	1.0
Yes	1.76 (1.50–2.06)
Prior diagnosis of syphilis	
No	1.0
Yes	1.96 (1.42–2.72)
HSV-1 antibody	
Absent	1.0
Present	0.78 (0.66–0.92)

NOTE. CI, confidence interval; OR, odds ratio.
[a] Adjusted for all other variables in table, in addition to study site, prior diagnosis of chlamydial infection, % of condom use with vaginal sex during the past 3 months, and history of same-sex partner.

after we adjusted for age, race or ethnicity, and number of lifetime sex partners, the odds of having HSV-2 infection were >4 times greater in women than in men. Likely contributing to this finding is the demonstrated higher efficiency of HSV-2 transmission from men to women, compared with that from women to men [16]. The larger exposed mucosal surface area in women, which may be more easily traumatized, could account for a large part of this difference in transmission [2]. However, lack of circumcision, an anatomic condition that increases mucosal surface area in men and that has been shown to increase the risk of HIV acquisition [17], was not associated with HSV-2 infection in a multivariate model. It has also been postulated [8] that high rates of HSV-2 among women may be partially explained by the fact that women are more likely to choose partners who are older than themselves [18] and who therefore have a greater risk of HSV-2 infection. However, we found that HSV-2 seroprevalence was generally higher among younger women than among considerably older men, indicating that choice of older male partners is unlikely to be the primary explanation for high rates of HSV-2 infection in women. For women in this study, the prevalence of HSV-2 was notably high even among adolescents and those with few lifetime sex partners. Thus, HSV-2 prevention strategies must start at an early age in populations with high rates of STD.

A second noteworthy finding was the higher seroprevalence of HSV-2 among black men and women than among other racial or ethnic groups, even when we controlled for other demographic and sexual-behavior characteristics. For any given number of lifetime sex partners, the adjusted odds of having HSV-2 infection were 2.5 times higher in blacks than in whites. This observation supports the idea that, with respect to HSV-2, the pool of potential partners is different for blacks and whites and that sexual networks may play a critical role in determining an individual's STD risk [19, 20]. Because the prevalence of HSV-2 is higher in blacks, and because sex partnerships tend to develop among members of the same race or ethnic group [18], blacks are likely to have a higher risk of

Table 3. Independent predictors of remaining undiagnosed with genital herpes among herpes simplex virus type 2 (HSV-2)–seropositive persons (n = 1686), by multivariate analysis.

Variable	Adjusted OR (95% CI)[a]
Sex	
Male	1.0
Female	1.51 (1.11–2.06)
Racial or ethnic group	
White	1.0
Black	2.17 (1.44–3.27)
Hispanic	0.74 (0.43–1.25)
Other	1.26 (0.70–2.27)
Age (years)	
14–19	1.0
20–24	1.50 (0.87–2.59)
25–29	1.53 (0.86–2.70)
30–39	1.60 (0.92–2.76)
≥40	2.86 (1.53–5.36)
Education	
Some college	1.0
High school graduate	0.99 (0.70–1.40)
Less than high school	1.29 (0.83–2.00)
Still in school	1.83 (1.01–3.34)
Site	
San Francisco	1.0
Baltimore	1.09 (0.67–1.77)
Denver	1.42 (0.94–2.15)
Long Beach	1.19 (0.75–1.89)
Newark	4.34 (2.33–8.10)
Diagnosis of gonorrhea at enrollment	
No	1.0
Yes	2.28 (1.36–3.84)
HSV-1 antibody	
Absent	1.0
Present	1.58 (1.16–2.14)

NOTE. CI, confidence interval; OR, odds ratio.
[a] Adjusted for all other variables in table in addition to prior diagnosis of chlamydial infection, ever having oral sex, and history of same-sex partner.

Table 4. Percentage of total study population with undiagnosed herpes simplex virus type 2 (HSV-2) infection, found only by serologic tests, according to age, race, and sex.

	Undiagnosed, %					
Race, sex	14–19 years	20–24 years	25–29 years	30–39 years	≥40 years	Overall
Black						
Male	13.8	29.8	38.3	37.2	56.1	34.2
Female	31.6	55.2	67.1	68.4	82.5	56.4
Nonblack						
Male	4.7	4.1	12.7	21.0	41.3	14.4
Female	17.4	21.5	28.1	43.1	54.6	29.4

NOTE. Data were calculated from percentage of HSV-2 seroprevalence and percentage of seroprevalent infections remaining undiagnosed and represent the potential yield, in the setting of sexually transmitted–disease clinics, of serologic screening to detect clinically undiagnosed HSV-2 infection.

coming into contact with an infected partner with each new partnership. In addition, recent work has shown that blacks who have had only 1 partner in the past year are much more likely to choose partners who have had ≥4 partners in the past year than are their white counterparts [19]. If replicated in other studies, this "dissortative" partner choice may be a major contributor to the high prevalence of HSV-2 in black STD clinic attendees.

For both sexes, past sexual behavior and STD history were predictors of HSV-2 infection, especially the number of lifetime sex partners and a prior history of gonorrhea or syphilis, as were both prostitution and prior or current diagnosis of trichomoniasis in women. Of note, after adjustment for other characteristics, such as age and total numbers of lifetime sex partners, we did not find an association between age at first intercourse and HSV-2 infection. This observation is consistent with that found in the general US population [8] and may have programmatic implications in that STD prevention efforts aimed at delaying first coitus may ultimately have a limited impact on prevention of HSV-2 infection. The association between HSV-2 infection and past STDs, although likely reflective of unmeasured behavioral factors, raises the interesting question of a possible biologic interaction. For example, it is possible that STDs such as syphilis, gonorrhea, and trichomoniasis could be cofactors for HSV-2 shedding or susceptibility, just as they are suspected to be for HIV [21, 22]. Unfortunately, we could not assess the very important potential interaction between HIV and HSV-2, because HIV-positive persons were excluded from Project RESPECT. The inverse association between HSV-1 and HSV-2 antibodies after adjustment for demographic and sexual behavior characteristics also suggests a potential biologic interaction between HSV-1 and HSV-2 [1, 2]. In a cross-sectional study such as this one, the timing and rates of new HSV-1 and HSV-2 infections are not known; however, our data suggest that HSV-1 may partially protect against HSV-2 infection.

As also was true in other studies [3–5, 8–11], the vast majority of our patients with HSV-2 infection (84.7%) had never been given a diagnosis of genital herpes, either previously or at the time of their enrollment visit. A prior diagnosis of herpes was based on the question "Have you ever been told by a doctor or nurse that you had genital herpes?" There may have been participants who suspected that they had genital herpes but who had never received a definitive diagnosis from a clinician. Thus, our estimates may be influenced by either access to health care or health care–seeking behavior and may underestimate the number of participants who were aware of having genital herpes. Indeed, it is possible that geographic variation in health care utilization might partially explain the association between remaining undiagnosed and 1 of the 5 sites (Newark) involved in the study. Nonetheless, lack of a definitive diagnosis for those who are infected and who may not take precautions to prevent transmission could contribute to ongoing spread of HSV-2 infection.

Because of this issue, HSV-2 serologic screening of selected populations at risk for STD has been discussed as a potential prevention strategy [23, 24]. Studies have shown that the majority of patients with previously "asymptomatic" HSV-2 infection can be taught to subsequently recognize clinical outbreaks [3, 25]; thus, screening would increase the likelihood that many subclinically infected persons would come to recognize lesions. Such knowledge would allow infected persons to avoid intercourse when herpetic lesions were present, to decrease the chance of transmission [3]. In fact, preliminary data indicate that knowledge of genital herpes is associated with delayed transmission of HSV to a sex partner [26]. Avoiding sex when one is symptomatic might also lead to a reduction in HIV transmission efficiency [6, 7], another potential benefit of an HSV-2 screening program. Furthermore, because a recent study of HSV-2–discordant couples has shown for the first time that condoms can prevent transmission of genital herpes [27], knowledge of HSV-2 infection detected by serologic screening might also facilitate prevention of herpes transmission, by condom use, even without recognition of symptomatic lesions. Our data indicate that, at the very least, the yield of a screening program in identifying undiagnosed HSV-2 infection in STD clinics would be substantial. Moreover, given the associations between HSV-2 infection and black race, female sex, and older age, combined with the increased likelihood that these groups will remain undiagnosed when infected, it follows that the yield of serologic screening in a particular clinical setting would partially depend on patient demographics. However, the degree of benefit of serologic screening in terms of clinical care and prevention has not yet been quantified, and there are potential concerns about the psychosocial and economic impact of screening [28, 29]. Thus, the role that newly licensed type-specific HSV-2 serologic tests play in HSV-2 prevention efforts should continue to be evaluated, with a focus on populations at greatest risk of undiagnosed infection.

The present study had several limitations. First, the study population consisted of selected patients, representing only 43% of those eligible, who enrolled in a randomized controlled trial conducted in 5 inner-city public clinics; thus, these findings may not be generalizable to all STD clinic patients. Second, the type-specific antibody test used in this analysis is no longer available, affecting the reproducibility of these findings in future seroprevalence studies. However, the sensitivity of the strip immunoblot assay for HSV-2 has been found to be >98%, and specificity >99%, compared with Western blot analysis [15]. Thus, our results are likely to be generally valid. Finally, this study was a secondary analysis of existing data and thus is not as strong as it would be if designed specifically to evaluate HSV-2 seroprevalence. Because it was a secondary analysis, we were unable to evaluate certain herpes-specific risks, such as whether a participant had ever had a sex partner with genital herpes or whether a participant had ever experienced genital sores or blisters.

Despite these limitations, the data from this large evaluation offer observations that will be important for future prevention efforts. First, the high seroprevalence rates among women and blacks, even among adolescents and those with few lifetime sex partners, indicate that HSV-2 prevention efforts must begin during early adolescence, before presentation for STD-related concerns and, ideally, even before the onset of sexual activity. Second, the high seroprevalence among blacks, even after adjustment for lifetime sexual exposure, implies that HSV-2 transmission may be influenced as much by sexual-network dynamics as by individual risk behaviors, potentially limiting the impact of prevention approaches aimed at changing individual behavior. Finally, the high rate of undiagnosed HSV-2 infection in this population likely contributes to ongoing transmission, highlighting the need for further evaluation of the risks and benefits of HSV-2 serologic screening as a prevention strategy.

Project RESPECT Study Group

Baltimore: Carolyn Erwin-Johnson, Andrew L. Lentz, Mary A. Staat, Dawn Sweet, Jonathan M. Zenilman (Principal Investigator [PI]). Denver: John M. Douglas (PI), Tamara Hoxworth, Ken Miller, William McGill. Long Beach: Ruth Bundy (co-PI), Laura A. Hoyt, C. Kevin Malotte, Fen Rhodes (PI). Newark: Michael Iatesta, Eileen Napolitano (co-PI), Judy Rogers, Ken Spitalny (PI). San Francisco: Gail A. Bolan (PI), Coleen LeDrew, Kimberly A. J. Coleman, Luna Hananel, Charlotte K. Kent. NOVA, Inc., Bethesda, Maryland: Robert Francis (PI), Christopher Gordon, Nancy Rosenshine (PI), Carmita Signes. Centers for Disease Control and Prevention: Sevgi Aral, Robert H. Byers, Beth Dillon, Martin Fishbein, Sandra Graziano, Mary L. Kamb, William Killean, James Newhall, Daniel Newman, Thomas A. Peterman, and Karen L. Willis.

Acknowledgments

We thank Rae Lynn Burke of Chiron for provision of the strip immunoblot reagents and equipment and Denise Brown for performance of the laboratory assays.

References

1. Nahmias AJ, Lee FK, Beckman-Nahmias S. Sero-epidemiological and -sociological patterns of herpes simplex virus infection in the world. Scand J Infect Dis Suppl 1990;69:19–36.
2. Corey L, Wald A. Genital herpes. In: Holmes KK, Sparling PF, Mardh PA, et al., eds. Sexually transmitted diseases. 3d ed. New York: McGraw-Hill, 1999:285–312.
3. Langenberg A, Benedetti J, Jenkins J, Ashley R, Winter C, Corey L. Development of clinically recognizable genital lesions among women previously identified as having "asymptomatic" herpes simplex virus type 2 infection. Ann Intern Med 1989;110:882–7.
4. Mertz GJ, Schmidt O, Jourden JL, et al. Frequency of acquisition of first-episode genital infection with herpes simplex virus from symptomatic and asymptomatic source contacts. Sex Transm Dis 1985;12:33–9.
5. Koutsky LA, Stevens CE, Holmes KK, et al. Underdiagnosis of genital herpes by current clinical and viral-isolation procedures. N Engl J Med 1992;326:1533–9.
6. Hook EW, 3rd, Cannon RO, Nahmias AJ, et al. Herpes simplex virus infection as a risk factor for human immunodeficiency virus infection in heterosexuals. J Infect Dis 1992;165:251–5.
7. Wald A, Link K. Risk of human immunodeficiency virus infection in herpes simplex virus type 2–seropositive persons: a meta-analysis. J Infect Dis 2002;185:45–52.
8. Fleming DT, McQuillan GM, Johnson RE, et al. Herpes simplex virus type 2 in the United States, 1976 to 1994. N Engl J Med 1997;337:1105–11.
9. van de Laar MJ, Termorshuizen F, Slomka MJ, et al. Prevalence and correlates of herpes simplex virus type 2 infection: evaluation of behavioural risk factors. Int J Epidemiol 1998;27:127–34.
10. Cowan FM, Johnson AM, Ashley R, Corey L, Mindel A. Relationship between antibodies to herpes simplex virus (HSV) and symptoms of HSV infection. J Infect Dis 1996;174:470–5.
11. Lowhagen GB, Jansen E, Nordenfelt E, Lycke E. Epidemiology of genital herpes infections in Sweden. Acta Derm Venereol 1990;70:330–4.
12. Austin H, Macaluso M, Nahmias A, et al. Correlates of herpes simplex virus seroprevalence among women attending a sexually transmitted disease clinic. Sex Transm Dis 1999;26:329–34.
13. Kamb ML, Fishbein M, Douglas JM Jr, et al. Efficacy of risk-reduction counseling to prevent human immunodeficiency virus and sexually transmitted diseases: a randomized controlled trial. Project RESPECT Study Group. JAMA 1998;280:1161–7.
14. Schmid DS, Brown DR, Nisenbaum R, et al. Limits in reliability of glycoprotein G–based type-specific serologic assays for herpes simplex virus types 1 and 2. J Clin Microbiol 1999;37:376–9.
15. Ashley RL, Wald A. Genital herpes: review of the epidemic and potential use of type-specific serology. Clin Microbiol Rev 1999;12:1–8.
16. Mertz GJ, Benedetti J, Ashley R, Selke SA, Corey L. Risk factors for the sexual transmission of genital herpes. Ann Intern Med 1992;116:197–202.
17. Quinn TC, Wawer MJ, Sewankambo N, et al. Viral load and heterosexual transmission of human immunodeficiency virus type 1. N Engl J Med 2000;342:921–9.
18. Laumann EO, Gagnon JH, Michael RT, Michaels S. Sexual networks. The social organization of sexuality: sexual practices in the United States. Chicago: University of Chicago Press, 1994:225–68.
19. Laumann EO, Youm Y. Racial/ethnic group differences in the prevalence of sexually transmitted diseases in the United States: a network explanation. Sex Transm Dis 1999;26:250–61.
20. Rothenberg R. How a net works: implications of network structure for the persistence and control of sexually transmitted diseases and HIV. Sex Transm Dis 2001;28:63–8.
21. Fleming DT, Wasserheit JN. From epidemiological synergy to public health policy and practice: the contribution of other sexually transmitted diseases to sexual transmission of HIV infection. Sex Transm Infect 1999;75:3–17.
22. Laga M, Manoka A, Kivuvu M, et al. Non-ulcerative sexually transmitted

diseases as risk factors for HIV-1 transmission in women: results from a cohort study. AIDS 1993;7:95–102.
23. Corey L. Raising the consciousness for identifying and controlling viral STDs: fears and frustrations—Thomas Parran Award Lecture. Sex Transm Dis 1998;25:58–69.
24. Corey L, Handsfield HH. Genital herpes and public health: addressing a global problem. JAMA 2000;283:791–4.
25. Wald A, Zeh J, Selke S, et al. Reactivation of genital herpes simplex virus type 2 infection in asymptomatic seropositive persons. N Engl J Med 2000;342:844–50.
26. Wald A, Baseman J, Selke S, et al. Sexual transmission of genital herpes simplex virus (HSV): a time-to-event analysis of risk factors associated with rapid acquisition [abstract 6]. In: Program and abstracts of the 2000 National STD Prevention Conference (Milwaukee). Washington, DC: Department of Health and Human Services, 2000.
27. Wald A, Langenberg AG, Link K, et al. Effect of condoms on reducing the transmission of herpes simplex virus type 2 from men to women. JAMA 2001;285:3100–6.
28. Handsfield HH, Stone KM, Wasserheit JN. Prevention agenda for genital herpes. Sex Transm Dis 1999;26:228–31.
29. Mindel A. Genital herpes—how much of a public-health problem? Lancet 1998;351:16–8.

AMERICAN
Family Physician
January 1991

Published by the American Academy of Family Physicians

Perinatal Transmission of Human Papillomavirus / 143 Antiviral Therapy / 197
Psychostimulants for Depression in the Medically Ill / 163
Upper Lobe Cavitary Disease / 187 Diagnosis of Developmental Disabilities / 132
Spontaneous Abortion / 175 Ketorolac / 207 Clinical Quiz / 31 Contents / 3
The Painful Shoulder / 119

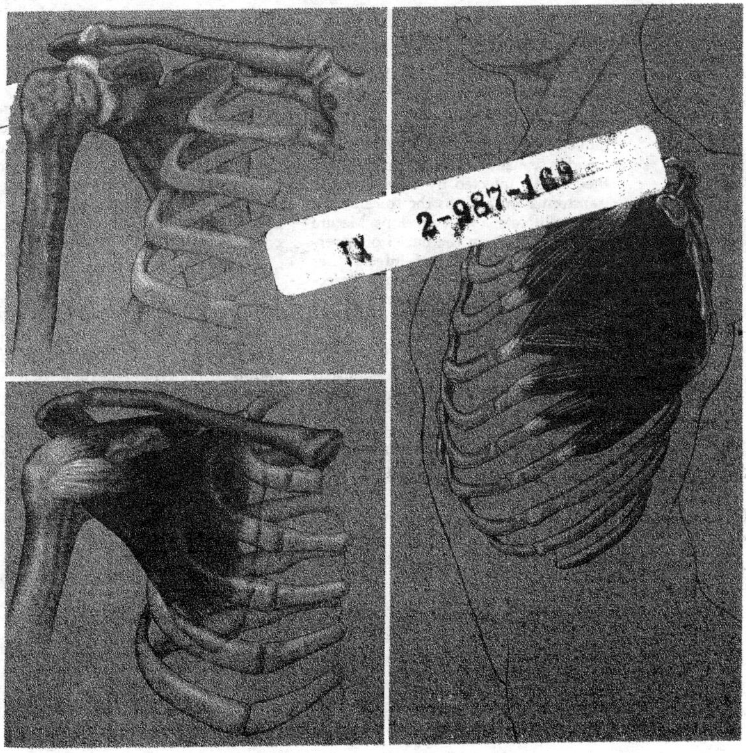

Perinatal Transmission of Human Papillomavirus

JAMES L. FLETCHER, JR., M.D., Medical College of Georgia, Augusta, Georgia

Human papillomavirus infection is probably the most prevalent sexually transmitted disease in the United States. In adults, it is associated with condylomata acuminata and with neoplastic changes ranging from dysplasia to carcinoma. Infected mothers may transmit human papillomavirus during the perinatal period; affected children face prolonged, difficult treatment for respiratory papillomatosis. Prevention of infection remains the best approach, since diagnostic and therapeutic methods are suboptimal.

The viral particles of human papillomavirus (HPV) were discovered in a cutaneous wart in 1949 and in a genital wart in 1969. HPV is a double-stranded DNA virus belonging to the papovavirus family.[1] At least 54 known types have been distinguished by DNA hybridization techniques[2]; types 6, 11, 16 and 18 have been found in sexually transmitted lesions. Epithelial cells infected by HPV undergo transformation and, as the transformed cells proliferate, a wart develops. Mature virus forms within the nuclei of superficial cells and, when shed, infects other cells, so that the cycle continues.[1] Infection may be followed by a latency period of many years.[2]

Epidemiology

Between 1966 and 1981, the estimated number of consultations for condylomata acuminata with office-based private physicians in the United States increased by 459 percent—from about 169,000 in 1966 to 946,000 in 1981. By comparison, genital herpes accounted for an estimated 295,000 consultations in 1981. HPV infections may be seriously underreported.[3] The total number of cases in the United States has been estimated at 12 million, with 750,000 new cases added each year.[4]

Most genital warts are found in young adults; in 1981, more than 65 percent of consultations for HPV involved patients 15 to 29 years of age. Condylomata acuminata are often encountered in family practice; in 1981, family physicians accounted for about 18 percent of the reported consultations by men and about 9 percent of those by women.[3]

Prevalence of infection varies with the population examined. A recent study in Baltimore[5] showed a 13 percent prevalence of HPV infection among 89 consecutive urban, sexually active female adolescents. West German investigators have estimated that about one-third of Western women of childbearing age may be infected with HPV and that one-third to one-half as many men are infected.[2]

Transmission

GENITAL LESIONS

The usual incubation period for HPV infection is one to three months. Warts can be found in all the classic genital sites and also in nongenital sites (e.g., oral cavity). Anal warts frequently occur in association with genital warts in women, less frequently so in men.[1] Penile warts are more common in circumcised than in uncircumcised men[6] and often involve the urethra. In women, warts tend to appear first at the posterior introitus and adjacent labia; perineal and anal extension occurs in about 20 percent of women with vulvar warts. Vaginal warts commonly involve the upper and lower thirds of the canal while sparing the middle third. Cervical warts may show the typical acuminatum morphology or may be flat lesions.[1]

Complications of condylomata acuminata in women include ulceration, hemorrhage, secondary infection and giant condylomas (lesions that appear benign histologically but behave clinically as if malignant). During pregnancy, condylomata acuminata often proliferate and enlarge to such an extent that decisions about labor and the route of delivery may be affected.[1,7,8]

Oncogenesis is the most feared adult complication. HPV has been shown to be associated with cancer (intraepithelial neoplasia and squamous carcinoma) of the penis, anus, vulva and cervix.[1,9] HPV types 16 and 18 appear to be most closely associated with cervical dysplasia and carcinoma; however, a recent study suggests that, since many women with normal Papanicolaou smears harbor HPV-16, a subtype of 16 may actually be responsible for neoplastic changes.[10]

A large and complicated French study[11] demonstrated a high prevalence (about 64 percent) of HPV-associated penile lesions among the sexual partners of women with cervical flat condylomata or cervical intraepithelial neoplasia. Visualization of lesions was enhanced in this study by colposcopy and the application of 5 percent acetic acid. Disturbingly, in about 43 percent of the men, HPV-associated macules and slightly elevated papules were observed only after the application of acetic acid. HPV DNA sequences were detected in 80 percent of the papules and 50 percent of the macules analyzed. In the Baltimore study of female adolescents,[5] the majority of papillomavirus infections were caused by HPV types associated with lower genital tract malignancies.

LARYNGEAL PAPILLOMATOSIS

HPV-associated disease is not limited to adults and adolescents. Genital warts have been reported in children born to mothers with condylomata acuminata, although such lesions are rare.[7] Much more serious is the inoculation of HPV into the upper respiratory tracts of infants born to affected mothers.

Infected infants may develop respiratory papillomatosis (*Figure 1*). Retrospectively, the presence of maternal condylomata acuminata has been reported in 55 to 65 percent of children with respiratory papillomatosis.[7] Although HPV infection does not appear to be associated with increased risk of spontaneous abortion, prematurity or other prenatal complications, its etiologic association with respiratory papillomatosis in infants and children now seems indisputable.[12-15]

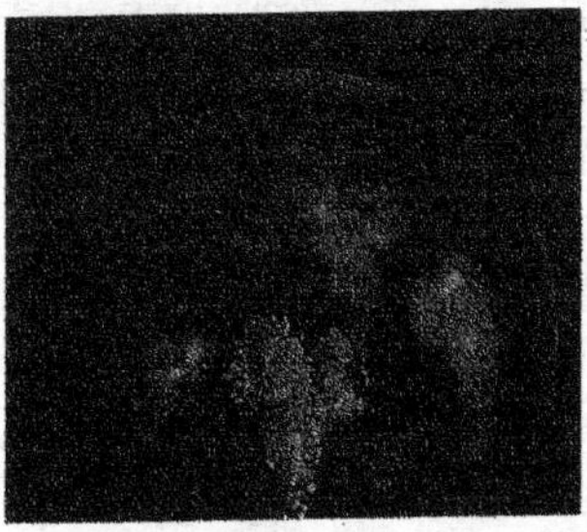

FIGURE 1. Laryngeal papillomatosis in an 18-month-old child.

The specifics of maternal-child transmission remain unknown. Understanding of the mechanisms is hampered by the fact that maternal lesions may be easily overlooked. Transmission typically follows vaginal delivery but has also been documented after cesarean section.[16] Estimates of the rate of transmission have been quite variable and are based on limited data.

The lifetime risk of developing laryngeal papillomatosis for children born to mothers with condylomata acuminata has been estimated as about one in 30.[7] Steinberg,[2] however, estimated a rate of one infant case per 1,000 infected mothers. This means that if the disease prevalence were about 20 percent among the approximately 5 million annual pregnancies in the United States and western Europe, about 1,000 affected babies could be expected each year. This may seem like a small number, but its importance is magnified by the devastation associated with juvenile respiratory papillomatosis—a disease without a consistently curative treatment, in which recurrence is the rule and lifelong morbidity and multiple operations result.[7]

The child with respiratory papillomatosis typically presents between two and three years of age, although the age of onset varies considerably and extends into adolescence. Papillomatosis follows an extremely variable course. Underlying factors that determine whether the disorder behaves in a benign or an aggressive fashion are not yet clear. Hoarseness and respiratory distress are the usual presenting features. The larynx, trachea and pulmonary tree may all be affected; the larynx may become completely obstructed.[2,17,18] Although one study showed no associated mortality among 23 patients followed from four to 45 years,[15] pulmonary involvement by papillomatosis may be severe.[19]

Diagnosis

Diagnosis of HPV infection is difficult. No tissue culture system is available. Electron microscopy is useful for detecting viral particles, and fluorescent or immunoperoxidase techniques stain the viral protein coat, but both of these techniques give a significant number of false-negative results. The definitive diagnostic technique is DNA hybridization (Southern blot), which detects both viral presence and type; however, this method is not feasible for most clinical laboratories.[2]

In the gynecologic clinical setting, condylomata acuminata may be detected by simple macroscopic or colposcopic inspection. Microscopic diagnosis may be made on a Pap smear or biopsy specimen; the finding of koilocytosis (halo cells) is diagnostic of HPV infection. However, Pap smears are relatively insensitive, yielding positive results in only about half of infected women.

Histologically, HPV is associated with changes that range from mild dysplasia to carcinoma in situ.[2] In fact, HPV may be the underlying diagnosis in many Pap smears reported as dysplasia.[1] It should also be noted that no current laboratory test is capable of detecting incubating condylomata acuminata.[3] Circulating antibodies to HPV can be detected by complement fixation in perhaps 50 percent of infected patients, but the finding is of little clinical use.[1]

Treatment

CONDYLOMATA ACUMINATA

For infected adults, treatment includes cytotoxic, cryosurgical and electrocautery therapies. Standard surgical excision is difficult because of the friability of the warts and their tendency to bleed. Cytotoxic agents include podophyllin, 10 to 25 percent, in tincture of benzoin, which may be applied once or twice weekly; if no regression has occurred by four treatments, alternative therapies should be considered. Podophyllin is best suited for small, external genital and perianal warts and probably should not be used to treat vaginal or intraurethral warts.[20,21] Because of its potential local and systemic toxicity, podophyllin therapy is contraindicated during pregnancy; fetal death and severe systemic maternal toxicity have been reported with the use of this agent during pregnancy.[7,22]

A 5 percent 5-fluorouracil (5-FU) cream (Efudex) may be effective for intraurethral warts, extensive vaginal warts, and lesions at other genital sites, but it can cause irritation.[1,21] This drug also is contraindicated during pregnancy, because of possible systemic absorption.[7,21]

Trichloroacetic acid is a caustic/astringent agent that may be applied topically to condylomatous lesions during pregnancy. A solution strength of 80 to 85 percent is probably optimal. For a single application, a 20 to 30 percent cure rate is all that can be expected; therefore, treatment may have to be repeated every seven to ten days.[7,20,21]

Cryosurgery or electrocoagulation/desiccation may be the treatment of choice during pregnancy, especially for cervical warts. Cryosurgery (applied for 30 to 60 seconds) is particularly useful for small warts.[1] Electrocoagulation/desiccation is contraindicated for lesions proximal to the anal verge.[20] Cryotherapy should be carried out with liquid nitrogen; use of a cryoprobe involves the risk of vaginal perforation and fistula formation.[20]

Treatment of cervical warts may be complicated, and patients with these lesions should undergo colposcopic examination. Management of pregnant patients with cervical warts should be carried out in consultation with an expert.[20]

Laser therapy (CO_2) has recently gained popularity. In some reports, a single treatment has resulted in effective ablation of visible lesions in 90 to 95 percent of women treated,[7] although extensive treatment of patients with subclinical disease (e.g., infection discovered by colposcopic examination) has been reported to be associated with significant side effects and histologic evidence of persistent infection.[23] Interferon alfa-2b (Intron A) has been approved for intralesional treatment of condylomata acuminata[24] and has also been used systemically.[25] Three clinical trials demonstrated modest intralesional efficacy with interferon alfa-2b, but the agent may hurt adolescent menstrual function and should not be used during pregnancy.[21,24]

Whatever treatment is chosen, it must be remembered that "therapy can be difficult, prolonged, and only marginally efficacious."[3(p308)] HPV infection may be multicentric and often cannot be seen on gross inspection.[26,27] It should also be apparent that current therapies focus on local treatment of what is actually regional pathology. Although various treatments

---

The Author

JAMES L. FLETCHER, JR., M.D.
is an assistant professor in the Department of Family Medicine at the Medical College of Georgia, Augusta. Dr. Fletcher graduated from Vanderbilt University School of Medicine, Nashville, Tenn., and served a residency in family medicine at the University of Connecticut Health Center, Farmington.

may eliminate visible lesions, the papillomavirus seems to be difficult to eradicate completely. Some investigators believe that HPV remains dormant in the skin and mucous membranes despite aggressive, destructive therapy, thus accounting for the high rate of recurrence.

RESPIRATORY PAPILLOMATOSIS

Treatment of respiratory papillomatosis in affected infants and children is surgical. Both standard excision and CO_2 laser treatment have been employed. Multiple procedures are the expectation. A recent multicenter trial showed no curative or substantial long-term benefit in 123 patients treated with leukocyte interferon.[28] Radiation therapy of lesions may result in malignant transformation, and tracheostomy is contraindicated because it may increase the risk of pulmonary disease.[2] In most cases, the frequency of surgery diminished with age, especially after puberty, but complete remission appears to be rare.[13]

Prevention

Screening of pregnant women for possible HPV infection is quite problematic. Such screening, coupled with an effective strategy for management, would be valuable in preventing neonatal transmission; however, currently available diagnostic methods and management remain suboptimal.

A Papanicolaou test and careful gross inspection for condylomatous lesions should be performed in all pregnant women. Abnormal Pap smear results should be followed up appropriately, probably in consultation with an expert. Exophytic warts should be treated with the goal of removing the lesions, but not of eradicating HPV.[20] Beyond these recommendations, routine screening for HPV infection lies within the realm of uncertainty. Recently, slide tests (e.g., ViraPap [Life Technologies, Inc., Gaithersburg, Md.]) for the detection of HPV DNA have become commercially available. Such tests, however, are fairly expensive, and their clinical practicality remains uncertain.

Cesarean delivery is recommended for women with genital warts large enough to produce mechanical difficulties with vaginal delivery, but routine operative delivery of women infected with HPV is not indicated, because of the relatively low rate of fetal transmission.[7,20] Careful postnatal maternal follow-up (e.g., Pap smears, colposcopy) is needed, as is prolonged follow-up of all children born to mothers with condylomata acuminata.

Final Comment

Infection with HPV is a common and potentially serious clinical event. Infected adults apparently face a significant risk of subsequent neoplastic disease. Children infected in the perinatal period face the prospect of respiratory papillomatosis and its prolonged, difficult treatment.

Diagnostic and therapeutic techniques remain suboptimal. Nonetheless, since HPV infection occurs in both sexes, with a peak incidence in 14- to 24-year-old persons, family physicians should be prepared to identify and manage this troublesome disease.

REFERENCES

1. Oriel JD. Genital warts. In: Holmes KK, ed. Sexually transmitted diseases. New York: McGraw-Hill, 1984:496-507.
2. Steinberg BM. Papilloma virus: effects on mother and child. In: Kundsin RB, Falk L, Hipp SS, eds. Impact on the fetus of parental sexually transmitted disease. New York: New York Academy of Sciences, 1988:118-28.

3. Condyloma acuminatum—United States, 1966-1981. MMWR 1983;32:306-8.
4. Goldsmith MF. 'Silent epidemic' of 'social disease' makes STD experts raise their voices [News]. JAMA 1989;261:3509-10.
5. Martinez J, Smith R, Farmer M, et al. High prevalence of genital tract papillomavirus infection in female adolescents. Pediatrics 1988;82:604-8.
6. Oriel JD. Natural history of genital warts. Br J Vener Dis 1971;47:1-13.
7. Schwartz DB, Greenberg MD, Dauod Y, Reid R. The management of genital condylomas in pregnant women. Obstet Gynecol Clin North Am 1987;14:589-99.
8. Reeves WC, Brinton LA, Garcia M, et al. Human papillomavirus infection and cervical cancer in Latin America. N Engl J Med 1989; 320:1437-41.
9. Daling JR, Weiss NS, Hislop TG, et al. Sexual practices, sexually transmitted diseases, and the incidence of anal cancer. N Engl J Med 1987;317:973-7.
10. Tidy JA, Vousden KH, Farrell PJ. Relation between infection with a subtype of HPV16 and cervical neoplasia. Lancet 1989;1(8649): 1225-7.
11. Barrasso R, De Brux J, Croissant O, Orth G. High prevalence of papillomavirus-associated penile intraepithelial neoplasia in sexual partners of women with cervical intraepithelial neoplasia. N Engl J Med 1987;317:916-23.
12. Hajek EF. Contribution to the etiology of laryngeal papilloma in children. J Laryngol 1956;70:166-8.
13. Cook TA, Brinschwig JP, Butel JS, Cohn AM, Goepfert H, Rawls WE. Laryngeal papilloma: etiologic and therapeutic considerations. Ann Otol 1973;82:649-55.
14. Quick CA, Watts SL, Krzyzek RA, Faras AJ. Relationship between condylomata and laryngeal papillomata. Ann Otol 1980;89:467-71.
15. Byrne JC, Tsao MS, Fraser RS, Howley PM. Human papillomavirus-11 DNA in a patient with chronic laryngotracheobronchial papillomatosis and metastatic squamous-cell carcinoma of the lung. N Engl J Med 1987;317: 873-8.
16. Shah K, Kashima H, Polk BF, Shah F, Abbey H, Abramson A. Rarity of cesarean delivery in cases of juvenile-onset respiratory papillomatosis. Obstet Gynecol 1986;68:795-9.
17. Kashima HK, Shah K. Recurrent respiratory papillomatosis: clinical overview and management principles. Obstet Gynecol Clin North Am 1987;14:581-8.
18. Brodsky L, Siddiqui SY, Stanievich JF. Massive oropharyngeal papillomatosis causing obstructive sleep apnea in a child. Arch Otolaryngol Head Neck Surg 1987;113:882-4.
19. Christiansen PL, Jorgensen K, Grontved A. Juvenile papillomatosis of the larynx. Acta Otolaryngol [Stockh] 1984;412(Suppl):37-9.
20. 1989 Sexually transmitted diseases treatment guidelines. MMWR 1989;38(Suppl):18-21.
21. Moscicki A-B. HPV infection in teenage girls. Med Aspects Hum Sexuality 1990;24:22-7.
22. Chamberlain MJ, Reynolds AL, Yeoman WB. Toxic effect of podophyllum application in pregnancy. Br Med J 1972;3:391-2.
23. Riva JM, Sedlacek TV, Cunnane MF, Mangan CE. Extended carbon dioxide laser vaporization in the treatment of subclinical papillomavirus infection of the lower genital tract. Obstet Gynecol 1989;73:25-30.
24. Alpha interferon for venereal warts. FDA Drug Bull 1988;Aug:19-20.
25. Interferon for treatment of genital warts. Med Lett Drugs Ther 1988;30:70-2.
26. Campion MJ. Clinical manifestations and natural history of genital human papillomavirus infection. Obstet Gynecol Clin North Am 1987;14:363-88.
27. Spitzer M, Krumholz BA, Seltzer VL. The multicentric nature of disease related to human papillomavirus infection of the female lower genital tract. Obstet Gynecol 1989;73: 303-7.
28. Healy GB, Gelber RD, Trowbridge AL, Grundfast KM, Ruben RJ, Price KN. Treatment of recurrent respiratory papillomatosis with human leukocyte interferon. Results of a multicenter randomized clinical trial. N Engl J Med 1988;319:401-7.

Sexually Transmitted Diseases Jan-Feb 1995

Condom Use to Prevent Incident STDs: The Validity of Self-Reported Condom Use

JONATHAN M. ZENILMAN, MD, CAROL S. WEISMAN, PHD, ANNE M. ROMPALO, MD, NANCY ELLISH, DRPH, DAWN M. UPCHURCH, PHD, EDWARD W. HOOK III, MD, AND DAVID CELENTANO, SCD

Background: Studies of sexual behavior and of interventions designed to reduce human immunodeficiency virus risk usually depend on self-report. Validation of self-reported condom use measures has not been previously reported in an urban population at high risk for sexually transmitted diseases and human immunodeficiency virus.

Methods: A prospective cohort study was performed in subjects recruited from sexually transmitted disease clinics in Baltimore. At enrollment, a questionnaire was administered that assessed human immunodeficiency virus risk factors and sexually transmitted disease history, and used a retrospective calendar to assess sexual events and condom use over the previous 30 days. Clinical evaluation was performed for sexually transmitted diseases. At follow-up 3 months later, the same procedures were repeated. Incident sexually transmitted diseases at follow-up were defined as new culture or serologically documented diagnoses of gonorrhea, chlamydia, syphilis, or trichomoniasis.

Results: In the 323 male and 275 female (total = 598) subjects who completed a follow-up visit, 21% reported using condoms for every act of sexual intercourse over the previous 30 days, 21% reported occasionally using condoms, and 59% reported not using condoms. At follow-up, 21% of subjects had new incident gonorrhea, chlamydia, syphilis, or trichomoniasis. Fifteen percent of the men who were "always" condom users had incident sexually transmitted diseases compared with 15.3% of "never users;" 23.5% of women who were "always" users had incident sexually transmitted diseases compared with 26.8% of "never" users.

Conclusions: In this high-risk population, self-reported condom use is not associated with lower sexually transmitted disease incidence. This finding suggests that self-reported condom use measures, even in a research setting, may be subject to substantial reporting bias.

Dr. Thomas Quinn provided chlamydia cultures for this study and helpful comments. Koren Waters assisted in preparation of the manuscript. This work was supported by grant AI29508 from NIH.

Dr. Zenilman is a Scholar of the American Foundation for AIDS Research (AmFAR Award 700322-12-RF).

Reprint requests: Jonathan M. Zenilman, MD, Division of Infectious Diseases-Ross 1159, Johns Hopkins University School of Medicine, 720 Rutland Avenue, Baltimore, MD 21205-2196.

Received for publication March 31, 1994, revised August 1, 1994, and accepted August 5, 1994.

From the Division of Infectious Diseases, Johns Hopkins University School of Medicine; Department of Health Policy and Management, Johns Hopkins University School of Hygiene and Public Health; and Preventive Medicine and Epidemiology, Baltimore City Health Department, Baltimore, Maryland.

NEARLY ALL STUDIES of human immunodeficiency virus (HIV) and sexually transmitted disease (STD) risk behaviors, including evaluations of interventions, rely upon self-reported measures of condom use as a major outcome variable.[1-18] However, the validity of these self-reports (that is, the extent to which the measures accurately reflect behavior) has not been evaluated.

The validity of self-reports is difficult to assess. Condom use under-reporting or over-reporting may occur because of embarrassment, perceptions of the researcher's expectations, problems with recall, or other factors.[1,2] For example, in many clinics that provide care for individuals at risk for STDs and HIV infection, condom use is heavily promoted, and patients may feel compelled to report they use condoms so they conform to the expectations of the clinical environment.

Most reported longitudinal studies of condom use have been in homosexual populations and have used crude measures of condom use.[11-14,17] These studies nonetheless suggest that condom use protects against STDs and increases as a result of behavioral interventions. With the epidemiology of the HIV epidemic shifting into heterosexual, inner-city populations,[19,20] understanding condom use patterns in these groups is crucial to developing effective interventions. Studies of heterosexuals attending STD clinics have focused on the knowledge, attitudes, and behaviors associated with self-reported condom use and have found varying rates of condom use and a trend toward increasing condom use over time.[4,18]

Previous attempts to validate condom use have focused on the community level by monitoring retail sales[21] or by collecting used condoms from sewers. At the individual level, studies have addressed reliability (that is, consistency of responses over time or between raters) more often than validity. For example, regular heterosexual partners are highly consistent in their retrospective reports of the frequency and types of sexual behaviors, including condom use, over a 30-day period.[22] The problem, of course, is that partners may both report inaccurate information. Validity at the individual level might be assessed indirectly through redemption of condom coupons[23] or by using biological markers such as STDs. Incident STDs also have been used as measures of high-risk, unprotected sexual behavior after HIV counseling interventions.[24,25]

In the present report, we assess the validity of self-reported condom use in a prospective observational study of high-risk clients of inner-city STD clinics, using incident STDs as biological markers. No previous studies have examined the relationship between self-reported condom use and incident STDs acquired during the same period for which condom use is reported.

Studies using STDs as outcome measures are methodologically complex. They require prospective evaluation of high-risk, often difficult-to-follow patient populations. They also require substantial logistical, technical, and laboratory support. In particular, accurate incident STD assessment in longitudinal studies requires comprehensive laboratory assessment for multiple STDs at each visit to detect asymptomatic cases. In this study, we examined the association between self-reported condom use and incident STDs for a sample of subjects interviewed and examined at two times in STD clinics.

Methods

Study Design and Sample

Condom use patterns and incident STDs were determined as part of a prospective study on the transmission and acquisition of STDs, which was described previously.[22] The study was conducted in two Baltimore City Health Department STD clinics. These clinics serve approximately 20,000 patients at 35,000 visits annually. Clinic attendees have high incidence rates of STD. Baltimore has one of the highest gonorrhea rates in the country,[26] and about half of all gonorrhea cases in the city are identified in these clinics. Confidential HIV counseling and testing is offered to attendees who have not been tested within the previous 3 months.[27] In 1992, over 18,000 HIV tests were performed, and the seroprevalence rate was 4%.

Eligible subjects were male and female clients presenting at the clinic for evaluation of symptoms, for a check-up, or as a sexual partner of another patient. All participants gave written informed consent, and the study was performed with the approval of The Johns Hopkins Joint Committee on Clinical Investigation. At the enrollment visit, each subject received a baseline interview administered by a study clinician. The interview measured STD symptoms and history, detailed sexual behaviors (including an inventory of sexual partners and condom use), attitudes about high-risk behaviors and condom use, (including self-efficacy for condom use), perceived HIV/STD risk, health care use, and alcohol and drug use.

After the interview, patients received a directed physical examination that included culture for *Neisseria gonorrhoeae*, *Chlamydia trachomatis*, and *Trichomonas vaginalis*. Wet mount examination of vaginal secretions was performed on all women. Patients with genital ulcers were evaluated for *Treponema pallidum* by dark-field microscopy. All subjects were evaluated serologically for syphilis using the rapid plasma reagin confirmed by fluorescent treponemal antibody tests. Individuals who consented to HIV testing (92% of participants) were evaluated using the standard enzyme-linked immunosorbent assay and Western blot algorithm.[28] Gonorrhea and chlamydia were diagnosed on the basis of a positive culture for *N. gonorrhoeae* or *C. trachomatis*. Syphilis was diagnosed using clinical criteria, dark-field lesion examination, and serologic tests.[29] *Trichomonas* was diagnosed on the basis of either a positive culture or wet mount exam.

After the initial visit, all subjects were given an appointment for a follow-up visit 3 months later. At the follow-up visit, an abbreviated form of the interview was administered, along with repeated physical examination and diagnostic tests.

Measures

The key independent variable was self-reported condom use during the 30-day period before the follow-up clinic visit. Data were obtained in the follow-up interview using a calendar devised for each subject (and shown to the subject by the interviewer), as described previously.[22] Subjects provided partner-specific information indicating on which days they had engaged in sexual activity, the type of sexual activity (vaginal, oral, or anal sex), the number of episodes of each type on each day, and whether a condom was used for each sexual encounter. The measure of condom use constructed from this information for this analysis was calculated by dividing the number of times condoms were used during vaginal and anal sex by the number of vaginal and anal sex acts reported with all partners. Thus, this measure sales[21] or by collecting used condoms from sewers. At the individual level, studies have addressed reliability (that is, consistency of responses over time or between raters) more often than validity. For example, regular heterosexual partners are highly consistent in their retrospective reports of the frequency and types of sexual behaviors, including condom use, over a 30-day period.[22] The problem, of course, is that partners may both report inaccurate information. Validity at the individual level might be assessed indirectly through redemption of condom coupons[23] or by using biological markers such as STDs. Incident STDs also have been used as measures of high-risk, unprotected sexual behavior after HIV counseling interventions.[24,25]

In the present report, we assess the validity of self-reported condom use in a prospective observational study of high-risk clients of inner-city STD clinics, using incident STDs as biological markers. No previous studies have examined the relationship between self-reported condom use and incident STDs acquired during the same period for which condom use is reported.

Studies using STDs as outcome measures are methodologically complex. They require prospective evaluation of high-risk, often difficult-to-follow patient populations. They also require substantial logistical, technical, and laboratory support. In particular, accurate incident STD assessment in longitudinal studies requires comprehensive laboratory assessment for multiple STDs at each visit to detect asymptomatic cases. In this study, we examined the association between self-reported condom use and incident STDs for a sample of subjects interviewed and examined at two times in STD clinics.

Methods

Study Design and Sample

Condom use patterns and incident STDs were determined as part of a prospective study on the transmission and acquisition of STDs, which was described previously.[22] The study was conducted in two Baltimore City Health Department STD clinics. These clinics serve approximately 20,000 patients at 35,000 visits annually. Clinic attendees have high incidence rates of STD. Baltimore has one of the highest gonorrhea rates in the country,[26] and about half of all gonorrhea cases in the city are identified in these clinics. Confidential HIV counseling and testing is offered to attendees who have not been tested within the previous 3 months.[27] In 1992, over 18,000 HIV tests were performed, and the seroprevalence rate was 4%.

Eligible subjects were male and female clients presenting at the clinic for evaluation of symptoms, for a check-up, or as a sexual partner of another patient. All participants gave written informed consent, and the study was performed with the approval of The Johns Hopkins Joint Committee on Clinical Investigation. At the enrollment visit, each subject received a baseline interview administered by a study clinician. The interview measured STD symptoms and history, detailed sexual behaviors (including an inventory of sexual partners and condom use), attitudes about high-risk behaviors and condom use, (including self-efficacy for condom use), perceived HIV/STD risk, health care use, and alcohol and drug use.

After the interview, patients received a directed physical examination that included culture for *Neisseria gonorrhoeae*, *Chlamydia trachomatis*, and *Trichomonas vaginalis*. Wet mount examination of vaginal secretions was performed on all women. Patients with genital ulcers were evaluated for *Treponema pallidum* by dark-field microscopy. All subjects were evaluated serologically for syphilis using the rapid plasma reagin confirmed by fluorescent treponemal antibody tests. Individuals who consented to HIV testing (92% of participants) were evaluated using the standard enzyme-linked immunosorbent assay and Western blot algorithm.[28] Gonorrhea and chlamydia were diagnosed on the basis of a positive culture for *N. gonorrhoeae* or *C. trachomatis*. Syphilis was diagnosed using clinical criteria, dark-field lesion examination, and serologic tests.[29] *Trichomonas* was diagnosed on the basis of either a positive culture or wet mount exam.

After the initial visit, all subjects were given an appointment for a follow-up visit 3 months later. At the follow-up visit, an abbreviated form of the interview was administered, along with repeated physical examination and diagnostic tests.

Measures

The key independent variable was self-reported condom use during the 30-day period before the follow-up clinic visit. Data were obtained in the follow-up interview using a calendar devised for each subject (and shown to the subject by the interviewer), as described previously.[22] Subjects provided partner-specific information indicating on which days they had engaged in sexual activity, the type of sexual activity (vaginal, oral, or anal sex), the number of episodes of each type on each day, and whether a condom was used for each sexual encounter. The measure of condom use constructed from this information for this analysis was calculated by dividing the number of times condoms were used during vaginal and anal sex by the number of vaginal and anal sex acts reported with all partners. Thus, this measure reflects consistency of condom use, or degree of exposure to STD transmission, during the last 30 days.

The objective outcome variable measured at the follow-up visit was having any one of the following incident STDs: syphilis, gonorrhea, chlamydia, or trichomoniasis. These infections diagnosed at the follow-up visit represented new infection since the enrollment visit, because routine testing by reference methods (i.e., culture for all except syphilis) was conducted at both visits. Subjects with infections diagnosed at the enrollment visit or with suspected exposure to an STD were treated immediately. In cases where infections were not clinically apparent at the enrollment visit (e.g., a positive culture result that is returned later), these patients were recalled for definitive treatment. Because treatment efficacy is greater than 95% with current regimens for syphilis, gonorrhea, chlamydia, and trichomoniasis, we can confidently assert that these infections diagnosed at follow-up visits represented new infections.

Herpes and human papillomavirus infection were not included in the measure of incident STDs because it was difficult to ascertain whether a clinical episode at the follow-up visit represented new infection or manifestations of a chronic, prevalent infection. Human immunodeficiency virus was not included because no seroconversions between enrollment and follow-up were identified in study subjects.

Statistical Analysis

Analyses were performed using PC-SAS 6.04 (SAS Institute, Cary, NC). Univariate and multivariate analysis was conducted separately for men and women. Gender differences were assessed using the chi-squared test or Fisher's exact test for cell size <5. Unconditional multiple logistic regression was used to estimate odds ratios and 95% confidence limits, using a diagnosis of "definite STD" (syphilis, gonorrhea, chlamydia, or trichomoniasis) at follow-up as the outcome variable. Covariates, in addition to condom use, considered in multiple regression analyses of disease status at follow-up, included disease risk factors such as number and types (regular, casual, new) of sexual partners in the last 30 days, frequency of anal and vaginal intercourse in the last 30 days, having an STD diagnosis at enrollment, and age. We also included substance use patterns within the past 30 days, including IV drugs, crack cocaine use, and alcohol use. Alcohol use was categorized as either more or less than twice weekly, a categorization that in our population has been shown to be associated with syphilis and HIV.[30] Length of time between enrollment and follow-up visit also was included as a covariate.

Results

The subjects of this analysis were 323 men and 275 women who were enrolled in the study between 1990 and 1992, made a follow-up clinic visit, and were sexually active during the follow-up period. On average, the follow-up visits occurred 4.4 months after the enrollment visit. Returning subjects (52% of the enrolled subjects) did not differ significantly from nonreturning subjects on a number of sociodemographic and behavioral variables relevant to this study. However, there was a tendency for employed women and men who were high school graduates to be more likely to return for follow-up visits. Table 1 describes the study subjects regarding sociodemographic variables and STD status at enrollment. Men were significantly older than women and were more likely to be black and currently employed. Only 3% of men and 1% of women reported anal intercourse.

The condom use pattern reported by these subjects for the 30 days before the follow-up visit is described in Table 2. Twenty-one percent of the subjects reported using condoms in all acts of vaginal and anal intercourse, 21% reporting using condoms some of the time (i.e., more than 0% but less than 100% of the time), and 59% using condoms in no acts of intercourse. Therefore, the measure was trichotomized for analysis (always used condoms, sometimes used condoms, never used condoms). In men and women, a self-report of always using condoms was associated with fewer sex

TABLE 1. Sociodemographic Characteristics of Subjects at Enrollment

Characteristics	Men (n = 323) %	Women (n = 275) %
Age*		
≤20	17.7	31.3
21–29	42.7	43.3
30–64	39.6	25.4
Race*		
Black	97.5	90.6
White	2.5	7.6
Other	—	1.8
Education		
<high school	33.9	40.1
High school or more	66.1	59.9
Marital status		
Never married	78.2	80.0
Married	7.5	8.0
Separated, widowed, divorced	14.3	12.0
Employment status*		
Not working	37.9	54.2
Currently working	62.1	45.8
Diagnosis of syphilis, gonorrhea, *Chlamydia* or *Trichomonas*		
Yes	31.3	36.4
No	68.7	63.6

* Sex difference is significant ($P < .05$) by the chi-square test.

TABLE 2. Self-Reported Condom Use In Sexual Activity, 30 Days Before Follow-up Clinic Visit

How Frequently Were Condoms Used During Sexual Acts?	Males (n = 323)		Females (n = 275)	
	No.	%	No.	%
None of the time	183	57	169	61
Some of the time	67	21	55	20
All of the time	73	23	51	19

partners and fewer sexual episodes per month (Table 3). In contrast, always using condoms was inversely associated with having had oral sex (i.e., subjects who reported having oral sex were less likely to report condom use during vaginal intercourse), and in men, having a regular sex partner.

We hypothesized that self-reported condom use should be inversely related to incident STDs. Subjects reporting always using condoms should have a significantly lower rate of disease than subjects who never use condoms or who use them some of the time. Table 4 shows the incidence rate of new STD according to self-reported condom use for men and women. (Incidence of gonorrhea, chlamydia, and syphilis were similar in both genders; women had higher rates of trichomoniasis, which accounts for their overall higher STD rates.) At enrollment, self-reported condom use was associated with a protective effect in women, but not men. There was no association between self-reported condom use and STD acquisition during follow-up for either gender. Results were not associated with circumcision state or use of contraception (in women).

In terms of specific diagnoses at follow-up, 0.5% (n = 3) of subjects were diagnosed with syphilis, 9.0% (n = 54) had gonorrhea, 6.2% (n = 37) had chlamydia, and 8.9% (n = 53) had *Trichomonas*. Included are 20 subjects with two or three diagnoses. Seventy-nine percent (n = 473) of subjects did not acquire any of these diseases during the follow-up period. We then evaluated the relationship between self-reported condom use and specific disease diagnoses at follow-up. Only one significant relationship was found. At the follow-up visit, none of 72 men who reported always using condoms had a diagnosis of chlamydia, compared with 16 of 251 (6.3%) of "sometimes" or "never users" (P = .015; Fisher's exact test).

Table 5 presents results of multiple logistic regression analyses, separately for men and women, regarding the determinants of incident STDs. In the models presented here, the objective was to examine the relative predictive importance of condom use (or lack of condom use) and other risk factors. Self-reported condom use in the previous 30 days was not found to be a significant predictor of protection from incident STDs for men or women. The only predictor that is statistically significant for both men and women was having an STD diagnosis at enrollment. This variable increased the odds of an incident STD by 3.11 for men and by 1.99 for women.

For men, other statistically significant predictors of incident STDs were having vaginal or anal intercourse nine or more times in the previous 30 days and making a follow-up clinic visit more than 3 months after the enrollment visit (i.e., later than was recommended by the clinic). This suggests that a new infection—rather than the study follow-up appointment—may have caused them to return. Thus, men who had more sexual activity, who had a STD diagnosis at enrollment, and who were less compliant with regard to return visits were at a higher risk for incident STDs.

For women, other significant predictors of incident STDs were engaging in oral or anal sexual activity within the last 30 days, IV drug use within the last 30 days, crack cocaine use within the last 30 days, and younger age.

One possible explanation for the failure of self-reported condom use to predict incident disease is that subjects might have been using condoms incorrectly. Therefore, we recomputed the regression models and

TABLE 3. Characteristics of Condom Users—Baltimore STD Transmission-Acquisition Study

	Condom Use							
	Male				Female			
	Never (%)	Sometimes (%)	Always (%)	P	Never (%)	Sometimes (%)	Always (%)	P
≥2 partners (past 30 days)	22	37	14	.028	8	20	6	.002
>9 sexual episodes past month	45	38	15	<.001	35	35	17	.006
Definite STD at visit 1	30	37	31	.539	36	38	37	.961
New partner (past 30 days)	20	31	21	.160	6	13	8	.285
Casual partner (past 30 days)	12	16	14	.677	7	13	10	.350
Regular partner (past 30 days)	87	84	72	.011	94	91	86	.182
Had oral sex	32	26	11	.003	34	25	12	.006

TABLE 4. Number and Percent of Individuals With STD Diagnosis* at Enrollment and Follow-up, by Self-Reported Condom Use† and Gender

	Condom Use							
	Males				Females			
	Enrollment		Follow-up		Enrollment		Follow-up	
	No.	%	No.	%	No.	%	No.	%
Never	64	32.0	28	15.3	67	39.6	45	26.8
Sometimes	21	29.6	16	23.5	17	28.3	13	23.1
Always	11	35.5	11	15.3	5	17.9	12	23.5
χ^2 trend	0.018		0.118		6.380‡		0.321	

* Diagnosis of syphilis, gonorrhea, *Chlamydia*, or *Trichomonas*.
† Condom use reported for each act of vaginal or anal intercourse, with all sex partners, during 30 days before visit.
‡ $P = 0.012$.

included a variable indicating whether the subject reported that a condom ever broke during sexual activity during the time for which condom use was reported. Although 17% of subjects reported at least one instance of breakage, this variable was not a significant predictor of disease for men or women.

Discussion

The results of this analysis demonstrate no significant relationship between self-reported condom use and incident STDs for male and female clients of STD clinics in Baltimore. Because self-reports of condom use frequently form the basis for assessing HIV risk-reduction interventions, our findings suggest an important deficiency in studies that rely on such self-reports.

If condoms protect against acquisition of STDs, there are at least three possible explanations for the failure to validate self-reported condom use using incident STDs. First, subjects may not be reporting their condom use behavior accurately because of recall bias. Recall could be affected among subjects who used drugs or alcohol during sexual activity. Although other researchers have noted that alcohol use reduces the level of condom

TABLE 5. Predictors of Incident STDs* by Gender

	Men (n = 322)		Women (n = 273)	
	Odds Ratio	95% CI	Odds Ratio	95% CI
Condom Use†				
Some of the time	1.50	0.68–3.30	0.69	0.30–1.56
All of the time	1.41	0.59–3.34	0.58	0.24–1.40
Two or more partners, last 30 days	1.20	0.45–3.19	1.58	0.41–6.09
Types of partners, last 30 days‡				
Casual partner	1.69	0.65–4.39	0.73	0.18–2.99
New partner	1.95	0.80–4.76	2.77	0.95–8.07
Frequency of intercourse, last 30 days§				
5–8 times	1.28	0.51–3.19	1.19	0.55–2.59
9+ times	2.55	1.12–5.80	0.89	0.42–1.91
Any oral or anal sex, last 30 days	0.87	0.41–1.84	0.44	0.20–0.97
Intravenous drug use, last 30 days	0.70	0.14–3.51	20.96	4.20–104.70
Cocaine use, last 30 days	0.46	0.04–5.34	5.01	1.16–21.66
Alcohol use, last 30 days	1.17	0.55–2.47	0.71	0.26–1.93
STD diagnosis at enrollment	3.11	1.64–5.88	1.99	1.06–3.73
Age‖				
21–29 years	0.62	0.26–1.48	0.42	0.21–0.84
30–64 years	0.70	0.27–1.78	0.25	0.10–0.62
Followup visit >3 months after enrollment	1.98	1.01–3.85	0.89	0.45–1.77

* Outcome variable is any of the following incident STDs at follow-up: syphilis, gonorrhea, *Chlamydia*, or trichomoniasis.
† Omitted reference category is "none of the time."
‡ Omitted reference category is regular partner only. A "regular partner" is defined as someone "you've been having sex with for longer than a month and that you have sex with often." A "casual partner" is someone "you've been having sex with for longer than a month but only have sex with occasionally." A "new partner" is someone "you've had sex with for the first time in the past 30 days."
§ Intercourse includes both vaginal and anal. Omitted reference category is fewer than five instances of intercourse.
‖ Omitted reference category is 14–20 years of age.
CI = confidence interval.

use,[31] validation of those reports has not been addressed. In our multivariate analysis, drug use significantly increased the odds of disease among women only.

Second, subjects may be reporting their actual condom use, but they may not be using condoms properly. That is, condoms may be breaking, falling off, being reused, or being put on after intromission has begun, thereby putting the subjects at risk for an STD. This and most other studies of condom use are limited in their ability to directly assess the technical skills required to use a condom. Except for one measure of condom breakage, which was not associated with disease status, we were unable to analyze the effects of proper condom use.

Third, patients may be misrepresenting their actual condom use. That is, although the majority of subjects (59%) reported they never used condoms, we suspect that at least some of the remaining subjects overestimated their actual condom use. In general, reports of high-risk behaviors or their preventive interventions may be contaminated by the social desirability of responses, especially within an environment that provides continuous educational messages. In the STD clinic setting, reporting use of condoms is likely to be perceived by subjects as the "right" answer. Latkin recently commented on a similar phenomenon in reports of high-risk IV drug use behaviors.[32] We suspect that there was misrepresentation because of social desirability, despite that patients were enrolled in an observational study that was not intended to modify behavior.

This study has several limitations. First, patients attending STD clinics may not be representative of the general population at risk, and the results may not be generalizable. However, we believe that this population, because of its demonstrated high-risk behaviors and high rates of STDs, including HIV, represents the group with the greatest need for intensive intervention. Furthermore, from a practical standpoint, the STD clinic contains one of the few populations where incidence rates of STD are high enough so that STDs can be used as biological validators of self-reported data. In populations where STD incidence is low, the sample sizes required become unmanageable.

Second, there may have been selection bias in determining who returned to the clinic for the follow-up visit and interview. Patients who became symptomatic may have been more likely to return for treatment and may have been more likely to misrepresent condom use. These two factors could have skewed our results toward increased STD incidence in reported condom users. Our data indicate, however, that there were no significant demographic or baseline risk profile differences between returners and nonreturners.

Third, at follow-up, condom use and sexual histories were measured only for the previous 30 days. Conceivably, asymptomatic or mildly symptomatic STDs that were acquired before the 30 day calendar period could have been misclassified as incident infections in those patients who reported consistent condom use. Incompletely treated STDs at enrollment, if they occurred, also could have been misclassified. However, we believe that these issues did not affect our results. In a recent review of the epidemiologic literature, Brunham estimated that the mean duration of infectivity for gonorrhea is 6 days and for chlamydia 18 days.[33] Our incidence rates of STDs (10–15% over 3 months) are similar to those reported earlier in retrospective and prospective studies of our patient population and in a prospective study of STD clients in Birmingham, Alabama.[34] Thus, carryover of untreated or partially treated infections do not appear to be an issue. Furthermore, especially in men, because >95% of gonococcal and >70% of chlamydia infections become symptomatic within 4 weeks, the vast majority of STD infections diagnosed at follow-up would have been acquired within the previous 30 days.

Although we demonstrated that prior infection with an STD at enrollment is an independent risk factor for infection at follow-up (Table 4), we believe this represents a manifestation of continued risk-taking behavior, similar to that seen epidemiologically in "core groups" or "repeaters."[35,36]

Our results demonstrate important limitations of current knowledge about the measurement of condom use. This is the first longitudinal study to demonstrate that self-reported condom use is not associated with rates of acquisition of STDs. Because valid measures of condom use are needed to assess risk status and changes in risk status over time, future research is needed to develop more accurate measures. Suggestions include conducting interviews in as "neutral" a context as possible (e.g., interviewing in a nonclinical setting or using machine-mediated interviewing techniques rather than live interviewers) so that subjects do not feel compelled to give socially desirable responses. Another suggestion is to include more extensive measures of the appropriateness of condom use (e.g., by requiring a demonstration of technical skills on a model and by including questions about condoms breaking, falling off, or being reused) so that reported use can be "weighted" according to the subject's skills.

References

1. Catania JA, Gibson DR, Chitwood DD, et al. Methodological problems in AIDS behavioral research: Influences on measurement error and participation bias in studies of sexual behavior. Psychol Bull 1990; 108:339–362.

2. Weller SC. A meta-analysis of condom effectiveness in reducing sexually transmitted HIV. Soc Sci Med 1993; 36:1635–1644.
3. Catania JA, Coates TJ, Stall R, et al. Prevalence of AIDS-related risk factors and condom use in the United States. Science 1992; 258:1101–1106.
4. Weinstock HS, Lindan C, Bolan G, et al. Factors associated with condom use in a high-risk heterosexual population. Sex Transm Dis 1993; 20:14–20.
5. CDC. Drug use and sexual behaviors among sex partners of injecting drug users—United States 1988–90. MMWR 1991; 40:855–860.
6. CDC. Condom use among male injecting drug users—New York City 1987–1990. MMWR 1992; 41:617–620.
7. CDC. Sexual behavior among high school students—United States, 1990. MMWR 1992; 40:885–888.
8. Moatti J-P, Bajos N, Durbec J-P, Menard C, Serrand C. Determinants of condom use among French heterosexuals with multiple partners. Am J Public Health 1991; 81:106–109.
9. Kost K, Forrest JD. American women's sexual behavior and exposure to risk of sexually transmitted diseases. Fam Plann Perspect 1992; 24:244–254.
10. CDC. Sexual behaviors of STD clinic patients before and after Earvin "Magic" Johnson's HIV-infection announcement—Maryland 1991–1992. MMWR 1993; 42:45–48.
11. CDC. Changes in sexual behavior and condom use associated with a risk-reduction program—Denver, 1988–1991. MMWR 1992; 41:412–415.
12. Kelly JA, Murphy DA, Roffman RA, et al. Acquired immunodeficiency syndrome/human immunodeficiency virus risk behavior among gay men in small cities. Arch Intern Med 1992; 152:2293–2297.
13. Valdiserri RO, Lyter D, Leviton LC, Callahan CM, Kingsley LA, Rinaldo CR. Variables influencing condom use in a cohort of gay and bisexual men. Am J Public Health 1988; 78:801–805.
14. Kelly JA, St Laurence JS, Brasfield TL. Predictors of vulnerability to AIDS risk behavior relapse. J Consult Clin Psychol 1991; 59:163–166.
15. CDC. Condom use and sexual identity among men who have sex with men—Dallas 1991. MMWR 1993; 23:7–14.
16. Schechter MT, Craib KJ, Willoughby B, et al. Patterns of sexual behavior and condom use in a cohort of homosexual men. Am J Public Health 1988; 78:1535–1538.
17. Silvestre AJ, Kingsley LA, Wehman P, Dappen R, Ho M, Rinaldo CR. Changes in HIV rates and sexual behavior among homosexual men 1984 to 1988/92. Am J Public Health 1993; 83:578–580.
18. Upchurch DM, Brady WE, Reichart CA, Hook EW III. Behavioral contributions to acquisition of gonorrhea in patients attending an inner-city sexually transmitted disease clinic. J Infect Dis 1990; 161:938–941.
19. Holmes KK, Karon JM, Kreiss J. The increasing frequency of heterosexually acquired AIDS in the United States, 1983–1988. Am J Public Health 1990; 80:858–862.
20. Nwanyanwu OC, Conti LA, Cieselski CA, et al. Increasing frequency of heterosexually transmitted AIDS in Southern Florida: Artifact or reality? Am J Public Health 1993; 83:571–573.
21. Moran JS, Janes HR, Peterman TA, Stone KM. Increase in condom sales following AIDS education and publicity, United States. Am J Public Health 1990; 80:607–608.
22. Upchurch DM, Weisman CS, Shepherd M, et al. Interpartner reliability or reporting of recent sexual behaviors. Am J Epidemiol 1991; 143:1159–1166.
23. Solomon MZ, DeJong W. Preventing AIDS and other STDs through condom promotion: A patient education intervention. Am J Public Health 1989; 79:453–458.
24. Zenilman JM, Erickson B, Fox R, Reichart C, Hook EW III. Effect of HIV Posttest Counseling on STD Incidence. JAMA 1992; 267:843–845.
25. Otten MW, Zaidi AA, Wroten JE, Witte JJ, Peterman TA. Changes in sexually transmitted disease rates after HIV testing posttest counseling, Miami, 1988 to 1989. Am J Public Health 1993; 83:529–533.
26. Centers for Disease Control. Sexually transmitted disease surveillance 1991. DHHS-USPHS-CDC. Atlanta, GA: CDC, 1992.
27. Erickson B, Wasserheit JN, Rompalo AM, Brathwaite W, Glasser D, Hook EW III. Routine voluntary HIV screening in the STD clinic clients: Characterization of infected clients. Sex Transm Dis 1990; 17:194–199.
28. CDC. Interpretation and use of the Western Blot assay for serodiagnosis of human immunodeficiency virus type 1 infections. MMWR 1989; 38(Suppl S-7):1–7.
29. Hutchinson CM, Rompalo AM, Reichart CA, Hook EW III. Characteristics of patients with syphilis attending Baltimore STD clinics. Arch Intern Med 1991; 151:511–516.
30. Zenilman JM, Hook EW III, Shepherd M, Smith P, Rompalo AM, Celentano D. Alcohol and other substance use in STD clinic patients: Relationship with STDs and prevalent HIV infection. Sex Transm Dis 1994;21:220–225.
31. Clapper RL, Lipsitt LP. A retrospective study of risk taking and alcohol-meditated unprotected intercourse. J Subst Abuse Treat 1991; 3:91–96.
32. Latkin CA, Vlahov D, Anthony JC. Socially desirable responding and self-reported HIV infection risk behaviors among intravenous drug users. Addiction 1993; 88:517–526.
33. Brunham RC, Plummer FA. A general model of sexually transmitted disease epidemiology and its implications for control. Med Clin N Am 1990; 74:1339–1352.
34. Louv WC, Austin H, Alexander WJ, Checks J. A clinical trial of nonoxynol-9 for preventing gonococcal and chlamydia infections. J Infect Dis 1988; 158:518–523.
35. Rothenberg RB. The geography of gonorrhea: Empirical evidence of core group transmission. Am J Epidemiol 1983; 117:688–694.
36. Rice RJ, Roberts PL, Handsfield HH, Holmes KK. Sociodemographic distribution of gonorrhea incidence: Implications for prevention and behavioral research. Am J Public Health 1991; 81:1252–1258.

13. Background on Virginity Pledge Study

TheMedicalInstitute
SCIENCE·CHARACTER·EDUCATION
P.O. BOX 162306 • Austin, TX 78716-2306
512.328.6268 • SALES 800.892.9484
FAX 512.328.6269 • medinstitute@medinstitute.org

For Immediate Release

Contact: Jeff Rosenberg
301-972-0646

Columbia Study of Virginity Pledges Reveals Much More About Teen Sexual Activity Than Media Reports Reveal, Notes The Medical Institute for Sexual Health

AUSTIN, TX (March 12, 2004) – "A just-released follow-up study about youth who signed virginity pledges reveals much more about the sexual health and sexual decision-making of American young people than what is being reported in the popular press," commented Joe S. McIlhaney, Jr., MD, Chairman and Founder of The Medical Institute for Sexual Health.

Dr. McIlhaney criticized advocates who seized upon the study who dismiss abstinence-education programs as ineffective. He also noted that the study, released Wednesday at a conference by Columbia University professor Dr. Peter Bearman, finds some important health effects of virginity pledges.

"First of all, we must realize that virginity pledges are not the same as abstinence-education. These programs generally include character and relationship education, skill-building to support healthy choices, information on sexually transmitted diseases (STD), and parent and teen communication skills.

"While the Columbia study looked only at virginity pledges and their impact on later sexual activity of youth, the study did find important health effects, most notably that teens who took the pledge delayed sexual debut an average of 18 months and, after becoming sexually active, had fewer sexual partners. This is important because the number of sexual partners is the number one risk factor for contracting an STD."

Dr. McIlhaney pointed out other important findings from the study:

- The percentage of those 18 to 24 years of age who had intercourse before marriage was 88 percent among pledge takers and 99 percent among non-pledge takers. Those who signed pledges were therefore 12 times more likely than non-pledge takers to be virgins at marriage.

- Twice as many pledge-takers were married by age 23 as compared to non-pledge takers – it is therefore very possible that sexual activity of many pledge-takers was with their fiancé.

- While the prevalence of STDs was essentially the same between the two groups – those who had not signed virginity pledges had slightly higher rates than those who did – it must be noted that STD rates in this study are for the period of the study only. Given the earlier age of sexual debut and higher number of sexual partners for youth who did not sign virginity pledges, it is reasonable to expect that these youth had more STD infections in the past than did pledge-takers.

- The Columbia study reports that, once sexually active, young people who had signed pledges were less likely to use condoms than young people who had not signed pledges. Yet the study reveals an almost equal STD rate among the two groups, raising questions about the effectiveness of condoms as an STD risk-reduction tool. It is interesting to note that of the group who used condoms the most, only 59 percent actually used condoms and that the group with the lowest condom use rate had the lowest STD rate.

The Medical Institute for Sexual Health is a non-profit educational organization established in 1992 to identify, evaluate, and communicate credible scientific data to promote healthy decisions and behavior. To learn more about The Medical Institute visit www.medinstitute.org

National Institute of Child Health & Human Development

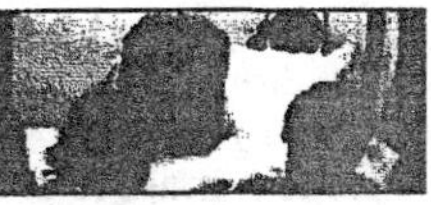

January 5, 2001

Virginity Pledge Helps Teens Delay Sexual Activity

Teens who pledged to remain a virgin until marriage began sexual activity much later than their peers who did not take such a pledge, according to an analysis of data from a study funded by the National Institute of Child Health and Human Development (NICHD) and several other Federal agencies. On average, teens who took a public or written pledge to remain abstinent until marriage delayed having sex about one-third longer than comparable teens who had not pledged, the analysis showed. However, the effectiveness of pledging depended on the student's age. Among older teens (18 and older), pledging had no effect. Among 16 and 17 year olds, pledgers delayed sex significantly compared to non-pledgers. Among the youngest teens, the effect of pledging depended strongly on the social environment of the teen's school.

Although the analysis showed that pledgers delayed sexual intercourse, it also indicated that among those teens who eventually did begin to have intercourse, pledgers were less likely to use contraception than were non-pledgers.

"This analysis shows that virginity pledges can be an effective tool for delaying sexual intercourse in the teenage years," said Duane Alexander, M.D., Director of the NICHD. "The analysis has provided sound, substantial information for educators and others who work with youth to take into account when planning interventions to help teens to avoid early sex and its associated risks."

The analysis, conducted by Peter S. Bearman, Ph.D., now of Columbia University, and Hannah Brückner, Ph.D., now of Yale University, appears in the January American Journal of Sociology. The researchers conducted their analysis on information from the National Longitudinal Study of Adolescent Health (Add Health), a comprehensive survey of 90,000 seventh through twelfth graders. The survey was designed to measure the effects of family, peer group, school, neighborhood, religious institution, and community on behaviors that promote good health. Detailed information about the survey is available http://www.cpc.unc.edu/addhealth http://www.cpc.unc.edu/addhealth. A summary of the survey and other explanatory materials are available at http://www.nichd.nih.gov/new/releases/adolescent.html. Dr. Bearman co-designed the Add Health survey while he was at the Carolina Population Center of the University of North Carolina at Chapel Hill (UNC-CH).

The study found that as of 1995, more than two and a half million adolescents had taken spoken or written pledges to remain virgins until they marry. The Southern Baptist Church began the pledge movement and it has since grown to include hundreds of church, school, and college chapters. The movement is loosely organized around more than 80 independent organizations that sponsor public pledges and rallies.

"Early sexual intercourse increases the risk for unwanted pregnancy and sexually transmitted diseases such as AIDS," said Christine Bachrach, Chief of NICHD's Demographic and Behavioral Sciences Branch. "The research by Drs. Bearman and Brückner highlights a potential strategy for prevention efforts that should be tested further in experimental studies."

The two researchers began by analyzing information from adolescents who were virgins when the Add Health survey began. The researchers compared the likelihood of later having sexual intercourse among both pledgers and non-pledgers. The researchers noted that pledgers and non-pledgers differed in many respects.

Compared to non-pledgers, pledgers were more likely to be religious, of Asian ancestry, to score lower on a verbal vocabulary test, and to be in a romantic relationship. They were also less advanced in pubertal development, on average, than were non-pledgers. Dr. Bearman noted that three of these factors, independent of the virginity pledge, are likely to result in adolescents delaying sexual intercourse: being more religious, of Asian Ancestry, and less advanced in pubertal development. However, the differences between pledgers and non-pledgers did not account for pledgers' greater success in delaying sexual activity. When compared to non-pledgers having these same three characteristics, pledgers still were more likely to delay sexual activity a third longer than were non-pledgers.

The researchers found that the effectiveness of pledging among the youngest teens depended on the characteristics of their school. In socially "open" schools-those in which students had a large number of friends and romantic ties outside the school-the effectiveness of pledging increased with the number of students who pledged. In fact, each one percent increase in the proportion of students pledging resulted in a two percent increase in delaying sexual intercourse. Pledgers appeared to need the social support of fellow pledgers in order to remain abstinent.

The researchers observed a very different effect in socially "closed" schools. In these schools-where most friendships and romantic ties occur within the school-a higher percentage of pledgers actually decreased the pledge's effectiveness. If comparatively few adolescents in these schools pledged, pledging was effective in delaying sexual intercourse. However, if 30 percent or more of the students pledged, pledgers were no more likely to delay sexual intercourse than were non-pledgers. The researchers theorized that the pledge may appeal to some students because it gives them a unique identity, apart from the crowd. After too many of their fellow students joined them in pledging, abstinence lost its special appeal. The researchers noted that socially closed schools are in the minority, composing only 30 percent of schools in the survey.

"Once the pledge becomes normative, it ceases to have an effect," Bearman and Bruckner wrote. "The pledge identity is meaningful, consequently, only if it is a minority identity, a common situation for identity movements."

The researchers also examined the consequences of breaking a pledge. Previous studies have found that girls who began having sex experienced a slight decrease in self-esteem. Teens who broke their pledges, however, suffered no greater loss of self-esteem than did non-pledgers who began having sexual intercourse.

###

14. Congressional Women's Caucus Letter of Support for HPV Education Law

Thursday, October 26, 2000

▶ PUBLIC HEALTH & EDUCATION

7 HUMAN PAPILLOMAVIRUS: Women's Caucus Urges Hastert's Support for Education Proposal

The Congressional Women's Caucus yesterday wrote a letter to House Speaker Dennis Hastert (R-Ill.) expressing its "support for language addressing the human papillomavirus." Stating that the caucus "recognize[s] that HPV is associated with nearly all cancers of the cervix," the letter continues, "[w]e support efforts to educate all Americans about HPV so that women can make fully informed choices that will affect their health." The caucus members also pledge their support of educating health care providers about HPV "so they are fully prepared to identify and care for those who are infected." They added, "We feel strongly that women need to be encouraged at all levels about the importance of regular pap smears, which can detect cervical cancer in its earlier stages." The letter concludes by asking for Hastert's support in enacting an HPV education and prevention proposal (Women's Caucus letter, 10/25). The group did not specify whether it supported any specific existing legislative proposals regarding HPV. Deborah Arrindell, senior director of public policy at the American Social Health Association, stated that "we support the efforts of Congress to increase education and awareness about HPV and emphasize the importance of screening. Increased awareness about HPV and cervical cancer prevention will reduce unnecessary deaths from this preventable cancer" (Ingrid Dries-Daffner, *Kaiser Daily Reproductive Health Report*, 10/25).

Congress of the United States
House of Representatives
Washington, DC 20515

October 25, 2000

The Honorable Dennis Hastert
The Speaker
H232 Capitol
Washington, D.C. 20515

Dear Mr. Speaker,

We are writing to express our support for language addressing the human papilloma virus (HPV) during these last days of the 106th Congress.

While the vast majority of HPV infections do not lead to serious problems, and only a small percentage can lead to cervical cancer, we recognize that HPV is associated with nearly all cancers of the cervix. In 1999, it was estimated that 12,800 cases of invasive cervical cancer would be diagnosed in the U.S. and that 4,800 women would die from cervical cancer. Unfortunately, most Americans have never even heard of HPV.

We support efforts to educate all Americans about HPV so that women can make fully informed choices that will affect their health. We also support efforts to educate health care providers about the disease so they are fully prepared to identify and care for those who are infected. Finally, we feel strongly that women need to be encouraged at all levels about the importance of regular pap smears, which can detect cervical cancer in its earlier stages.

Education and awareness about HPV is extremely important. We urge your support for these efforts and look forward to working with you to enact an HPV education and prevention proposal this year.

We thank you for your consideration.

Sincerely,

Carolyn B. Maloney
Sue Kelly
Louise M. Slaughter
Sue Myrick
Lois Capps
Connie Morella

The Honorable Dennis Hastert
Page 2

Carolyn McCarthy Jo Ann Emerson

Anna G. Eshoo Tillie K. Fowler

Carolyn Cheeks Kilpatrick Jan Schakowsky

Juanita Millender-McDonald Donna M. Christensen

Julia Carson

15. ACOG's Opposition to HPV Education Law

Condom Cover-up: "Safe-sex" advocates are manipulating the medical accuracy debate

March 2, 2004 (Updated: March 18, 2004)

by Jerry Gramckow

They called a meeting for supporters of medically inaccurate sex education and no one showed up. Can't imagine why. So, next they held a reception for proponents of fear-based sex education. Empty room. Hmm.

In a July 2002 speech, Planned Parenthood President Gloria Feldt stated that first on her federation's five-point agenda for the 21st century is to codify **"medically accurate"** sexuality education. "We can harness our power to advance our agenda by working together with one vision, one goal, one set of issues, one message spoken by many voices," Feldt stated.[1]

Planned Parenthood has been behind numerous efforts to introduce and pass so-called "medically accurate" sex education bills at the federal level and in many states—in some states where the bills have failed, they have been introduced again and again.

Speaking before the California State Assembly in 1999, Katherine Kneer, CEO of Planned Parenthood Affiliates of California, said, "Despite overwhelming public support for responsible sex education, we continue to find some school districts in California adopting medically inaccurate and fear-based sex education curricula that endanger young people."[2]

By labeling their version of sex education "medically accurate" and their opposition's version inaccurate and "fear based," Planned Parenthood and friends had captured the strategic high ground in the cultural war of words. After all, what parents would want their kids to learn a fear-based and medically inaccurate form of sex education?

What parents would want their kids to learn a fear-based and medically inaccurate form of sex education?

However, with the recent (but long-delayed) government admission that condoms are not effective in preventing the spread of human papillomavirus (HPV),[3] the medical accuracy mantra is boomeranging back at the "safe-sex" crowd. Now, the same people and organizations that have regularly rolled out bills and initiatives requiring "medical accuracy" in sex education are demanding that the latest and most accurate condom studies be concealed.

Every year 5.5 million Americans contract HPV, a sexually transmitted virus that can lead to cervical, penile and anal cancer. In fact, several studies have concluded that *HPV is the leading (some say only) cause of cervical cancer.*

So why do Planned Parenthood and other "safe sex" promoters want to hide these medically accurate facts? Quite simply, because they fear that exposure to the truth about HPV will lead to an erosion of public confidence in condoms—and condom promotion is, after all, the foundation for "safe sex."

History of the HPV/condom cover-up

When Congressman Tom Coburn (R-OK) introduced the Breast and Cervical Cancer Treatment Act in 1999, "safe-sex" advocates quickly went on the defensive. Julie Scott, field representative for the American College of Obstetricians and Gynecologists (ACOG) stated, "HPV should not be singled out. Just as you should not single out HIV."

ACOG continued to encourage condom use for HPV prevention, despite the fact that the National Cancer Institute had concluded, "Condoms are ineffective against HPV...."[4]

In 2000, ACOG boasted it "worked closely with the Senate to ensure that the HPV provisions were not included in the Senate [version of Coburn's] bill."[5]

To address the Senate opposition, Rep. Coburn sent a letter to Senator Tom Harkin "clarify[ing] any confusion" about his HPV proposal. Coburn's letter responded to a *CongressDaily* article that claimed the provision "requires a warning label on condoms stating that they do not protect against the spread of HPV." Senator Harkin had called such a label a "sticking point" for the bill. Coburn explained that the bill's language did not call for a warning label; instead the provision "merely states that the FDA must ensure that the existing condom labels are 'medically accurate and not misleading.'" Coburn added, "It also directs the CDC to conduct studies to determine the prevalence of HPV and develop HPV prevention and education programs for the public and health care providers."[6]

On July 31, 2000, Lifestyle condoms claimed in a press release about its new "succulent flavors" condoms that, "According to the Centers for Disease Control and Prevention, the proper and consistent use of latex condoms is the most effective way to prevent the spread of such diseases as HIV, AIDS and HPV."[7] In response to the Lifestyle press release, the Physicians Consortium wrote the following as part of a letter to Ansell Healthcare (parent company of Lifestyle condoms):

> Your publicity campaign for LifeStyle condoms has all the appearances of ignoring science for the sake of selling a product. For years the public health community and condom industry have been reluctant to disclose the truth about the inability of condoms to prevent the spread of HPV, and to a lesser degree, chlamydia and herpes genitalis—type 2. Please send us any documentation from the CDC that supports your public statements. Absent such documentation, we can only consider your promotional activities to be an irresponsible threat to the health of millions of women.[8]

"Under **Coburn's proposal**, HPV cases would be reported confidentially to state health departments in an effort to monitor the epidemic, identify at-risk populations and analyze any changes in transmission. Coburn said that the CDC already requires physicians to report cases of 58 infectious diseases, however it does not extend that requirement to HPV, which the CDC estimates affects 45 million Americans and is responsible for 99.7% of all cervical cancers. In a related amendment, Coburn would require condom packages to feature a warning label in the same style as those on tobacco and alcohol products. Coburn suggests the following warning: 'The National Cancer Institute has found that condoms are ineffective in preventing the transmission of the human papillomavirus, the cause of cervical cancer.'"
National Cervical Cancer Coalition, **http://www.nccc-online.org/news_0054.htm**

In her reply to the Physicians Consortium, Ansell's regional director wrote the following: "Our public relations firm prepared the release and *mistakenly included HPV*among the diseases for which latex condoms provide protection [emphasis added]."[9]

"Our public relations firm prepared the release and mistakenly included HPVamong the diseases for which latex condoms provide protection.

Three days after the letter to the Physicians Consortium, Lifestyle Condoms issued another press release with no direct reference to condoms as being protective against HPV, instead inferring that condoms make sex "safe and responsible," but not openly correcting its error in the previous press release. The Physicians Consortium followed with letters to Ansell and to the Food and Drug Administration (FDA) making clear that Lifestyle's amended press release did nothing to erase the misinformation of the first release.[10]

Deborah Wolf, at the FDA's Office of Compliance Center for Devices and Radiological Health then wrote in a November 17, 2000, letter to Ansell, "Ansell's second press release does not adequately correct the misinterpretation created by the first press release."[11]

In December 2000, the Physicians Consortium filed a Freedom of Information Act Request with the Department of Health and Human Services, calling for "Any and all additional correspondence and guidance provided to said condom manufacturers dealing with issues of implementation, correspondence from condom manufacturers and any and all industry trade groups, and any and all correspondence between federal agencies relating to said guidance."[12]

In a February 2001 letter to Congressman Coburn, the FDA stated that Ansell/Lifestyle's removal of the HPV reference from its press release (without directly acknowledging its earlier misstatement) was an "appropriate" revision.

In July of 2001 the National Institute of Allergy and Infectious Diseases, National Institutes of Health and the U.S. Department of Health and Human Services released a report the agencies had sat on for a year. "Scientific Evidence on Condom Effectiveness for Sexually Transmitted Disease (STD) Prevention" reported that condoms are approximately 85 percent effective in preventing the spread of HIV and somewhat effective in preventing female-to-male transmission of gonorrhea.

Beyond that, the top public health specialists in the nation concluded in the report that evidence is insufficient to cite condoms as being effective in preventing the spread of any of the other 25 or more STDs. Regarding HPV, "the Panel concluded that there was no epidemiologic evidence that condom use reduced the risk of HPV infection...."

Even with a Capitol building press conference calling for the resignation of CDC Director Jeffrey P. Koplan, this landmark report got little mainstream media attention.

The silence persists

The CDC released its HPV report (the one saying it cannot recommend condoms as a primary prevention method against HPV transmission) on February 4, 2004. Nearly four weeks later, among major media outlets, only *The Washington Times* had reported on the CDC finding and its report to Congress.

"Despite the fact that it is the most common sexually transmitted virus in the United States, over three-fourths of the respondents in a recent poll have never heard of HPV. CDC, the federal agency charged with disease prevention, provides no guidance to states on how to curtail the spread of HPV or leadership to health care providers on how to counsel or even recognize those with the virus. Because of this failure, thousands will die every year and millions more will become infected and pass the disease onto others. In addition, the organization which claims to advocate for women's health, the American College of Obstetricians and Gynecologists (ACOG), has aggressively opposed Congressional efforts to educate the public about HPV." **IWF Alert on Condom Warning Labels** 6/13/2000

Independent Women's Forum

Take action (The CDC report on HPV is available as a PDF at **http://www.cdc.gov/nchstp/dstd/HPVInfo.htm**)
Write a letter to your local newspaper's editor, asking when he or she will assign a reporter to write about the CDC's HPV report.
Call local radio call-in shows and discuss the CDC's HPV report.
Take a copy of the CDC's HPV report to a school board meeting and insist the school's sex education program informs students of condom ineffectiveness against HPV.
Write to your local, state and federal representatives and insist they support truly medically accurate sex education that includes the HPV report and the findings of the multi-agency report "Scientific Evidence on Condom Effectiveness for Sexually Transmitted Disease (STD) Prevention" (available as a PDF at **http://www.niaid.nih.gov/dmid/stds/condomreport.pd**).

---

[1]"Winning with Agenda Discipline," Planned Parenthood Federation of America "Speeches" Web site, **http://www.plannedparenthood.org/about/thisispp/president.html**

[2]"California State Assembly Approves Bill that Sets New Standards for Sex Education in Schools," PPAC: News Stories, Planned Parenthood Affiliates of California, 6/3/1999, **http://www.ppacca.org/news/read.asp?ID=75**

[3]"The available scientific evidence is not sufficient to recommend condoms as a primary prevention strategy for the prevention of genital HPV infection." REPORT TO CONGRESS, Prevention of Genital Human Papillomavirus Infection, p. 4 **http://www.cdc.gov/std/HPV/2004HPV%20Report.pdf**

[4]Letter from Richard D. Klausner, Director of National Cancer Institute to Tom Bliley Jr., Chairman of the House Commerce Committee, February 16, 1999.

[5]ACOG Legislative News, 10/6/2000

[6]The Kaiser Daily Reproductive Health Report, 10/25/2000 (also see HPV Update -- October 2000 Date: Sun, 29 Oct 2000 15:59:41 -0500, October 2000, **http://www.beyondaids.org/hpvupdate.html**)

[7]http://www.physconsortium.com/pdfs/aoacu_press_release_07_31_00.pdf

[8]Physicians Consortium letter to Mr. Harry Boon, CEO, Ansell Healthcare, August 30, 2000, **http://www.physconsortium.com/pdfs/aoacu_pc_to_ansell_08_30_00.pdf**

[9]Letter from Kerry A. Hoffman, Regional Director, Ansell Personal Healthcare, September 8, 2000,
http://www.physconsortium.com/pdfs/aoacu_ansell_to_pc_09_08_00.pdf

[10]Lifestyles Condoms press release, September 11, 2000,
http://www.physconsortium.com/pdfs/aoacu_amended_press_release_09_11_00.pdf

[11]Letter from Deborah Wolf, FDA, to Harry Boon, CEO of Ansell Healthcare, Nov. 17, 2000,
http://www.physconsortium.com/pdfs/aoacu_fda_to_ansell_11_17_00.pdf

[12]Physicians Consortium letter to United States Department of Health and Human Services, **http://www.physconsortium.com/pdfs/aoacu_pc_to_foia_officer_12_11_00.pdf**

Kaiser Daily HIV/AIDS Report

Monday, October 25, 1999

PUBLIC HEALTH & EDUCATION

HPV: Coburn Will Offer Amendments on Tracking, Condom Warning Labels Despite ACOG Protest

The Breast and Cervical Cancer Act of 1999 -- which would allow states to provide low-income women who do not qualify for Medicaid with access to cervical and breast cancer screening and treatment -- is slated for a House Commerce Committee mark up Thursday, and Rep. Tom Coburn (R-OK) said he will offer his amendments to the bill, despite protests from the American College of Obstetricians and Gynecologists and other women's health groups regarding his recent statement that sexual abstinence outside of marriage is the only way to protect against the human papilloma virus. His proposed amendments to the bill, sponsored by Reps. Rick Lazio (R-NY) and Anna Eshoo (D-CA), include mandates that the CDC conduct "sentinel surveillance" as well as other studies to determine the prevalence of HPV in various regions. HHS would then be required provide Congress with the best strategies for prevention and how to make HPV a "reportable disease" within two years. Finally, Coburn will propose that warning labels be placed on condoms alerting users "that they do not effectively prevent the transmission of HPV and that HPV can cause cervical cancer."

ACOG's Beef

In a letter responding to Coburn's statement on HPV prevention, Drs. Ralph Hale, ACOG's executive vice president, and William Hoskins, president of the Society of Gynecologic Oncologists, assert that they "agree with [Coburn] that HPV is a major public health concern and that more information should be available to help stop transmission of this disease." However, they were "alarmed" by Coburn's abstinence stance, and in particular, his "suggestion that all women with HPV will get cervical cancer, and that by avoiding HPV, women can absolutely avoid cervical cancer." Hale and Hoskins argue that "all men and women engaged in sexual intercourse, whether in or outside of marriage, are in danger of transmitting and receiving HPV." Further, they assert that "married couples are not shielded from this disease anymore than anyone else," because research "has proven that HPV can lie dormant and undetected in individuals and can be unknowingly transmitted to a sexual partner, including a spouse." They maintain that "while there are millions of women infected with HPV, only a small percentage of these women will ever develop significant cervical neoplasia, leading to cervical carcinoma." Hale and Hoskins conclude by requesting that Coburn alter his legislative proposals. Writing in response, Coburn maintained that virtually all cervical cancer is caused by HPV, and said that ACOG should offer some specific changes to his amendments. "What has ACOG done [to address HPV]? Zero," Coburn said, adding that the issue has become controversial because "it's not politically correct" to suggest abstinence. And he maintains, "You cannot have sex safely outside marriage." Roland Foster, Coburn's senior legislative assistant, said Coburn had not received a response from ACOG regarding specific recommendations or changes to his amendments (Amanda Wolfe, *Kaiser Daily Report*, 10/25).

Kaiser Daily HIV/AIDS Report

((●))

Kaiser Daily HIV/AIDS Report

Thursday, October 28, 1999

POLITICS & POLICY

HPV: Coburn Amendments Folded Into Breast and Cervical Cancer Treatment Act; Markup Scheduled Today

Amendments Rep. Tom Coburn (R-OK) proposed to the Breast and Cervical Cancer Treatment Act concerning the connection between cervical cancer and the human papillomavirus will be included in this morning's scheduled House Commerce Committee markup, despite the continued objections of the American College of Obstetricians and Gynecologists. The measure would allow states to extend Medicaid coverage for breast and cervical cancer-related treatments for certain low-income women diagnosed through the CDC's early detection program. Coburn's amendments direct the CDC to begin tracking and reporting HPV, as well as implement an HPV research and education program. He is also seeking HPV-related condom warning labels stating that condoms are not effective against HPV, and that HPV can result in cervical cancer. ACOG opposes the warning label, asserting that it will deter condom use and further spread other preventable STDs, such as HIV.

Poison Pens?

In a series of letters, ACOG lobbed criticism at Coburn for his suggestion that abstinence was the only method to prevent HPV, and expressed concern that the congressman has not "made clear that not all women diagnosed with HPV will develop cervical cancer." ACOG maintains that while specific strains of HPV may cause cervical cancer, scientific data also suggests that smoking, failure to obtain regular cytologic screenings and immunosuppression also could impact a woman's chances for developing the disease. However, in a subsequent letter to Coburn, ACOG and the Society of Gynecologic Oncologists said they were willing to work with Coburn in crafting legislative proposals that would address HPV and its connection to cervical cancer. As evidence of their opposition to the proposed condom label, ACOG sent out another letter this week assuring committee members they were "still committed" to the HPV issue, and as the legislation moved forward, they would continue to seek approval to change the language of the bill.

Condoms Still Work

Julie Scott, ACOG's federal representative, said, "HPV should not be singled out. Just as you can't single out HIV." Instead, the group suggested that the label inform consumers about the effectiveness of condoms against disease transmission and should utilize "medically accurate," up-to-date research. Scott added that the label should be crafted "delicately," so as not to discourage all condom use. ACOG wants to ensure that women don't receive the wrong message about condoms, she said, and that they understand that condoms still are critical for protecting against STDs including HIV. Scott added, "If you put out a fear message, that will only lead to huge problems." Scott also advocated that HPV be clearly defined, to avoid confusion with HIV, and that women should understand that not all cases of HPV lead to cervical cancer. ACOG's current patient education concerning HPV "still encourages condom use," telling women that some cases of HPV can be prevented by using condoms, and encourages regular screenings and PAP tests, Scott said, adding that if the language remains unchanged after the committee markup, "That doesn't mean the issue is over." But Roland Foster, Coburn's senior legislative aide, dismissed the group's proposal as "a desperate attempt by ACOG to save face on an issue they have been AWOL on" (Amanda Wolfe, *Kaiser Daily Report*, 10/28).

Kaiser Daily HIV/AIDS Report

((●))

Tom A. Coburn, M.D.
Press Release

FOR IMMEDIATE RELEASE
October 28, 1999

Contact: Michael Schwartz
(202) 225-2701

Coburn Asks 'Where's ACOG?' as Cancer Bill Is Approved

WASHINGTON — The House Commerce Committee unanimously approved legislation intended to fight cervical and breast cancer, despite the opposition of the American College of Obstetricians and Gynecologists to a cancer-prevention amendment proposed by Rep. Tom A. Coburn (R-OK), a physician who specializes in family practice and obstetrics.

The bill, jointly sponsored by Reps. Rick Lazio (R-NY) and Anna Eshoo (D-CA), authorizes treatment for uninsured women diagnosed at federally-funded health centers with breast or cervical cancer.

During negotiations on the bill, Coburn noted that the primary cause of cervical cancer has been identified as human papillomavirus (HPV), a sexually transmitted disease. He urged that, in addition to providing treatment, the legislation should also emphasize prevention, and the sponsors accepted an amendment authored by Coburn to fight the spread of HPV.

The Coburn amendment requires the Centers for Disease Control to study the prevalence of HPV infection and to carry on educational activities about HPV among health care providers and the public. It also directs the Food and Drug Administration to develop a warning label for condom packages to advise consumers that the National Cancer Institute has found condoms to be ineffective in preventing the transmission of HPV.

While the Coburn amendment was accepted by both Republicans and Democrats on the Commerce Committee, it was opposed by the American College of Obstetricians and Gynecologists (ACOG).

"ACOG has been AWOL in the fight to protect women's health in recent years," charged Coburn. "For some reason, they have taken the position that ignorance is better than knowledge. When we proposed that pregnant mothers be tested for HIV so they would get treatment and not pass the virus on to their babies, ACOG came out in favor of ignorance. When we proposed testing newborn babies so we could get the same benefits, ACOG came out in favor of ignorance. Now that we have achieved a consensus in favor of shedding light on the HPV epidemic, ACOG is still in favor of ignorance.

"It is very disappointing that the organization most directly concerned with the health of American women has not done what it could have done to help prevent disease. I hope that when we take our next step in Congress to improve women's health, ACOG will be pulling with us instead of against us."

— 30 —

Kaiser Daily HIV/AIDS Report

Friday, October 29, 1999

POLITICS & POLICY

HPV: Committee Clears Breast and Cervical Cancer Treatment Act; Adds Coburn Amendments

The House Commerce Committee yesterday unanimously approved the Breast and Cervical Cancer Treatment Act including Rep. Tom Coburn's (R-OK) amendments to address HPV. The bill would allow states to extend Medicaid coverage for breast and cervical cancer-related treatments for certain low-income women diagnosed through the CDC's early detection program. Under the bill, the federal government would reimburse states for at least 75% of the treatment costs for women diagnosed in the federal screening programs who are ineligible for Medicaid but are under age 65, lack health insurance and have incomes up to 250% of the poverty line (Rich, *National Journal News Service*, 10/28). The measure was delayed for several weeks while Reps. Rick Lazio (R-NY) and Anna Eshoo (D- CA), the bill's sponsors, worked out an agreement with Coburn, settling on amendments that call for the CDC to track HPV cases and create a public assistance program, as well as direct the FDA to create a label on condom packages to warn users that condoms do not effectively prevent HPV and that HPV can cause cervical cancer (Rovner, *CongressDaily/A.M.*, 10/29). In her introductory remarks before the committee, Eshoo called the amendments a "good compromise" and one she believed the entire committee could accept (Amanda Wolfe, *Kaiser Daily Report*, 10/29). In earlier committee meetings, Rep. Henry Waxman (D-CA) was wary of adding Coburn's amendments and had called for further research on HPV. Asserting that he "strongly" supported the bill, Waxman still expressed concern about the condom label. He said that in informing people of the fact that condom use may not block the transmission of HPV, "we want to be sure that we do not end up with an unintended effect of confusing people about the situations when condoms do work -- in HIV transmission to name only one, and actually reduce their use. I fear that the requirements that both the label and all labeling include information on HPV can result in so much information on a small package that it reduces the effectiveness of any information" (Waxman release, 10/28). Waxman is not alone is his criticism of the amendments. Coburn, who has drawn the ire of the American College of Obstetricians and Gynecologists, lashed out at the group yesterday for not supporting his condom label proposal, saying, "It is very disappointing that the organization most directly concerned with the health of American women has not done what it could have done to help prevent disease. I hope that when we take our next step in Congress to improve women's health, ACOG will be pulling with us instead of against us" (Coburn release, 10/28).

Kaiser Daily HIV/AIDS Report

((●))

Tom A. Coburn, M.D.
Press Release

FOR IMMEDIATE RELEASE
May 9, 2000

Contact: John Hart
(202) 225-2701

COBURN VOTES TO CREATE CONDOM WARNING LABELS

Criticizes American College of Obstetricians and Gynecologists for HPV cover-up

(Washington, D.C.) — U.S. Representative Tom Coburn (R-OK), a practicing physician, today voted for the Breast and Cervical Treatment Act, H.R. 4386, a bill that includes a provision requiring the creation of condom warning labels which will state that condoms do not prevent the transmission of HPV (human papillomavirus) and that HPV can cause cervical cancer. The condom warning label provision enjoys bipartisan support and was one of the HPV prevention measures passed unanimously in the House Commerce Committee last fall.

"HPV, like smoking, is deadly. The link between HPV and cervical cancer is as undeniable as the link between smoking and lung cancer but most Americans have never heard of HPV. Congress has an obligation to educate the American people about the risk of contracting this dreaded virus. Condom warning labels will save lives and end the conspiracy of silence surrounding HPV," Coburn said.

HPV is the most common sexually transmitted disease and is the cause of virtually all cases of cervical cancer. The virus is present in 99.7 percent of all cervical cancers according to a study published last year in the Journal of Pathology. Five thousand women die from cervical cancer every year.

Many sexually active Americans believe that using a condom will protect them from STDs, but this is not the case with HPV. According to Dr. Richard Klausner, the Director of the NCI, "condoms are ineffective against HPV because the virus is prevalent not only in mucosal tissue (genitalia) but also on dry skin of the surrounding abdomen and groin, and can migrate from those areas into the vagina and cervix."

— more —

The American College of Obstetricians and Gynecologists is the only health care advocacy organization to oppose educating the public about HPV. Organizations such as the Medical Institute for Sexual Health, the Independent Women's Forum, and the Institute for Youth Development all support the HPV provisions in H.R. 4386.

"As a practicing physician who has cared for countless young women with this horrible disease, I was dismayed that AGOG has actively lobbied against HPV education and prevention efforts. ACOG doesn't dispute the facts about the link between HPV and cervical cancer; they simply prefer to keep women in the dark about this potential killer. In short, ACOG is AWOL in the war against HPV.

"There is no evidence to support ACOG's claim that condom warning labels will discourage condom use and place women at greater risk of HIV infection. Every year, more women die of HPV-related cancer than AIDS. In addition, ACOG's aggressive opposition to congressional efforts to even educate the public about HPV shows that they are more interested in protecting their safe sex ideology than the health of women," Coburn said.

###

Independent Women's Forum

May 12, 2000

IWF Congratulates the US House of Representatives for passage of the Breast and Cervical Cancer Treatment Act

The Independent Women's Forum congratulates the House of Representatives for passage of the Breast and Cervical Cancer Treatment Act on May 9th. This bill will guarantee treatment for women diagnosed with breast and cervical cancer. It will also highlight one of the causes of cervical cancer: a little known yet very widespread and often deadly virus called human papillomavirus, or HPV.

Twenty-four million Americans are believed to be infected with HPV. While everyone infected with HPV will not develop cancer, every year 15,000 cases of cervical cancer are diagnosed and 5,000 women die from the disease.

Despite the fact that HPV is so pervasive and claims thousands of lives every year, most Americans have never heard of the disease.

The Breast and Cervical Cancer Treatment Act would make cervical cancer prevention a priority. It does this by requiring the Centers for Disease Control and Prevention to develop educational materials for health care providers and the public regarding HPV. It directs the CDC to determine the prevalence of the disease. And it requires condom packages to include educational information that HPV is the cause of cervical cancer and that condoms do not prevent the transmission of HPV.

This is an extremely important point to note. Many sexually active Americans think that using a condom will protect them from sexually - transmitted diseases. Unfortunately, this is not the case with HPV. According to the National Cancer Institute, the evidence that condoms do not protect against HPV is so definitive that "additional research efforts by NCI on the effectiveness of condoms in preventing HPV transmission is not warranted." The American Cancer Society has concurred, stating "research shows that condoms cannot protect against infection with HPV."

The Independent Women's Forum is dismayed that the American College of Obstetricians and Gynecologists (ACOG) has actively lobbied against HPV prevention efforts. ACOG, which should represent the health care needs of women, in this case is acting to keep women uninformed about this potential health risk. ACOG is the only health care advocacy organization to oppose educating women and the American public about HPV.

Additionally, U.S. Reps. Henry Waxman (D-CA), Connie Morella (R-MD), Louise Slaughter (D-NY) and Diane DeGette (D-CO) spoke against the HPV education provisions during the House debate. These members of Congress and ACOG owe women an explanation as to why they think women should be ignorant about a disease that could take their lives.

FRIDAY, MAY 12, 2000 · USA TODAY

Label would warn of risk in 'safe' sex

Cigarettes have warning labels. So do lawn mowers and ladders. Now, if Rep. Tom Coburn, R-Okla., has his way, condoms will, too.

The House voted 421-1 Tuesday for a bill that includes obstetrician Coburn's proposal to require warning labels on condom packages. The labels would state that condoms do not prevent transmission of the human papillomavirus (HPV). Studies have shown that certain types of HPV cause cervical cancer.

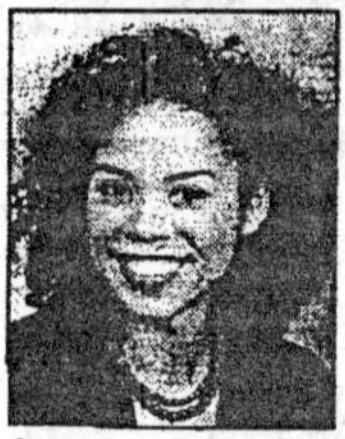

Commentary
By Amy M. Holmes

Startling as the idea is, condom warning labels make sense. The National Cancer Institute states that condoms are "ineffective" in stopping the spread of HPV. The public deserves to know there is no such thing as safe sex.

Curiously, the American College of Obstetricians and Gynecologists has tried to defeat Coburn's plan. It contends that warning the public of the dangers of HPV will discourage condom usage across the board — despite the absence of scientific or anecdotal evidence to support the claim. The other lobby against labels is, unsurprisingly, the condom manufacturing industry. Both groups, it seems, would rather maintain the "safe sex" myth than prevent cervical cancer, which kills 5,000 American women every year.

One lobbyist even told Coburn's aides that HPV tracking, public education and warning labels discriminate against women. The logic or illogic? Women are more likely than men to be counted as HPV positive, because women seek gynecological care more often.

The inconvenient fact, however, is that cervical cancer does discriminate — as does breast cancer, ovarian cancer and osteoporosis. In the interest of women's health, women have a right, and the Centers for Disease Control and Prevention has an obligation, to understand the risks of HPV and effective methods to halt its progress.

The real issue is the politics surrounding safe sex. After two decades of safe-sex education — correct and consistent use of latex condoms — the human papillomavirus has surfaced as an awkward and unfortunate refutation of the notion that it is possible for educated adults to eliminate the risks of sexual activity.

But surely, risking one's reproductive future should be a greater fear than falling off a ladder. Four of the six House members who spoke against the warning-label provision were female. Politics does indeed make strange bedfellows — and bedfellows strange politics.

Amy M. Holmes is a policy analyst for the Independent Women's Forum in Washington and a Fox News Channel contributor.

Government Relations and Outreach

Contact:

Government Relations Staff
General Information
(202) 863-2509
(202) 488-3985 - fax

Mailing Address:
PO Box 96920
Washington, DC
20090-6920

Grassroots Program
(202) 863-2505
(202) 479-0238 - fax
keycontact@acog.org

Like our Website?
Send Comments to:
govtrel@acog.org

Human Papillomavirus (HPV)

Make Decisions about Human Papillomavirus Based on Sound Medicine, Rather than Politics

Human papillomavirus (HPV) is a complex public health problem that deserves attention. While the vast majority of HPV infections do not lead to serious problems, a very small percentage can lead to cervical cancer. In order to respond to this linkage between HPV and cervical cancer, legislation addressing this complex public health issue was put forward by certain members of Congress last fall. However, before enacting policies that may be quite costly yet have a limited impact on improving the overall health of American women, a review of what is known about cervical cancer and HPV, and what further research scientists need to conduct before establishing global policies needs to take place.

What is human papillomavirus?

Human papillomavirus (HPV) is the name of a group of viruses that includes more than 100 different types, of which approximately 30 are sexually transmitted. HPV is usually spread from skin-to-skin contact during vaginal, anal, or oral sex with someone who has this infection. Currently, HPV is the most common sexually transmitted disease in America. An estimated 80 percent of sexually active people contract it at some point in their lives. However, most cases resolve on their own.

Only a small fraction of women with HPV are at high risk for cervical cancer.

Most types of HPV are quite specific in the sites they can invade and the pathology they can cause. Certain types of HPV cause warts on the hands or feet, while some genital strains cause visible genital warts. Some, however, are high risk and lead to cervical cancer. In fact, one out of a thousand women with HPV ends up with invasive cervical. It is important to keep in mind that cervical cancer is preventable treatable, and curable. Some genital strains of HPV most strongly associated with cervical cancer are types 16, 18, 31, and 45. These are known as "high-risk" types, not because they usually or frequently cause cancer – in fact, cervical cancer is a rare disease in the United States today, but because, in the infrequent event that cancer does develop, it can almost always be traced back to one of those types. In other words, infection with high-risk types appears to be "necessary" for the development of cervical cancer, it is not "sufficient" in that the cancer does not develop in the vast majority of infected women.

In 1999, it was estimated that 12,800 cases of invasive cervical cancer would be diagnosed in the U.S. and that 4,800 women would die from cervical cancer. According to the National Cancer Institute, about half of women with newly diagnosed cervical cancer have never had a Pap smear, and another 10 percent have not had a smear in the past five years.

What is the appropriate public health response to HPV?

All women who are sexually active should continue to get yearly Pap smears. Efforts to increase access to and insurance coverage of Pap tests should be supported. They remain the most cost-effective safeguard against cervical cancer. Pap smears detect abnormal cells present on the surface of the cervix. Because cervical cancer most commonly takes 10 years to 20 years or more to develop, it can almost always be prevented through the early detection and treatment of abnormal cervical cells.

Recently, the federal Food and Drug Administration approved a test manufactured by the Digene Corporation that used DNA to test for HPV. However, it was approved as a secondary screening tool, meaning that it should be used only after a woman has had an ambiguous or abnormal Pap test. In order to detect whether or not a woman has a "high-risk" strain of HPV that could potentially lead to cervical cancer. This test was not approved as a substitute for a Pap test. Currently, HPV testing is not recommended by the American College of Obstetricians and Gynecologists as a primary screening tool for women in the United States. ACOG does recommend that sexually active women and women age 18 and older have an annual Pap test and pelvic examination.

Along these lines, the Centers for Disease Control acknowledged the usefulness of HPV testing as an option for use with women with the lowest level of abnormal Paps – referred to as ASCUS (atypical squamous cells of undermined significance.) CDC has also suggested more research be conducted to determine the usefulness of HPV testing as a primary screen in targeted high-risk groups and for use as a primary screen in developing countries.

What does the HPV language in the Breast and Cervical Cancer Prevention and Treatment Act seek to achieve and is it good public health policy?

The legislative language related to HPV that was authored by Representative Tom Coburn (R-OK) and included by in the popular Breast and Cervical Cancer Treatment Act (H.R. 1070) during the House Commerce Committee's mark-up last fall has generated some concern in the public health community.

Coburn's amendment calls for the CDC to conduct sentinel surveillance of the prevalence of specific types of HPV. Given the many unanswered questions about the virus, such research may shed important light on the disease. However, public health experts take issue with the amendment's directive to the

Department of Health and Human Services to outline further steps toward making HPV a reportable disease. Such action may not be warranted given that most cases resolve on their own and only a very small proportion lead to cervical cancer. In fact, CDC concluded in a December 1999 report, "Prevention of Genital HPV Infection and Sequelae," that "routine disease reporting of all genital HPV infections or for any specific types is not recommended at this time."

The Coburn amendment's further directive to HHS "contractors, grantees, and subgrantees" to specifically state the effectiveness or lack of effectiveness of condoms in preventing the transmission of HPV, herpes and other sexually transmitted diseases in all informational materials related to condoms or sexually transmitted diseases" seems problematic and wasteful.. Also of concern is Coburn's condom labeling provision, which would amend the federal food, drug, and cosmetic act to require condom labels to state that "they do not effectively prevent the transmission of the human papillomavirus and that such virus can cause cervical cancer."

These two provisions could easily be misinterpreted by the general public, which remains largely unaware of HPV. First, it could deter condom use, despite their effectiveness against a range of STDs, including HIV. In addition, the warning label would not make clear that there are a number of types of HPV, of which only a small number can lead to cervical cancer. In addition, the label would not help educate women about cervical cancer and that it can be eliminated before it starts through regular pap tests.

What does makes sense as a public health response to HPV?

Since HPV has been causally linked to cervical cancer, it is being debated whether HPV testing should be used more routinely or even instead of a Pap test. However, at this time, primarily because the large majority of cervical lesions disappear on their own, HPV as a primary screen for young women is unlikely to become the standard of care in this country. However, whether routine HPV testing is beneficial to high-risk populations, women who do not get routine Pap tests regularly, older women, and women in developing countries who do not have access to Pap tests, should be investigated.

Research that may prove useful to policymakers would answer some of the following questions:

- What are the factors that activate the virus and which other factors (genetics, smoking, oral contraceptive use), increase risk?
- Is the "cleared" virus is suppressed or eliminated?
- To what degree do condoms decrease risk of the transmission or acquisition?
- Can HPV be transmitted asexually?
- What is the natural history of the disease?

- Is it possible or desirable to test men for the disease?
- How useful is HPV testing prior to Pap?
- What are the benefits/drawbacks of knowing HPV status?
- What are the legal issues regarding partner disclosure?

Other research that may prove useful could focus on primary prevention methods, including vaccines, condoms, and microbicides. Increased funding for programs to increase patient and provider awareness and to assess and improve the effectiveness of behavioral interventions may also be worthwhile.

NFPRHA, 5/00

Top Back Home E-mail Us

Government Relations and Outreach

Contact:

Government Relations Staff
General Information
(202) 863-2509
(202) 488-3985 - fax

Mailing Address:
PO Box 96920
Washington, DC
20090-6920

Grassroots Program
(202) 863-2505
(202) 479-0238 - fax
keycontact@acog.org

Like our Website?
Send Comments to:
govtrel@acog.org

Human Papillomavirus (HPV)

Issue Overview

The House of Representatives overwhelmingly passed legislation to allow states to provide Medicaid coverage to women who have been found to have breast or cervical cancer under the CDC screening program for uninsured women. ACOG is supportive of the legislation, but has major concerns regarding a provision that was added to the bill to address human papillomavirus (HPV).

The HPV provision, opposed by ACOG and other medical and health care organizations, was introduced by Rep. Tom Coburn (R-OK). This provision would require the government to develop a mandatory reporting system for HPV and would require condom labels that read "condoms do not effectively prevent the transmission of human papillomavirus and that such virus can cause cervical cancer."

With ACOG's assistance, Reps. Henry Waxman (D-CA), Connie Morella (R-MD), Diana DeGette (D-CO), Nita Lowey (D-NY), and Louise Slaughter (D-NY) spoke against the HPV provision during floor debate. ACOG advocates instead for an effective educational policy to inform men and women about HPV--what it is, how it's contracted, how to be screened, and how to get treatment. The Senate has yet to take up this legislation, and ACOG is working to educate Senators on the best public health policy regarding HPV and other STDs, including HIV/AIDS.

Top Back Home E-mail Us

ACOG Legislative News Home Page

Legislative News

<FEDERAL> Legislative News 10/6/00

Contact:
Federal Legislative Staff
PO Box 96920
Washington, DC 20090
govtrel@acog.org
State Legislative Staff
PO Box 96920
Washington, DC 20090
stateleg@acog.org

Headlines include: Score 1! ACOG Wins Major Victory for Preventive Care, Score 2! Breast and Cervical Cancer Treatment Act Passes Senate, and Rep. Coburn Legislation to Restrict Distribution of RU-486

- **Score 1! ACOG Wins Major Victory for Preventive Care**
- **Score 2! Breast and Cervical Cancer Treatment Act Passes Senate**
- **Rep. Coburn Legislation to Restrict Distribution of RU-486**

Score 2! Breast and Cervical Cancer Treatment Act Passes Senate A Final Push Can Make it Law!!

Urge your Representative to support the Senate-passed HR 4386.

The Breast and Cervical Cancer Treatment Act unanimously passed the Senate yesterday. This important legislation allows states to provide Medicaid coverage for the treatment of women diagnosed with breast or cervical cancer under the Centers for Disease Control and Prevention (CDC) screening program for uninsured women. The Senate bill now carries the same number as the House bill, HR 4386.

Because the Senate-passed bill is different than the one passed in the House last year, it has to be approved by the House before the President can sign it into law. The major difference between the House and Senate versions of the bill concern human papilloma virus (HPV). These provisions, by Rep. Tom Coburn (R-OK), would require the government to develop a mandatory reporting system for HPV and would require condom labels that warn that condoms do not protect against HPV. ACOG worked closely with the Senate to ensure that the HPV provisions were not included in the Senate bill.

What you can do: A clean bill, WITHOUT THE HPV PROVISIONS, must be signed into law. You can help determine which version goes to the President. Contact your Representative today and urge him or her to support the Senate-passed HR 4386.

Click here to view a letter sent in support of Senate-passed S. 662.

Call the U. S. Capitol Switchboard and ask to speak to your Member of Congress: (202) 224-3121.

Tom A. Coburn, M.D.
Press Release

FOR IMMEDIATE RELEASE
December 5, 2000

Contact: John Hart
(202) 225-2701

COBURN SAYS CDC FAILING TO CONTROL STD EPIDEMIC

(Washington, D.C.) -- U.S. Representative Tom Coburn, M.D. (R-OK), a practicing physician, believes that a report issued today by the Centers for Disease Control and Prevention (CDC) finding that sexually transmitted diseases (STDs) are on the rise in the United States indicates that the agency has failed to live up to its name and new leadership is needed.

With the exception of syphilis, the CDC has found rates of nearly every other STD are on the rise. The report states that 15 million Americans become infected every year with an STD, half of which are incurable viral infections, and such incurable STDs affect 65 million Americans.

"Syphilis has declined precisely because it has been addressed in a traditional public health context, which includes contact tracing, reporting and treatment," according to Dr. Coburn. "The other diseases have increased because there is no real strategy to prevent their spread. Treatment rather than prevention is the new paradigm for disease control. If this was a report card, the CDC is failing," Coburn concluded.

Coburn also pointed out that the CDC report claims 5.5 million Americans are infected each year with human papillomavirus (HPV), which can cause cervical cancer. "The fact is that the CDC has no idea how many people are infected with this disease that kills 5,000 women every year because the CDC does not require HPV reporting. Furthermore, the CDC and others entrusted with protecting women's health such as the American College of Obstetricians and Gynecologists (ACOG) have done nothing to educate women about HPV. In a very shameful manner, ACOG has actually aggressively combated congressional attempts to educate the public about HPV."

"The U.S. has spent tens of billions of dollars on STDs over the last several years and yet, with the exception of syphilis, we have made no progress," Coburn stated. "The reason is simple -- the truth has been withheld. Most Americans have never even heard of HPV and contrary to the safe sex mantra, which has been promulgated for decades, condoms do not protect against HPV."

"No amount of money can ever end the scourge of STDs, only real leadership and honesty will protect the health of Americans," Coburn concluded.

###

kaisernetwork.org
Health Policy As It Happens

Kaiser Daily HIV/AIDS Report

Tuesday, December 19, 2000

National Politics & Policy

HPV Education and Prevention Provision Receives Congressional Approval

Congress on Friday approved a human papillomavirus education and prevention program as part of the FY 2001 HHS appropriations bill. The provision requires that the CDC:

- Determine the prevalence of HPV in the United States;
- Develop and distribute educational materials to the public and health care professionals regarding "HPV prevention, modes of transmission, the link between HPV and cervical cancer, the effectiveness or lack of effectiveness of condoms in preventing HPV and the importance of regular Pap smears";
- Ensure that "all educational and prevention materials prepared for the public by the federal government and its grantees regarding HPV and other sexually transmitted diseases (STDs) contain 'medically accurate information regarding the effectiveness or lack of effectiveness' of condoms in preventing HPV infection."

The provision, drafted by Rep. Tom Coburn (R-Okla.) also requires the FDA to "re-examine" condom labels to determine whether they are "medically accurate" in addressing the effectiveness of condoms in preventing STDs, including HPV. HPV causes "virtually all cervical cancer" and has been linked to oral cancer, skin cancer and cancer of the vagina, penis and anus (Coburn release, 12/14).

Biotech Business Week
March 29, 2004
SECTION: EDITOR'S CHOICE; Pg. 6

HUMAN PAPILLOMAVIRUS: Data demonstrate **HPV** testing catches more serious cervical disease

A growing body of data demonstrating the ability of HPV (human papillomavirus) testing to identify women at high risk of cervical cancer more accurately than the most advanced type of Pap test was presented at an international medical conference in Mexico City, announced Digene Corp. (DIGE).

In recognition of these research findings, some experts are recommending that the HPV test replace the Pap as the first-line tool for cervical cancer screening, particularly in low-resource countries in the developing world.

Speaking as an invited lecturer at the 21st Annual Papillomavirus Conference & Clinical Workshop, professor Jack Cuzick, PhD, head of epidemiology for Cancer Research U.K. at Queen Mary's College in London, said: "The general principal is that screening should be performed as infrequently as possible using the best available test. There is no doubt that the HPV DNA test is more sensitive than cytology (Pap testing). This has been shown in every study conducted, using both conventional and liquid-based cytology." Cuzick concluded that the available evidence supports a recommendation that the high-risk HPV DNA test be used as the primary tool for cervical cancer screening, with the Pap performed only in women who test positive for the human papillomavirus - which causes virtually all cases of cervical cancer. To further research this proposal, he announced he is planning a European primary-screening study involving one million women.

Digene's DNAwithPap Test is the only test for high-risk types of HPV approved by the U.S. Food and Drug Administration (FDA). It is approved in the United States for use in conjunction with the Pap test in women age 30 and older, as well as for follow-up evaluation in women whose Pap results are uncertain.

In a study from the Netherlands, involving more than 44,000 women followed for 2 years to date, 5.2% of 574 women who were HPV-positive but had normal Pap results were found to have serious cervical disease (cervical intraepithelial neoplasia CIN grade 2 or 3), compared to 0.07% of 3,029 women who were HPV-negative and had normal Paps.

In the developing world, challenges such as civil strife and poverty make it unlikely that women can be screened more than one or twice in their lifetimes - making the use of one, highly sensitive test a critical success factor. Thomas Wright Jr., MD, Associate professor of Pathology at Columbia University Medical Center, reported on the results of a 4-year, approximately 4000-woman study in

Capetown, South Africa, in which women were screened and immediately treated - in the same office visit - if they were HPV positive.

This approach reduced cervical disease in the study population by 78%, compared to those women who were monitored for an additional 6 months. "HPV plus treatment appears to be safe and clinically effective. Now we need data that extends beyond 6 months and that look at cost- effectiveness in these low-resource regions," concluded Wright.

Evan Jones, chairman and CEO of Digene, noted that the corporation recently announced a partnership with the Program for Appropriate Technology (PATH) to develop a customized version of its HPV DNA test for low-resource countries. "The growing body of evidence showcased at this conference further demonstrates the high sensitivity of HPV testing and its practical value in a variety of settings over time. Now we need to focus on making it as broadly available as possible."

Remarks before FDA Microbiology Devices Panel

March 8, 2002

Thank you for the opportunity to provide the recommendations of the American College of Obstetricians and Gynecologists on HPV testing. I am Mary Mitchell, ACOG's director of clinical practice in the areas of gynecology, primary care, and ethics. I have no personal financial involvement with Digene or Cytyc. Both companies are members of our Friends of AOCG program for industry.

ACOG's recommendations on HPV DNA testing appear in *Guidelines for Women's Health Care.* This week we are releasing the second edition of *Guidelines,* and these recommendations are from that edition.

First, HPV testing as a primary screen. We believe that HPV testing lacks the specificity necessary to be a useful screening test for cervical cancer or its precursors, because the vast majority of women with HPV DNA detected from cervical lavages would be cytologically normal. Second, HPV testing for triage purposes. HPV testing with identification of specific HPV types may be of value in the triage of certain subsets of patients. Before it can be recommended for routine clinical use, however, we believe that its use along with cytology must be evaluated prospectively in a clinical trial.

Guidelines for Women's Health Care derives its recommendations from ACOG's Committee on Gynecologic Practice and other established authorities. Although the second edition has just been published, the content was finalized before last year's significant events regarding cervical cytology and HPV testing. Thus, *Guidelines* does not reflect the baseline results of the ALTS trial or the September 2001 consensus conference sponsored by the American Society for Colposcopy and Cervical Pathology. The Committee on Gynecologic Practice is currently reevaluating ACOG's position on HPV DNA testing. Should it develop new recommendations based on these recent data, the new guidelines would be published in our journal *Obstetrics & Gynecology*.

In summary, ACOG recognizes that laboratory tests for the detection and typing of HPV infections are currently available in many areas of the country. At this time, it does not appear that such testing is clinically useful.

On behalf of ACOG, I thank you for the opportunity to provide this information. I am happy to answer any questions.

New Test Helps Spot Cervical Cancer

But Doctors Worry It Raises False Alarms, Sexual Issues
How to Know if You Need It

By Laura Johannes

The Wall Street Journal via Dow Jones

IT'S EXPENSIVE. It raises awkward questions about sexual fidelity. And it infuriates many gynecologists.

But a new test called the DNA Pap could catch more cases of cervical cancer before it's too late. The DNA Pap has received an important nod from a U.S. Food and Drug Administration advisory panel, and while it hasn't been approved by the FDA, a regulatory loophole already allows gynecologists to give it to women who ask for it. The question is: Will doctors use the test?

The DNA Pap is a two-in-one process that combines the standard Pap test with a test for the human papilloma virus, which causes cervical cancer. The DNA Pap's effectiveness means some women who test negative may not need to get tested again for several years -- potentially eliminating the hassle of making an annual trip to the gynecologist.

Critics say that routine screening for HPV will unnecessarily alarm women who have the virus, because only a fraction of those with HPV will ultimately get cancer. Also, the DNA Pap costs more -- as much as $60, compared with a basic Pap test for between $7 and about $30 -- and insurers may be reluctant to cover it. Meanwhile, widespread testing for HPV will put pressure on doctors to raise a touchy subject that many haven't ever discussed with patients: the link between cervical cancer and a sexually transmitted virus.

The new test is aimed at a weak point in the current cancer-screening system: The standard Pap test, a visual examination of cells, catches only 50% to 60% of precancerous abnormalities. Since cervical cancer grows slowly, there's a good chance that even if a woman gets one faulty reading, her diseased cells will be detected in her next Pap test. But that doesn't always happen. Proponents of the DNA Pap say it could prevent many of the nearly 2,000 deaths that occur annually in U.S. women who had a standard Pap test at least once in the past five years.

The HPV test, which looks for virus genes in cells, is already used to clear up ambiguous Pap-test results. Now Digene Corp., which developed the combined HPV-Pap test, is seeking to market it for routine use in women over 30 -- about 35 million of whom currently get the Pap test each year. Until it gets a green light from the FDA, Digene can't market the test for routine screening, but federal law allows doctors to use commercially available drugs or tests in any way they see fit.

Many gynecologists, however, oppose the idea of using the new test routinely. The DNA Pap test would likely come up positive in 5% of women over 30, according to Digene. But fewer than 10% of those women would get cervical cancer, even if they got no follow-up medical treatments, says Tom Wright, director of gynecologic pathology at Columbia University's College of Physicians and Surgeons in New York. For this reason, the American College of Obstetricians and Gynecologists testified to the FDA panel in March that Digene's test is "not clinically useful."

Many physicians also fear that testing for HPV, which often has no symptoms, could raise delicate social questions. What worries doctors most is the prospect of explaining to married women that they may have been infected by their husbands; the virus, which is almost always transmitted sexually, doesn't usually survive in the body for more than two years. Some doctors fear that hidden infidelities could surface. There is no test on the market that detects the virus in men.

Like many doctors, Eugene Washington, chairman of the department of gynecology at the University of California at San Francisco, doesn't tell patients about the role of HPV in causing abnormal Paps, because he feels the information would upset them. Even so, he says, some women find out about the link and then focus on where they got the virus. "They want a Pap smear every six months and they want their husbands to use condoms," he says.

Should you ask for the DNA Pap test? It may be a good idea for those who can afford to pay out of pocket. But women who get the test will face an array of decisions.

Some women may test positive for HPV but have no visible abnormalities on their Pap. Digene, which will be acquired by Cytyc Corp., a company that markets an easier-to-read version of the Pap, says it plans to recommend that these women come back six to 12 months later for another DNA Pap. J. Thomas Cox, who heads the gynecology clinic at the University of California in Santa Barbara and is on the committee that will set the American Cancer Society's guidelines, believes women who consistently test positive for HPV should get colposcopies, in which a doctor examines the cervix, even if their Paps appear normal.

Those guidelines will likely be hotly debated, because colposcopies are expensive, ranging from $200 to $1,000. In addition to the high initial cost of the DNA Pap, insurers could face increased claims for colposcopies, biopsies and other treatments, says Alan Garber, a professor of health policy and medicine at Stanford University.

For insurers to pay for the DNA Pap, "they will need pretty definitive evidence that it improves outcomes," says Dr. Garber, an adviser to the Blue Cross Blue Shield Association, a nonprofit group of insurers. Digene argues that the test saves money by making colposcopies unnecessary for women with ambiguous Paps who test negative for HPV.

An advantage that may appeal to insurers is that the DNA Pap can be given to some women less often. If a woman has a clean test and is in a monogamous relationship, her doctor may feel she can wait a few years between screenings; the test will provide assurance that she isn't at high risk. Already, researchers in Europe are studying the possibility of using the HPV test every eight years instead of the Pap.

--- Q. What does HPV cause? A. Depending on the type of HPV, it can cause genital warts, cervical cancer and, in rare cases, penile cancer and vulvar cancer.

Often, it has no obvious symptoms.

Q. How many different types of HPV are there? A. More than 100, of which 25 are commonly found in the genital areas. Thirteen of those cause cervical cancer.

Q. How do you get it? A. It is generally transmitted by sexual intercourse. It can also happen during nonpenetrative sexual activity. In rare cases, transmission has been reported through unclean public areas, such as a tanning bench.

Q. How common is it? A. An estimated 5% to 10% of women over 30 are infected with HPV at any given time. No data are available on male infection rates.

Q. How do you treat it? A. Researchers are studying promising drugs to treat HPV, but none are FDA-approved. In 90% of women, HPV disappears within two years of infection. In rare cases, it can linger in the body for decades.

Source: Interview with Thomas Wright, Columbia University College of Physicians and Surgeons

16. American Cancer Society

TOM A. COBURN, M.D.
2d District, Oklahoma

COMMITTEE ON COMMERCE
SUBCOMMITTEES:
HEALTH AND ENVIRONMENT
ENERGY AND POWER

Congress of the United States
House of Representatives
Washington, DC 20515–3602

215 State Street, Suite 815
Muskogee, OK 74401
(918) 687-2533
(918) 682-8503 (Fax)

120 S. Missouri, Room 105
Claremore, OK 74017
(918) 341-9336
(918) 341-9437 (Fax)

34 "A" Street N.E., Room 202
Miami, OK 74354
(918) 542-5337
(918) 542-5367 (Fax)

September 20, 2000

Mr. Daniel E. Smith
National Vice President
Federal and State Government Relations
American Cancer Society
701 Pennsylvania Avenue, N.W., Suite 650
Washington, DC 20004-2608

Dear Mr. Smith,

As a cancer survivor and a practicing physician, I am writing to once again enlist your support to ensure the passage of the Breast and Cervical Cancer Treatment Act this year. Enactment of this bill is crucial for many low-income women diagnosed with breast or cervical cancer because it will guarantee life saving treatment under the Medicaid program.

As you know, this bill was overwhelming approved, 421- 1, by the House of Representative in May. Unfortunately it has lagged in the Senate due in large part to the opposition of a small minority of Senators who oppose the House-passed cervical cancer prevention provisions, which I authored with Congresswoman Anna Eshoo.

Unanimously approved by the Commerce Committee, the Coburn/Eshoo cancer prevention provisions seek to address the underlying cause of cervical cancer, which is infection with the human papillomavirus (HPV). It will do this through increased education and research regarding HPV, including a national campaign to educate health care providers and the public about HPV.

As you know, nearly 13,000 new cases of invasive cervical cancer will be diagnosed and 4,600 women will die from this disease this year alone. Some researchers estimate that non-invasive cervical cancer is about 4 times as common as the invasive type. Nearly all of these cases are a direct result of infection by a number of specific strains of HPV. This virus is present in 99.7 percent of all cervical cancers according to a study published last year in the Journal of Pathology.

While not everyone infected with HPV will develop cancer, the virus has also been linked to oral cancer and cancer of the vagina, prostate, penis and anus, as well as genital warts. At least 24 million Americans are infected by HPV according to the National Cancer Institute (NCI). Many of those infected, however, have no visible symptoms. And despite the fact that it is the most common sexually transmitted virus in the United States, over three-fourths of the respondents in a recent poll have never heard of HPV.

Many sexually active Americans think that using a condom can protect them against all STDs. This is not the case with HPV. According to Dr. Richard Klausner, the Director of the NCI,

429 Cannon House Office Building
Washington, DC 20515
(202) 225-2701 Fax: (202) 225-3038

E-mail: rep.coburn@mail.house.gov
Web site: www.house.gov/coburn

the evidence that condoms do not protect against HPV is so definitive that "additional research efforts by NCI on the effectiveness of condoms in preventing HPV transmission is not warranted."

The federal Centers for Disease Control and Prevention (CDC) provides no guidance on how to curtail the spread of HPV or leadership to health care providers on how to counsel— or even recognize— those with the virus. Because of this vacuum of leadership, thousands will continue to die every year and millions more will become infected and pass this potentially deadly virus onto others.

The Coburn/Eshoo proposal would make HPV and cervical cancer prevention a priority. It would do this by directing the CDC to determine the prevalence of HPV, specifically what populations is the disease most affecting, and to develop and disseminate educational materials for the public and health care providers regarding HPV. It would also require condom labels to state the facts that condoms do not prevent the transmission of HPV and that HPV can cause cervical cancer.

Unfortunately, because a handful of Senators oppose telling the public the truth about HPV, the Breast and Cervical Cancer Treatment Act has been stalled in the Senate. I can not explain why these Senators oppose ensuring that women have the medical facts that can protect their health and save their lives. I do know, however, that with very few days remaining in this legislative session that unless these Senators drop their opposition to educating the public about HPV, all of the hard work you have done to move this bill forward will have been for nothing. And the countless women who would have benefitted from improved access to cancer treatment will once again be left to fend for themselves.

What can we do to make sure this bill does become law this year?

It is quite simple. We must first educate the Senators who oppose HPV education the truth about this horrible virus and that continuing to keep women and health care providers in the dark about HPV and its consequences is not in the best interest of public health or women's health. We must then also convince the Senate to take up the House bill, as passed in May, immediately.

Because of your history of support for policies and legislation to increase cancer awareness and to reduce risks associated with cancer, I would request your help in meeting these two goals before Congress recesses in October.

Thank you again for your leadership on this issue. I look forward to working with you to ensuring that all women have access to life saving cancer treatment and to information regarding HPV that could save their lives.

Sincerely,

Tom

Tom A. Coburn, M.D.
Vice Chair
Commerce Subcommittee on Health and Environment

AMERICAN CANCER SOCIETY® Hope. Progress. Answers.

National Government Relations Office

September 25, 2000

The Honorable Tom Coburn
U.S. House of Representatives
Washington, DC 20510

Dear Representative Coburn:

On behalf of the more than 18 million volunteers and supporters of the American Cancer Society (ACS) we are writing to thank you for your recent correspondence and express our appreciation for your commitment to seeing the "Breast and Cervical Cancer Treatment Act" become law. We agree with you that immediate enactment of this measure is critical to providing life-saving treatment to those women diagnosed with breast and cervical cancer under the Centers for Disease Control and Prevention's (CDC) National Breast and Cervical Cancer Early Detection Program (NBCCEDP).

Since its inception, the NBCCEDP has provided necessary breast and cervical cancer screening, outreach and case management services to assist high-risk, low-income, and medically-underserved women. The program builds on existing public health infrastructure at both the local and state level and is unique in its ability to involve the private sector, health care providers, and members of the community in the outreach and delivery of services to women at risk for cancer. To date, more than 1.3 million women have been screened, thousands of breast and cervical cancers have been diagnosed, and thousands of women have ultimately received treatment for cancer -- making a real difference in each of their lives.

Given the current state of science and technology, the Society, and other leading medical organizations, maintain that the best way to reduce cervical cancer incidence and mortality is to ensure that women receive regular cervical cancer screenings and to ensure that those diagnosed with cervical cancer, or known precursor lesions, receive timely, quality treatment. We know that regular screening for cervical cancer would have made a difference in the lives of those 4,600 women who tragically will lose their battle with cervical cancer this year. Since a majority of cervical cancer deaths occur among women who lack a regular source of health care and therefore fail to receive regular, or even a single cervical cancer screening, more emphasis should be placed on strategies that provide access to important early detection technology to those individuals who are medically underserved. The NBCCEDP is a successful means for reaching out to those populations at risk, but it unfortunately is able to reach less than 15% of the eligible population. This limitation is due primarily to lack of adequate resources for the program.

701 PENNSYLVANIA AVE., N.W., SUITE 650, WASHINGTON, DC 20004-2608 • PHONE (202) 661-5700 • FAX (202) 661-5750

Please know that we appreciate your efforts to bring increased attention to and awareness of issues related to the relationship between cervical cancer and the Human Papilloma Virus (HPV). As you note in your letter dated September 20, 2000, while HPV is believed to be an important risk factor for cervical cancer, most people who are positive for HPV will not develop this disease. Irrespective of HPV status, it is critical that all women receive cervical cancer screening according to the Society's guidelines so as to ensure that changes in the cervix and cervical cancer are caught at the earliest possible stage. We have strong data about the positive impact that widespread regular use of the Pap smear has had on reducing cervical cancer deaths. Between 1955 and 1992, the number of cervical cancer deaths declined by an incredible 74% -- a public health success primarily due to increased regular use of the Pap smear. The Society joins with you in believing that women should be better educated about what is known about the relationship between HPV and cervical cancer and that women should have a greater understanding of the vital importance of regular screening for cervical cancer. The Society believes that any such public health education campaign should be evidenced-based, and should be balanced and appropriate with regards to what is known about the range of sexually transmitted diseases and the risk factors associated with them.

We agree that the CDC is the federal agency best suited to identify those populations most at risk for HPV infection and that disease surveillance and public health education are appropriate activities in which the CDC should be engaged with regards to cervical cancer and HPV. However, there is no scientific consensus with regards to the effectiveness of condom use in preventing the transmission of HPV. Nor is there any general agreement on the impact that condom labeling would have on reducing HPV infection. Additionally, we are concerned that without ensuring that additional resources are made available for a new public health awareness initiative related to HPV and cervical cancer, the CDC will be unable to adequately and appropriately address this important issue.

The Society urges that Congress take the following steps to ensure that all women have adequate access to quality cervical cancer screening and follow-up care:

- Appropriate $215 million for FY 2001 for the NBCCEDP;
- Enact the "Breast and Cervical Cancer Treatment Act" – a needed complement to the NBCCEDP to ensure women served by the NBCCEDP receive timely, quality cancer care;
- Authorize and appropriate funding to the CDC to conduct scientific research on public health communication strategies related to HPV and cancer – such efforts will help ensure that any future public health campaign on the issue is effective and evidence-based;
- Ensure that any new public health campaign conducted by the CDC on HPV and cervical cancer is authorized and appropriated the funding necessary to ensure its success;
- Pass the "Cancer Screening Coverage Act" (HR 1285/S 1641) – this measure ensures that enrollees in private health plans have access to the full range of breast, cervical, colorectal, and prostate cancer according to the Society's guidelines; and
- Provide Medicare coverage for three consecutive annual Pap smears to establish the baseline recommended by the consensus of leading medical organizations for determining subsequent intervals for Pap testing – this will allow health care providers and women to establish cervical health status and decide future cervical cancer screening needs.

Again, we thank you for your interest in securing enactment of the "Breast and Cervical Cancer Treatment Act." We are hopeful that we can work together to find ways to reduce cervical cancer incidence and mortality and identify the best ways to both educate women about the risks of cervical cancer and develop science-based methods to reduce those risks.

Should you have any questions or require additional information, please feel free to contact me or Wendy Selig, Managing Director Federal Government Relations (202/661-5700).

Sincerely,

Daniel E. Smith

Daniel E. Smith
National Vice President, Federal and State Government Relations

TOM A. COBURN, M.D.
2D DISTRICT, OKLAHOMA

COMMITTEE ON COMMERCE
SUBCOMMITTEES:
HEALTH AND ENVIRONMENT
ENERGY AND POWER

Congress of the United States
House of Representatives
Washington, DC 20515–3602

215 State Street, Suite 815
Muskogee, OK 74401
(918) 687–2533
(918) 682-8503 (Fax)

120 S. Missouri, Room 105
Claremore, OK 74017
(918) 341–9336
(918) 341–9437 (Fax)

34 "A" Street N.E., Room 202
Miami, OK 74354
(918) 542–5337
(918) 542–5367 (Fax)

September 29, 2000

Mr. Daniel E. Smith
National Vice President
Federal and State Government Relations
American Cancer Society
701 Pennsylvania Avenue, N.W., Suite 650
Washington, DC 20004-2608

Dear Mr. Smith,

Thank you for your prompt response to my letter requesting your support with efforts to educate the Senate about the need for inclusion of cervical cancer prevention and education in the Breast and Cervical Cancer Treatment Act and the necessity for prompt passage of this very important legislation.

While I appreciate your comments in support of better education and surveillance regarding the human papilloma virus (HPV) and cervical cancer, I am bewildered by several of your other statements.

First, you state that "there is no scientific consensus with regards to the effectiveness of condom use in preventing the transmission of HPV." This is inaccurate and contradicts your own organization's position. The American Cancer Society's website emphatically states that "recent research shows that condoms ("rubbers") cannot protect against infection with HPV." In April 1996, the National Institutes of Health (NIH) Consensus Development Conference Statement on Cervical Cancer concluded that "the data on the use of barrier methods of contraception to prevent the spread of HPV is controversial but does not support this as an effective method of prevention." And according to Dr. Richard Klausner, Director of the National Cancer Institute (NCI), the evidence that condoms do not protect against HPV is so definite that "additional research efforts by NCI on the effectiveness is not warranted."

Dr. Klausner pointed out that "condoms are ineffective against HPV because the virus is prevalent not only in mucosal tissue (genitalia) but also on dry skin of the surrounding abdomen and groin, and can migrate from those areas into the vagina and cervix." Your website echoes these observations, stating that "HPV can be passed from person to person with any skin-to-skin contact with any HPV-infected area of the body, such as skin of the genital or anal area not covered by the condom. The absence of visible warts cannot be used to decide whether caution is warranted, since HPV can be passed on to another person even when there are no visible warts or other symptoms."

Your letter also states that "the best way" to reduce cervical cancer incidence is to ensure that women receive regular cervical cancer screening. While I agree that regular screening and treatment

429 Cannon House Office Building
Washington, DC 20515
(202) 225–2701 Fax: (202) 225–3038

PRINTED ON RECYCLED PAPER

E-mail: rep.coburn@mail.house.gov
Web site: www.house.gov/coburn

for those diagnosed with cancer is extremely important, I believe your conclusions are not the best possible medical advice for avoiding cervical cancer. Diagnosis is not disease prevention. It is merely disease detection.

As a practicing physician, I believe that the best medical advice I can provide is promoting positive behaviors which actually prevent disease. In regards to lung cancer, for example, the public health community agrees that we should advocate abstaining from smoking. I think you would agree that to prevent lung cancer we should emphasize the danger of smoking rather than focusing on the need for regular lung cancer screening. The same logic should hold true for preventing other forms of cancer, including cervical cancer.

The 1996 NIH consensus statement concluded that we can be successful "reducing the rate of HPV infection by encouraging changes in the sexual behavior of young people." I agree with the NIH consensus and believe that cancer advocates and the public health community should place a greater emphasis on advocating behavior changes. Obviously, abstinence is the most effective life style to prevent HPV and cervical cancer. The federal Centers for Disease Control and Prevention (CDC) has reported that a majority of high school students are now sexually abstinent. Policy makers and public health advocates should support this positive behavior in the same manner that we have united to educate adolescents about the dangers of cigarettes, alcohol and drugs.

While I agree with you that regular screening is vital to reducing cervical cancer mortality, screening is not enough. If a woman is diagnosed with cancer of the cervix, or even a precancerous condition, she will still require surgery and remains at risk for future irregularities that could result in cancer. We should not minimize the discomfort, anxiety, potential impact on fertility and other possible related complications. I have had the misfortune of diagnosing countless women and young girls with such conditions, many too late to save.

No woman, and especially no adolescent girl, should have to suffer a similar fate because she was denied the medical knowledge and advice that could have protected her health or saved her life.

Your statement that there is not "any general agreement on the impact that condom labeling would have on reducing HPV infection" seems to miss the intent of the proposal. Currently, condom labels read "if used properly, latex condoms are effective against pregnancy, AIDS and other STDs." This statement is inaccurate because it implies condoms can prevent HPV infection, which they do not according to the NIH consensus statement, the Director of the NCI and the ACS website. A recent press release from LifeStyles Condoms claimed that "the proper and consistent use of latex condoms is the most effective way to prevent the spread of such diseases, including HIV, AIDS and HPV (human papaloma virus)." This statement is not only deceptive, it is a lie.

Would we be content allowing the tobacco companies to print similar misleading labels on cigarettes? I would hope not.

The Food and Drug Administration currently requires birth control pills to state that oral contraceptives (COCs) do not prevent sexually transmitted diseases and that "some reports indicate a statistical association between COC use and cervical cancer." Why would we not require condom labeling to contain similar information?

This label is not only about prevention, it is about awareness. Why should anyone be denied the medically accurate facts that will allow them to make a truly informed decision that could impact their health? The claims of the condom manufacturers and Planned Parenthood and their associates that telling the truth will discourage condom use altogether and lead to increases in HIV/AIDS and other sexually transmitted diseases is unfounded. There is no scientific data or anecdotal evidence to support these claims.

There is, however, plenty of evidence to indicate that the present conspiracy of silence has been effective in hiding the truth and allowing the epidemic to spread. Despite the fact that every year 15,000 cases of cervical cancer are diagnosed, 5,000 women die from the disease and hundreds of thousands of other women will be diagnosed and treated for pre-cancerous conditions related to HPV, over three-fourths of the respondents in a recent poll have never heard of HPV.

I would like to once again applaud your dedicated efforts to ensure treatment access to all who are diagnosed with cancer and your efforts to promote healthy behaviors. I would, however, once again urge you to undertake a campaign against HPV and cervical cancer similar to the American Cancer Society's efforts against smoking. After all, the link between smoking and lung cancer is as conclusive and definitive as the link between HPV and cervical cancer. I think it is particularly important to target adolescents with messages that promote life styles that emphasize risk avoidance.

I am troubled that there seems to be some confusion about the scientific data regarding HPV and a vacuum of leadership in addressing the epidemic, so I have decided to request that Commerce Committee Chairman Thomas Bliley, Jr., hold a hearing to bring the scientific community together and reach some consensus on these issues. I would hope that you would be willing to participate with this effort and do everything possible to educate the public about HPV.

Thank you again.

Sincerely,

Tom A. Coburn, M.D.
Vice Chair
Commerce Subcommittee on Health and Environment

Enclosures

HUMAN PAPILLOMAVIRUS (HPV)

WHAT ARE HPVs?

Human papillomaviruses (HPVs) are a group of more than 70 types of viruses. They are called papillomaviruses because they tend to cause warts, or *papillomas,* which are benign (noncancerous) tumors. Different types of HPVs cause the common warts that grow on hands and feet and those that develop in the mouth and genital area. Genital HPVs can be passed from one person to another through sexual intercourse and oral or anal sex.

Genital HPVs may cause warts to appear on or around the genitals and anus of both men and women. In women, visible warts may also appear in the cervix. This type of a "genital wart" is known technically as *condyloma acuminatum* and is generally associated with two HPV types, numbers 6 and 11. Because these genital warts rarely develop into cancer, HPV-6 and HPV-11 are often referred to as "low-risk" viruses. Other sexually transmitted HPVs have been linked with genital or anal cancers in both men and women. These are called "high risk" HPV types and include HPV-16, HPV-18, HPV-31, HPV-45, as well as some others. High risk HPV types aren't usually contained in visible warts. Both high-risk and low-risk types of HPVs can cause the growth of abnormal cells in the cervix.

PREVENTING HPV INFECTION

Limiting your number of sexual partners and avoiding sex with people who have had many other sexual partners decreases your risk of exposure to HPV. HPV infection does not always produce warts or other symptoms, so a person may be infected with, and pass on, HPV without knowing it. Recent research shows that condoms ("rubbers") cannot protect against infection with HPV. This is because HPV can be passed from person to person with any skin-to-skin contact with any HPV-infected area of the body, such as skin of the genital or anal area not covered by the condom. The absence of visible warts cannot be used to decide whether caution is warranted, since HPV can be passed on to another person even when there are no visible warts or other symptoms. HPV can be present for years with no symptoms. It is still important, though, to use condoms to protect against AIDS and other sexually transmitted diseases that are passed on through some body fluids.

HOW IS HPV INFECTION DIAGNOSED?

Diagnosis of cell abnormalities related to HPV infection is currently based on using a microscope to find abnormal cells in Pap test specimens or biopsy specimens. Several different terms have been used to describe the abnormal cells that may be seen in Pap smears. In the Bethesda system (one system used to report the results of Pap smears), precancerous conditions are called low-grade and high-grade squamous intraepithelial lesions. Squamous cells are thin, flat cells resembling fish scales that are found in the tissue that forms the surface of the skin, cervix, vagina, mouth, throat and several other organs. Other terms sometimes used to describe these abnormal cells are dysplasia and intraepithelial neoplasia. Depending on the organ involved intraepithelial neoplasia may be given more specific names, such as cervical intraepithelial neoplasia (CIN), vulvar intraepithelial neoplasia (VIN), or vaginal intraepithelial neoplasia (VAIN).

HPV TESTING

About 20 years ago, researchers began developing tests to detect DNA from HPVs and determine the specific HPV type causing a patient's infection. Early HPV DNA tests were quite costly, and doctors were not convinced that test results would provide useful information to guide their treatments. Recent studies suggest that a new test called the Hybrid Capture HPV Test may be useful and cost-effective in determining which women whose Pap tests detect a mild cellular abnormality called *atypical squamous cells of undetermined significance* (ASCUS) should undergo further testing by *colposocpy* (viewing the cervix through a binocular magnifying instrument).

TREATMENT OF HPV INFECTION

Although there is currently no cure for a papillomavirus infection, the warts and abnormal cell growths these viruses cause can be removed or destroyed by cold cautery (freezing that destroys tissue), hot cautery (burning warts off with an electric instrument), and laser treatment (surgery with a high-intensity light), as well as conventional surgery. In addition, two powerful chemicals (podophyllin and trichloroacetic acid) will destroy genital warts when applied directly to them. Imiquimod cream has also been recently approved by the Food and Drug Administration (FDA) as an effective drug treatment for external genital and perianal warts. Imiquimod works by stimulating the immune system to fight the virus.

Only a small percentage of women with certain types of abnormal cells resulting from HPV infection will develop cancer if these cells are not removed or destroyed. Studies suggest that whether a person will develop cancer depends on a variety of factors that act together with HPVs. These factors include smoking, decreased resistance to infection, and infection with other viruses, such as human immunodeficiency virus (HIV). In any case, frequent Pap tests and careful medical followup, with tissue biopsies and treatment if necessary, can help ensure that the mild abnormalities in the cervix caused by HPV infection do not develop into cancer.

Some resistant cases of HPV infection have been treated with interferon, a substance that can boost the action of the immune system.

HPV VACCINES

Vaccines for preventing and treating cervical cancer and other HPV-related cancers are being developed and tested. Some of these vaccines are intended to produce immunity to HPV, so that women who are exposed to these viruses will not develop infections that persist for a long time. Instead, a woman's immune system will destroy the virus before an infection becomes fully established. Other vaccines are intended for women with established HPV infections, to help their immune systems destroy the virus and cure the infection before a cancer develops.

Still other vaccines are meant to help people who already have advanced genital cancer that has recurred or metastasized. Substances called *tumor suppressor gene products* are produced by normal cells to prevent them from growing too rapidly and becoming cancers. Two proteins (E6 and E7) produced by high-risk HPV types can interfere with the functioning of p53 and Rb, known tumor suppressor gene products. Some HPV vaccines attempt to produce an immune reaction to the E6 and E7 proteins that specifically contribute to the abnormal cell growth of HPV-related cancers. It is hoped that this immunity will kill the cancer cells or stop them from growing.

REFERENCES

Ackerman S. HPV Myths and Misconceptions [American Social Health Association Web site]. 1998; Available at: www.ashastd.org/hpv/hpvmyth.html. Accessed November 10, 1999.

PDQ database. Human papillomavirus infection and cervical cancer. Bethesda, Md: National Cancer Institute; 1999. Available at

cancernet.nci.nih.gov/Cancer_Types/Cervical_cancer.shtml#genetics.

Murakami M, Gurski KJ, Steller MA. Human papillomavirus vaccines for cervical cancer. *Journal of Immunotherapy.* 1999; 22(3):212-8

Published: 03/06/2000

I want to know.

Fill in the boxes below to receive information updates for this cancer type.

Email address:

First, M.I., & Last Names:

SUBMIT

Do Condoms Protect Against HPV Infection?

According to the scientific experts, the answer is a resounding and conclusive

'NO.'

"Condoms are ineffective against HPV because the virus is prevalent not only in mucosal tissue (genitalia) but also on dry skin of the surrounding abdomen and groin, and it can migrate from those areas into the vagina and the cervix. Additional research efforts by NCI on the effectiveness of condoms in preventing HPV transmission are not warranted."

NATIONAL CANCER INSTITUTE

Excerpt from a February 19, 1999 letter to House Commerce Committee Chairman Tom Bliley from Dr. Richard D. Klausner, Director of the National Cancer Institute at the National Institutes of Health

AMERICAN CANCER SOCIETY

"Recent research shows that condoms ("rubbers") cannot protect against infection with HPV. This is because HPV can be passed from person to person with any skin-to-skin contact with any HPV-infected area of the body, such as skin of the genital or anal area not covered by the condom. The absence of visible warts cannot be used to decide whether caution is warranted, since HPV can be passed on to another person even when there are no visible warts or other symptoms. HPV can be present for years with no symptoms."

Excerpt from the American Cancer Society website (www.cancer.org).

"The data on the use of barrier methods of contraception to prevent the spread of HPV is controversial but does not support this as an effective method of prevention. ... Reducing the rate of HPV infection by encouraging changes in the sexual behavior of young people and/or through developing an effective HPV vaccine would reduce the incidence of this disease."

National Institutes of Health Consensus Development Conference Statement on Cervical Cancer, April 1-3, 1996

17. Government Spending on "Safe" Sex and Abstinence

Backgrounder

Published by The Heritage Foundation

No. 1718
January 14, 2004

Government Spends $12 on Safe Sex and Contraceptives for Every $1 Spent on Abstinence

Melissa G. Pardue, Robert E. Rector, and Shannan Martin

Early this year, Congress will work to renew welfare reform by reauthorizing the Temporary Assistance for Needy Families (TANF) program. As part of this process, Congress will also seek to reauthorize the Title V abstinence education program that was created, along with TANF, in the original 1996 welfare reform act, the Personal Responsibility and Work Opportunity Reconciliation Act (PRWORA). It is expected that advocates of "safe sex" programs will use the welfare reform debate as an opportunity to push for additional federal funding for comprehensive sex education and contraception promotion programs in the name of reducing the occurrence of teen pregnancy and out-of-wedlock childbearing.

In fact, programs promoting contraceptive use already receive very large amounts of government funding. In 2002, the federal and state governments spent an estimated $1.73 billion on a wide variety of contraception promotion and pregnancy prevention programs.[1] More than a third of that money ($653 million) was spent specifically to fund contraceptive programs for teens.[2]

1. For a detailed description of funding sources, see Table 1 and Appendix. Unless otherwise noted, FY 2002 figures were used in all cases because they were the most accurate and comprehensive data available.
2. See Republican Study Committee, "2002 Federal Sex-Ed/ Contraception vs. Abstinence Funding," September 6, 2002, at *www.house.gov/burton/RSC/Abstinence4.PDF.*

Talking Points

- Total government spending for abstinence was only $144.1 million in FY 2002, but total government spending on family planning, safe sex, and contraceptive promotion was $1.73 billion in the same year: in other words, $12 on contraception services and promotion for each dollar spent on abstinence.
- Similarly, government spending on family planning, safe sex, and contraceptive promotion for teens in FY 2002 was $653 million, but total spending for teen abstinence was only $144.1 million: nearly $4.50 on contraception services and promotion for teens for each dollar spent on abstinence.
- These spending priorities are exactly the opposite of what parents in the United States say they want taught to their teens. In a recent Zogby poll, an overwhelming majority—85 percent—of parents said that the emphasis placed on abstinence for teens should be equal to or greater than the emphasis placed on contraception

This paper, in its entirety, can be found at: *www.heritage.org/research/family/bg1718.cfm*

Produced by the Domestic Policy Studies Department

Published by The Heritage Foundation
214 Massachusetts Ave., NE
Washington, DC 20002–4999
(202) 546-4400 heritage.org

By contrast, programs teaching teens to abstain from sexual activity received only an estimated $144.1 million in the same year. Overall, government spent $12 to promote contraception for every dollar spent to encourage abstinence. In addition, most contraceptive promotion or comprehensive sex-ed curricula contain material that is alarming and offensive to most parents.

This funding asymmetry seems out of line with general social priorities. Early sexual activity has harmful effects on the health, psychological well-being, and long-term life prospects of teens, and these harmful effects will be reduced only slightly by contraceptive use.

Regrettably, relatively few teens receive a clear message about the harmful effects of early sexual activity; few are taught that society expects teens to delay sexual activity. Instead, most safe sex/comprehensive sex-ed programs send the clear, if implicit, message that society expects and condones teen sexual activity. The main message is that it's okay for teens to have sex as long as they use condoms.

Any new monies devoted to preventing pregnancy should be directed not to amply funded contraception programs, but to abstinence education programs that teach teens to delay sexual activity, reveal the harm caused by casual sex with multiple partners, and help young people to prepare for fidelity, intimacy, and healthy marriage.

Government Funding for Contraceptive Promotion and Services

Government-funded contraceptive programs promote the use of contraception for two purposes: to prevent unwanted pregnancy and to reduce the risk of infection by sexually transmitted diseases (STDs). To meet these goals, government contraceptive programs may provide contraceptive services, promote and encourage contraceptive use, or both.

A substantial amount of government funding is devoted to encouraging and facilitating contraceptive use among teens. Programs pursuing this goal are often called safe sex programs, comprehensive sex-ed programs, or STD prevention programs. These programs are also misleadingly characterized as "abstinence plus" or "abstinence first" programs although, in fact, they contain little or no abstinence content.[3]

Federal Funding

The federal government currently supports contraceptive programs to prevent pregnancy and STDs through eight separate funding streams. These include Medicaid; Temporary Assistance for Needy Families (TANF); Title X Family Planning; Indian Health Service funding; the Division of Adolescent School Health (DASH) of the Centers for Disease Control and Prevention (CDC); the Social Services Block Grant (SSBG); the Community Coalition Partnership Program for the Prevention of Teen Pregnancy; and the Preventive Health and Health Services Block Grant.

Medicaid Family Planning Funding

The Medicaid program is administered through the Center for Medicaid Services (CMS) in the Department of Health and Human Services (HHS). Established through the Social Security Amendments of 1965, Medicaid is the third largest source of health insurance in the United States and the largest source of funding for health-related services for America's poorest families. It is a joint federal and state program, with eligibility standards, benefits packages, payment rates, and administration established by each individual state under the same broad federal guidelines. Because it is a means-tested program, eligibility for Medicaid is based on a combination of income and resource standards.

According to federal law, the provision of family planning services and supplies is a mandatory component of the Medicaid program; such services must be provided by all states. The federal government reimburses Medicaid family planning services at a 90 percent matching rate—a rate far higher than that for most medical services. (The 90 percent matching rate means that the federal government pays for 90 percent of the costs of family planning services provided by the states through Medicaid.)

The government defines Medicaid family planning services as follows:

> Family planning services are those provided to prevent or delay pregnancy or to otherwise

3. See Advocates for Youth, "The Future of Sexuality Education: Science or Politics?" *Transitions*, Vol. 4, No. 3 (March 2001), p. 4.

Table 1 B1718

2002 Government Funding for Contraception Promotion/Pregnancy Prevention Programs*

Program Title and Administering Agency	A. Total Funding for Family Planning, Safe Sex, and Contraception Promotion (ALL AGES)	B. Total Funding for Family Planning, Safe Sex, and Contraception Promotion Excluding Ancillary Medical Services (ALL AGES)	C. Total Funding for Family Planning, Safe Sex, and Contraception Promotion Excluding Ancillary Medical Services (TEENS ONLY)
FEDERAL FUNDING			
Federal Medicaid Funding for Family Planning Services (CMMS)	$834.2 million	$555.6 million	$42.2 million
Federal TANF Funding for Pregnancy Prevention (ACF)	$307.7 million	$307.7 million	$204.9 million
Federal Funding for Title X Clinics (OPA)	$265 million	$176.6 million	$58.8 million
Indian Health Services (IHS)	$119 million	$119 million	Unknown
Division of Adolescent School Health (DASH)	$38.1 million	$38.1 million	$38.1 million
Social Services Block Grant (ACF)	$23.8 million	$23.8 million	Unknown
Community Coalition Partnership Program for the Prevention of Teen Pregnancy (CDC)	$13.1 million	$13.1 million	$13.1 million
Preventive Health and Health Services Block Grant (CDC)	$3.4 million	$3.4 million	Unknown
Total Federal Funding	**$1.60 billion**	**$1.24 billion**	**$358 million**
STATE AND LOCAL FUNDING			
State Funding Allocated to Teen Pregnancy Prevention	$295.5 million	$295.5 million	$295.5 million
State Funding for Title X Clinics	$318.0 million	$211.8 million	$70.5 million**
State Medicaid Funding for Family Planning Services	$92.7 million	$61.7 million	$4.7 million**
State and Local Funding for STD/HIV Prevention General Sex Education	Unknown	Unknown	Unknown
Total State and Local Funding:	**$631 million****	**$494 million****	**$295 million****
Total Government Funding for Contraception Promotion	**$2.23 billion**	**$1.73 billion**	**$653 million**

Source: See Appendix.

* All funding figures use FY 2002 amounts (the most recent year for which most data are available) except where indicated in the program description in the text.

**The $70.5 million for state Title X spending for family planning for teens and the $4.7 million in state funds for teens under Medicaid both overlap with the $295.5 million estimate of state funds for "Teen Pregnancy Prevention." To prevent an overcount of spending, the double-counted $75.2 million has been omitted from the state and local spending total for contraceptive promotion in columns A, B, and C.

Table 2 B1718

2002 Government Funding for Family Life/Abstinence Programs*

Program Title and Administering Agency	A. Total Program Costs	B. Total Program Cost Excluding Unrelated Spending (ALL AGES)	C. Total Program Cost Excluding Unrelated Spending (TEENS ONLY)
Title V Abstinence Program Federal Block Grants (HRSA)	$43.4 million	$43.4 million	$43.4 million
SPRANS Abstinence Education Community-based Grants (HRSA)	$40 million	$40 million	$40 million
Title XX Adolescent Family Life Demonstration and Research Program (OPA)	$12 million	$12 million	$12 million
TANF Funding for Abstinence	$16.2 million	$16.2 million	$16.2 million
State Funding for Abstinence Education	$32.5 million	$32.5 million	$32.5 million
Total Government Abstinence Funding	**$144.1 million**	**$144.1 million**	**$144.1 million**

Source: See Appendix.

* All funding figures use FY 2002 amounts (the most recent year for which most data are available) except where indicated in the program description in the text.

> control family size. Counseling services, laboratory tests, medical procedures, and pharmaceutical supplies and devices are covered if they are provided for family planning purposes.... Only items and procedures *clearly* provided or performed for family planning purposes may be matched at the 90 percent rate. The 90 percent matching rate is *not* available for procedures that are performed for medical reasons.[4]

The types of contraceptive services offered through Medicaid are determined by the individual states. Currently, most state Medicaid programs offer a wide variety of contraceptive services, including oral contraceptives, condoms, diaphragms, spermicides, natural family planning, sponges, cervical cap, vaginal film, and sterilization through vasectomy or tubal ligation. In many states, Medicaid family planning funds are also used to support school-based clinics.

Medicaid is the largest source of publicly funded family planning services in the United States.[5] Due to federal waivers, Medicaid funds available for family planning have increased very rapidly in the past several years, reaching $926.9 million in fiscal year (FY) 2001.[6] Of this amount, 90 percent ($834 million) was federal.[7] An estimated $63 million in federal funds went to pregnancy prevention and contraception services among teens.[8]

Calculating the cost of contraceptive services funded through Medicaid is complicated by the fact that Medicaid "family planning" charges often include such ancillary medical services as gynecological exams, pap smears, STD tests, and pregnancy tests. Medicaid rules are clear that these services are not fundable as family planning if they are provided independently or for purposes other than pregnancy prevention.

However, if these services are routinely integrated as part of the contraceptive service provided to individuals, they could be counted as family planning expenses. For example, if a clinic performs gynecological exams and pap smears as a routine procedure when providing contraceptives to individuals, these services could be included as part of overall family planning costs.

The share of overall Medicaid family planning expenditures resulting from these ancillary medical services is unknown. For purposes of this paper, we have estimated that two-thirds of Medicaid family planning costs covers contraceptives per se, while one-third covers ancillary medical services.[9] Thus, excluding expenditures for ancillary services, we estimate that federal Medicaid expenditures for contraceptive services were $555 million in 2002 (two-thirds of $834 million). Expenditures for teens were $42 million. These reduced figures, excluding ancillary medical costs, are included in columns B and C of Table 1.

Temporary Assistance for Needy Families

The Temporary Assistance for Needy Families program was created as part of the 1996 Personal

4. Chryl Andrews and Tracey Orloff, *State Medicaid Coverage of Family Planning Services*, National Governors' Association, December 1995, p. 2 (emphasis in original).
5. *Ibid.*
6. Total family planning expenditures for FY 2001 are according to preliminary internal CMS documents provided by congressional staff. Documents are available upon request from the authors. See also Medicaid information in Appendix.
7. In Table 1, the federal Medicaid expenditures for family planning ($834.2 million) and state Medicaid expenditures ($92.7 million) are presented separately.
8. Based on Medicaid's FY 2000 report, which shows that 7.6 percent of Medicaid family planning expenditures went to fund services for youth. The estimate of $63 million for teen services in 2001 assumes that the 7.6 percent share of family planning spending is relatively constant and would apply to 2001 spending as well. See Table 7, "Medicaid Expenditures—Fiscal Year 2000," at *www.dhhs.state.sc.us/NR/rdonlyres/ea5iyls55hidbqvgvj3amti6uqke4cbibb2nnyd3m5y5n4ic3qlxn27u4lsvcdapbmolbv6yjozpcj/208200partial.pdf.*
9. The authors have been unable to obtain information on the share of Medicaid family planning funds allocated to ancillary medical services and would welcome further research or information on this topic to better understand the allocation of resources.

Responsibility and Work Opportunity Reconciliation Act. TANF is operated by the Administration for Children and Families (ACF) within the Office of Family Assistance in the Department of Health and Human Services.

One of the major goals of the TANF program is to reduce out-of-wedlock childbearing; therefore, states are free to use federal TANF funds for pregnancy prevention. According to TANF financial data, 37 states spent federal TANF funds on pregnancy prevention in FY 2002. Overall, some 2 percent of federal TANF expenditures ($323.9 million) was spent on pregnancy prevention programs in that year.[10] State approaches to preventing teen pregnancy can be divided into several categories, including sex education curricula, reproductive health services, youth development programs, media campaigns, efforts to prevent repeat teen births, and multiple component interventions.

A small amount of TANF pregnancy prevention funds was spent on abstinence education. Eight states—Florida, Illinois, Kentucky, Louisiana, New Mexico, Pennsylvania, South Carolina, and Virginia—clearly describe funding of abstinence education as part of their formal TANF state plan. However, contacts with abstinence educators at the state level suggest that relatively little TANF funding is actually going to abstinence.

Based on a survey of state TANF plans and contacts with abstinence educators, we estimate that, overall, no more than 5 percent of TANF pregnancy prevention funds was channeled into abstinence education.[11] On the basis of that estimate, 95 percent of federal TANF pregnancy prevention funds ($307.7 million) would have been spent on contraceptive-based pregnancy prevention, and 5 percent ($16.2 million) would have been spent on abstinence, in 2002. These figures appear in column A of Table 1.

According to the TANF *Fifth Annual Report to Congress*, "Most pregnancy prevention programs have focused on teenagers."[12] Our analysis assumes, therefore, that two-thirds of federal TANF spending on contraceptive-based pregnancy prevention was directed to teen programs and services. This would mean that $204.9 million was spent on contraception promotion for teens through the TANF program in 2002.[13] This figure appears in column C of Table 1.

Title X Family Planning

The Title X program is operated by the Office of Population Affairs (OPA) within the Office of Public Health and Science in the Department of Health and Human Services. It is the only federal program exclusively focused on the provision of family planning services on a nationwide basis. Grants are provided for voluntary family planning services through the family planning program, established by the Public Health Service Act of 1970.

Title X funds are allocated among 10 regional offices, which then award grants and monitor services among a national network of community-based clinics, state and local health departments, hospitals, university health centers, Planned Parenthood affiliates, independent clinics, and public and nonprofit agencies. The program supports a nationwide network of more than 4,600 clinics that provide reproductive health services to approximately 4.4 million people each year. In nearly 75 percent of counties in the United States, at least one provider of contraceptive services is funded by the Title X family planning program.

---

10. See U.S. Department of Health and Human Services, Administration for Children and Families, FY 2002 TANF Financial Data, at *www.acf.dhhs.gov/programs/ofs/data/tableA_break_2002.html*. TANF financial reports also show $293 million in pregnancy prevention spending as part of state Maintenance of Effort spending under TANF. These expenditures, financed by state rather than federal revenue, are likely to overlap with state spending figures for Title X and for teen pregnancy prevention described below. For this reason, we have excluded them in the spending figures in Table 1. See *www.acf.dhhs.gov/programs/ofs/data/tableB1_2002.html*.

11. The authors are engaged in an ongoing communication with abstinence leaders in order to obtain a firmer estimate of TANF funding for abstinence.

12. TANF, *Fifth Annual Report to Congress*, February 2003, pp. II-11.

13. *Ibid.*

The program is designed to provide access to a broad range of family planning methods and services. It provides Food and Drug Administration–approved methods of contraception, contraceptive supplies, and information to all who want or need them, with priority given to low-income persons aged 15 to 44. In addition to contraceptive services and related counseling, Title X–supported clinics also provide preventive health services, including breast and pelvic examinations; cervical cancer, STD, and HIV screenings; and pregnancy testing and counseling.

Despite the fact that legal authorization for the program expired in 1985, Congress continues to appropriate money for Title X. Federal appropriations for this program for 2002 totaled $265 million.[14] This figure appears in column A of Table 1. As in the case of the Medicaid program, our analysis assumes that one-third of Title X funding goes for ancillary medical services such as gynecological exams and pap smears; this would leave $177 million of federal Title X funding to promote contraception services.[15] According to the U.S. General Accounting Office, roughly one-third of the program's clients are teens. Therefore, in 2002, roughly $59 million was spent on teen pregnancy prevention and contraception.[16] These figures appear in columns B and C of Table 1.

Direct Health Care Services for American Indians and Alaskan Natives

Health care services for American Indians and Alaskan Natives are administered by Indian Health Services (IHS) within the Department of Health and Human Services. The IHS is responsible for providing health services to members of federally recognized tribes as part of the special government-to-government relationship between the federal government and Indian tribes. As the principal federal health care provider and health advocate for Indian people, it currently provides health services to approximately 1.5 million American Indians and Alaska Natives who belong to more than 557 federally recognized tribes in 35 states.

The IHS provides teenage pregnancy programs through a wide array of community-based services and programs. Teen pregnancy prevention activities are provided through the hospitals and clinics, as well as local community and school-based adolescent health care centers. Services provided for teens include pregnancy testing and counseling, family planning counseling, and contraceptive education.[17]

In 2002, out of $3.06 billion that was available for direct health care services for American Indians and Alaskan Natives, $119 million was spent on pregnancy prevention efforts.[18] This figure appears in columns A and B of Table 1. It is unknown how much of that funding is specifically directed to teens, although, according to an HHS document, "Many IHS programs aim to improve the health of Indian children and adolescents."[19]

Division of Adolescent School Health

The Division of Adolescent School Health (DASH) is operated by the Centers for Disease Control and Prevention in the Department of Health and Human Services. DASH exists to support the development and implementation of health promotion policies and programs that address priority health risks among youth.

14. See Office of Family Planning, "Funding History Table, FY 1971–2002", at *http://opa.osophs.dhhs.gov/,titlex/ofp-funding-history.html.*

15. The authors have been unable to obtain information on the specific allocation of Title X funds and would welcome further research or information on the breakdown of Title X funds in order to better understand where the resources are being spent.

16. See U.S. General Accounting Office, *Teen Pregnancy: State and Federal Efforts to Implement Prevention Programs and Measure Their Effectiveness*, GAO/HEHS-99-4, November 1998, p. 34. See also "Background on the Federal Title X Program," Republican Study Committee *Policy Brief*, April 2003, at *www.house.gov/burton/RSC/TitleX03PB.doc.*

17. Information provided by Congressional Research Service.

18. See Republican Study Committee, "2002 Federal Sex-Ed/Contraception vs. Abstinence Funding."

19. *Federal Grants Manual for Youth Programs: A Guide to Youth Risk Behavior Prevention Funding*, Vol. I, U.S. Department of Health and Human Services, 1999, p. 227.

DASH provides funding and technical support for coordinated school health programs, HIV prevention, teen pregnancy prevention, and the prevention of STDs and other related diseases. It supports national, state, and local organizations, including national nongovernmental organizations that work with and target various populations; state and local education agencies; a nationwide network of training centers that help teachers in every state provide HIV education within coordinated school health programs; demonstration centers that train policymakers and program managers; and universities.

DASH expenditures for 2002 were $47.6 million, all of which went to programs for teens.[20] Our analysis assumes that 80 percent of that sum ($38 million) went to support safe sex and contraceptive programs for teens. This figure appears in columns A, B, and C of Table 1.[21]

Social Services Block Grant

The Social Services Block Grant is operated through the Administration for Children and Families in the Department of Health and Human Services. The program exists to enable each state to furnish the social services that are best suited to the needs of its residents. General Block Grant funds may be used to provide services directed toward one of the following five goals specified by law: to prevent, reduce, or eliminate dependency; to achieve or maintain self-sufficiency; to prevent neglect, abuse, or exploitation of children and adults; to prevent or reduce inappropriate institutional care; and to secure admission or referral for institutional care when other forms of care are not appropriate.

The program was designed to consolidate federal assistance to states for social services into a single grant, increase state flexibility in using social service grants, and encourage each state to furnish services related to its five goals. States and other eligible jurisdictions determine their own social services programs and receive grant awards quarterly on a fiscal-year basis.

Family planning services are included in the program's goals and are defined as "educational, comprehensive medical or social services or activities, which enable individuals, including minors, to determine freely the number and spacing of their children and to select the means by which this may be achieved."[22] Services available include contraceptive services, counseling and education, reproductive health care, and fertility services.

The Social Services Block Grant received $1.7 billion in 2002 appropriations, of which $23.8 million was used for pregnancy prevention programs.[23] This figure appears in columns A and B of Table 1. While the amount specifically directed toward teen pregnancy prevention efforts is unknown, states are encouraged to use the funds received under this block grant to offer special services to at-risk youths.

Community Coalition Partnership Programs for the Prevention of Teen Pregnancy

Community Coalition Partnership Programs for the Prevention of Teen Pregnancy (CCPP) is operated from and funded by the Centers for Disease Control and Prevention in the Department of Health and Human Services. It is a consortium of several agencies whose aim is to reduce pregnancies among high-risk adolescents through outreach programs in 11 states among 13 different communities.[24]

Initiated in 1995, the program awards grants to communities in order to mobilize resources to support comprehensive teen pregnancy prevention programs. It also provides support for national nongovernmental education organizations to help schools implement teen pregnancy prevention programs.[25] In FY 2002, $13.1 million was spent on

20. See Republican Study Committee, "2002 Federal Sex-Ed/Contraception vs. Abstinence Funding."

21. See *www.cdc.gov/nccdphp/dash/index.htm.*

22. *Federal Grants Manual for Youth Programs: A Guide to Youth Risk Behavior Prevention Funding*, Vol. I, p. 114.

23. See Republican Study Committee, "2002 Federal Sex-Ed/Contraception vs. Abstinence Funding."

24. For a list of the 13 communities, see *www.cdc.gov/reproductivehealth/tpartner.htm.*

25. See National Campaign to Prevent Teen Pregnancy, "Breaking Ground: Lessons Learned from The Centers for Disease Control and Prevention's Community Coalition Partnership Programs for the Prevention of Teen Pregnancy," December 2003 at *www.teenpregnancy.org/resources/data/pdf/BreakingGround.pdf.*

community coalition pregnancy prevention programs, all of which focused on teenagers.[26] This figure appears in columns A, B, and C of Table 1.

Preventive Health and Human Services Block Grant

The Preventive Health and Health Services (PHHS) Block Grant is administered through the Centers for Disease Control and Prevention in the Department of Health and Human Services. Grants awarded through this program provide states with funds to improve their residents' quality of life and reduce high-risk behaviors and activities. This program serves as the primary source of funding to states for health education and risk-reduction activities. The PHHS Block Grant provides states with flexibility to tailor disease prevention and health promotion programs to their health priority needs while enabling states to implement new programs and respond to unexpected emergencies.

The PHHS Block Grant is the primary source of flexible funding that gives states the latitude to fund any of 265 national health objectives identified in the nation's Healthy People 2010 health improvement plan, including family planning and pregnancy prevention services. Its funding is used to support, among other things, clinical services, preventive screening, laboratory support, public education, data surveillance, and program evaluation.

Because of the variance in the allowable uses of the funds, no two states allocate their block grant resources in the same way, and no two states provide similar amounts of funding to the same programs or activities. A strong emphasis is being placed on adolescents, communities with little or poor health care services, and disadvantaged populations. The states depend on this block grant to support public health funding where no other adequate resources are available.

In FY 2002, PHHS Block Grants totaled $134.9 million, a portion of which went toward pregnancy prevention efforts.[27] In that year, states used $1.4 million to fund maternal and child health programs and family planning programs. Additionally, states used $2.03 million on sexually transmitted disease programs, emphasizing contraception. In total, the PHHS Block Grant provided at least $3.4 million to states for contraceptive and pregnancy prevention programs, many of which were likely to have been directed at teens, although the specific amount is unknown.[28] This figure appears in columns A and B of Table 1.

State and Local Funding

State Funding for Programs to Prevent Teen Pregnancy

Many states have large-scale programs to reduce teen pregnancy that are funded by state revenues. Most of these programs focus on encouraging or facilitating contraceptive use among teens.

One survey published by the Urban Institute found that states spent $328.3 million of their own revenues on teen pregnancy prevention programs in 1999.[29] The survey found that 44 states had specific policies to provide contraceptive services to teens; 28 states had specific pregnancy prevention programs in public schools. More recent data on state spending to prevent teen pregnancy are not available, but it seems unlikely that funding has fallen below the 1999 levels.

It is likely, however, that some state teen pregnancy prevention funds were used to support abstinence education. Our estimates assume that 10 percent of teen pregnancy funds went to abstinence

26. See Advocates for Youth information on CCPP at *www.advocatesforyouth.org/publications/coststudy/investments.htm*. See also Republican Study Committee, "2002 Federal Sex-Ed/Contraception vs. Abstinence Funding."
27. See National Center for Chronic Disease Prevention and Health Promotion, "Preventive Health and Health Services Block Grant: PHHS Block Grant Appropriations History," at *www.cdc.gov/nccdphp/blockgrant/history.htm*.
28. See "Preventive Health and Health Services Block Grant: National Allocation of Funds by Healthy People, 2000/2010 Health Problem," at *www.cdc.gov/nccdphp/blockgrant/hp2010.htm*.
29. Richard Wertheimer, Justin Jager, and Kristin Moore, "State Policy Initiatives for Reducing Teen and Adult Nonmarital Childbearing: Family Planning to Family Caps," Urban Institute *New Federalism Paper*, Series A, N. A-42, November 2000, at *www.urban.org/UploadedPDF/anf_a43.pdf*.

programs, while 90 percent ($296 million) was used to support contraceptive-oriented programs and services. This figure appears in columns A, B, and C of Table 1.

State Funding for Title X Family Planning Clinics

Title X clinics are supported by a variety of funding sources.[30] In 1999, for every $1.00 received by clinics in direct federal Title X funds, state and local governments provided an additional $1.20.

Assuming that a similar spending ratio continued in subsequent years, we estimate that Title X clinics would have received $318 million in state and local funding in 2002. This figure appears in column A of Table 1. As in the case of federal Title X funds, we estimate that a third of this spending went to ancillary medical services; this would leave $212 million in state and local of funds for contraceptive services in Title X clinics.[31] This figure appears in column B of Table 1.

As noted above, one-third of Title X spending is for teens. Roughly $71 million in state and local Title X contributions went to provide contraceptives to teens in 2002. This figure appears in column C of Table 1.

State Funding for Medicaid Family Planning Services

Under the Medicaid program, states pay 10 percent of family planning costs. In 2002, state Medicaid spending on family planning came to $93 million. This figure appears in column A of Table 1. Assuming that one-third of this spending was for ancillary reproductive health services such as gynecological exams and pap smears, direct spending on contraceptive services would have been $62 million. This figure appears in column B of Table 1. Of that sum, approximately $5 million would have gone to contraceptives for teens.[32] This figure appears in column C of Table 1.

State TANF Matching Funds for Pregnancy Prevention

States are required to contribute matching or "maintenance of effort" (MOE) funds to the Temporary Assistance for Needy Families program; these expenditures are financed by state rather than federal revenue. TANF financial reports for FY 2002 show that $293 million in state TANF Maintenance of Effort funds was allocated to pregnancy prevention.

These expenditures are likely to overlap considerably with state spending figures for Title X and for teen pregnancy prevention, described above. Because of the overlap, state TANF MOE spending on pregnancy prevention has not been included in the spending figures in Table 1.[33]

State and Local Funding for STD and HIV Prevention, Safe Sex, and General Sex Education

State governments also place a heavy emphasis on STD and HIV prevention among teens. In 1999, 41 states had a specific state policy requiring or encouraging HIV education in the public schools; 35 states required or encouraged STD education in the schools.[34]

Nearly all STD/HIV education programs place a heavy emphasis on encouraging contraceptive use and "safe sex." In addition, most public school systems use state and local funds to provide general sex

30. In 1999, Title X grantees reported $737.9 million in total revenues. Of that sum, 25 percent came directly from the federal Title X program, 12 percent came from other federal sources, 14 percent from Medicaid reimbursements, 29 percent from state and local governments, and 20 percent from patient fees and other sources. See U.S. Department of Health and Human Services, Office of Population Affairs, Office of Family Planning, "OFP References: Government Performance Results Act (GPRA)," at *http://opa.osophs.dhhs.gov/titlex/ofp_references.html*.

31. As noted previously, the authors have been unable to obtain information on the specific allocation of Title X funds and would welcome further research or information on the breakdown of Title X funds to clarify how resources are being spent.

32. This sum represents 7.6 percent of $62 million. See note 8.

33. See U.S. Department of Health and Human Services, Administration for Children and Families, FY 2002 TANF Financial Data, at *www.acf.dhhs.gov/programs/ofs/data/tableB1_2002.html*.

34. Wertheimer *et al.*, "State Policy Initiatives."

education; most sexuality education has a contraceptive orientation. Figures on state and local funding for STD/HIV education and general sex education are not available, but given the widespread official policies supporting these programs, funding is likely to be substantial.

Abstinence Education Programs

Funding for abstinence education is far more limited and recent than funding for contraceptive services and promotion. There are only four federal programs that fund abstinence education.

Title V Abstinence Funding

A major source of abstinence funding is the Section 510 Abstinence Education Grant Program, found in Title V of the Social Security Act, established under the 1996 welfare reform legislation. Administered as block grants by the Health Resources and Services Administration (HRSA) of the Department of Health and Human Services, Title V funds provide abstinence education and, at the option of states, mentoring, counseling, and adult supervision to promote abstinence from sexual activity, with a focus on those groups who are most likely to bear children out of wedlock.

These programs encourage teen abstinence as preparation for healthy adult marriage. Grants are awarded to states based on the proportion of all low-income births in the entire country that occurred among their residents, and states can use these funds either to create abstinence education programs or to augment existing programs.

Congress authorized $50 million per year in Title V grants for FY 1998 through FY 2002.[35] However, as California has consistently elected not to receive Title V funds, actual spending has been less than that amount. In 2002, the federal government spent a total of $43.4 million to fund Title V abstinence programs.[36] This figure appears in columns A, B, and C of Table 2.

In 1999, states provided direct service to 1.28 million young people with Title V funds; two-thirds of these clients were age 14 or younger. The low numbers of high school students receiving abstinence education is in line with the states' apparent practice of focusing primarily on contraceptive promotion in high schools.[37]

SPRANS Abstinence Funding

Funding for abstinence programs is also available through the Title V Special Projects of Regional and National Significance (SPRANS) program, administered by the Health Resources and Services Administration of the Department of Health and Human Services. Included in SPRANS is the Community-based Abstinence Education Project Grant Program, which provides direct grants for public and private entities to develop and implement abstinence-only education programs for adolescents of ages 12 through 18 in communities throughout the United States.

In FY 2002, SPRANS received $40 million for the Abstinence Education Project Grant Program. This sum was increased to $55 million in FY 2003.[38] This figure appears in columns A, B, and C of Table 2.

Title XX Adolescent Family Life Demonstration and Research Program

In addition, abstinence education funding is available through the Title XX Adolescent Family Life Demonstration and Research Program in the Office of Population Affairs within the Office of Public Health and Science in the Department of Health and Human Services. Enacted in 1981 as part of the Public Health Services Act (P.L. 97-35),

35. See U.S. Department of Health and Human Services, Health Resources and Services Administration, Maternal and Child Health Bureau, fact sheet, "Section 510 Abstinence Education Grant Program," April 2002, at *ftp://ftp.hrsa.gov/mchb/abstinence/statefs.pdf.*

36. Figures supplied by HHS Health Resources and Services Administration.

37. U.S. Department of Health and Human Services, Health Resources and Services Administration, Maternal and Child Health Bureau, *2000 Annual Summary for the Abstinence Education Provision of the 1996 Welfare Law P.L. 104-193, Section 510 of Title V of the Social Security Act,* July 2002, at *ftp://ftp.hrsa.gov/mchb/abstinence/annualrpt00.pdf.*

38. See "Consolidated Appropriations Resolution, 2003," P.L. 108-7, February 20, 2003.

Title XX provides funding for a variety of adolescent health programs.

Total funding for Title XX in FY 2002 was $28.9 million. Of this amount, only an estimated $12 million was directed toward teen abstinence programs.[39] This figure appears in columns A, B, and C of Table 2.

TANF Funding for Abstinence

As noted previously, states spent $323.9 million of federal TANF funds on pregnancy prevention in FY 2002. Based on a review of state TANF plans and contacts with abstinence leaders, we estimate that approximately 5 percent of that sum ($16.2 million) went to abstinence education. This figure appears in columns A, B, and C of Table 2.

State Funding for Abstinence

State governments are required to match federal funding for the Title V abstinence program at a 75 percent rate. Funding from any source—state, local, or private—can be used in the match.

Abstinence educators report that a large portion of Title V matching funds takes the form of in-kind contributions made by local abstinence organizations backed by private donations. Our analysis assumes, however, that state funding for abstinence in 2002 was roughly $32.5 million, or 75 percent of federal funding for Title V. This figure appears in columns A, B, and C of Table 2.

Overall Spending On Pregnancy Prevention, Safe Sex, and Contraception Promotion Compared to Abstinence

Overall spending totals are shown in both Tables 1 and 2. Total government spending allocated to family planning, pregnancy prevention, safe sex, and contraceptive promotion was approximately $2.23 billion in 2002.[40] However, these figures are likely to be substantially below real expenditure totals, since figures on state and local spending on STD/HIV prevention and general sex education are not available. Individual program spending figures are shown in column A of Table 1.

As noted in the prior discussion, accurate spending estimates are complicated by the fact that some portion of family planning spending in the Medicaid and Title X programs goes to ancillary medical services such as gynecological exams and pap smears. We have attempted to adjust for this in column B of Table 1. In that column, federal and state spending totals for Medicaid and Title X have been reduced by one-third to exclude estimated costs of ancillary medical services. After this adjustment, total government spending on pregnancy prevention, safe sex, and contraceptive promotion is estimated to have been $1.73 billion in 2002.

Expenditures on teens, with a similar adjustment, are shown in column C of Table 1. After adjustment, total spending on teens for pregnancy prevention, safe sex, and condom promotion is estimated to have been $653 million in 2002. Summary spending figures are shown in Chart 1.

An overall comparison of spending on pregnancy prevention and safe sex compared to abstinence is shown in Chart 2. Total government spending on family planning, safe sex, and contraceptive promotion (after the exclusion of funding for ancillary medical services and non-related expenditures) was $1.73 billion for adults and teens combined. By contrast, total spending for abstinence was only $144.1 million. Thus, the government spent $12 on contraception services and promotion for each dollar spent on abstinence.

A similar disparity exists in funding for teens. Total government spending on family planning, safe

39. See U.S. Department of Health and Human Services, Office of Population Affairs, Office of Adolescent Pregnancy Programs, "Funding History Table, FY 1982–2002," at *http://opa.osophs.dhhs.gov/titlexx/oapp-funding-history.html.*

40. The estimates for total spending on family planning, safe sex, and contraceptive promotion in columns A, B, and C of Table 1 are complicated by the fact that there is overlap in the spending figures for state and local programs. Specifically, both state spending on teens in the Title X program ($70.5 million) and state spending on teens in Medicaid ($4.7 million) are likely to be duplicated in the overall category of "state funds allocated to teen pregnancy prevention." To avoid duplicate counting, state spending on teens in Title X and Medicaid (a total of $75.2 million) has been subtracted from the government spending totals in columns A, B, and C of Table 1. Consequently, the total spending figures will be slightly less than the sum of the individual program totals.

Chart 1 B1718

Government Spending on Family Planning, Safe Sex, Contraceptive Services and Promotion: FY 2002

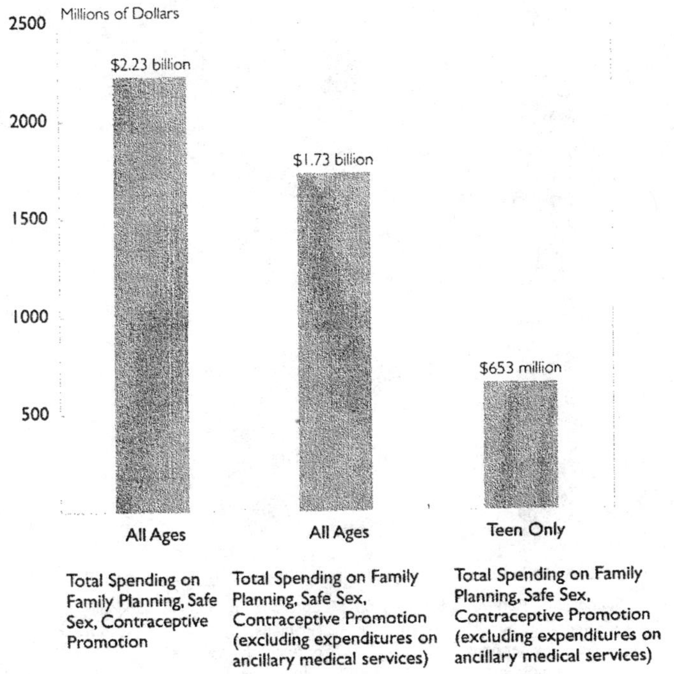

Sources: See Table 1 and Appendix.

Chart 2 B1718

Government Funding for Contraceptive Services and Promotion Compared to Abstinence Education: FY 2002

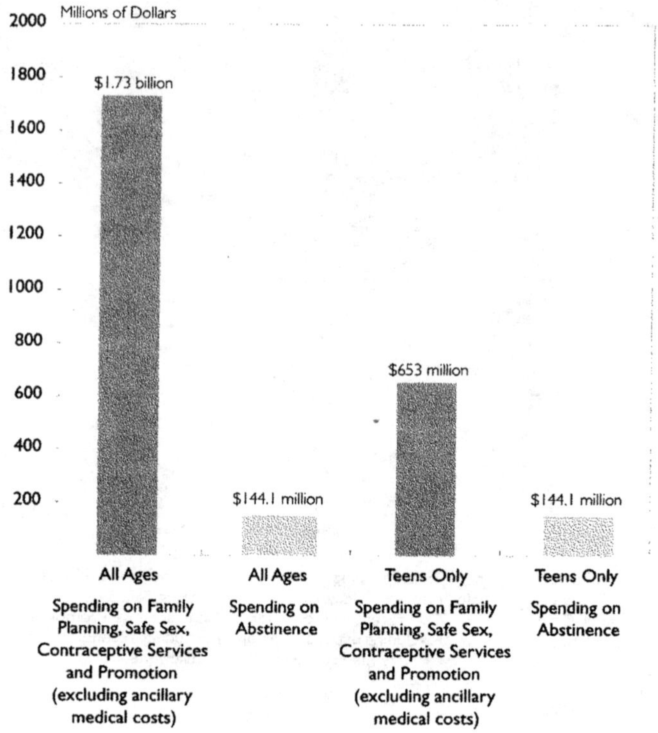

Sources: See Tables 1 and 2 and Appendix.

sex, and contraceptive promotion for teens (after the exclusion of funding for ancillary medical services and non-related expenditures) was $653 million. By contrast, total spending for teen abstinence was only $144.1 million. Thus, the government spent nearly $4.50 on contraception services and promotion for teens for each dollar spent on abstinence.

However, these spending priorities are exactly the opposite of what parents in the United States say they want taught to their teens. In a recent Zogby poll, only 8 percent of parents surveyed said they believe that teaching teens how to use a condom is more important than teaching teens to abstain from sexual activity. Instead, an overwhelming majority—85 percent—of parents said that the emphasis placed on abstinence for teens should be equal to or greater than the emphasis placed on contraception. (see Table 3).[41]

Table 3 B1718

Question from December 2003 Zogby Poll

Which of the following statements is closest to your view?

A. Teaching teens to abstain from sexual activity is more important than teaching teens to use condoms when having sex- 44%

B. Abstinence for teens and condoms for teens should have equal emphasis- 41%

C. Teaching teens how to use condoms when having sex is more important than teaching about abstinence- 8%

D. Government and the schools should promote neither abstinence for teens nor condoms for teens- 7%

E. Not sure- 1%

Source: Zogby International Poll of a Representative National Sample of Parents, taken in December 2003.

Uncertainties in Estimates

The figures in Table 1 involve a number of uncertainties. The largest of these is the share of Medicaid and Title X family planning funding that goes to ancillary medical services such as gynecological exams and pap smears. These procedures are often treated as essential components of the provision of contraceptives. Therefore, they could reasonably be included as a component of the overall cost of contraceptive services.

However, our analysis has assumed that ancillary medical costs represented one-third of total family planning costs in the Medicaid and Title X programs, and we excluded these ancillary medical costs from the contraceptive spending totals in columns B and C of Table 1 and from the comparisons in Chart 2. Others may estimate that the costs of these ancillary services are higher or lower than our figures.

A second major uncertainty or inaccuracy is the absence of figures for state and local spending on HIV/STD prevention and general sex education.[42] This sum is likely to be considerable, but information is not available at the present time.

Other smaller uncertainties exist. The amount of TANF funding directed to abstinence education is uncertain, as is state and local funding for abstinence. However, contacts with abstinence educators suggest that the funds received from these sources are limited.

Clearly, it would be possible to produce estimates for contraceptive and abstinence spending that are somewhat higher or lower than the figures in Tables 1 and 2. However, no matter how the figures were adjusted, it would be extremely difficult to produce figures that contradicted the primary finding that government funding for contraceptive services and promotion is many times greater than funding for abstinence education.

For example, if spending on ancillary medical services were assumed to be two-thirds of family planning totals in the Medicaid and Title X pro-

41. Zogby International Poll of a representative national sample of parents, taken in December 2003.

42. Most sex education in the United States that is not explicitly abstinence education has a strong contraceptive orientation.

grams, rather than one-third as our analysis assumes, total government spending on contraception would still remain at $1.36 billion and $603 million for teens. The overall spending figure would be still be 10 times higher than spending on abstinence, and the teen spending figure would still be four times higher.

Efforts to Expand Contraceptive Funding

Despite the large current imbalance between contraceptive funding and abstinence funding, strong efforts exist to further expand contraceptive funding and to reduce or eliminate funding for abstinence. For example, as part of the welfare reform reauthorization process, Representative Henry Waxman (D–CA) joined with many other liberals on the House Energy and Commerce Committee in an unsuccessful effort to abolish the existing Title V abstinence education program and replace it with new sex education funding that state bureaucracies could use for either safe sex or abstinence programs. Since the public health bureaucracies that would control the allocation of these funds are largely wedded to the "safe sex" approach and are hostile to abstinence education, the net effect of this legislative change, had it been enacted, would have been to eliminate a substantial portion of the abstinence education funds that are currently available.

Similarly, the Family Life Education Act (H.R. 3469), sponsored by Representative Barbara Lee (D–CA), seeks to provide $100 million per year in new funding for "comprehensive sexuality education" programs. Advocates of this type of legislation often try to solicit support by claiming that safe sex or comprehensive sex-ed programs support abstinence. They frequently mislabel these programs as "abstinence plus" or "abstinence first" curricula.

These terms, however, are very misleading; most "abstinence plus" curricula contain little or no abstinence content.[43] Typically, comprehensive sex-ed curricula contain only a few token sentences on abstinence in a text devoted almost exclusively to promoting condom use. In reality, most of these curricula convey the message that society expects and condones widespread teen sexual activity; none conveys the message that society expects young people to avoid sexual activity throughout their teen years.

Another effort to expand funding for contraceptive education is the Work and Family Act,[44] co-sponsored by Senators Evan Bayh (D–IN) and Tom Carper (D–DE). This bill would provide $50 million to states' contraceptive programs to prevent teen pregnancy. The bill's contraceptive programs are labeled "abstinence first." However, as noted above, safe sex curricula are habitually passed off as "abstinence" curricula because they contain a few token references to abstinence. Advocates of the Bayh–Carper legislation have been unable to explain how "abstinence first" programs would differ from existing comprehensive sex-ed/safe sex programs.

Finally, as part of his overall TANF reauthorization bill, the Work, Opportunity and Responsibility for Kids Act (WORK) Act, Senator Max Baucus (D–MT) included a new program to provide $50 million per year in funding for safe sex and contraception education. The sex education provisions of this bill closely followed those of the Bayh–Carper Work and Family Act. The Baucus WORK bill was passed by the Senate Finance Committee in the summer of 2002 but was never brought to the Senate floor.

Sex-Ed Curricula Materials Deeply Offensive to Parents

As noted above, given the popularity of abstinence education among parents, safe sex and comprehensive sex-ed programs are often misleadingly labeled "abstinence plus" or "abstinence first." Advocates of these curricula will disingenuously assert they are pro-abstinence because they contain a few perfunctory references to abstinence among materials that are overwhelmingly devoted to encouraging contraceptive use.

In addition, safe sex/comprehensive sex-ed curricula generally contain materials that are deeply offensive to most parents. Most government-funded safe sex programs contain explicit demonstrations of contraceptive use, especially condoms. Often, comprehensive sex-ed programs require middle school students to practice unrolling condoms on dildos or

43. Based on a forthcoming Heritage Foundation content analysis of comprehensive sex-ed, "abstinence plus," and "abstinence first" curricula.

44. S. 2524, 107th Congress.

bananas, and they have students practice shopping for condoms.

For example, the sex education program "Focus on Kids" teaches middle school and high school students that "there are other ways to be close to a person without having sexual intercourse.... The list may include body massage, bathing together, masturbation, sensuous feeding, fanaticizing watching erotic movies, reading erotic books and magazines."[45] This program is widely promoted by the Centers for Disease Control.

Another well-known "abstinence plus" sex-ed curriculum promoted at the CDC is "Be Proud! Be Responsible!" This curriculum has students engage in homosexual role-playing; it also encourages middle school and high school students to "think up a sexual fantasy using condoms" and to "use condoms as a method of foreplay." Students as young as 13 years old are taught to "act sexy/sensual when putting condoms on, hide them on your body and ask your partner to find it" and "tease each other manually while putting the condom on."[46]

Another aggressively promoted CDC "abstinence-plus" program, "Becoming a Responsible Teen (B.A.R.T.)," has students practice putting condoms on a plastic phallus. In addition, students receive instruction about using condom lubricants and are told to "find something around the house or at a convenience store to use as a substitute." If they "don't have a water-based lubricant handy," they are told that "grocery store lubricants...grape jelly, maple syrup, and honey" can serve as substitutes.[47]

Conclusion

Early sexual activity has manifold harmful effects. Teens who are sexually active are more likely to be depressed and are more likely to attempt suicide.[48] Beginning sexual activity at a young age greatly increases the probability of becoming infected with sexually transmitted diseases. Girls who begin sexual activity at an earlier age are far more likely to have abortions.[49]

Women who begin sexual activity at an early age are far more likely to become pregnant and give birth out of wedlock and to be single mothers. Since single mothers are far more likely to be poor, early sexual activity is linked to higher levels of child and maternal poverty.[50]

Early sexual activity seriously undermines the ability of girls to form stable marriages as adults. When compared to women who began sexual activity in their early 20s, girls who initiated sexual activity at ages 13 or 14 were less than half as likely to be in stable marriages in their 30s. Beginning sexual activity at an *older* age, however, is linked to higher levels of personal happiness in adult years.[51]

Abstinence education programs seek to encourage a delay in sexual activity.[52] Abstinence is widely popular, and many evaluations show that abstinence education programs can substantially reduce teen sexual activity. Despite this, there is currently relatively little government funding for abstinence education.

Total government spending for abstinence was only $144.1 million in FY 2002. By contrast, total government spending on family planning, safe sex, and contraceptive promotion was $1.73 billion in

45. Physicians Consortium, "Sexual Messages in Government-Promoted Programs and Today's Youth Culture," April 2002.

46. *Ibid.*

47. *Ibid.*

48. Robert E. Rector, Kirk A. Johnson, Ph.D., and Lauren R. Noyes, "Sexually Active Teenagers Are More Likely to Be Depressed and to Attempt Suicide," Heritage Foundation *Center for Data Analysis Report* No. 03-04, June 3, 2003.

49. Robert E. Rector, Kirk A. Johnson, Ph.D., Lauren R. Noyes, and Shannan Martin, *The Harmful Effects of Early Sexual Activity and Multiple Sexual Partners Among Women: A Book of Charts*, The Heritage Foundation, June 26, 2003.

50. *Ibid.*

51. *Ibid.*

52. By contrast, comprehensive sex-ed programs accept teen sexual activity and do not seek to promote a significant delay in initial sex activity. These programs, for example, do not urge young people to avoid sexual activity during their high-school years.

the same year. In other words, the government spent $12 on contraception services and promotion for each dollar spent on abstinence.

A similar disparity exists in funding for teens and youth. In FY 2002, government spending on family planning, safe sex, and contraceptive promotion for teens was $653 million. By contrast, total spending for teen abstinence was only $144.1 million. Thus, the government spent nearly $4.50 on contraception services and promotion for teens for each dollar spent on abstinence.

This term, the Senate will act to renew welfare reform by reauthorizing TANF. This legislation will also include reauthorization of the Title V abstinence program. As part of TANF reauthorization, it is likely that some in the Senate will seek to establish new funding for safe sex/contraceptive promotion programs. Given the alarming content of most comprehensive sex-ed programs, and given the current funding imbalance between contraceptive promotion and abstinence, efforts to increase contraceptive programs for teens would be dangerously counterproductive.

—Melissa G. Pardue is Harry and Jeanette Weinberg Fellow in Social Welfare Policy in the Domestic Policy Studies Department, Robert E. Rector is Senior Research Fellow in Domestic Policy Studies, and Shannan Martin is Research Assistant in Welfare Policy at The Heritage Foundation.

Appendix:

Spending Calculations

Medicaid: Federal Family Planning Funding

Medicaid spending on family planning has expanded very rapidly in recent years due to federal waivers that have allowed states to expand the number of beneficiaries. In FY 2000, Medicaid expenditures on family planning were $577.6 million; of that total, 7.6 percent went to services for youth. See Table 7 at *www.dhhs.state.sc.us/NR/rdonlyres/ea5iyls55hidbqvgvj3amti6uqke4cbibb2nnyd3m5y5n4ic3qlxn27u4lsvcdapbmol bv6yjozpcj/208200partial.pdf.* According to preliminary internal Center for Medicaid Services (CMS) documents provided by congressional staff, total Medicaid family planning expenditures rose to $926.9 million in FY 2001. (These documents are available from the authors upon request.) Of this amount, some 90 percent ($834.2 million) was federal spending; this figure appears in column A of Table 1. Our analysis assumes that one-third of Medicaid family planning spending goes to ancillary medical services, leaving two-thirds ($555.6 million) for contraceptive services in 2001. Of the total of $555.6 million, we estimate that some $42.2 million (7.6 percent) went to services to teens, based on historic spending patterns.

Federal TANF Funding for Pregnancy Prevention (ACF)

According to 2002 TANF Financial Data available at *www.acf.dhhs.gov/programs/ofs/data/tableA_break_2002.html*, $323.9 million (2 percent of total federal TANF expenditures) was spent on pregnancy prevention efforts. Our estimate assumes that 95 percent of this funding goes to contraceptive promotion and 5 percent to abstinence education ($307.7 million and $16.2 million, respectively). According to the TANF *Fifth Annual Report to Congress*, "Most pregnancy prevention efforts have focused on teenagers." The estimate of $204.9 million in funding for contraception for teens in column C of Table 1 assumes that 66.6 percent of $307.7 million in TANF contraceptive funds went to teens.

Federal Funding for Title X Clinics (OPA)

According to the Office of Family Planning in the Office of Population Affairs at the Department of Health and Human Services, federal funding for the Title X program was $265 million in FY 2002. See *http://opa.osophs.dhhs.gov/titlex/ofp-funding-history.html*. Our estimate assumes that one-third of Title X funding was used for ancillary medical services, leaving $176.6 million available for contraception promotion; this figure appears in column B of Table 1. Estimated funding for teens appears in column C of Table 1. According to the General Accounting Office, approximately one-third of the program's funding is for teens. See *Teen Pregnancy: State and Federal Efforts to Implement Prevention Programs and Measure Their Effectiveness*, GAO/HEHS-99-4, November 1998, p. 34. See also "Background on the Federal Title X Program," Republican Study Committee *Policy Brief*, April 2003, at *www.house.gov/burton/RSC/TitleX03PB.doc*. One-third of $176.6 million is $58.8 million, spent on teen pregnancy prevention. See also "Surveillance of Family Planning Services at Title X Clinics and Characteristics of Women Receiving These Services, 1991," at *www.cdc.gov/epo/mmwr/preview/mmwrhtml/00053549.htm*.

Division of Adolescent School Health (DASH)

Funding for the DASH program in FY 2002 was $47.6 million, all of which went to programs for teens. Our estimate assumes that 20 percent of DASH funding went to general reproductive health services, leaving $38 million available for contraception promotion programs for teens. See *www.cdc.gov/nccdphp/dash/index.htm*. See also Republican Study Committee, "2002 Federal Sex-Ed/Contraception vs. Abstinence Funding," September 6, 2002, at *www.house.gov/burton/RSC/Abstinence4.PDF*

Social Services Block Grant (ACF)

The Social Services Block Grant received $1.7 billion in 2002 appropriations, of which $23.8 million was used for pregnancy prevention programs. While the amount specifically directed to teen pregnancy prevention efforts is unknown, states are encouraged to use this money to offer special services to at-risk youth. See "2002 Federal Sex-Ed/Contraception vs. Abstinence Funding" at *www.house.gov/burton/RSC/Abstinence4.PDF.*

Community Coalition Partnership Program for the Prevention of Teen Pregnancy (CDC)

According to the CDC, $13.1 million was spent on pregnancy prevention programs in 2002 under the Community Coalition Partnership program. All of this funding was directed to programs for teenagers. See *www.cdc.gov/nccdphp/drh/up_adolpreg.htm.*

Preventive Health and Health Services Block Grant (CDC)

According to figures available at *www.cdc.gov/nccdphp/blockgrant/hp2010.htm*, states spent roughly $3.4 million in Preventive Health and Health Services Block Grant funds on contraceptive services and related programs in FY 2002. This sum includes $2.03 million on programs to prevent sexually transmitted diseases (the majority of which are contraception promotion programs); $882,893 on family planning services; and $518,390 on Maternal, Infant, and Child Health programs. No data were available to determine what proportion of that funding was spent on teen contraception promotion.

State Funding Allocated to Teen Pregnancy Prevention

According to a study published by the Urban Institute, states reported spending $328.3 million of their own revenues on teen pregnancy prevention in 1999. See Richard Wertheimer, Justin Jager, and Kristin Moore, "State Policy Initiatives for Reducing Teen and Adult Nonmarital Childbearing: Family Planning to Family Caps," November 2000, at *www.urban.org/UploadedPDF/anf_a43.pdf.* More recent data are not available. Our estimate assumes that 10 percent of these funds may go to abstinence education, leaving $295.5 million (in column B of Table 1) for programs with a contraceptive focus.

State Funding for Title X Clinics

Title X clinics are supported by a variety of funding sources. In 1999, Title X grantees reported $737.9 million in total revenues. Of that sum, 25 percent came directly from the federal Title X program, 12 percent came from other federal sources, 14 percent came from Medicaid reimbursements, 29 percent came from state and local governments, and 20 percent came from patient fees and other sources. See "Government Performance Result Act (GPRA)" at *http://opa.osophs.dhhs.gov/titlex/ofp_references.html.*

In 1999, for every $1.00 received by clinics in direct federal Title X funds, state and local governments provided an additional $1.20. Our estimates assume that a similar spending ratio continued in subsequent years. This means that Title X clinics would have received $318 million in state and local funding in 2002. As in the case of federal Title X funds, we estimate that a third of this spending went to ancillary medical services. This would leave $212 million in state and local funds for contraceptive services in Title X clinics. This figure appears in column B of Table 1. As noted above, one-third of Title X spending is for teens. Roughly $71 million in state and local Title X contributions went to provide contraceptives to teens in 2002.

State Medicaid Funding for Family Planning Services

Medicaid spending on family planning has expanded very rapidly in recent years due to federal waivers that have allowed states to expand the number of beneficiaries. According to preliminary internal CMS documents provided by congressional staff, total Medicaid family planning expenditures rose to $926.9 million in FY 2001. Of this total, 10 percent ($92.7 million) was state spending; this figure appears in column A of Table 1. Our analysis assumes that one-third of Medicaid family planning spending goes to ancillary medical services, leaving two-thirds ($61.7 million) for contraceptive services in 2001. Of that $61.7 million total, we estimate that some $4.7 million (7.6 percent) went to services to teens based on historic spending patterns.

Total Spending figures for Contraception Promotion

The figures for total state spending on contraception promotion are slightly less than the sum of the individual program totals because of overlap in the funding for some individual programs. Specifically, the $70.5 million for state Title X funding for teens and the $4.7 million for state Medicaid funding for teens overlap with the $295.5 million in "State Funds Allocated to Teen Pregnancy Prevention." Consequently, the duplicated amount of $75.2 million has been subtracted from all the spending totals in columns A, B, and C of Table 1.

Title V Abstinence Program Federal Block Grants (HRSA)

See Section 510 of Title V fact sheet at *ftp://ftp.hrsa.gov/mchb/abstinence/statefs.pdf.*

SPRANS Abstinence Education Community-based Grants (HRSA)

See SPRANS Community-based Abstinence Education Project Grant Program fact sheet at *ftp://ftp.hrsa. gov/mchb/abstinence/cbofs.pdf.*

Title XX Adolescent Family Life Demonstration and Research Program (OPA)

According to the Office of Adolescent Pregnancy Programs, total funding in FY 2002 for Title XX was $28.9 million. The estimate assumes that only $12 million of those funds was spent on abstinence programs, all of which are directed at teens. See *http://opa.osophs.dhhs.gov/titlexx/oapp-funding-history.html.*

TANF Funding for Abstinence

According to 2002 TANF Financial Data available at *www.acf.dhhs.gov/programs/ofs/data/tableA_break_2002.html*, $323.9 million (2 percent of total federal TANF expenditures) was spent on pregnancy prevention efforts. Our estimate assumes that 5 percent of this funding ($16.2 million) went to abstinence education.

State Funding for Abstinence Education

The figure $32.55 million equals the state match in the Title V abstinence funds (75 percent of federal Title V spending). This figure is also consistent with our assumption that some 10 percent of the $328.3 million in state funds for pregnancy prevention went to abstinence. See "State Funding Allocated to Teen Pregnancy Prevention," above.

18. UK "Comprehensive" Sex Education Outcomes

BBC NEWS
Published: 2004/03/15

Teen pregnancy plan 'a disaster'

Teenage pregnancies have risen fastest in areas where the government has tried to reduce them, campaigners say.

Teenagers should be taught the benefits of not having underage sex rather than being given the means to have sex, Family and Youth Concern says.

President Valerie Riches called the government's efforts to cut teenage pregnancy a "disaster".

The Department of Health says access to contraception is just part of its strategy to combat teenage pregnancy.

They seem to be actively urging young people to have sex with the free availability of contraception

Valerie Riches
Family & Youth Concern

In a booklet entitled Sex Education or Indoctrination published on Monday the group claims the government's efforts to half pregnancies in under-18s by 2010 are not working.

Earlier this month, it was revealed latest figures showed that the number of teenagers becoming pregnant had increased by 2.2%.

The number of under-18s who became pregnant in England and Wales rose from 40,966 in 2001 to 41,868 in 2002, according to government statistics.

'No questions asked'

Mrs Riches said areas with special programmes to tackle the problem had seen a rise in teenage pregnancies, citing increases of 22.4% in Torbay and 16.4% in Cornwall

"They seem to be actively urging young people to have sex with the free availability of contraception, no questions asked and with parents out of the loop," she said.

She said the "vast majority" of youngsters did not want to have sex and that girls, in particular, felt under pressure to "give it away".

"Until our sexual educators overcome their phobia about abstinence and their obsession with sexual expression, they are unlikely to make any positive progress", she added.

A Department of Health spokesman said providing access to contraception should be seen "in the overall context" of the government's teenage pregnancy and sexual health strategies.

"This includes helping young people to resist pressure to have early sex through improved sex and relationship education.

"It also includes improving knowledge of risks of unprotected sex, increasing early uptake of contraceptive and sexual health advice by sexually active young people and involving parents and the wider community", he added.

Story from BBC NEWS: http://news.bbc.co.uk/go/pr/fr/-/1/hi/health/3510962.stm

SUNDAY TELEGRAPH(LONDON)
March 14, 2004, Sunday
SECTION: News Pg. 12

Teen pregnancies increase after sex education classes

Pounds 15m scheme to give advice and free contraceptives has 'encouraged children to have sex' and caused a rise in pregnancies of up to 34 per cent, says report

BY DAVID BAMBER Home Affairs Editor

TEENAGE PREGNANCIES have risen fastest in areas of the country where the Government has specifically targeted resources to reduce them, a new survey has revealed.

The report, to be published tomorrow, says that the explicit sex education leaflets and free condoms provided to under-age girls by the Government schemes have simply encouraged them to have sex.

The report, Sex Education or Indoctrination?, from the Family Education Trust, an independent think-tank, claims that there is a direct link between giving young people such sex education and a rise in live births.

Official figures released last week showed that teenage pregnancies in England rose year-on-year by more than 800, despite the pounds 15 million spent by the Government on strategies to reduce them.

There has also been a 62 per cent increase in the number of cases of sexually transmitted diseases among young people aged 19 and under, rising from 25,143 cases in 1997 to 40,821 in 2002.

The Government's Teenage Pregnancy Unit, established in 1999, said that pregnancies among under-18s rose from 38,439 in 2001, of which 46 per cent were aborted, to 39,286 in 2002. Abortion statistics for 2002 are not yet available. The figures relate to pregnancies among 15- to 17-year-olds - no national statistics are kept on girls of 14 and below.

Teenage pregnancy rates in Britain remain the highest in western Europe. One in every 10 babies born in England is to a teenage mother.

The Government's aim is to reduce teenage pregnancies by 50 per cent by 2010, with an interim target of a 15 per cent reduction by the end of this year.

The Family Education Trust report analyses areas where the Teenage Pregnancy Unit have set up programmes to reduce the number of girls falling pregnant. The unit's strategy involves more explicit sex education in schools, often conducted by nurses without teachers present; free condoms; and sending birthday cards when girls reach 14 asking them to attend confidential health checks without their parents.

The trust discovered, however, that in most places the strategy had backfired. According to the Government figures, one target area, Cornwall, saw a 17 per cent rise in teenage pregnancies between 2001 and 2002 (from 306 to 359); Torbay rose 22 per cent (from 92 to 113); and Haringey eight per cent (from 281 to 310). In York teenage pregnancies rose by 34 per cent (from 93 to 125) over the same period and in Solihull by 17 per cent (from 121 to 142).

In some targeted areas, there was a decrease. In Rotherham pregnancies decreased by eight per cent (from 258 to 235) and in Bury by three per cent (from 156 to 150).

The author of the report, Valerie Riches, a former social worker, said: "The Government's teenage pregnancy strategy is based on the premise that it is unrealistic to expect young people to abstain from sex. They have embarked on a damage-limitation exercise dependent on condom use and the use of the morning-after pill.

"The figures show, however, that it might be wiser to support the majority in abstinence and demonstrate to the minority the physical, emotional and psychological benefits of delaying sex until marriage."

She is deeply critical of the material used by the Teenage Pregnancy Unit, especially of a guide for girls produced by the Family Planning Association, a charity that is partly funded by the Government.

One guide, called "4 Girls", tells teenagers how to obtain contraception, explains sexually transmitted diseases, and gives reassuring advice about sex. Another leaflet tells young girls: "Contraceptive advice and supplies are free to everyone. It doesn't matter how old you are . . . there's no right age to have sex."

Mrs Riches said: "The Family Planning Association sows confusion in a child's mind about right and wrong and presents only one moral absolute - the use of condoms."

The report points out that the promotion of abstinence among young people in America has lead to a drop in teenage pregnancies by 10 per cent.

Anne Weyman, the chief executive of the FPA, defended her charity's advice. She said: "Good sex and relationships education is most effective as a multi-faceted approach, from within home, school and healthcare settings.

"Studies have shown that abstinence education doesn't work, it makes young people more vulnerable, because they don't have the knowledge to protect themselves against pregnancy or sexually transmitted infections."

A spokesman for Cathy Hamlyn, the head of the Teenage Pregnancy Unit, part of the Department for Education and Skills, said: "The teenage pregnancy strategy is the first cross-government strategy to tackle our unacceptably high rates of teenage pregnancy.

"The strategy helps people to resist pressure to have early sex through improved sex and relationship education and supporting parents in talking to children about these issues."

Sunday Times (London)
March 14, 2004, Sunday
SECTION: Home news; News; 10

Pregnancies rise after sex classes

BYLINE: Chris Johnston

MAKING sex education in schools more explicit has increased teenage pregnancies rather than reducing them, according to a report.

In schools where pupils have been given free condoms, more sex education, and girls have been invited to have confidential health checks, schoolgirl pregnancies have risen by up to 34%.

The Family Education Trust, which promotes "responsible attitudes to marriage and family life", has found the number of pregnancies has increased in areas targeted by the government's Teenage Pregnancy Unit.

Quoting official figures the trust reveals the pregnancy rate in one target area, Cornwall, rose from 306 schoolgirl pregnancies in 2001 to 359 in 2002 -a 17% increase. Torbay in Devon saw a 22% rise from 92 to 113, Solihull in the Midlands 17% (121 to 142), and York 34% (93 to 125).

However, the pregnancy rate did fall in some areas. In Rotherham, South Yorkshire, there was a 9% decline from 258 to 235 and 4% in Bury, Lancashire, from 156 to 150.

The report, Sex Education or Indoctrination?, written by a former social worker, Valerie Riches, claims that sex education is being used as a "manipulative tool to replace the influence of parents with the authority of the state".

She is highly critical of the material used by the Teenage Pregnancy Unit, in particular a guide for girls produced by the Family Planning Association.

"It sows confusion in a child's mind about right and wrong and presents only one moral absolute -the use of condoms," Riches said.

"The government's teenage pregnancy strategy is based on the premise that it is unrealistic to expect young people to abstain from sex. They have embarked on a damage-limitation exercise dependent on condom use and the morning-after pill."

Anne Weyman, chief executive of the Family Planning Association, defended her charity's advice and said numerous studies had indicated that promoting abstinence did not work.

"It makes young people more vulnerable," she said. because they don't have the knowledge to protect themselves against pregnancy or sexually transmitted infections."

A spokesperson for the Teenage Pregnancy Unit said the strategy helped resist the pressure to have sex too early by improving sex and relationship education.

Press Association
March 15, 2004, Monday
SECTION: HOME NEWS

TEENAGERS SHOULD BE TAUGHT SEXUAL ABSTINENCE, SAYS CAMPAIGNER

BYLINE: Lyndsay Moss, Health Correspondent, PA News

Teenagers should be taught the advantages of not having underage sex rather than being given the means to help them, a sexual health campaigner said today.

Valerie Riches, president of Family & Youth Concern, said teaching the benefits of abstinence would work better in schools than promoting safe sex and handing out free condoms and the morning-after pill.

She branded the Government's strategy to tackle teenage pregnancy "a disaster" and said ministers had made matters worse.

Mrs Riches outlines her controversial views in a report Sex Education or Indoctrination? which is published today.

The booklet claims that the Government's efforts to half pregnancies in under-18s by 2010 were not working, with figures showing a 0.7% increase between 2001 and 2002.

Mrs Riches, a former social worker, said in areas where special programmes were operating to specifically tackle the problem teenager pregnancies were actually rising - by 16.4% in Cornwall and 22.4% in Torbay.

"They seem to be actively urging young people to have sex with the free availability of contraception, no questions asked and with parents out of the loop," she said.

Mrs Riches said abstinence education programmes in the US had seen a 19% fall in teenage pregnancies during the 1990s and urged the Government to stress the "advantages of restraint".

"If we are to tackle rising sexual disease and teenage pregnancies, schools need to first focus on the future and see the advantages of restraint and teach children to respect their gift of fertility.

"Fertility is a wonderful thing. They don't need to abuse it."

Mrs Riches said that most under-16s were not having sex and it was not "the norm".

"The vast majority of youngsters don't want to do it (have sex).

"They think they are obliged to, and girls in particular are under pressure to just give it away," she said.

Asked what ministers should do now, Mrs Riches said: "They need to take a good hard look at what they are doing and reverse their policies.

"Instead of saying to youngsters we are going to supply the methods to try to make you not make people pregnant, they should be teaching why it is good not to have sex."

She added: "Until our sexual educators overcome their phobia about abstinence and their obsession with sexual expression, they are unlikely to make any positive progress."

A Department of Health spokesman said: "A key aim of the Government's teenage pregnancy strategy is to reduce rates of unintended pregnancy and provision of good quality contraceptive services play a major part in achieving this.

"Health professionals can provide contraception to young people under 16 provided they are satisfied that the young person is competent to understand fully the implications of any treatment and to make a choice of the treatment involved."

He added: "Improving access to emergency contraception should be seen in the overall context of the Government's teenage pregnancy and sexual health strategies.

"This includes helping young people to resist pressure to have early sex through improved sex and relationship education, improving knowledge of risks of unprotected sex, increasing early uptake of contraceptive and sexual health advice by sexually active young people and involving parents and the wider community."

Anne Weyman, chief executive of the Family Planning Association (fpa), said: "We have always believed that parents play a vital role in educating their children about sex and relationships.

"In fact fpa deliver programmes empowering parents to talk to their children about sex, as they often find it a difficult subject to discuss.

"Good sex and relationships education is most effective as a multi-faceted approach, from within the home, schools and health care settings."

19. HPV and Gay and Lesbian Health

Serving the lesbian, gay, transgender & bisexual communities

GayHealth™

Lesbians Often Misinformed About HPV, Cervical Cancer Risk

by GayHealth Staff

Women who have sex with women (WSW) are sometimes not informed about their risks for HPV, cervical cancer, and are often told they don't need regular Pap tests, according to a study published in the August issue of the Health Promotion Journal of Australia.

"The disturbing thing is that most women who are given this advice received it from a doctor."

</TD< tr>

"Among more than 400 lesbians surveyed about their Pap screening behavior, nine percent were told that they didn't need a Pap test," said the lead author of the study Adrienne Brown from the Cancer Council of Victoria. "The disturbing thing is that most women who are given this advice -- 89 percent of the them -- received it from a doctor," said Ms. Brown.

Regular Pap screenings can save your life. Early detection is key to fighting cervical cancer. "The reason for alarm is that most women who die from cervical cancer have not had regular Pap tests," according to Kate Broun, Manager of PapScreen Victoria.

HPV does not require penetration to pass between partners, it spreads between sexual partners during close skin to skin contact. Research shows that HPV is transmitted sexually between female partners.

Results from international research suggests that as many as one in five lesbians who've never had sex with men are being infected with HPV, a press release from the Health Promotion Journal of Australia stated.

You should have your first cervical screening within about three years of your first sexual encounter or by the age of 21. Most women between the ages of 21 and 30 should have a Pap test at least once a year, according to the latest recommendations from the American College of Obstetrics and Gynecology. Women over 30 may require screenings less often.

There is evidence that 90 percent of the most common type of cervical is preventable with two yearly screening, however only two thirds of Australian women are doing so.

Lesbians having regular Pap smears were much more likely to visit health care providers who knew about their sexual orientation, and who were sensitive to gay and lesbian health needs compared to those not having regular pap tests.

Research has demonstrated that HPV is not the only sexually transmitted infection WSW need to worry about.

In a study published in the October 2000 issue of the Journal of Sexually Transmitted Diseases, WSW demonstrated a significantly higher prevalence of bacterial vaginosis (BV), hepatitis C, and HIV risk behaviors compared to non-WSW. "The assumption that women who engage in sex with other women are not at risk of STIs is clearly incorrect," said Katherine Fethers, M.D., lead author of the study from the Sexual Health Unit at Alice Springs Hospital in Australia.

A total of 1,408 women who reported ever having sex with another woman were compared with 1,423 women who had never had sex with a woman. The women had all attended the Sydney Sexual Health Center between 1991 and 1998. Only seven percent of the WSW or 283 women reported no sex with a male in the past 12 months (exclusive WSW) -- 25 percent of these WSW reported never having had sex with a man.

For more information about Pap screenings visit the Web site PapScreen Victoria at www.papscreen.org. There is a link in the sidebar.

Updated: Wednesday, August 20th 2003

Serving the lesbian, gay, transgender
& bisexual communities

GayHealth™

Inadequate Screening Puts WSW at Risk for Cervical Cancer

by Sarah Albert

Women who have sex with women (WSW) are often not adequately screened for human papillomavirus (HPV), a sexually transmitted disease (STD) that can lead to cervical cancer, according to a study published in the June 2001 issue of the *American Journal of Public Health.*

HPV is the "first proven transmittable STD among women who've never had sex with men."

HPV is particularly worrisome for lesbians and bisexual women because it is "so ubiquitous, and it causes cancer," Jeanne M. Marrazzo, M.D., M.P.H., the study's lead author, told GayHealth.com. "And it is the first proven transmittable STD among women who've never had sex with men."

In February of 1998, Dr. Marrazzo and colleagues from the University of Washington in Seattle, WA recruited 248 women who reported having had sex with other women within the prior year. All participants volunteered their medical and sexual histories, and gave cervical and vaginal specimens for analysis. Eighty percent of participants reported having had sex with men at least once, and 23 percent reported having had sex with men within the prior year. Participants' median age was 32, and 88 percent were Caucasian -- not as young or ethnically diverse a group as the researchers had hoped, due to a lack of funding for recruitment, Dr. Marrazzo noted.

The study uncovered disturbing news. Pap tests -- which can detect cervical cancer in its early stages -- were performed less often and later in life among WSW who had not had sex with men. Reasons for not getting regular Pap tests included lack of health insurance, a belief that the tests were unnecessary and prior adverse experiences. "We didn't ask specifically about the adverse experiences. A description line has been added to the study," said Dr. Marrazzo. It would be an interesting study to look only at what types of negative experiences WSW have had with Pap exams, she says. Dr. Marrazzo has heard reports from patients about providers treating them differently after they disclose that they are gay or bisexual.

In addition, nine percent of WSW who hadn't had a Pap test in over two years said their doctors told them -- erroneously -- that they didn't need the test if they weren't sexually active with men. This incorrect medical advice put the health of these women at risk. "There is a huge need for education" about cervical cancer and Pap tests, said Dr. Marrazzo, who added that many providers operate "without specific guidelines" for gynecological care of WSWs, which adds a further stumbling block to proper care.

Next, the researchers analyzed the women's specimens. They detected HPV DNA in 13 percent of participants, of whom 74 percent had cancer-causing strains. Overall, 25 participants (10 percent) had abnormal Pap tests, four participants had high-grade pre-cancerous lesions and seven participants had low-grade pre-cancerous lesions. Most of the abnormalities occurred in WSW who reported never having had sex with men, or who had had sex with men a year or more prior to the study. "The population we studied was not very sexually active," noted Dr. Marrazzo.

To counter the dangerous notion that woman-on-woman sex carries no risk of STDs, the study authors called for efforts to educate providers and WSW patients about gynecological health. The authors also recommended that all women -- regardless of sexual history -- get routine Pap tests according to standard guidelines.

In the U.S., cervical cancer is the second most common form of cancer in women, and the most common in younger women. It used to be one of the deadliest cancers, but with the advent of the Pap test, there has been a 74 percent drop in cervical cancer deaths from 1955 to 1992. When detected at an early stage, invasive cervical cancer is one of the most successfully treatable cancers, according to the American Cancer Society.

Updated: Wednesday, June 6th 2001

Serving the lesbian, gay, transgender & bisexual communities

GayHealth™

Anal Cancer: A "Wake-up Call" for Gay Men

by Jon Garbo

Men who have sex with men, especially those with HIV, are at considerably higher risk for anal cancer than the general population, according to a study presented by Stephen Goldstone, M.D., F.A.C.S., medical director of GayHealth.com. Of men who have sex with men referred to surgeons for treatment of benign anorectal diseases, 68 percent with HIV and 45 percent without HIV had high-grade dysplasia, a precursor to anal cancer. The study was presented June 26 at the American Society of Colon and Rectal Surgeons in Boston, Mass.

Statistics show that the rate for anal cancer in men (without HIV) with same-sex partners is roughly the same as the rates of cervical cancer in women before pap smears became routine. Men with HIV and same sex partners, however, have approximately twice the incidence of anal cancer than their HIV-negative counterparts. Routine pap smears have decreased the incidence of cervical cancer from 40 to 50 per 100,000 women to approximately 8 per 100,000, studies estimate.

"The alarming rise in anal cancer in gay men is a wake-up call to the gay community and to healthcare providers worldwide," says Dr. Goldstone.

The higher incidence of cancer is attributed to infection with a cancer-causing strain of human papillomavirus (HPV) through receptive anal intercourse. Approximately 95 percent of gay men with HIV and 65 percent of gay men without HIV have HPV in their anal canals or the surrounding skin, says to Dr. Goldstone. HPV is responsible for causing cervical cancer in women, and genital warts in both sexes.

"The average gay man should be screened to find out if he has abnormal cells, and should be treated if he does," says Dr. Goldstone. Gay men with anorectal problems, especially anal warts, should go see their doctors for screenings. "It's not enough to just treat anal warts. They are a marker that you may have something more serious going on," Dr. Goldstone warns. Gay men with HIV should have an anal pap smear every year, or more often if their test results are abnormal, recommends Dr. Goldstone. Men without HIV with normal test results should have an anal pap smear every two to three years. These screenings should commence when a patient becomes sexually active.

Participants included 200 men who have sex with men referred by primary care physicians to surgeons in New York City. Seventy-nine percent were referred for treatment of condyloma (a benign strain of genital warts caused by HPV), 20 percent for non-condylomatous anorectal disease (including hemorrhoids, fissures and anal itch), and two percent for abnormal anal pap smears. Participants received a rectal exam as well as a general physical. The mean age of participants was 38.8. Sixty-six percent reported having HIV, while 34 percent said they did not have the virus.

For some men, being in the closet may be a stumbling block for getting screened, but it's only part of the problem. "There are plenty of men who are 'out,' including those with HIV who see their doctors every month or two, who don't get screened," says Dr. Goldstone. "Doctors need to start taking human papillomavirus seriously. They must start screening their gay male patients for anal cancer with pap smears and rectal examinations," Dr. Goldstone adds.

To screen for anal cancer, doctors pass a swab into the rectum and examine collected cells under a microscope. Treatment for pre-cancerous anal lesions varies from simple in-office procedures, such as freezing the cells or applying a topical cream, to surgery, if the lesions are widespread. Treatment is very effective in removing lesions, but "the problem is that they may come back in other areas, so you need to be watched very carefully," says Dr. Goldstone.

Updated: Monday, June 26th 2000

Serving the lesbian, gay, transgender
& bisexual communities

GayHealth™

HPV: Next Threat To Gay Men's Health?

by Stephen E. Goldstone, M.D., F.A.C.S.

There are close to one hundred different types of human papillomavirus (HPV), causing everything from common hand and plantar warts to esophageal and laryngeal cancer. But why are they a particular problem for men who have sex with men? Approximately 20 different types of HPV can infect your ano/genital area causing those pesky genital warts known as condyloma. Around 65 percent of men who don't have HIV and 95 percent of gay men with HIV carry HPV in their anal canals, and most don't even know they have it. Not all HPV is created equally. Types 6 and 11, for example, cause typical genital warts, while types 16 and 18 are far more dangerous. In women, types 16 and 18 are known to cause cervical cancer, and in men we are now seeing anal cancer caused by these infections.

The glands in your anal canal are very similar to the glands found in a woman's cervix, a place the virus loves to infect -- talk about getting in touch with your feminine side. Normal anal cells reproduce several times and then die. But, when they are infected with HPV 16 or 18 they can reproduce uncontrollably. With time, mutations in these cells accumulate, and slowly a cancer emerges. That's the bad news. The good news is that it takes many years for an infected cell to become a cancer and the vast majority of cells will never reach that stage because your body's own natural defenses kill them. If precancerous cells that escape your immune system are discovered by your doctor before they become full blown cancer, the problem is easily treated.

Welcome to 2000: The male Pap smear

So how do we find the problem? We get in touch with our feminine side, that's how! Women have long been conditioned to have pap smears of their cervix, a procedure by which a tiny "Q-tip" like swab collects cells from their cervix and a doctor looks at those cells under a microscope. If the cells are abnormal, take bizarre shapes or have more than one nucleus, for example, a woman may have dysplasia (a precancerous cellular change). Dysplasia is graded as being normal, a little abnormal or atypical, low grade (a more moderate change) or high grade, which is thought to be precancerous. In the high grade cases doctors aggressively treat the condition by freezing or removing the abnormal areas. This type of screening and treatment has drastically reduced the incidence of cervical cancer.

Doctors are now learning to apply these same principles for cervical dysplasia to the anal canals of men who have sex with men. Doctors now advise men get an anal pap smear every two to three years, or every year for men with HIV. Keep in mind that even if your doctor puts his finger in your anus he probably won't feel dangerous areas until they have grown large and require more radical treatment; the same is true if your doctor uses a scope to examine your rectum. Acetic acid (vinegar) is a crucial tool used during a proper visual examination because it turns suspicious areas white and makes it easier for doctors to see them. However, a visual inspection can't replace the pap smear, which can find precancerous cells before they are visible with the naked eye!

Even an anal pap smear that shows high grade dysplasia does not mean that you will definitely develop an anal cancer if you aren't treated. Doctors think that only about 10 percent of men with high grade dysplasia will eventually develop cancer. Since no one can predict who will ultimately end up with a cancer, most doctors advise that all high grade dysplasias be removed. This treatment can usually be performed in your doctor's office and is relatively pain free. Men who have HIV are at a greater risk for ultimately developing an anal cancer.

Common genital warts usually don't become cancer because they are caused by HPV types 6 and 11. It's infections with HPV types 16 and 18 that we have to worry about. These infections don't resemble typical warts; they are flatter and often inside your anal canal. If you have anal warts and your doctor just treats the ones on the outside, he or she may miss a more dangerous infection on the inside. Moreover, treating your warts alone is not enough. By doing this, your doctor can leave you with the more dangerous precancerous areas that lack the typical warty appearance.

Pretty much everybody's been exposed

Many men infected with HPV are infected with multiple types. You may have HPV 6 and 11 (which cause common warts) and HPV 16 and 18 (which slowly turn your cells toward cancer), at the same time. Some men can clear the virus through their own natural immunity, but many don't. If you've had genital warts in the past, you should ask your doctor for an anal pap smear to be sure you don't have a problem brewing. If you've never had warts, it doesn't mean you are safe. Remember, more than half of all gay men unknowingly carry this virus

I know you're thinking that you've never had sex with a man who had warts on his penis so you must be safe. Wrong! The virus grows ten times better in your anus than it does on a penis. It is possible for your partner to carry the virus on his penis where it didn't grow and put it inside your anus where it does grow.

You're probably also thinking you're safe if you've only had protected anal sex. Wrong again! HPV is spread by skin to skin contact. You can get HPV from rubbing your penis against his anus (or vice versa) during foreplay without a condom. It gets worse. A condom doesn't cover the base of his shaft, scrotum or pubic area (unless your partner is inside a plastic bag) and these are all areas where the virus can lurk and contact your exposed skin during sex. Fingers and toys can also transport the virus between partners. Although the virus rarely grows on your fingers, one partner can deposit HPV on your anus where it will grow.

HPV is a growing health threat for gay men, but it can be effectively treated. Knowledge is power and what you don't know can definitely hurt you. Visit your doctor and ask for a pap smear. If he or she says it isn't necessary or doesn't know how to do it, find a doctor who can.

Updated: Wednesday, June 6th 2001

Serving the lesbian, gay, transgender & bisexual communities

GayHealth™

Nearly 40% of Gay and Bi Men Infected with Dangerous Strain of HPV

by GayHealth Staff

Thirty-eight percent of men who have sex with men (MSM) may be infected with HPV-16 compared with eight percent of heterosexual men and 19 percent of women, according to the Centers for Disease Control and Prevention (CDC).

You may have heard about the human papillomavirus (HPV) or genital warts; you might even know that most sexually active MSM have some form of HPV, but HPV-16 is a strain associated with 50 percent of all cervical cancer cases.

"While there is significant research on the link between HPV-16 and cervical cancer, much less is known about the impact of HPV on anal and reproductive tract cancers in gay and bisexual men," said Stuart Berman, M.D., head of CDC's STD epidemiology and surveillance branch. "These new findings begin to provide information about the transmission of this STD in this population."

The data, which is the first national data concerning the prevalence of HPV-16 among MSM, was presented at the National STD Prevention Conference held in San Diego March 4 to 7.

In April of 2000, Stephen E. Goldstone, medical director of GayHealth.com issued a report concerning the alarming increase in the rate of anal cancer among gay men. Dr. Goldstone attributes the rise in this cancer to HPV.

"The incidence of cervical cancer in women has plummeted because of aggressive screening and early treatment," said Stephen E. Goldstone, M.D. "HPV is a major health threat that all gay men need to know about in order to stem the rise of anal cancer."

The CDC findings were based on a sample of 83 MSM surveyed from 1988 to 1994 in the CDC's National Health and Nutrition Examinations Survey (NHANES). The data is preliminary, and more MSM focused research is needed, according to the CDC.

Updated: Thursday, March 7th 2002

Serving the lesbian, gay, transgender & bisexual communities

GayHealth™

Reuters Health - April 10, 2000

Gay Men May Benefit from Cancer Screen

NEW YORK, Apr 10 (Reuters Health) -- Homosexual men may benefit from routine screening for anal cancer, in much the same way that women benefit from routine Pap smears for cervical cancer, according to a New York surgeon.

In a study of 200 male homosexuals who were referred for surgery to treat anal warts or other relatively benign conditions, Dr. Stephen Goldstone, a general surgeon in New York City, found that 53% had precancerous lesions of the anus. Five patients were diagnosed with cancer, including 4 men who were HIV positive.

Overall, 131 men in the study were HIV infected, according to the report presented at the 4th International Congress on Papillomavirus in Human Pathology, held in Paris, France.

"Anal Pap testing can be used as a screening tool for anal cancer," Goldstone told Reuters Health in an interview prior to the meeting. He suggests Pap testing for any individual participating in anal sex. In Pap tests, cells are collected and looked at under a microscope for signs of cancerous changes.

Human papillomavirus (HPV) is a sexually transmitted organism that can cause genital warts or be completely symptom-free. Certain strains of HPV are known to increase the risk of dysplasia -- abnormal looking cells -- and cancer of the cervix in women.

"All men who have sex with men should be screened for human papillomavirus and dysplasia every year if HIV positive and every 2 to 3 years if HIV negative," Goldstone said. He added, however, that a test can determine if HPV is the type that can increase the risk of cancer, although "this (test) is not FDA-approved for men."

People at risk for anal HPV infection can visit the website www.GayHealth.com, which "offers health information specific to gay, lesbian, and bisexual individuals and will eventually include physician referral," Goldstone said. Goldstone serves as medical director to the website.

Updated: Friday, April 14th 2000

Serving the lesbian, gay, transgender
& bisexual communities

GayHealth™

Beyond the Anal Pap Smear

by Stephen E. Goldstone, M.D., F.A.C.S.

Physicians are feeling the crunch of time with patients more each day. Now there is yet another procedure that can help keep your patients healthy -- the anal Pap smear.

Current recommendations published by Goldie et al. document the cost effectiveness of this simple technique in prolonging life. According to Dr. Sue Goldie men with HIV who have sex with men should have an anal Pap smear every year while HIV-negative men should have one every two to three years -- provided the results are normal.

If you start smearing all the men who come to your office, what will you find?

Excellent prevalence studies carried out by Palefsky et al. and Kiviat et al. conducted in San Francisco and Seattle, respectively document surprisingly similar findings. Over 90 percent gay men with HIV carry HPV while about 65 percent of HIV-negative men carry it. They also documented that about 40 percent of HIV-positive men and 20 percent HIV-negative men carried type 16, which is considered to be a high risk oncogenic form of HPV. Palefsky et al. found that in routine screening, 40 percent of HIV-positive men and 79 percent of HIV-negative men had normal anal cytology by Pap smear, while 36 percent of positive men and seven percent of negative men had either low grade or high grade cytology.

As with abnormal cervical cytology, abnormal anal cytology requires further investigation with a type of colposcopy called high resolution anoscopy and biopsy of suspicious lesions. Palefsky et al. found that five percent of HIV infected men had biopsy proven HSIL while only 0.4 percent of HIV negative men had it.

It is important to regularly screen your patients, for even when normal at base line they can either become newly infected with HPV or have progression of disease. In the San Francisco cohort they noted that over two years 52 percent of HIV + men progressed from normal to either low grade or high grade dysplasia. For HIV-negative men, the rate of progression was slower with only 17 percent going from normal to low or high grade dysplasia. Those men with low grade lesions at baseline had a high risk of progressing to high grade dysplasia within 2 years (62 percent of HIV-positive and 36 percent of HIV-negative men). Regression from low grade disease was found in 50 percent of HIV-negative men and only 5 percent of HIV-positive men.

Those of us who care for men who have sex with men -- especially those infected with HIV -- are seeing dramatic and disturbing increases in anal cancer rates. As it is with cervical cancer and many other cancers, screening and early detection is our best means to combat this deadly disease.

For more in depth information I urge you to read the following articles:

Goldstone S. Anal dysplasia in men who have sex with men. The Aids Reader 9: 204 –208, 220, 1999. (Also available on Medscape)

Palefsky Jm, Holly EA, Ralston MI, et al: Anal squamous intraepithelial lesions in HIV-positive and HIV-negative homosexual and bisexual men: Prevalence and risk factors. J Acquir Immune Defic Syndr Hum Retrovirol. 17: 320 – 326, 1998.

Palefsky JM, Holly EA, Ralston MI, et al: Prevalence and risk factors for human papillomavirus infection of the anal canal in human immunodeficiency virus (HIV) – positive and HIV-negative homosexual men. J Infect Dis. 177:362-377, 1998.

Palefsky Jm, Holly EA, Hogeboom CJ, et al: Virologic, immunologic, and clinical parameters in the incidence and progression of anal squamous intraepithelial lesions in HIV- positive and HIV-negative homosexual men. J Acquir Immune Defic Syndr Hum Retrovirol 17: 314-319, 1998.

Kiviat NB, Critchlow CW, Holmes KK: Association of anal dysplasia and human papillomavirus with immunosuppression and HIV infection among homosexual men. AIDS 7: 43-49, 1993.

Goldie SJ, Kuntz KM, Weinstein MC, et al. Cost-effectiveness of screening for anal squamous intraepithelial lesions and anal cancer in HIV-negative homosexual and bisexual men. Amer J of Med 108: 634-641, 2000.

Goldie SJ, Kuntz KM, Weinstein MC, et al. The clinical-effectiveness and cost-effectiveness of screening for anal squamous intraepithelial lesions and anal cancer in HIV-positive homosexual and bisexual men. JAMA 281: 1822-1829, 1999.

Updated: Wednesday, December 20th 2000

Serving the lesbian, gay, transgender
& bisexual communities

GayHealth™

How To Do An Anal Pap Smear

by Stephen E. Goldstone, M.D., F.A.C.S.

Why do it?

Relax, it's easy. This simple test can be performed right in your office just like a cervical pap smear. An anal pap smear is critical to the health and wellness of your patients because it can help predict a potentially dysplastic anal lesion. A landmark study by Dr. Joel Palefsky et al (J of Infec Dis, 1998), in which anal canals of over 600 men who have sex with men were tested for HPV, found 61 percent of men without HIV and 93 percent of men with HIV carry HPV, and many contain oncogenic strains of the virus. Goldie, et al, Jama, 1999, showed that a yearly anal pap smear in men with HIV who have sex with men is an extremely cost effective test, more so than a yearly chest x-ray and annual pap smear in women. Men without HIV should have pap smears every two to three years.

The Procedure

You can do the pap smear with your patient on his side or in a knee-chest position. Perform the pap smear before you do a digital exam, which will put lubricant into his rectum and possibly remove loose, dysplastic cells. You won't need to use the wooden spatula that comes with most kits -- that will only give your male patients splinters! Gently spread his buttocks with one hand while holding a dacron swab or cyto brush in the other. Place your fingers as close to his anus as possible, so that when you spread his buttocks, anoderm spouts out. You cannot use lubricant on the swab or brush because this will distort the smear, making it more difficult for the cytologist to give an accurate reading. Moistening the swab or brush may make it less scratchy and decrease patient discomfort. Either way, it is a quick test and patients don't usually complain. I find that most men prefer a dacron swab because it is far less irritating than a cytobrush. Don't use cotton applicators as they hold onto the cells and prevent easy transfer to the slide.

Gently insert the swab or brush an inch or two into your patient's anus. I find that you can insert it until just after the end of the swab or brush disappears. Remember, you must push the swab above the squamo/columnar junction (where the squamous cells transition with columnar epithelium, usually at the dentate line) to be sure you sample the entire anus. The transition zone is also the most common site of dysplasia. If your brush or swab meets resistance, change your angle of insertion until it passes easily. If you encounter hemorrhoids, it may be difficult to find the actual anal opening and you might need several attempts. Once successfully in, twirl your brush or swab while moving it in and out several times. Remove it and immediately roll it across a microscope slide. (Be sure you label the slide with the patient's name.) Finish by spraying cytology fixative across the slide, as you would any routine pap smear. You must work quickly to prevent air drying and distortion of cellular architecture. Don't worry about feces or blood, the cytologist can read through it. As an alternative to preparing the smear on a slide, you can use a Thin-Prep cytology kit. In this case, you drop the swab or brush into the cytolyte solution and swish it around to transfer cells from swab or brush to the liquid. Discard the brush or swab and send the fluid to the cytologist. Thin-Prep has the advantage of decreasing air drying artifact. Finish every exam with a digital rectal.

The Lab

Send the specimen to your laboratory with a requisition for anal cytology. **Do not send it as a routine pap smear.** (I have rarely had a problem with insurance companies covering the test and I usually give a diagnosis of rectal bleeding or HPV -- after all, who hasn't experienced rectal bleeding?) If your cytologist feels uncomfortable reading an anal pap smear, tell them to apply the same criteria they would when grading a cervical pap. Results are generally reported as benign, ASCUS (atypical), low grade or high grade. Any abnormal pap smear should be investigated by anoscopy with magnification and acetic acid. You must be biopsy abnormal areas and ablate high grade dysplasia.

The Condyloma Connection

Whenever you have a patient with external condyloma or feel nodules on rectal exam, look inside. A standard anoscope works well. Insert the scope into your patient's anus. Remove the obterrator and pass a cotton applicator wrapped in a single 4X4 gauze soaked in slightly diluted vinegar down the barrel (three parts vinegar to one part water). Remove the anoscope while leaving the vinegar soaked swab in for 5 minutes. Remove the swab and reinsert the anoscope for a good look. The vinegar makes it easier to see HPV lesions which turn white. Frequently, men who have sex with men and have condyloma on the outside also have a severe case on the inside their anorectal canal. It is not enough to treat external condyloma alone! You can be missing the more dangerous dysplastic internal lesions. High grade dysplastic lesions usually don't look like condyloma. They tend to be flatter and resemble plaque.

Good luck with this new and exciting technique. Just tell your patient's to bend over and go for it. If you have any question, please write to me at GayHealth.com and I'll get back to you as quickly as I can.

Updated: Monday, September 24th 2001

News

back to news search ▲ back to news hitlist

Posted: 10 May 2004

eMail this article to a friend

Michael Carter

Pap smears may not accurately detect high-grade pre-cancerous anal lesions

Pap smears may not be an accurate predictor of high grade precancerous anal lesions that can lead to the development of anal cancer, according to a US study published in the May 15th edition of *Clinical Infectious Diseases*, which is now available on-line. Recently there has been much discussion about the value of offering Pap smears to HIV-positive gay men who have anal HPV infection, particularly as several studies have indicated that not only are HIV-positive men at an increased risk of anal cancer, but that HAART does not appear to reduce the risk. These findings underline the importance of closely monitoring individuals with abnormal anal cells.

Investigators from Boston paired the cytology results from 153 gay men attending an anal dysplasia clinic with histology results obtained from high resolution anoscopy. A total of 100 men (65%) were HIV-positive and the remaining 53 (35%) were HIV-negative. Cytology samples were obtained by swabbing or scraping the anus and rectum, whilst the histology samples were obtained by obtaining a tissue sample by biopsy.

Analysis of the paired results indicated that Pap cytology tests were not an accurate predictor of high grade precancerous anal lesions (anal intraepithelial neoplasia, AIN), and that a third of the Pap smears categorised by cytology as "low-grade" (AIN I) were in fact found to be "high-grade" (AIN III) when the histology results from an anal biopsy were studied.

The investigators note that their data "independently confirm a substantial incidence of histologically proven high-grade anal dysplasia in [gay men] who present with minimally abnormal anal Pap smear findings." No association between the presence of high-grade lesions and HIV status was found.

The investigators conclude that "abnormal anal cytological findings of any grade should suggest the possibility of high-grade histological findings."

Further information on this website

French study shows HAART no benefit against HPV or pre-cancerous anal lesions - news story

Anal cancer bad news for HIV-positive gay men even in HAART era, but incidence is rare - news story

Recent news

- HPV infection more common in HIV-positive women who smoke
- Pap smears may not accurately detect high-grade pre-cancerous ana lesions
- Prednisolone delays CD4 T-cell decreases in chron HIV infection
- Lipodystrophy associated with high levels of interleukin-18
- BCG vaccine against TB still works after 60 years says long-term follow-up study
- French report finds kidne toxicity on tenofovir to b rare and reversible

Pap smear

Reference

Panther LA et al. *High resolution anoscopy findings for men who have sex with men: inaccuracy of anal cytology as a predictor of histologic high-grade anal intraepithelial neoplasia and the impact of HIV serostatus*. Clinical Infectious Diseases 38 (on-line edition), 2004.

back to news search | ▲ back to news hitlist ▲

News

back to news search ▲ back to news hitlist

Posted: 30 March 2004

eMail this article to a friend

Michael Carter

French study shows HAART no benefit against HPV or pre-cancerous anal lesions

<

Improved immune function after treatment with HAART does not lead to the regression of pre-cancerous anal lesions in HIV-positive men, or to the clearance of human papilloma virus (HPV) infection, according to a French study published in the February edition of *Sexually Transmitted Diseases*. Investigators also found that neither infection with HPV nor the presence of pre-cancerous lesions was related to current or lowest-ever CD4 cell count. Numerous studies have now shown that HAART does not lead to an improvement in pre-cancerous anal lesions, or anal cancer.

Between summer 1999 and October 2000, 45 HIV-positive men who had taken at least six months of protease inhibitor-containing HAART were recruited to a cross-sectional study at the Hôpital Européen Georges Pompidou in Paris. Swabs were obtained for anal cytology and HPV testing, and then, within two months of the anal swabbing, investigators recorded the CD4 cell count and viral load for the individuals. Information on each individual's nadir CD4 cell count prior to commencing HAART was also recorded.

Of the 45 anal cytology samples obtained, 32 (71%) were abnormal, including 22 cases of low-grade pre-cancerous lesions, anal intraepithelial neoplasia (AIN) and six cases of high-grade AIN. A further four individuals had abnormal anal cytology of undetermined severity.

A total of 36 men were infected with HPV (80%), with 22 of these men infected with an HPV type known to be associated with a high risk of cancer. In addition, the investigators established that infection with multiple types of HPV was common, affecting 20 men (56%).

The presence of pre-cancerous anal lesions was not significantly different in men who had a CD4 cell count above or below 250 cells/mm^3 at enrolment (p=0.7). Furthermore, the investigators did not find any difference in the prevalence of pre-cancerous lesions when they stratified individuals according to their nadir CD4 cell count (above or below 150 cells/mm^3, p=0.3) prior to starting HAART, or according to the magnitude of their CD4 cell increase after starting treatment with HAART (above or below 150 cells/mm^3, p=0.3).

"No significant difference was observed between patients with and without anal HPV infection or between patients with or without abnormal cytology with regard to median CD4 cell count, median nadir of CD4 cell count, median increase in CD4 cell count,

Recent news

- HPV infection more common in HIV-positive women who smoke
- Pap smears may not accurately detect high-grade pre-cancerous ana lesions
- Prednisolone delays CD4 T-cell decreases in chron HIV infection
- Lipodystrophy associated with high levels of interleukin-18
- BCG vaccine against TB still works after 60 years says long-term follow-up study
- French report finds kidne toxicity on tenofovir to b rare and reversible

To receive a weekly ema update from aidsmap, featuring the latest news and additions to the site, click here.

median viral load... and median duration of previous protease inhibitor regimen," write the investigators.

They add, "our data suggest that immune restoration under HAART is not associated with a decrease in the prevalence of anal HPV or [A]IN." They conclude that the prevalence of HPV infection and AIN in HIV-positive gay men has remained unchanged since the introduction of HAART, and express concern that "if HAART exhibits no or little effect on the restoration of specific immunity against HPV, there would be more time for [AIN] to progress to cancer. This could in turn lead to an increase in anogential cancer among men and women receiving HAART, because they would be living longer."

Further information on this website

Human papilloma virus - overview

Consistent condom use associated with regression of CIN and clearance of HPV in Dutch studies - news story

Anal cancer bad news for HIV-positive gay men even in HAART era, but incidence is rare - news story

Reference

Piketty C et al. *High prevalence of anal squamous intraepithelial lesions in HIV-positive men despite use of highly active antiretroviral therapy*. Sexually Transmitted Diseases 31: 96 – 99, 2004.

back to news search | ▲ back to news hitlist ▲

News

back to news search ▲ back to news hitlist

Posted: 19 January 2004

eMail this article to a friend

Michael Carter

Anal cancer bad news for HIV-positive gay men even in HAART era, but incidence is rare

Anal cancer occurs more frequently in HIV-positive gay men, doesn't respond to HAART, is difficult to treat, has a poor outcome, but is, thankfully, rare, according to data from the largest UK HIV cohort presented to a forum on HIV and cancer on January 17th organised by London University's Wolfson Institute.

Since 1986, 8,640 individuals have been enrolled into the Chelsea and Westminster HIV cohort, providing over 40,000 patient years of follow-up. A total of 26 cases of invasive anal cancer have been diagnosed during this period, 25 of them in gay men (the remaining case being in a heterosexual woman).

Although a pre-HIV US study showed that gay men were 33 times more likely to develop anal cancer, data from the Chelsea and Westminster cohort showed that the incidence of anal cancer was even higher in HIV-positive individuals, at 60 cases per 105 patient years of follow-up, against 0.5 cases per 105 patient years in the age and sex matched Thames Cancer registry. This finding was consistent with a US study which found that gay HIV-positive men had a risk ratio of developing anal cancer of 66.

Unlike the AIDS-defining cancers Kaposi's sarcoma and non-Hodgkin's lymphoma, the development of anal cancer was not linked to severe immune suppression, the median CD4 cell count of individuals presenting with anal cancer being 206 cells/mm^3.

The incidence of anal cancer has not fallen with the introduction of HAART ($p>0.05$). Since 1996, 67% of individuals diagnosed with malignancy have been taking HIV therapy, and 28% (18 individuals) have had a viral load below 50 copies/mL.

Clinicians at the Chelsea and Westminster used chemoradiotherapy to treat anal cancer in 22 individuals, surgery in two patients with small cancerous lesions, with the remaining two patients, who had advanced HIV disease, receiving palliative care only. A total of eleven patients died, seven of anal cancer and four of an AIDS-defining condition.

This provided a two-year survival rate of 47%. Further, the prognosis of patients with anal cancer in the Chelsea and Westminster cohort has not improved since the use of HAART. Neither CD4 cell count, use of HAART, history of a prior AIDS-defining illness, nor length of HIV diagnosis of prognostic value.

To further enhance these data, the London investigators pooled their findings with of US clinicians. This provided the investigators with information on a total of 46 individuals. The findings were consistent with those from the 26 London patients. A

Recent news

- HPV infection more common in HIV-positive women who smoke
- Pap smears may not accurately detect high-grade pre-cancerous ana lesions
- Prednisolone delays CD4 T-cell decreases in chron HIV infection
- Lipodystrophy associated with high levels of interleukin-18
- BCG vaccine against TB still works after 60 years says long-term follow-up study
- French report finds kidne toxicity on tenofovir to b rare and reversible

To receive a weekly ema update from aidsmap, featuring the latest news and additions to the site, click here.

of individuals died of anal cancer within a year of diagnosis and the 66% one-year survival rate continued to decline with time.

The bad news didn't end there. Screening for anal cancer appears to be of no particular value.

A pilot programme to detect cancers and precancerous cells in the anus - anal intraepithelial neoplasma (AIN) – was conducted at the Chelsea and Westminster Hospital. A total of 156 screens were conducted on 100 patients. All individuals with AIN were infected with the HPV virus, which causes genital and anal warts. Certain strains of HPV, particularly HPV-16, have been associated with an increased risk of cancer. However, the London investigators found that no particular strain of HPV was associated with the presence of AIN, suggesting that infection with any strain of HPV increased the risk of precancerous cells developing.

Furthermore, no correlation was found between the presence of AIN and either CD4 and CD8 cell count, or HIV viral load.

To see if HAART had an impact on the AIN, 23 gay men were assessed six months after starting HIV therapy. The grade of AIN went down in 35% of individuals, remained stable in 43%, and become worse in 22%. Changes in CD4, CD8, or viral load after starting HAART were not related to alterations in the grade of AIN.

Difficulties in the management of AIN were also encountered by the Chelsea and Westminster clinicians. The use of surgery to remove the precancerous lesions left 50% of individuals in uncontrollable pain for over three weeks, and 75% experienced a recurrence of AIN within three years.

Further information on this website

Anal cancer risk high in all HIV-positive men regardless of sexual behaviour - news story

Genital warts - factsheet

ATU September 2002

Reference

Bower M. *HIV associated anal cancer and anal intraepithelial neoplasma.* Oral presentation, AIDS-related cancer forum, Wolfson Institute for Biomedical Research, University College London, January 17th, 2004.

back to news search | ▲ back to news hitlist ▲

20. Miscellaneous Documents

October 5, 2000

The Honorable Tom Coburn
United States House of Representatives
Washington, D.C. 20515

Dear Representative Coburn:

I would like to thank you for your continued efforts to educate men and women across the country about the human papillomavirus (HPV). I, unfortunately, am one of the thousands of women who contracted this virus through, what I thought was, "safe sex."

I contracted this virus through my *first* sexual encounter three years ago, when I was 25 years old. Imagine my horror when, at my first gynecological visit, I was informed that I had a sexually transmitted disease – a disease I had never heard of. "Not me!" was my arrogant response. STDs, in my mind, were associated only with promiscuous, morally deviant individuals. This is not the case. It can happen to anyone.

I have always been a healthy, athletic, and morally principled individual. I am a college-educated woman and the daughter of a nurse and a doctor! Unfortunately, I made a poor choice – a poor, *uneducated* choice. I blame no one but myself for the consequences of my actions, but can't help but wonder if I would have made a different choice if the facts had been previously laid out before me. The physical and mental effects of this virus, and the stigma surrounding it, are devastating. I have experienced debilitating depression and low self-esteem. It has taken three years to gain back some semblance of self-respect, but the shame still lingers.

Support for an HPV education program is NOT an endorsement for sexual promiscuity; it is, rather, and endorsement for abstinence. Women AND MEN need to know that condoms do not protect against HPV. Women need to know that HPV can be linked with 90% of cases of cervical cancer. Women need to know that cervical cancer is the second-deadliest form of cancer in the world. I know this now…I wish I had known then.

This is not an easy subject to discuss, and I hope you will understand my desire for privacy. If this letter will help you persuade your colleagues that this is a real issue that affects real people, then this exercise is not in vain. I am not a constituent, but rather a citizen who appreciates what you are doing, and prays for your success. Thank you for being a voice for those of us too ashamed to speak for ourselves.

Sincerely,

An Appreciative Citizen

Thank you.

University Wire

February 27, 2001

College Nurse: "Most Cases of Herpes and HPV Are Contracted While Wearing a Condom"

Sixty-five million people are living with incurable sexually transmitted diseases (STDs) in the U.S., according to the Center for Disease Prevention and Control. This is a frightening reality that college students everywhere are facing, and many are under the illusion that a condom is giving them ultimate protection from everything.

"People think they're protected when they use a condom, but they're not," said Marlene Hjeldness, a nurse practitioner at the University of North Dakota's Student Health. "Most cases of herpes and HPV (human papillomavirus) are contracted while wearing a condom. Condoms are only good for HIV and diseases only spread by the body fluids, there is no protection against the herpes and warts that are on the skin where the condom doesn't cover."

Hjeldness said giving a student a positive test result is very hard thing to do. "Most of the girls seek a female nurse when they come in," she said. "They are in shock, tearful and crying. We give them all the pamphlets we have and tell them they can be treated here for it. I always tell them that they can come and talk to me anytime. It is unfortunate, but most girls don't want to talk to their friends about it."

Hjeldness said she feels alcohol plays a major role in the spread of STDs on college campuses. "Alcohol removes all inhibitions," she said. "Most girls will say things like 'I never would have done that if I wasn't drunk,' 'I never would have slept with him.' They are very saddened by the incident, and now they have an STD."

At UND, the most common STDs diagnosed are chlamydia, the human papillomavirus (HPV) and herpes.

Chlamydia is one of the most common STDs diagnosed around the country and at Student Health, particularly in men. This disease is difficult to detect, as it is often asymptotic. If symptoms do occur, they consist of burning urination and discharge. Chlamydia is responsible for 200,000 cases of infertility each year in the U.S., and is the leading cause of blindness in underdeveloped countries. There are four million reported cases of chlamydia each year in the U.S. In North Dakota alone there were 934 reported cases in 1999-2000. Of these, 158 of them were in Grand Forks, and the highest number of them, 397, were reported in people ages 20-24. The second highest was 307 in youths ages 15-19.

HPV is another one of the most common STDs in the country, causing genital warts. It is estimated that as many as 24 million Americans are currently infected with the reoccurring virus. The disease most commonly causes small warts on the genitals and in women is often closely associated with the development of cervical cancer and other genital cancers. The main problem with HPV is that it too will often have no symptoms. At UND's Student Health, there were 58 cases of genital warts diagnosed on campus in the last year alone.

There were also seven cases of Herpes Simplex diagnosed at student health this past year. There are two strains of the virus: Herpes I and Herpes II. Herpes I is what occurs as cold sores found on the mouth. These reoccur less than Herpes II, which is the same sort of blistering, but on the genitals. Herpes is the fastest-growing STD in America. Some statistics say that one in every six Americans carries the virus and a total of half a million are infected each year. Early symptoms of the herpes virus consist of tingling, itching and burning in the genital area, and are followed by redness and painful blisters. One of the biggest problems with herpes is that a person may not even know that they have it, because it is often symptomless. It is said that upward of 60 percent of herpes carriers don't even know they have it. Also, according the United States Health Department, one quarter of Americans over the age of 15 are infected with the herpes virus.

There were also 81 reported cases of gonorrhea across the state, with its frequency lying in the 15-24-year-old range. "Most (men) come in because their partner told them to, or because they got a call from the state," said Mark Christenson, M.D., at Student Heath.

All positive diagnoses of chlamydia, gonorrhea, syphilis and hepatitis B are reported to the North Dakota Public Health Department. At this point the carrier of the STD is required by law to report the names of their past partners to the health department. The past partners will then be confidentially contacted by the health department and informed that they have been in contact with someone who tested positive for the disease. This is a part of the ongoing effort to control the spread of STDs in the country.

Student Health reports that it has had no positive HIV or syphilis tests in years. "As a whole we've been lucky here at UND," Christenson said.

It is important for someone diagnosed with an STD to get treatment because oftentimes the person can slip into depression or withdrawal, and avoid relationships in general. Hjeldness feels that education is key. "I think the problems start when the kids are young," she said. "We have to educate kids at a young age so they know about these things when they get to college. The education also needs to continue at the college level, because this is when the kids are becoming infected."

"I know it sounds impossible, but abstinence is the only safe way," Hjeldness said. "It's the only way we're going to start getting this problem under control."

Partner reduction is crucial for balanced "ABC" approach to HIV prevention

James D Shelton, Daniel T Halperin, Vinand Nantulya, Malcolm Potts, Helene D Gayle, King K Holmes

Behaviour change programmes to prevent HIV have mainly promoted condom use or abstinence, while partner reduction remains the neglected component of ABC

The key to preventing the spread of HIV, especially in epidemics driven mainly by heterosexual transmission, is through changing sexual behaviour. Interest has been growing in an "ABC" approach in which A stands for abstinence or delay of sexual activity, B for be faithful, and C for condom use (box).[1] Although "be faithful" literally implies monogamy, it also includes reductions in casual sex and multiple sexual partnerships (and related issues of partner selection) that would reduce higher risk sex. While most of the often polarised discussion surrounding AIDS prevention has focused on promoting abstinence or use of condoms,[w1 w2] partner reduction has been the neglected middle child of the ABC approach.

ABC of sexual behaviour change

A = abstinence or delay of sexual activity
B = be faithful (including partner reduction and avoiding high risk partners)
C = condom use, particularly for high risk sex

Epidemiological importance of partner reduction

It seems obvious, but there would be no global AIDS pandemic were it not for multiple sexual partnerships. The rate of change of sexual partners—especially concurrent partners—is a crucial determinant in the spread of sexually transmitted infections,[w3] including HIV.[2] Moreover, HIV viral load and therefore infectiousness is dramatically higher during the early (acute) stage of HIV infection,[3] so transmission would be particularly heightened by partner change among newly infected people. Transmission of HIV is also facilitated by the presence of other sexually transmitted infections, especially ulcerative ones.[w4] Hence, increased risk of other sexually transmitted infections from multiple partnerships further magnifies the spread of HIV.

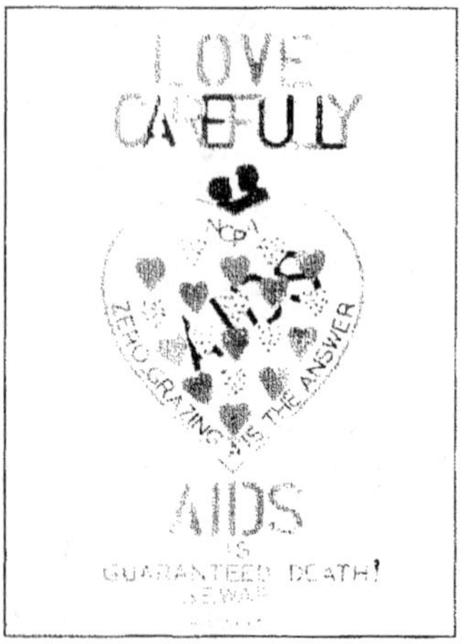
LOVE
CAREFULLY
ZERO GRAZING IS THE ANSWER
AIDS
IS
GUARANTEED DEATH!

Fig 1 Poster from Uganda's AIDS Control Programme in the late 1980s

Role in HIV prevention successes

Partner reduction seems to have been pivotal to success in two countries heralded for reversing their HIV epidemics, Thailand and Uganda. Thailand's "100% condom" approach in brothels is widely credited with reversing its more concentrated epidemic. However, this intervention was also followed by a striking reduction (about a twofold decline between 1990 and 1993) in the proportion of men who reported engaging in commercial and other casual sex.[4-6]

In Uganda, where the estimated prevalence of HIV in adults has fallen from about 15% to 5% during the past decade,[7] each component of the ABC approach probably had an important role. However, the least recognised element, partner reduction, was perhaps the key.

It is difficult to reconstruct the events that occurred during the late 1980s and early 1990s, when the rate of new infections was falling in Uganda.[5-7 w5] With respect to abstinence, Demographic and Health Surveys between 1989 and 1995 show that age at sexual debut increased by less than one year,[6] and the proportion of single women aged 15-24 who reported sex during the previous year fell by about a third. Such changes were clearly important, but alone probably cannot account for the large national decline in HIV infection across all age groups.

In the same surveys, ever use of condoms increased from 1% to 6% for women, and by 1995 had reached 16% among men.[7] In the 1989 and 1995 surveys conducted by WHO's Global Programme on

References w1-w10 and a figure with data for Uganda are on bmj.com

Editorial by Wilson

Bureau for Global Health, US Agency for International Development, 1300 Pennsylvania Avenue, Washington, DC 20523-3700, USA
James D Shelton *senior medical scientist, office of population and reproductive health*
Daniel T Halperin *senior technical adviser, office of HIV/AIDS*

Global Fund for AIDS, Tuberculosis and Malaria, Geneva, Switzerland
Vinand Nantulya *senior adviser*

University of California, Berkeley 94720 USA
Malcolm Potts *Bixby population professor*

Bill and Melinda Gates Foundation, Seattle, WA 98102, USA
Helene D Gayle *director of HIV, tuberculosis, and reproductive U*

Center for AIDS and Sexually Transmitted Diseases, University of Washington, Seattle 98104, USA
King K Holmes *director*

Correspondence to: D Halperin dhalp@worldwidedialup.net

BMJ 2004;328:891-4

AIDS, which sampled a more urban population, reported ever use of condoms was substantially higher, increasing from 7% to 20% in women and from 15% to 30% in men.[8] Especially in such a generalised epidemic, however, these levels of condom use were still relatively modest, and ever use encompasses much more than the correct and consistent use of condoms required to prevent HIV infection.[8 9] Therefore, although condom use probably contributed, it seems unlikely to account for the dramatic fall in HIV incidence in the late 1980s and early 1990s. By 2000, Uganda had one of the highest levels of reported condom use for non-regular partners in Africa,[6] which probably supported the continuing stabilisation of the epidemic in the later 1990s.

But evidently even more important changes in sexual behaviour had occurred in Uganda. In the face of the then pervasive national campaign to encourage sticking to regular partners ("zero grazing," fig 1), reported multiple partner behaviour dropped noticeably. The Global Programme on AIDS surveys found that the proportion of men with one or more casual partners in the previous year fell from 35% in 1989 to 15% in 1995, and the proportion of women from 16% to 6%.[5-7] Notably, the proportion of men reporting three or more non-regular partners fell from 15% to 3% (see bmj.com).[6]

Because people with large numbers of sex partners are most likely to spread sexually transmitted diseases, such changes are profound. Indeed, modelling of HIV interventions in rural Uganda suggests that such degrees of partner reduction could have had a substantial effect on incidence.[10 w6] Although a direct causal link cannot be definitively established between the campaign to promote monogamy and partner reduction, and the concomitant fall in the incidence of HIV, it seems likely that it was critical to the success in Uganda.[5 7]

Other examples of partner reduction

Partner reduction has also occurred in other places. Many people, including gay men in Europe and the United States,[1 5 11] seem to have responded to the threat of AIDS by reducing their number of partners. Demographic and health surveys in 29 developing countries in the 1990s asked individuals if they had done anything to avoid AIDS.[w7] Almost 80% of men and 50% of women reported that they had. The commonest reported change by far was restricting activity to one partner, followed by reducing numbers of partners, avoiding prostitutes, and adopting condom use. However, such survey findings were one time, retrospective responses, and therefore may not accurately represent changes in behaviour over time.

Other data provide more direct evidence of such behavioural change. Surveys from Cambodia, where prevention efforts seem to have reduced HIV infection,[12 w8] indicate the proportion of men who reported paying for sex has fallen greatly (fig 2).[13] In Zambia, the prevalence of HIV reportedly fell among urban young women during the 1990s.[6 12 14] At about that time there was a large reduction in casual and multiple partner sex[6 15] in the presence of faith based and other grassroots efforts to promote delay of sexual

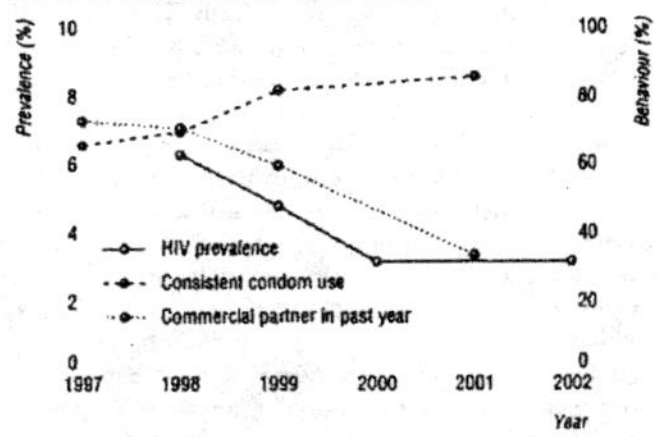

Fig 2 HIV prevalence and reported use of condoms and commercial sex among police in Cambodia, 1997-2002. The method for asking about condom use changed in 1999, which accounts for part of the increase from 1998 to 1999

debut among young people and monogamy for those who were sexually active. More recently, HIV prevalence has declined in Addis Ababa, Ethiopia,[w9] where large reductions in commercial and other casual sex have been reported among male factory workers.[16] And in the Dominican Republic, where HIV also seems to have abated,[12 17] men have reported partner reduction in addition to increased condom use with sex workers.

Implications for behaviour change programmes

Our analysis of the importance of partner reduction and monogamy rests largely on ecological and other observational evidence, including self reported behavioural findings. Nevertheless, the overall patterns and associations seem consistent and logical and suggest that partner reduction could have a major effect. Yet it is still given little attention in most HIV prevention programmes, despite its epidemiological importance and apparent behavioural "acceptability." We believe it is imperative to begin including (and rigorously evaluating) messages about mutual fidelity and partner reduction in ongoing activities to change sexual behaviour. Formative research should identify which changes are feasible for each audience, and programmes should then build on behaviour changes that people already seem willing to make.

Moreover, it seems important and feasible to promote monogamy and partner reduction alongside abstinence and use of condoms. People seem generally able to grasp that the root problem with HIV transmission is risky sex and adopt the behaviour that best fits their circumstances. We have a public health responsibility to help people understand the strengths and limitations of each component and not promote one to the detriment of another. For example, although abstinence may be a viable option for many young people, for others it may be an unrealistic expectation. Likewise, even though prospective studies have shown that condoms reduce risk by about 80-90% when always used,[9 w1] in real life they are often used incorrectly or inconsistently.[8 9] They should therefore not be advertised in a manner that leads to overconfidence or risky behaviour.

Importantly, evidence from both Thailand and Uganda indicates not only that individual behaviour changed but also that group norms of behaviour were altered.[1 7 18] In Uganda, a combination of explicit and repeated presidential pronouncements and the committed engagement of faith based organisations, the governmental apparatus, the military, the health system, and community based and mass communications—all in the context of the stark reality of people dying from AIDS—seem to have achieved a "tipping point" so that avoiding risky sex has become the community norm. This experience supports the need for reinforcing messages from multiple sources. In addition, most of the behaviour change approaches originated within Uganda (and similarly within Thailand),[1 5 7] suggesting external assistance should reinforce such locally developed approaches.

Of course, HIV prevention must extend beyond the ABC approach. Other behaviour changes such as avoiding the particularly risky practice of unprotected anal intercourse are important,[19] as are efforts to reduce risk from intravenous drug use, promote safe injection practices in healthcare settings, expand access to voluntary counselling and testing, and treat other sexually transmitted infections, especially in high risk populations. In addition, it is imperative to continue efforts to develop an effective AIDS vaccine, develop safe microbicides so that women can directly lower their risk, explore increased availability of male circumcision,[20 w10] and remain open to other new tools in the fight against the pandemic. How all these components are optimally promoted and deployed depends on many factors, including the stage and nature of a given epidemic and the particular subpopulations at risk. Additional research is necessary to maximise the impact of partner reduction and other interventions. Rather than arguing over the merits of abstinence versus condoms, it is time for the international community to unite around a balanced, evidence based ABC approach.

We thank Bernard Branson, Martha Campbell, Ward Cates, Kate Crawford, Paul Delay, Nomi Fuchs, Edward Green, Douglas Kirby, Anne Peterson, William Phillips, Glenn Post, Jeff Spieler, and John Stover for their useful comments.

Contributors and sources: The authors are all experts in HIV prevention with long experience in the developing world, and VN was involved in the early AIDS prevention efforts in Uganda. The two principal authors, DH and JS, developed the original concept from their review of published and unpublished evidence on what epidemiological and programmatic factors seem to have contributed to successful HIV prevention outcomes, particularly in Africa and southeast Asia. The other authors contributed importantly in reformulating and revising the paper.

Competing interests: None declared.

"The horror of Slim [AIDS] is forcing people to change social habits … In Bugolobi, a young housewife with three children declared, with a gleam in her eye, "My husband stays at home much more. And I encourage him to do so by enthusiastically keeping him informed of the latest gossip about Slim victims."

New Vision newspaper,
Kampala, Uganda, 1987 Oct 23:10

Summary points

Controversy in AIDS prevention has primarily centred on abstinence versus condoms

Meanwhile, partner reduction has had an important role in countries that have cut HIV infections

Locally developed behaviour change approaches are often most effective in altering social norms

Abstinence, monogamy, and condom use should be promoted in an evidence based, mutually supportive way

1 Green E. A plan as simple as ABC. *New York Times* 2003 Mar 1.
2 Garnett GP. The basic reproduction rate of infection and the course of HIV epidemics. *AIDS Patient Care STDs* 1998;12:435-49.
3 Pilcher CD, Tien HC, Eron JJ, Vernazza PL, Leu SY, Stewart PM, et al. Brief but efficient: acute HIV infection and the sexual transmission of HIV. *AIDS* (in press).
4 Mills S, Benjarattanaporn P, Bennett A, Pattalug RN, Sundhagul D, Trongsawad P. HIV risk behavioral surveillance in Bangkok, Thailand: sexual behavior trends among eight population groups. *AIDS* 1997;11(suppl 1):S43-51.
5 Low-Beer D, Stoneburner RL. Behaviour and communication change in reducing HIV: is Uganda unique? *African J AIDS Res* 2003;2:9-21. www.hsph.harvard.edu/hcpds/PublicationsWeb/Low-Beer1.pdf (accessed 29 Jan 2004).
6 Bessinger R, Akwara P, Halperin DT. *Sexual behavior, HIV and fertility trends: a comparative analysis of six countries; phase I of the ABC study.* Chapel Hill, NC: Measure Evaluation, 2003. www.cpc.unc.edu/measure/publications/special/ (accessed 20 Jan 2004).
7 Hogle J, Green EC, Nantulya V, Stoneburner R, Stover J. *What happened in Uganda? Declining HIV prevalence, behavior change, and the national response.* Washington, DC: USAID, 2002. www.usaid.gov/pop_health/aids/Countries/africa/uganda_report.pdf (accessed 29 Jan 2003).
8 Ahmed S, Lutalo T, Wawer M, Serwadda D, Sewankambo NK, Nalugoda F, et al. HIV incidence and sexually transmitted disease prevalence associated with condom use: a population study in Rakai, Uganda. *AIDS* 2001;15:2171-9.
9 Hearst N, Chen S. *Condoms for AIDS prevention in the developing world: a review of the scientific literature.* Geneva: UNAIDS, 2003. www.usp.br/nepaids/condom.pdf (accessed 29 Jan 2004).
10 Robinson R, Mulder DW, Auvert B, Hayes RJ. Modelling the impact of alternative HIV intervention strategies in rural Uganda. *AIDS* 1995;9:1263-70.
11 Rotello G. Sexual ecology: AIDS and the destiny of gay men. New York: Dutton, 1997.
12 UNAIDS. *Report on the global HIV/AIDS epidemic 2002.* Geneva: WHO, 2002. www.unaids.org/Unaids/EN/Resources/Publications/Corporate+publications/Report+on+the+global+HIV_AIDS+epidemic+2002+.asp (accessed 30 Jan 2004).
13 National Center for HIV/AIDS, Dermatology and STDs. *Behavioral sentinel survey (BSS) V: sexual behavior among urban sentinel groups, Cambodia 2001.* Phnom Penh: NCHADS, 2003.
14 Fylkesnes K, Musonda RM, Sichone M, Ndhlovu Z, Tembo F, Monze M. Declining HIV prevalence and risk behaviors in Zambia: evidence from surveillance and population-based surveys. *AIDS* 2001;15:907-16.
15 Agha S. Declines in casual sex in Lusaka, Zambia: 1996-1999. *AIDS* 2002;16:291-3.
16 Mekonnen Y, Sanders E, Aklilu M, Tsegaye A, Rinke de Wit TF, Schaap A, et al. Evidence of changes in sexual behaviours among male factory workers in Ethiopia. *AIDS* 2003;17:223-31.
17 Green EC, Conde A. Sexual partner reduction and HIV infection. *Sex Trans Inf* 2000;76:145.
18 VanLandingham M, Trujillo L. Recent changes in heterosexual attitudes, norms and behaviors among unmarried Thai men: a qualitative analysis. *Int Fam Plann Perspect* 2002;28:6-15.
19 Halperin DT, Padian NS, Palefsy J, Shiboski SC. High level of HIV-1 infection associated with anal intercourse: A neglected risk factor in heterosexual AIDS prevention. International AIDS Conference, Barcelona, July 2002. www.aids2002.com/Program/ViewAbstract.asp?id=/T-CMS_Content/Abstract/200206290751215051.xml (accessed 29 Jan 2004).
20 Bailey RC, Plummer FA, Moses S. Male circumcision and HIV prevention: current knowledge and future research directions. *Lancet Inf Dis* 2001;1:223-31.

(Accepted 19 January 2004)

Competing interests: FH was a member of the board and chairperson of ASH Ireland and is their current spokesperson. He was also a member of the board of the European Network on Smoking Prevention.

1 *Public Health (Tobacco) Acts 2002 and 2004*. Dublin: Stationery Office, 2004.
2 *Tobacco (Health Promotion and Protection) Regulations 1995*. Dublin: Stationery Office, 1995.
3 Department of Health. *Working together for cleaner air. Developing smoke free policies in the workplace*. Dublin: Health Promotion Unit, 1994.
4 California Environmental Protection Agency. *Health effects of exposure to environmental tobacco smoke*. Sacramento: California Environmental Protection Agency, 1997.
5 Department of Health and Children. *Quality and fairness. A health system for you*. Dublin: Stationery Office, 2001. www.doh.ie/hstrat/index.html (accessed 1 Apr 2004).
6 Department of Health and Children. *Towards a tobacco free society: report of the tobacco free policy review group*. Dublin: Stationery Office, 2000. www.doh.ie/publications/tobacco.html (accessed 1 Apr 2004).
7 Joint Committee on Health and Children. *A national anti-smoking strategy. A report on smoking and health*. Dublin: Houses of the Oireachtas, 1999.
8 Joint Committee on Health and Children. *Second interim report of the subcommittee on health and smoking*. Dublin: Houses of the Oireachtas, 2001.
9 Repace J. Right to life overrides right to smoke. *Irish Times* 2002;Feb 11.
10 Allwright S, McLoughlin JP, Murphy D, Pratt I, Ryan MP, Smith A. *Report on the health effects of environmental tobacco smoke (ETS) in the workplace*. Dublin: Office of Tobacco Control/Health and Safety Authority, 2002. http://69.20.28.11/article.asp?article=34 (accessed 1 Apr 2004).
11 National and united force representing at least 1.1 million people living in Ireland fully endorse smoking ban and welcome date. www.smokefreeatwork.ie/news/detail.asp?id=10 (accessed 18 Feb 2004).
12 Smokers say publicans should obey the smoking ban. www.otc.ie/article.asp?article=145 (accessed 4 Nov 2003).

Partner reduction and the prevention of HIV/AIDS

The most effective strategies come from within communities

Education and debate p 891

In an era of increasingly complex HIV/AIDS analyses and responses, Shelton et al reaffirm the simple truth that without multiple sexual partnerships, an HIV epidemic would not occur and that by extension partner reduction is the most obvious, yet paradoxically neglected, approach to the prevention of HIV (p 891).[1] They note that in the ABC model for preventing AIDS/HIV (abstinence, or deferred sexual inception—A, be faithful, or partner reduction—B, and condom use—C), sexual deferral and condom use have persuasive advocates but partner reduction does not.

Their analysis of the vital part played by partner reduction in reducing HIV infection in Western gay communities, Uganda, and Thailand is timely. We face a crisis in HIV prevention. The successes in Uganda and Thailand occurred 15 years ago, and in the intervening period no national declines of similar clarity or scope have occurred. Similarly, in HIV prevention research, the heady days of the Mwanza sexually transmitted infections trial were succeeded by the disappointing findings (albeit explicable) in the more ambitious Rakai sexually transmitted infections trial, the Masaka triplet IEC (information, education, and communication) and sexually transmitted infections trial, and most distressingly, the recent Mwanza adolescent trial.[2-4] Shelton et al's analysis may help to infuse new life into HIV/AIDS prevention. Their argument that partner reduction is the potential centrepiece of a unified ABC approach is good common sense—and good epidemiology.

Whether the ABC approach addresses the needs of women is debatable, with commentators arguing that many women are unable to negotiate relationships based on abstinence, faithfulness, or condom use.[11] The enduring contribution of gender inequalities, including economic inequality and gender violence, to women's vulnerability to HIV is incontrovertible. Yet it is intriguing that some of the steepest declines in HIV infection levels in Uganda seem to have occurred among women, particularly young women, putatively the most powerless members of society. Shelton et al present evidence that where HIV prevalence has declined among pregnant women (Uganda, Thailand, Zambia, Ethiopia, Cambodia, and the Dominican Republic) the primary reported behaviour change has been partner reduction and monogamy by men, especially older men. Uganda's experience shows that achieving sexual deferral and partner reduction among men, particularly older men, may create safer environments for women, particularly young women. Community norms that proscribe older men having sexual relationships with younger women may be especially protective. A successful ABC approach that reduces HIV infection among women, particularly young women, is a vital element of a broader gender response. Uganda's ABC approach was reinforced by practical measures to increase women's participation in higher education and political life and to protect women from gender violence and sexual coercion.

Analysis of factors contributing to behaviour change in Uganda and elsewhere is even more challenging than the reaffirmation of partner reduction. Contexts as disparate as California, Uganda, and Thailand share unnerving similarities.[2-10] Above all, HIV prevention responses were rapid, endogenous, inexpensive, and simple.[8 9] They were based on the premise that communities, however disparate, have within themselves the resources and capital to reverse this epidemic. They preceded large scale exogenous assistance and occurred largely without the involvement of specialist agencies. They were locally led, by gay leaders and activists in California and by political, religious, and community leaders in Uganda. They promoted changes in community norms, thus creating enabling and protective environments long before the concept gained currency. They stressed simple messages and actions and in doing so achieved declines in HIV infection that preceded the growth in HIV services, including distribution of condoms and voluntary counselling and testing. They relied on interpersonal communication channels and networks, rather than mass media.[8 9 11]

Remarkably they combined high fear approaches with openness and the capacity to rise above discrimination and to integrate prevention and care effectively.[8 9] In doing so they created a context in which people perceived high personal risk of HIV infection and a personal proximity to the epidemic (measured, for example, by the extent to which we know people who have died of AIDS) that many communities with equally high HIV infection levels have not yet attained.

BMJ 2004;328:848-9

Despite our lament that behaviour change is slow, they achieved rapid declines in risky sexual behaviour and HIV infection. The slowest element was our capacity to recognise the rapidity and extent of these changes. They unified personal values and societal messages to achieve conviction and consistency. As AIDS educators, we often publicly promote approaches that we would not countenance in our own personal lives, such as the notion that it is acceptable for our spouses or children to have multiple partners, provided condoms are used. In Uganda, emphasis on the primacy of partner reduction resonated with community perspectives.

Partner reduction is good epidemiology, not good ideology, and we must ensure that the ABC approach remains sufficiently scientifically grounded to withstand shifting ideological sands. Happily epidemiology's insights are diverse enough to affront all our ideologies in equal measure. While Uganda's achievements imply a major role for partner reduction, data from, for example, Nairobi, Abidjan, Accra, many other cities in Africa, and large swathes of Asia support a major focus on making sex work safe, through rights based legal reform, enhanced sexual health care, and promotion of condoms. Similarly, the epidemics in the former Soviet Union and much of Asia cry out for a major commitment to comprehensive initiatives to reduce harm to injecting drug users.

We are indebted to Shelton et al for calling attention to the importance of partner reduction and its possible determinants and the implications for our programmes. We must also recognise that many communities have not developed similarly effective local responses, and respond with improved epidemiological and social research to ensure we understand what happened in Uganda and elsewhere. We require this to communicate persuasively with hesitant communities and to improve our ability to facilitate and nurture effective local responses. In short, we must foster endogenous responses founded primarily on the resources, capital, and leadership within communities while enhancing research to ensure these responses are understood, evaluated, and illuminated by science.

David Wilson *senior monitoring and evaluation specialist*

Global HIV/AIDS Program, World Bank, 1818 H Street N.W, Washington, DC 20433, USA (dwilson@worldbank.org)

The findings, interpretations, and conclusions expressed in this paper are entirely those of the author. They do not necessarily represent the view of the World Bank, its executive directors, or the countries they represent.

Competing interests: None declared.

1 Shelton JD, Halperin DT, Nantulya V, Potts M, Gayle H, Holmes KK. Partner reduction is crucial for balanced "ABC" approach to HIV prevention. *BMJ* 2004;328:891-4.
2 Grosskurth H, Mosha F, Todd J, Mwijarubi E, Klokke A, Senkoro K, et al. Impact of improved treatment of sexually transmitted diseases on HIV infection in rural Tanzania: randomized controlled trial. *Lancet* 1995;346:530-6.
3 Wawer MJ, Sewankambo NK, Serwadda D, Quinn TC, Paxton LA, Kiwanuka N, et al. Control of sexually transmitted diseases for AIDS prevention in Uganda. *Lancet* 1999;353:525-35.
4 Kamali A, Carpenter L, Whitworth J, Pool R, Ruberantwari A, Ojwiya A. Syndromic management of sexually-transmitted infections and behaviour change interventions on transmission of HIV-1 in rural Uganda: a community randomized trial. *Lancet* 2003;361:645-52.
5 Obasi A. Assessment of validity and reliability of survey data on sexual behaviour: evidence from studies of young people in Africa. Workshop on measurement of sexual behaviour in the era of HIV/AIDS. London, 4-6 September 2003.
6 Kmietowicz Z. Women are being let down in efforts to stem HIV/AIDS. *BMJ* 2004;328:305.
7 McKusick L, Horstman W, Coates T. AIDS and sexual behavior reported by gay men in San Francisco. *Am J Public Health* 1985;75:493-6.
8 Low-Beer D, Stoneburner R. Behaviour and communication change in reducing HIV: Is Uganda unique?" *Afr J AIDS Res* 2003;2:1-13.
9 Green EC. *Rethinking AIDS prevention.* Westport, CT: Praeger Press, Greenwood Publishers, 2003
10 Hanenberg RS, Rojanapithayakorn W, Kunasol P, Sokal D. Impact of Thailand's HIV-control programme as indicated by the decline in sexually transmitted diseases. *Lancet* 1994;344:243-5.
11 Kaginuba K. What happened in Uganda. Paper presented at the XIIIth International Conference on AIDS in Kenya, Nairobi, Kenya, 21-26 September 2003.

Minimally invasive parathyroidectomy

Heralds a new era in the treatment of primary hyperparathyroidism

Primary hyperparathyroidism is a more prevalent condition than many perceive. The overall incidence is 25 per 100 000 of the United Kingdom's population.[1] However, in women over the age of 45 it may affect one in 500, and more than 1% of postmenopausal women have raised serum concentrations of calcium.[2] Parathyroidectomy is the treatment of choice in symptomatic primary hyperparathyroidism. It cures fatigue and the bone, abdominal, urological, and mental symptoms associated with hypercalcaemia. Parathyroidectomy also results in a quantifiable improvement in health related quality of life.[3] Additionally a 25 year follow up of patients with untreated "asymptomatic disease" showed a notable increase in cardiovascular deaths compared with age matched normocalcaemic controls.[2] Support for an operative approach is further provided by lack of an effective medical treatment and the cost and doctor hours involved in the follow up of conservatively managed patients.

BMJ 2004;328:849-50

Traditionally parathyroidectomy involves a collar incision, bilateral exploration of the neck, identification of all four parathyroid glands, and removal of the diseased gland or glands. This approach, in experienced hands in large volume centres, has enabled cure rates of up to 97% with minimal morbidity, although a cure rate of 70% probably reflects general surgical practice more faithfully.[4,5] More than 80% of patients with primary hyperparathyroidism have a solitary adenoma, removal of which guarantees cure. In the 1980s a unilateral approach (through a collar incision) was advocated, based on the principle that removal of the single abnormal gland in the presence of an identified ipsilateral normal gland avoided the need for a contralateral exploration.[6] Despite its enthusiasts this approach failed to gain universal support because of concerns over the reliability of the localisation procedures available at the time and the possible presence of undetected double adenomas or asymmetrical hyperplasia.

BBC NEWS

Promiscuity 'fuelling HIV spread'

More needs to be done to persuade people to have fewer sexual partners, according to leading HIV experts.

They said encouraging people to have fewer partners would result in fewer HIV infections.

Writing in the British Medical Journal, they said little effort has gone in to tackling the issue in recent years.

They said the message appears to have been lost, as campaigns put the emphasis on abstaining from sex or using condoms.

The experts, who include officials from the Global Fund for Aids, the Bill and Melinda Gates Foundation and the US Agency for International Development, said efforts in some countries to address the issue had paid off.

The 'ABC' sexual health strategy

A bstinence or delay of sexual activity
B e faithful and reduce partner numbers
C ondom use

HIV infection rates have fallen from 15% to 5% in Uganda over the past decade. The experts said a nationwide campaign encouraging people to stick with regular partners contributed to the fall.

They said similar campaigns in Thailand, Cambodia, Ethiopia and the Dominican Republic have shown similar results.

"It seems obvious but there would be no global Aids pandemic where it not for multiple sexual partnerships," they said.

"The rate of change of sexual partners - especially concurrent partners - is a crucial determinant in the spread of sexually transmitted infections."

ABC approach

The experts called for an "ABC" approach to improving sexual health - advocating abstinence, being faithful and condom use.

They said this would ensure that the message that fewer sexual partners reduces the risks of HIV was not lost.

"Rather than arguing over the merits of abstinence versus condoms, it is time for the international community to unite around a balanced, evidence-based ABC approach," they said.

There would be no global Aids pandemic where it not for multiple sexual partnerships
HIV experts

In an accompanying editorial, David Wilson, a member of the World Bank's global HIV/Aids programme, welcomed the report.

"Their argument that partner reduction is the potential centre-piece of a unified ABC approach is good common sense."

However, he said the "A,B,C" approach may not work everywhere, particularly in communities where women are often forced to have sex against their will.

In another article, researchers in Canada said abstaining from sex is the best way of protecting against HIV and other sexually transmitted infections.

Stephen Genuis, an associate professor at the University of Alberta, said studies have shown a link between having sex at an early age and having many sexual partners.

"Although partner reduction is a critical and often overlooked component in the ABC strategy, we believe that delayed sexual debut for young people should be the first step in programmes to prevent sexually transmitted infections."

The UK charity Terrence Higgins Trust expressed doubts about the ABC strategy.

"I take the idea of promoting monogamy with a large pinch of salt," said Will Nutland, its head of gay men's health promotion.

"What has worked in Uganda doesn't necessarily translate to London.

"In some societies would people really be able to implement this, where women don't necessarily have control over their sexual encounters."

If you'd like to comment on this piece please send your comments using the postform below.

This postform has just been published. Your comments will appear here shortly.

Story from BBC NEWS:
http://news.bbc.co.uk/go/pr/fr/-/1/hi/health/3610487.stm

Published: 2004/04/08 23:40:33 GMT

United Press International
May 9, 2004 Sunday

Study links promiscuity, prostate cancer

DATELINE: FLINT, Mich., May 9 (UPI)

A study at the University of Michigan finds that men with gonorrhea and those with many sexual partners are more likely to get prostate cancer.

The Flint Men's Health Study results were presented Sunday to the American Urological Association annual meeting in San Francisco.

The study is part of an effort to find out why African-American men are twice as likely to develop and die from prostate cancer.

Researchers at the University Health System asked 703 black men without prostate cancer and 129 men with the disease about their sexual habits, including number of partners, frequency of intercourse, age of first intercourse and history of sexually transmitted disease.

The group found that men with more than 25 sexual partners in the course of a lifetime are 2.5 times as likely to be diagnosed with prostate cancer than men with five or fewer partners. They also discovered that 65 percent of the men with prostate cancer had a history of gonorrhea, while only 51 percent of those without prostate cancer had suffered from the disease.

Some cervix treatments up pregnancy risk

Last Updated: 2004-05-04 16:00:20 -0400 (Reuters Health)

NEW YORK (Reuters Health) - Certain treatments for a precancerous lesion of the cervix significantly increase the odds of premature rupture of membranes occurring during a subsequent pregnancy, a new study shows.

Specifically, the risk applies to women with cervical intraepithelial neoplasia (CIN) who undergo a so-called loop electrosurgical excision procedure (LEEP) or laser cone therapy to remove the abnormal tissue on the cervix.

Reporting this finding in the Journal of the American Medical Association, the investigators say "careful consideration should be given to treatment of CIN in women of reproductive age, especially when treatment might reasonably be delayed or targeted to high-risk cases."

CIN is often diagnosed and treated during childbearing years, but whether CIN treatments increase the later risk of preterm delivery is unclear, Dr. Lynn Sadler from the University of Auckland in New Zealand and colleagues explain in their report.

To investigate, they reviewed the delivery outcomes over a 12-year period of 1078 women with CIN, 652 who underwent laser or LEEP treatment and 426 who were not treated.

According to the medical records, almost 14 percent of women delivered prematurely. The rate of premature rupture of membranes (PROM) was 6 percent.

CIN treatment with a laser or LEEP did not significantly increase in the risk of preterm delivery, the team reports. In contrast, the risk of PROM was roughly doubled for women who underwent these treatments.

The amount of cervical tissue removed is an important factor, Sadler's team found.

This study underscores "the importance of targeting treatment to women at high risk of progression," the authors conclude.

SOURCE: Journal of the American Medical Association, May 5, 2004.

Roche

Diagnostics

April 12, 2004

The Honorable Mark Souder
Chairman
Criminal Justice, Drug Policy and Human Resources Subcommittee
Government Reform Committee
U.S. House of Representatives
B-373 Rayburn House Office Building
Washington, DC 20515

Dear Chairman Souder:

On behalf of Roche Diagnostics, we are pleased to submit a written statement on the diagnosis of HPV and its association with cervical cancer. As one of the leading diagnostic manufacturers in the world we have extensive experience researching this issue in both the United States and around the globe. Based on the testimony you received during the most recent hearing, I hope you will also find this statement informative.

We hope you will consider entering this statement into the official record. If you have any questions, feel free to contact me at (202) 216-1109.

Sincerely,

David Nichols
Director, Federal Government Affairs

Roche Diagnostics
Operations, Inc.

9115 Hague Road
PO Box 50416
Indianapolis, IN 46250-0416

Tel.+1-800-428-5074

Roche

Diagnostics

Criminal Justice, Drug Policy and Human Resources Subcommittee Hearing

"Cervical Cancer and Human Papillomavirus"

March 11, 2004 at 1:00 p.m.
2247 Rayburn House Office Building, Washington DC

Written Statement by Roche Diagnostics

For More Information:
David Nichols
Director, Federal Government Affairs
(202) 216-1109
david.nichols@roche.com

Roche Diagnostics Operations, Inc.
9115 Hague Road
PO Box 50416
Indianapolis, IN 46250-0416
Tel.+1-800-428-5074

Criminal Justice, Drug Policy and Human Resources Subcommittee Hearing

"Cervical Cancer and Human Papillomavirus"

March 11, 2004 at 1:00 p.m.
2247 Rayburn House Office Building, Washington DC

Statement by Roche Diagnostics

Honorable Mark Souder, Rep. Cummings, and members of the Committee, Roche Diagnostics is the global leader of in-vitro diagnostic tests with a uniquely broad product portfolio. We supply a wide array of innovative testing products and services to researchers, physicians, patients, hospitals and laboratories worldwide. Roche Diagnostics' North American headquarters are in Indianapolis, Indiana. Roche Molecular Diagnostics, or (RMD), has its global headquarters for research, development and marketing in Pleasanton, California.

RMD is striving to become recognized as a premier provider of a comprehensive panel of diagnostics focused on serving women's health needs. Using the power of PCR (polymerase chain reaction) technology, our Women's Health business area plans to offer tests to help ensure a woman's reproductive health and manage common diseases where early detection can impact better outcomes. We believe we have a tremendous opportunity, both to significantly improve women's health testing, and to universally help women lead better and healthier lives.

The World Health Organization has identified cervical cancer as the second most common cause of female mortality worldwide. Every year as many as 500,000 women are affected by cervical cancer. Nearly 300,000 die due to the disease. As a screening test for cervical cancer, 160 million Pap tests are performed annually worldwide, including 50 to 60 million in the US and 44 million in Europe. However, the sensitivity of the Pap test (including thin-prep technology) alone in identifying women with precursors of cervical cancer is only 80 percent and high-grade cervical cancer is rarely found directly on a single Pap test.

Virtually all (99.8 percent) cervical cancers are caused by specific types of a sexually-transmitted virus called human papillomavirus (HPV.) Of the 100 different genotypes of HPV, at least 13 high-risk genotypes have been shown to be oncogenic (i.e., capable of causing pre-cancerous and cancerous changes in cells). These are now considered to be the causal agents of cervical cancer.

During the last decade, Roche has provided linear array research reagents for HPV to dozens of leading cancer investigators worldwide. This assistance to the world research community has been invaluable in characterizing the epidemiology and identification of HPV genotypes associated with cervical cancer. Research findings on HPV and cervical cancer conducted with the aid of Roche's HPV linear arrays have been published in many leading peer-reviewed journals.

As an important milestone in its Women's Health portfolio, RMD expects to provide a CE-Marked diagnostic kit in the European Union by May 2004. This product will be the first PCR-based reagent for the detection of HPV and is being designed to identify all 13 high-risk genotypes of HPV. Besides the CE-IVD product, RMD is also developing a PCR-based linear array test that identifies 37 HPV genotypes, including the most common high- and low-risk anogenital genotypes. This linear array test, will serve as a follow-up on positive results, and offer genotype information that will assist physicians with treatment decisions.

In response to the recognized urgency of testing for HPV and cervical cancer, government organizations, cancer research groups, and specialty physician organizations have developed or are considering guidelines that incorporate HPV testing to improve standards of care. Guidelines from various organizations endorse HPV testing as an important component of routine cervical examination for women age 30 and older. By combining HPV testing with Pap testing, women at high risk for development of pre-cancerous and cancerous lesions can be identified, thereby improving the choice of appropriate follow-up and individualized treatment.

We at Roche know that determining which women with abnormal Pap tests are at risk for cervical cancer and choosing the best treatment presents a major public health challenge. Roche supports programs that educate health care providers and patients about HPV transmission and testing. The American College of Obstetricians and Gynecologists, the American Society for Colposcopy and Cervical Pathology, The American Cancer Society, the National Cancer Institute, and the Association of Reproductive Health Professionals have all updated their guidelines to include HPV DNA testing as part of routine cervical cancer testing for women age 30 and older.

When HPV DNA testing is performed following inconclusive or ASC-US (atypical squamous cells of undetermined significance) Pap results, it is estimated that one-half of the 2 million U.S. patients with equivocal Pap results will be HPV DNA-negative. These women will not require follow-up with further, often more invasive examinations. They will be spared needless worry and precious health care dollars will be saved.

Roche expertise on HPV testing is available to the committee and we look forward to providing any additional information the committee may be interested in.

###